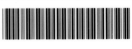

A DICTIONARY OF THE
HISTORY OF
SCIENCE

A DICTIONARY OF THE
HISTORY OF
SCIENCE

ANTON SEBASTIAN

The Parthenon Publishing Group
International Publishers in Medicine, Science & Technology

NEW YORK   LONDON

Also published by Parthenon Publishing from this author:
A Dictionary of the History of Medicine (ISBN 1-85070-021-4)
Dates in Medicine (ISBN 1-85070-095-8)

Published in the USA by
The Parthenon Publishing Group Inc.
One Blue Hill Plaza, PO Box 1564
Pearl River, NY 10965, USA

Published in the UK and Europe by
The Parthenon Publishing Group Limited
Casterton Hall, Carnforth
Lancs LA6 2LA, UK

Library of Congress Cataloging-in-Publication Data
A dictionary of the history of science / [edited by] Anton Sebastian.
     p. cm.
    Includes bibliographical references.
    ISBN 1-85070-418-X
     1. Science—History—Dictionaries. 2. Technology—History—Dictionaries.
   I. Sebastian, Anton.

   Q124.8 .D525 2000
   503—dc21   00-057428

British Library Cataloguing in Publication Data
A dictionary of the history of science
   1. Technology – History – Dictionaries
   I. Sebastian, Anton
   609'.03

   ISBN 1-85070-418-X

Copyright © 2001 The Parthenon Publishing Group

Typeset by Martin Lister Publishing Services, Carnforth, UK
Printed and bound by Butler & Tanner Ltd., Frome and London, UK

Preface

In writing and researching the *Dictionary of the History of Medicine* over the past 10 years I became involved in the history of other sciences and was motivated to write this book. The aim of this book is to give a brief historical understanding of the world around us on a scientific basis, so that we can relate to and appreciate it. I believe this book will also be of use to scientists and teachers who wish to give a historical perspective to their subject. I also hope that it will serve as an incentive and provide motivation to science students.

Science was borne out of man's struggle for survival, and the first elements of technology were stone implements used for the purpose of hunting, over two million years ago. Man's first lessons on anatomy and physiology were learnt through hunting. Making fire in order to keep warm and cook food was probably one of man's earliest discoveries. The elements of astronomy were probably discovered in his attempts to study and predict the weather. His earliest classification in botany was presumably in the identification of poisonous and non-poisonous plants for food. Through these experiences he developed a love and understanding of nature, which he started to express through his Stone Age cave paintings. Construction and architecture probably became established around ten thousand years ago with the first walled cities such as Jericho. At the same time, man learnt to domesticate animals in order to establish a reliable and steady source for food. These were the beginnings of the dairy and food industry. His knowledge of scientific principles in construction is reflected in the pyramids of Egypt and the remains of Indus Valley cities. Around 600 BC, Thales who is now regarded as the first philosopher tried to explain nature on an intellectual basis. Other Greek philosophers such as Anaximander and Anaximenes who followed put their thoughts in a logical sequence in understanding nature. Pythagoras believed that numbers rather than elements formed the principles of all things. As early as 400 BC, Democritus realized that everything in nature consisted of atoms. Up to the time of the British philosopher and statesman Francis Bacon in the 17th century, explanations of natural phenomena were based on conjecture derived from observations, or purely a matter of logical argument. Bacon set a new trend by conducting experiments to test theories, and this new culture, known as inductive reasoning, formed the basis for transition from natural philosophy to modern science. William Whewell in England in the 19th century developed this concept and popularized the term *science* in his *History of the Inductive Sciences, from the Earliest to the Present Time.*

In order to appreciate what we have today, we need to understand the contribution of human thought to the genesis of things around us. Most facets of everyday life are taken for granted today, and we are happy as long as what we have serves us well. Many scientists today, in their hurry to achieve, start where their predecessors finished and do not have the time nor the interest to know the history of something that they are going to spend the rest of their lives studying. In doing so, they fail to understand and appreciate the trend of human thought in science over the past thousands of years. I once met a physician and diabetician who had published over 100 papers on diabetes and yet did not know the meaning or the origin of the word *diabetes*. To me it was a disappointing and sad encounter. Teachers in schools and universities who discard history in their teaching help to propagate such superfluous and uninspired knowledge. If we have to be downright practical why do we sometimes bother to dress our food on the plate and light candles for dinner? We might as well be equally pragmatic, forget our esthetic or romantic instincts and do without the décor. Science without history presents a similar scenario. It fails to create an appetite for knowledge and fails to appeal. Isaac Newton indulged in history with his work such as *The Chronology of Ancient Kingdoms Amended.* The well-respected physician William Osler combed Europe for the important old books on medicine. As we all know, scientific classics continue to give an aura to the human race. William Harvey's *De Mortu Cordis* and *De Fabrica* of Vesalius are still a pride of medical profession. Aristotle's *Historia Animalorum* signifies the founding of biology. Newton's

Principia and Francis Bacon's *Novum Organon* are scientific classics. They are invaluable to science just as much as *Mona Lisa* is to art. Can we dissociate ourselves from these historical classics just because they are not of any direct practical application?

The momentum in the progress of science has been exponentially gathering over the past millennium. The modern period in the last four centuries has given proof and explanation to logical thought developed over the past few thousand years. Rutherford and other 20th century atomic scientists have gone beyond proving the atomic theory of Democritus and have unleashed the atomic energy. The theory of permutation of metals held by the alchemists became a reality with discovery of radioactive elements that could be transformed into one another. The observational astronomy by the ancient Babylonians and Greeks was transformed into a modern science through the discovery of the telescope. The planets that were observed by these ancient astronomers are now within our physical reach. Gregor Mendel's laws of heredity have culminated in genetic engineering and the Human Genome Project. The alchemist's pursuit of eternal youth is being continued through the studies to identify the locus for aging in the chromosome. All these reveal that over millions of years man has essentially not changed in his fundamental thought processes or his aspirations to discover. History is a journey through these long corridors of time where we occasionally pause to appreciate man's ingenuity, perseverance and dedication, which have all contributed to our advanced state of technology and to the comforts of life.

Selection of topics for this book has been difficult as no pursuit is exclusively an art or science. Is an architect a scientist or artist? Both. I consider art mainly the ability to illustrate while science provides the explanation and the means to carry out the expression. Both disciplines overlap to a great extent and one may find this reflected within these pages. In addition, medical history has been excluded, as it is another vast field that has been covered in a previous book of mine.

I would like to add that this book has been compiled from a wide range of sources, both ancient and contemporary. Consequently, I have attempted to draw often differing strands of opinion together to obtain the most accurate definitions. This, however, has its own limitations when obtaining the truth, since books, despite often rigorous review, are always subjective (and rightly so). Moreover, history is sometimes a difficult topic to document as contemporary texts can often benefit from hindsight, while historic texts can be dictated by hearsay and the political views of the time. Information that is genuine is always valued, and I have attempted to the best of my abilities to ensure that the book is as accurate as my sources allow. The readers' views are valuable to the future editions and, should there be any important omissions or errors, feedback sent via the publisher would be greatly appreciated.

Lastly I dedicate this book to my son Kevin and daughter Chuchi as a symbolic gesture to the future generation who I hope will look back at the past before they step forward.

Anton Sebastian
October 2000

Anton Sebastian, MBBS, MRCP, is a consultant physician in general medicine with a lifelong interest in the history of science and medicine. He has developed one of the finest private collections of antiquarian books in these fields, currently totaling well over 3000 volumes, including many original editions dating from as early as the 16th century. Following the completion of his postgraduate training at Charing Cross Hospital, London and Kingston Hospital, Surrey, he has held a number of appointments both in the United Kingdom and overseas. He is currently a consultant physician at Royal Victoria Hospital, Dundee.

A

Abacus [Greek: *abax*, slab] First mechanical counting device developed from the practice of writing on a board or slab covered with sand, or counting pebbles. Several races including the Chinese, the Aztecs, the Greeks, the Etruscans and the Egyptians developed their own devices to deal with numbers. The ancient Greek abacus, made of a series of holes with matching counting-pegs, may have alternatively derived its name from its resemblance to a *bachus* or wall cupboard with a linear arrangement of cups. The old Semitic word *abaq* for sand suggests a Hebrew origin. The only extant early Greek abacus, in the form of a marble table, discovered on the Island of Salamis in 1846, is currently exhibited in Athens. A reference to a Chinese abacus, made of balls threaded on frames, is found in a Chinese text dating back to AD 1593. It suggests that the Chinese abacus was known in AD 200. The early Greek abacus was copied by the Romans and was reintroduced into Europe by **Gerbert** or Pope Sylvester II (*c.* 940–1003) of Aurillac, France around AD 970. **Adelard of Bath** (1090–1150) wrote an early treatise, around 1130, on the rules of the abacus. During medieval times in Europe, the abacus with some modifications was known as *mensa Pythagorica*. An Italian mathematician, **Leonardo Fibonacci** (*c.* 1172–1250) of Pisa, wrote a *Book of the Abacus* (*Liber Abaci*) in 1202. *See numbers.*

Abbe, Cleveland (1838–1916) *See meteorology.*

Abbe, Ernst (1840–1905) *See contact lenses, electron microscope, microscope, phase contrast microscopy, Zeiss, Carl.*

Abbe's Law *See electron microscope.*

Abbot, Charles Greely (1872–1973) An American physicist from Wilton, New Hampshire, who lived for 100 years. He served as director of the Astrophysical Observatory at the Smithsonian Institution from 1907 to 1944, and invented a device for converting solar energy to power. He published *The Sun* (1907) and *The Earth and the Stars* (1925).

Abdera A town of Hispania on the shores of the Mediterranean near the mouth of the Nessus, supposed to have been built by Abderus, the son of Mercury. This town was the birthplace of the Greek philosopher and scientist, **Leucippus** (*c.* 500 BC) and his pupil **Democritus** (460–370 BC).

Abegg, Richard Wilhelm Heinrich (1869–1910) A German chemist from Danzig who recognized the chemical significance of electrons. In 1897 he proposed that the outer electron shell governed the chemical properties of the atom. He also did important work on osmotic pressures and the freezing points of dilute solutions. Abegg died in a ballooning accident at Koszalin in Poland. *See valency.*

Abel Tester A device for testing the flash-point of petroleum, invented by a London chemist **Sir Fredrick Augustus Abel** (1827–1902). He also introduced a new method for making gun-cotton and was knighted in 1883.

Abel, Sir Fredrick Augustus (1827–1902) An English chemist from Woolwich and student of **August Wilhelm von Hofmann** (1818–1892) at the Royal College of Chemistry in London, where he became an assistant in 1846. He published a *Handbook of Chemistry* in 1853 at the age of 26 in collaboration with the Scottish chemist, **Sir James Dewar** (1843–1923). Abel invented cordite which was adopted as the standard explosive by the British Army in 1891. He published *Gun-cotton* (1866), *Electricity Applied to Explosive Purposes* (1884) and several other treatises. *See Abel tester, explosives.*

Abel, John Jacob (1857–1938) An eminent biochemist from Cleveland, Ohio who graduated from the University of Michigan and studied under the foremost scientists in Austria and Germany before he returned to America in 1891 to become the professor of therapeutics at the University of Michigan. After a brief period in this post, he was called to Johns Hopkins University as the first professor of pharmacology at the age of 36. His contributions include the construction of the first membrane for artificial kidneys (1913), the extraction of epinephrine (1899) and the identification of posterior pituitary hormone and hirudin (1910). He isolated specific amino acids from the blood and determined the molecular weight of cholesterol. He was the first to obtain a crystalline form of insulin, in 1926.

Abel, Niels Henrik (1802–1829) A Norwegian mathematician who was the first to demonstrate that an algebraic solution of the general equation of the fifth degree is impossible. *See Abel–Ruffini theorem, elliptic functions.*

Abel–Ruffini Theorem Useful in evaluating the sum of a number of integrals which have the same integrand, but different limits. Proposed by a Norwegian mathematician, **Niels Henrik Abel** (1802–1829) in 1826. It had been stated earlier by an Italian mathematician, **Paolo Ruffini** (1765–1822) in Modena in 1798.

Abelson, Philip Hauge (b 1913) *See fossils, neptunium.*

Abercrombie, Sir Leslie Patrick (1879–1957) An English architect who was mainly responsible for town replanning in London in 1944. He was instrumental in planning several new post-war towns elsewhere in England.

Aberration [Latin: *ab,* from + *errare,* to wander] Defect in an image produced by an optical system, due to the failure of light rays refracted by a lens or reflected by a mirror to meet at the same point. It is corrected by the use of an achromatic lens. *See achromatic lens.*

Aberration of Light [Latin: *ab,* from + *errare,* to wander] Its occurrence in astronomy due to the earth's motion was first observed in 1727 by an English astronomer, **James Bradley** (1693–1762). It denotes the difference in an apparent position of a star from the position it would have had if the earth were stationary. Bradley used his finding to discover the nutation of the earth's axis and measure the velocity of light.

Abraham, Edward Penley (b 1913) *See Fleming, Alexander.*

Abraham, Max (1875–1922) *See electron.*

Absolute Zero [Latin: *absolutus,* complete; Arabic: *sifr,* zero] A temperature of zero on the Kelvin scale. This is equivalent to a temperature of minus 273.15 degrees Celsius or minus 459.67 degrees Fahrenheit. Since temperature is a measure of the kinetic energy of particles, absolute zero is the total absence of movement, in which electrons would have to be below their ground states. This is impossible to achieve in the quantum world, but closely approximated 1960 at the Cryogenics Laboratory at Pennsylvania State University under the direction of a British-born physicist, **John G. Aston** (1902–1990).

Absorption of Heat by Glass [Latin: *ab,* from + *sorbeo,* suck in] **Robert Hooke** (1635–1703) discovered that glass absorbed radiant heat, and his findings were advanced by M de La Roche of France, who, in 1812, demonstrated the loss of heat by radiation and conduction through a glass medium.

Absorption Spectra [Latin: *specter,* appearance] **Sir Isaac Newton** (1642–1727) described the production of a spectrum in his book *Opticks.* In 1752, **Thomas Melvill** (1726–1753), a Scottish scientist of Glasgow University, observed that metals did not give continuous spectra, owing to interruption by lines. Similar dark bands in the spectrum of sunlight were first observed by **William Hyde Wollaston** (1766–1822) in 1802. A German physicist and optician **Joseph von Fraunhofer** (1787–1826) in 1814 studied this phenomenon further and mapped about 400 dark lines (Fraunhofer lines). **Sir John Fredrick William Herschel**

(1792–1871) in 1823 suggested that the lines observed by Melvill could be used to detect various metals, by identifying the type of spectrum they emitted. **Robert Bunsen** (1811–1899) and **Gustav Robert Kirchhoff** (1824–1887) concluded in 1829 that the dark lines were due to the absorption of certain spectra by the atmosphere. **Anders Jonas Ångström** (1814–1874), a Swedish physicist from Lodgo, listed about 1000 Fraunhofer lines in his map of the *Normal Solar Spectrum* published in 1868. *See spectroscopy.*

Abu-Masher or **Albumazer** (787–885) *See tides.*

Academia de Ciencias Mathematicas Founded by Philip II of Spain, at Madrid in 1575.

Académie Royale des Sciences The initial base for a French academy was established by a group of eminent mathematicians and philosophers including **René Descartes** (1596–1650), **Blaise Pascal** (1623–1662), **Pierre de Fermat** (1601–1665), **Edmé Mariotte** (1620–1684) and **Pierre Gassendi** (1592–1655) in Paris in the mid-17th century. The academy was initiated as a regular institution by the French statesman **Jean-Baptiste Colbert** (1619–1683) under the sponsorship of Louis XIV in 1666. The French literary writer, **Bernard le Bovier de Fontenelle** (1657–1757) served as its secretary for 40 years. The Paris Observatory was established as a part of the Académie des Sciences in 1667 and its building was completed in 1672. The Académie was reorganized in 1699 and abolished in 1793. It was replaced by the Institut National des Sciences et des Arts in 1795.

Academy A term derived from the academia, a grove in Athens where **Plato** (428–348 BC) taught his pupils. According to Greek mythology, Helen, a beautiful woman, was carried off from Sparta by Theseus. Her two brothers Castor and Pollux went in search of her and a farmer, Academus, put them on the right track. Following this, the grove on the farm of Academus became protected, and it was named Academy. The academies of Plato and **Aristotle** (384–322 BC) continued for several centuries until they were closed by Emperor Justinian in AD 529. The modern term academy, borrowed from this source, denotes a place of learning. The Academy of the Secrets of Nature in Italy was the first of the scientific societies to be established, around 1450. Although it consisted of men who made discoveries in physical science, it was suspected of advocating magic and illicit arts, and was banned by Pope Paul III. The Accademia Del Cimento (Academy of Experiment), one of the first important scientific academies, was founded in Florence by Grand Duke Ferdinand II and his brother Leopold of Tuscany, in 1657. Although it lasted for only 10 years, within this time it boasted a string of distinguished members including **Evangelista Torricelli** (1608–1647), **Giovanni Alfonso Borelli** (1608–1679) and **Nicolaus Steno** (1638–1687), who made significant contributions in experimental science. The academy, at the time of closure, left a volume on *Natural Experiments*. The Berlin Academy was formed in 1700 after three decades of effort by the mathematical genius **Gottfried Wilhelm Leibniz** (1646–1716). Another important Academy of Sciences, at St Petersburg in Russia, was founded by Peter the Great in 1724. The Schemnitz Mining Academy, the first technical college in the world, was founded at Schemnitz, Hungary in 1733. This was followed by academies at Göttingen (1751), Munich (1759) and Stockholm (1786). The Royal Danish Academy of Sciences was founded by Christian IV in Copenhagen in 1742. The National Academy of Sciences in America was first founded as a private organization dedicated to science, and was given a charter by Congress in 1863, with **Alexander Dallas Bache** (1806–1867) as its first president. He was succeeded by **Joseph Henry** (1797–1878) in 1867. *See Accademia dei Lincei.*

Accademia dei Lincei of Rome. Named after the lynx, an animal with keen vision. The organization was formed by **Duke Federigo Cesi** (1585–1630) in 1603 to serve as a forum for stimulating scientific discussions. The astronomer and physicist **Galilei Galileo** (1564–1642) was one of the founder members of this first scientific society.

Accademia del Cimento [Academy of Experiment] Initiated in Florence, Italy by two of Galileo's pupils **Vincenzo Vivianni** (1622–1703) and **Evangelista Torricelli** (1608–1647) and established under the sponsorship of Grand Duke Ferdinand II and his brother Leopold of Tuscany in 1657. It was closed in 1667.

Acceleration [Latin: *accelerare*, to hasten] Rate of increase in the velocity of a moving body. A Greek philosopher, **Strato of Lampsacus** (Turkey), conducted experiments in 340 BC and came to the conclusion that bodies accelerate when they fall. **John Buridan** (*c.* 1300–1358) of Paris studied the cause of acceleration of falling bodies. The uniform acceleration of a falling or rolling body regardless of its weight was studied by **Galilei Galileo** (1564–1642). An English physicist and mathematician, **George Atwood** (1746–1807) investigated the motion of falling objects with his 'fall machine'. *See dynamics, motion.*

Accelerator *See antiproton, boson, cyclotron, particle accelerator.*

Accountancy A profession for dealing with accounts related to commercial or official business. **Leonardo Fibonacci**

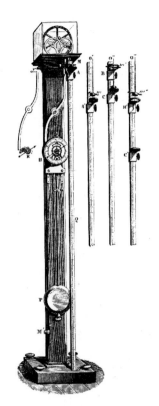

Figure 1 Atwood's fall machine. Atkinson, E. *Elementary Treatise on Physics*. London: Longmans, Green, and Co, 1872

(*c.* 1172–1250) of Pisa in 1202 wrote on the problems of calculating interest, and estimating the cost of commodities after accounting for expenses and exchange rates. The first book on commercial arithmetic, by Borghi, was published in Venice in 1484. In 1522 **Adam Riese** (1489–1559) published the first important work on commercial arithmetic in Germany entitled *Rechnung auff der Linier*. The English mathematician **Cuthbert Tonstall** (1474–1559), who wrote the first printed book on arithmetic in England, initially became interested in the subject when he had to verify his accounts with goldsmiths who in those days also acted as bankers. An Italian mathematician, **Niccolò Fontana Tartaglia** (1499–1557) of Venice published *Tratato di numeri et misure* (1556–1560), which contained a complete account of business mathematics used by the Venetian merchants. A table of compound interest by a German mathematician, **Christoff Rudolf** (b 1500), is found in *Exempel-Büchlin* published in 1540. Accountancy became established in the 16th century although the first society in Great Britain formed in Edinburgh was given a Royal Charter only in 1854. The Royal Institute for Chartered Accountants in England and Wales was founded in London in 1870. A Scottish economist and mathematician in

Edinburgh, **Robert Hamilton** (1753–1829), published some early works on the subject including *An Introduction to Merchandise* (1777) and *A System of Arithmetic and Book-Keeping* (1788). The Society of Incorporated Accountants and Auditors was established in 1885, and the Corporation of Accountants was formed in 1891. The London Association of Certified Accountants was founded in 1905.

Accumulator   A secondary battery or storage cell capable of storing electrical energy in the form of chemical energy. A German physicist, **Johann Wilhelm Ritter** (1776–1810) from Silesia discovered its principle in 1803. The first primitive device made of rolled lead sheets in sulfuric acid was constructed by a French physicist, **Gaston Plante** (1834–1889) in 1860. *See battery.*

Acetic Acid [Latin: *acidus*, sour]   First prepared by a German alchemist and physician, **Georg Ernst Stahl** (1660–1734). It was synthesized independently by **Adolf Wilhelm Hermann Kolbe** (1818–1884), a German professor of chemistry at Leipzig, in 1848.

Acetylene, now ethylene.   The effect of an electric spark within a glass ball containing carbon electrodes and hydrogen gas was demonstrated by Marcell Morren, Dean of the science faculty of Marseilles, in 1859. He named the hydrocarbon 'carbonized hydrogen', as it resembles coal gas during combustion. This was probably the first description of acetylene, although Edmund Davy claimed to have observed it earlier in 1836. It was demonstrated in 1860 by **Pierre-Eugène Marcellin Berthelot** (1827–1907) who re-named it acetylene. The safety of acetylene in an acetone solution was discovered by a French chemist, **Georges Claude** (1870–1960). A German chemist, **Friedrich Wöhler** (1800–1882), obtained it from calcium carbide around 1828. Further work on acetylene in 1929 by a Belgian-born American chemist, **Julius Arthur Nieuwland** (1878–1936) led to the discovery of artificial rubber.

Achard, Franz Karl (1753–1821)   *See beet sugar.*

Acheson, Edward Goodrich (1856–1931)   *See carborundum, graphite.*

Achromatic Lens [Greek: *a*, without + *chroma*, color]   Used for overcoming chromatic aberration in optical instruments. It is a combination of lenses made from materials of different refractive indexes, constructed in such a way as to minimize chromatic aberration. The possibility of making an achromatic combination of lenses was first suggested by a Scottish mathematician, **David Gregory** (1659–1708). A Swedish scientist, **Samuel Klingenstierna** (1698–1765), communicated a similar idea to a London instrument maker **John**

Dolland (1706–1761) in 1755. It was first produced around 1729 by **Chester More Hall** (1703–1771) of More Hall Essex who used it in the construction of a telescope around 1730. Hall failed to publish or patent his invention; the first patent for it was obtained by Dolland in 1755. The achromatic objective was also mentioned in 1807 by **Harmanus van Deijl** (1738–1809) who was of Danish origin. It was adapted for the microscope by an Italian physicist, **Giovanni Battista Amici** (1786–1863) of Modena in 1812. **Joseph Jackson Lister** (1786–1869), the father of **Lord Joseph Lister** (1827–1912) used two achromatic lenses to cancel each other's negative aberration in 1830.

Acid–Base Theory   The definition of an acid, a substance that gives off a proton in solution, and a base as a substance that accepts the proton (proton acceptor), was proposed by a Danish chemist **Johannes Nicolaus Brønsted** (1879–1947), a professor of chemistry at Copenhagen, in 1928. The part played by electrons in the formation of acids and bases was studied by an American physical chemist, **Gilbert Newton Lewis** (1875–1946) of Weymouth, Massachusetts, who published *Thermodynamics and the Free Energy of Chemical substances* with Merle Randall in 1923.

Acidity or pH [Latin: *acidus*, sour]   One of the earliest references to natural pigments as acid–alkali indicators was made in 1666 by **Robert Boyle** (1627–1691) during his observations on the change of color, related to acidity in syrup of violets. Litmus, derived from the plant *Roccella tinctoria* and other lichens, has been and still is used as a measure of acidity or alkalinity. Cochineal, another indicator of acidity, is obtained from an insect. Anthocyanin from tulips and other flowers was noted to change color, according to different levels of acidity or alkalinity, by the German chemist **Richard Willstätter** (1872–1942). E. Philip Smith used this finding to determine the pH of cell sap. Modern dyes as indicators of pH were introduced around 1909 by a Danish biochemist, **Søren Peter Lauritz Sørenson** (1868–1939) of Copenhagen. An American chemist, **William Mansfield Clark** (1884–1964) developed a reliable range of titration indicators for acidity and published *The Determination of Hydrogen Ions* in 1920. The colorimetric method for determining pH was introduced in the early 20th century.

Acids [Latin: *acidus*, sour]   The acidic properties of substances were attributed to various phenomena in the past. A Swiss alchemist and physician, **Paracelsus** (1493–1541) described a hypothetical substance *acidum primogenium*, as a cause of acidity. **Antoine Laurent Lavoisier** (1743–1794) thought that oxygen in various substances was responsible for their acidic properties. Nitric acid, known to the Arabs from AD 900, was prepared under the name *aqua fortis* by an alchemist, Raymond Lully, in 1287. The acids were first recognized as a group of compounds on a chemical basis in the 16th century. **John Rudolph Glauber** (1604–1668), one of the last of the German alchemists, obtained pure forms of sulfuric acid and nitric acid around 1640. The acids were first arranged in order of their affinity for certain bases in 1718 by a French physician, **Etienne François Geoffroy** (1672–1731). A Swedish apothecary and chemist **Carl Wilhelm Scheele** (1742–1786) discovered nitrous acid in 1774. **Henry Cavendish** (1731–1810) demonstrated its chemical nature in 1785. The modern theory of proton donors for acids was proposed by **Johannes Nicolaus Brønsted** (1879–1947), a Danish professor of chemistry at Copenhagen, in 1928. *See acid–base theory, acidity, Brønsted theory*.

Ackermann, Rudolph (1764–1834) *See lithography*.

Acoustics [Greek: *akouein,* to hear] Study of the generation, properties and reception of sound. The theory of acoustics was initiated by a Greek mathematician, **Archytas of Tarentum** (428–347 BC). He distinguished harmonics from arithmetical and geometrical progressions. The Roman architect **Marcus Pollio Vitruvius** (*c.* AD 100) in his work *On Architecture* dealt with acoustics and musical sounds in relation to the theater. The vocal organs in animals in relation to their muscle supply was studied by an Italian physician, **Bartolomeo Eustachio** (1520–1574). **Giovanni Benedetti** (1530–1590) discovered the relationship between pitch and frequency. A French natural philosopher, **Marin Mersenne** (1588–1648), was the first to determine the frequency of a musical note and show that raising a note an octave doubles its frequency. A French mathematician, **Joseph Sauveur** (1643–1716) from La Fleche first used the term acoustics in his work related to tones of the musical scale, in 1701. An Italian-born French mathematician, **Joseph Louis Lagrange** (1736–1813) gave a complete solution to the problem of the mathematical description of a vibrating string and explained echoes, beats and compound sounds. A German physicist and musical performer, **Ernest Florens Friedrich Chladni** (1756–1827) of Wittenberg is regarded as one of the founders of the science of acoustics. He discovered the longitudinal vibrations in a string or rod and studied the vibration of plates in relation to their shape and weight, and published *Traité d'acoustique* in 1809. A French physicist and physician, **Felix Savart** (1791–1841) devised an instrument, Savart's wheel, for determining the number of vibrations corresponding to a note of any pitch. In 1843 **Georg Simon Ohm** (1789–1854), a German professor of physics at

Nuremberg (1833–1849), demonstrated that the human ear recognizes only sinusoidal waves as pure tones in its analysis of any periodic sound into its component tones. Further research on acoustics in relation to sense organs, especially the ear, was conducted by a German physiologist and anatomist, **Ernst Heinrich Weber** (1795–1878) and his brother **Wilhelm Eduard Weber** (1804–1891), at Göttingen in 1825. **Sir Charles Wheatstone** (1802–1875), an English physicist who started his career as a musical instrument maker, studied sound and invented a sound magnifier or microphone. The resonance theory of hearing was proposed by a German physiologist and physicist, **Hermann Ludwig Ferdinand von Helmholtz** (1821–1894). The vibration microscope used for studying the visual resultant of two harmonic motions was invented by a French physicist, **Jules Antoine Lissajous** (1822–1880). He developed Lissajous figures for the visual demonstration of vibrations that produce sound waves. A German physicist, **Karl Rudolph Koenig** (1832–1901) invented a clock for determining absolute pitch, and a manometric flame for the study of air vibrations. A mechanical device for photographically recording sound waves was invented by an American physicist, **Dayton Clarence Miller** (1866–1941) of Ohio, who became an expert in architectural acoustics. Photographic study of sound waves reflected from objects of various shapes was carried out by an American physicist, **Robert Williams Wood** (1868–1955) of Concord, Massachusetts. An English physicist, **Lord John William Strutt Rayleigh** (1842–1919), published a *Theory of Sound* (1877–1878). Acoustics was established in 1898 as a science in architecture by an American physicist, **Wallace Clement Ware Sabine** (1868–1919) of Richwood, Ohio. He used acoustic principles to design the Symphony Hall in Boston. *See echo, musical theory, sound*.

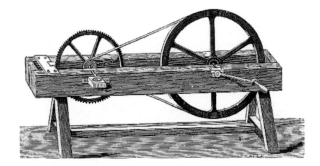

Figure 2 Savart's wheel for determining the number of vibrations that correspond to a musical note of any pitch. Lardner, Dionysius. *Handbook of Natural Philosophy, Electricity, Magnetism, and Acoustics*. London: Walton and Maberley, 1856

Acre   The first English statute defining an acre as 4840 square yards was passed in 1305.

Acrylic Paint   Consisting of acrylic vinyl copolymers, this was first produced by the British company, Reeves Ltd, in 1964.

Actinium [Greek: *aktis,* ray] An element with atomic number 89 discovered by a French chemist, André Debierne in 1899.

Actinometer [Greek: *actis*, ray + *metron,* measure] An instrument for measuring the heat from the sun, invented by **Sir John Fredrick William Herschel** (1792–1871) in 1825. It was improved by **Robert Bunsen** (1811–1899) and **Sir Henry Enfield Roscoe** (1833–1915) in 1856. Roscoe studied under **Thomas Graham** (1805–1869) in London before he became a professor at Owen's College, Manchester.

Ada   A high-level computer-programming language named after **Countess Augusta Ada Lovelace** (1815–1852) who was a mathematician and the daughter of the English poet, George Gordon, Lord Byron (1788–1824). She was a friend of the computer pioneer **Charles Babbage** (1792–1871), and translated an Italian work on Babbage's computer, entitled *Sketch of the Analytical Engine* in 1843.

Adair, John (*c*. 1655–1722)   *See cartography.*

Adam, James (1730–1794)   *See Adam, Robert.*

Adam, Neil Kensington (b 1891)   *See surface chemistry.*

Adam, Robert (1728–1792)   A Scottish architect from Kirkcaldy who established his firm in London in 1758. He designed several important buildings in London and became famous for his interior designing based on classical Roman and Greek styles. His brother **James Adam** (1730–1794) designed the Glasgow Infirmary in 1792.

Adams, George (1750–1795)   The son of a scientific instrument maker in London who wrote *Essays on the Microscope* (1787).

Adams, Sir John Bertram (1920–1984)   *See cyclotron.*

Adams, John Couch (1819–1892)   *See Neptune.*

Adams, Walter Sydney (1876–1956)   *See Mount Wilson Observatory.*

Adams, William Bridges (1797–1872)   An English inventor from Madeley, Staffordshire who took out over 32 patents relating to locomotives, carriages, roads and bridges. The fish-plate which is widely used for jointing rails was invented by him in 1846. *See railway.*

Adamson, Robert (1821–1848)   *See calotype process.*

Adanson, Michel (1727–1806)   *See botany.*

Adaptation   A process by which an organism adjusts to its environment in order to survive. *See evolution, Lamarck, Jean Baptiste Antoine de Monet, Chevalier de.*

Addiscombe College   Established near Croydon in England for the scientific training of the members of the East India Company in 1809. The college closed in 1861.

Adelard of Bath (1090–1150)   *See abacus, Euclid, vision.*

Ader, Clement (1841–1926)   *See airplane.*

Aeliophile   An early form of steam engine. *See steam engine.*

Aepinus, Franz Ulrich Theodosius (1724–1802)   *See electromagnetic theory.*

Aerial [Latin: *aer,* air] A Russian physicist, **Alexander Stepanovich Popov** (1859–1905) was the first to use a suspended wire as an aerial during his experiments on wireless telegraphy in 1897. **Guglielmo Marchese Marconi** (1874–1937) in 1901 used a kite to raise an aerial in Newfoundland for receiving messages from Cornwall. *See wireless telegraphy.*

Aerial Photograph   The first aerial photograph was taken by **Gaspard Felix Tournachon** (1820–1910) from an air balloon, the *Nadir,* as it flew over Paris in 1858. Aerial photography in England was pioneered by an archaeologist, **Osbert Guy Stanhope Crawford** (1886–1957). He published *Wessex from the Air* in 1928. **John Kenneth Sinclair Saint Joseph** (b 1912) of Worcestershire also used the method for archaeological surveying in England.

Aerodynamics [Latin: *aer,* air + Greek: *dynamis,* power] The study of forces exerted by air or other gases in motion on bodies such as land vehicles and aircraft moving at speed through the atmosphere. An English pioneer in the field of aviation, **Sir George Cayley** (1771–1857) of Scarborough was the first to study aerodynamics; he wrote a book on the behavior of objects in motion through air. A Russian pioneer of rockets, **Konstantin Eduardovich Tsiolkovsky** (1857–1935), was the first to propose the principles of aerodynamics, in 1892. He built several fan engines to determine the atmospheric friction exerted on a moving vehicle. He built the first wind tunnel, in Russia, in 1891. One of the first works on the subject, entitled *Experiments in Aerodynamics,* was published by an American aeronautical engineer, **Samuel Pierpont Langley** (1834–1906) of Roxbury, Massachusetts in 1891. He built models that flew in 1890. A Belgian, Camille Jenatzy, built the first aerodynamically designed land vehicle, which achieved a speed of 60 miles per hour in 1899. **André Gustav Citroën** (1878–1935) and **Walter Percy Chrysler** (1875–1940) were the first two car makers to produce aerodynamically designed cars. The German engineer and pioneer in aeronautics, **Otto Lilienthal** (1848–1896), studied the designs of various gliders and flying machines and published *Bird Flight as a Basis of Aviation* in 1889. The two American brothers, **Orville Wright** (1871–1948) and **Wilbur Wright** (1861–1912) of Dayton, Ohio, during their development of gliders constructed a wind tunnel and compiled accurate tables of lift and drag for different wing configurations. The science of aerodynamics was further developed by the Hungarian physicist, **Theodore von Karman** (1881–1963). He emigrated to America in 1926 and came to be regarded as the father of modern aerodynamics. Karman applied the science of aerodynamics to airplanes and founded the Aerojet Engineering Corporation in 1942. Further pioneering work was carried out by a German physicist, **Ludwig Prandtl** (1875–1953) of Freising, Bavaria who gave an explanation for induced drag. Most of the aerodynamic shapes of modern aircraft are due to the work of Karman and Prandtl. An English physicist, **Lord Frederick Alexander Lindemann** or **Viscount Cherwell** (1886–1957) was the first to develop the mathematical theory of aircraft spin. A Russian engineer, **Andrei Nikolaevich Tupolev** (1888–1972), one of the founders of the Central Institute of Aerodynamics in Moscow, designed several military aircraft and the ill-fated first supersonic passenger jet *Tu 144*.

Aerogel [Latin: *aer*, air + French: *gélatine*, jelly] A substance with a remarkable property of thermoinsulation. First produced in 1932 by an American, S. S. Kristler, by replacing a fluid solvent with gas.

Aeronautics [Latin: *aer*, air + Greek: *nautes*, sailor] *See aerodynamics, airplane, air balloon, ejection seat, jet engine.*

Aeroplane *See airplane.*

Aerosol The production of a fine suspension of droplets of liquid or solids in a gas (aerosol) was first suggested by Erik Rotheim of Norway in 1926. A device to achieve this was invented by an American, Julius S. Khan, in 1939. The commercial use of aerosol insecticide was introduced by L. D. Goodhue and W. N. Sullivan of America in 1941.

Aethrioscope [Greek: *atheros*, clear + *skopein*, to view] An instrument to measure radiation in the sky invented in 1819 by a Scottish physicist and professor of natural philosophy at Edinburgh, **Sir John Leslie** (1766–1832) from Largo, Fifeshire.

Affinity [Latin: *affinitas*, nearness] A term introduced into chemistry by the Dominican priest and scientist, **Albertus Magnus** (1192–1280). A Flemish chemist and physiologist, Franciscus Sylvius or Franz de la Böe (1614–1672) was one of the first to realize the significance of chemical affinity. The electrical nature of chemical affinity was suggested by the English chemist **Sir Humphry Davy** (1778–1829) in his work *On Some Chemical Agencies of Electricity* in 1807. In 1783 a Swedish chemist, **Torbern Olof Bergman** (1735–1784), compiled extensive affinity tables for acids and bases. The French chemist **Claude Louis Compte de Berthollet** (1748–1822) demonstrated that the temperature and concentration of reagents affected chemical affinity. An English chemist, **Henry Edward Armstrong** (1848–1937) suggested the concept of residual affinity, due to residual charge, after chemical combination. A French-born Swiss chemist, **Alfred Werner** (1866–1919), developed this theory, and proposed the modern theory of coordination bonds between molecules. *See bonds, valency.*

Agardh, Carl Adolf (1785–1859) *See diatoms.*

Agassiz, Alexander Emmanuel (1835–1910) Swiss-American engineer and son of **Jean Louis Rodolphe Agassiz** (1807–1873). He improved the apparatus for oceanic studies and made a complete study of deep-water animals and plants of the Caribbean and Pacific on the ship *Albatross* in 1880. *See oceanography.*

Agassiz, Jean Louis Rodolphe (1807–1873) A Swiss paleontologist from Motier-en-Vuly, who emigrated to America in 1846. He developed the theory of the Ice Age. He was an opponent of Darwinian evolution and an advocate of the recapitulation theory. *See Ice Age, zoology.*

Agnesi, Maria Gaetana (1718–1799) One of the first female mathematicians to gain fame before the 19th century. She was born in Milan and educated privately by her father who was a professor of mathematics. Her *Istituzioni analitiche* (1784) became a standard mathematical textbook in Italy.

Agricola, Georgius or **Georg Bauer** (1494–1555) A German mineralogist, metallurgist and physician born at Glauchau in Saxony. He studied at the Universities of Bologna, Leipzig and Venice, and wrote several treatises on medicine, geology, weights, measures and metals. He was official physician to Joachimsthal in Bohemia, a mining district, where he did most of his work on metallurgy. His *De Re Metallica,* published in 12 books in Basel in 1555, was the first systematic work on metallurgy. He published a book on physical geology, *De Ortu et Causis Subterraneorum* in 1546. *See bismuth, borax, boron, early printed science books, flint tools,* *fluorine, fossils, geology, metallurgy, mineralogy, stone age, ventilation, water pump.*

Agricultural Chemistry *See agriculture, fertilizers.*

Agricultural Instruments The plough is the oldest agricultural instrument. It was known to the Chinese from 3500 BC. Bronze ploughs were used in Vietnam around 1600 BC. The first combine-harvester was made in Roman Gaul. It consisted of a cart pulled through standing cereal by an ox or horse. It had knives on the front to cut the corn, and a device to knock the grain out of the ears of corn. An English inventor **Jethro Tull** (1674–1741) of Basildon experimented with ploughing instruments and developed a two-wheeled plough. He also invented a seed-drill with the function of drilling holes for sowing and covering seeds. A 'mould-board' which turned the soil after it was cut, was patented in England in 1730. The threshing machine, one of the most useful instruments for farmers, was invented by a Scottish millwright **Andrew Meikle** (1719–1811) in 1787. His father **James Meikle** (1690–*c.* 1719) was known for his invention of fanners for winnowing grain, and a barley mill. Joseph Boyce patented a mechanical reaper in England in 1799. A Scottish agriculturalist **James Anderson** (1739–1808), who had a farm in Aberdeenshire, invented a two-horse plough without wheels, known as the Scotch plough. An English agricultural instrument maker **Robert Ransome** (1753–1830) of Norfolk produced the first cast-iron plough in 1785. In 1789 he founded the Orville Works at Ipswich for making agricultural implements. A more efficient steel plough was invented in 1830 by John Deere of Illinois. A Scottish engineer, **James Smith** (1789–1850) of Perthshire, invented a subsoil plough for 'thorough drainage'. Corn was cut with a sickle and scythe for many centuries until the invention of the reaping machine by a Scottish clergyman **Patrick Bell** (1799–1869), from Dundee, in 1826. An improved version of the reaper was invented by an American inventor from Virginia **Cyrus Hall McCormick** (1809–1884) in 1831. He developed it and began manufacturing it on a larger scale in 1847. McCormick is also known for inventing a plough in 1831. Around the same time a successful reaping machine was independently invented by an American Quaker inventor, **Obed Hussey** (1792–1860) who patented his device before McCormick. A medical practitioner from Hertford County, North Carolina, **Jordan Richard Gatling** (1818–1903) devised a steam plough (1857) and a machine for sowing seeds (1850). Steam-powered tractors for ploughing started to be used in the late 19th century. The first tractor to use a moving tread was developed by the Holt Company of California in 1908, and the first gas-propelled harvester was introduced by the same

Company in 1910. The Agricultural Research Council was established in England in 1931. A machine called a crop stripper was invented in Australia in 1845. It was drawn by a team of horses and, as it moved, the revolving blades geared to the wheels stripped the wheat, which was then mechanically shoveled into wagons. The crop strippers were exported to the United States and were developed into harvesters in 1917. Tractors with an internal combustion engine were first produced by John Froelich of Iowa, in 1892. The first successful one was known as the Ivel tractor, with a medium-powered internal combustion engine, and was built by a British engineer, Dan Albone, in 1902. A farm tractor that controlled the depth of plowing through a hydraulic system was invented by an Irish engineer **Henry George Ferguson** (1884–1960) from Hillsborough, County Down. His invention of automatic draft-control for tractors (Ferguson tractors) played an important role in mechanizing British agriculture during the 1940s.

Agriculture [Greek: *agros*, field + Latin: *cultus*, cultivated] Wheat and barley were cultivated in Canaan [Israel] in 9000 BC and the ancient Greeks probably learnt their farming methods from them. An ancient village found near Nineveh, Iraq shows evidence of agriculture around 9000 BC. Rice and potatoes were cultivated in Peru around 8000 BC and maize was cultivated in the Tehuacan valley of Mexico in 7000 BC. Hesiod, a Greek poet in the 8th century BC, gave a description of the three principal parts of the plough. Rice was grown by the Yang Shao farmers in China around 4000 BC. A primitive form of plough, the ard, was known to the Chinese in 3500 BC. They also developed practices such as planting crops in rows, hoeing weeds and applying manure around 500 BC. An early farming site found in 1935 at Henbury in Devon, England has now been dated around 4000 BC. The Egyptians as early as 5000 years ago had a system of irrigation to utilize the water from the Nile River for agriculture. One of the first treatises on agriculture, *De Re Rustica* in 12 books, was written by a Roman **Lucius Junius Moderatus Colomella** (*c.* AD 100). It included the characteristics of arable and pasture lands, the culture of vines and olives, gardening and the care of domestic animals. Agricultural science in England was popularized by **Arthur Young** (1741–1820) of London who published several works including *The Farmer's Letters to the People of England* (1767) and *The Farmer's Tour through the East of England* (1771). He started the *Annals of Agriculture* (1794–1815). A Scottish politician and a pioneer of agricultural improvement, **Sir John Sinclair** (1754–1835), established the Board of Agriculture in 1793. A French chemist, **Jean Baptiste Joseph Dieudonné Boussingault** (1802–1887), was the

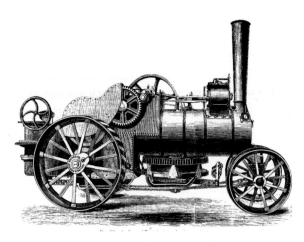

Figure 3 A steam-powered tractor used for ploughing. Guillemin, Amédée. *The Applications of Physical Forces.* London: Macmillan and Co, 1877

first to demonstrate inorganic nitrogen and phosphorus as soil fertilizers. The first experimental farm for agriculture in the world was founded by an English agriculturist, **Sir John Bennet Lawes** (1814–1900) at Rothamsted in England in 1843. He patented the first artificial manure, a superphosphate, in 1842. Pioneering work in England on nitrogen fertilizers was done by **Sir Joseph Henry Gilbert** (1817–1901) from Hull. The Royal Agricultural Society in England gained its charter in 1838 and began publishing its own journal in 1840. The first scientific agricultural laboratory was built at the Rothamsted Experimental Farm in 1885, and was manned by 40 agricultural scientists headed by **Sir John Edward Russell** (1872–1965) from Gloucestershire, in 1912. Russell also published *Soil Conditions and Plant Growth* in 1912. The Board of Agriculture in England was established in 1889. Haber's process for making a cheap fertilizer by extracting nitrogen from the air in order to make ammonia was invented by a Polish professor of physical Chemistry (1906–1911) at Karlsruhe, **Fritz Haber** (1868–1934) in 1908. The practice of crop rotation and the use of leguminous plants were advocated by an agricultural scientist, **George Washington Carver** (1860–1943) from Missouri. *See agricultural instruments, agronomy, animal husbandry, dairy farming, fertilizers, soil science.*

Agrippa, Marcus (*c.* 63–12 BC) Roman commander and statesman who defeated Mark Antony at Actium in 31 BC. *See water supply.*

Agronomy [Latin: *agros,* field + Greek: *nomia,* to arrange or classify] Science of soil management and crop rotation. **Sir Richard Weston** (1591–1672) from Sutton in Surrey was one of the pioneers of crop rotation in England. He studied

ley farming (rotation of crops and grass) in Europe and introduced the method into England. The four-course rotation system, which enabled the keeping of livestock during the winter and improved the productivity of the land, was developed in England by an agriculturist, **Charles Townshend** (1674–1738) of Norfolk. This system became popularly known as the Norfolk System. A pioneer in the field and professor of chemistry at the Sorbonne (1839), **Jean Baptiste Joseph Dieudonné Boussingault** (1802–1887), published *Mémoires de chimie agricole et de physiologie* (1854) and *Agronomie chimie agricole, et physiologie.* The practice of crop rotation and the use of leguminous plants in America were advocated by an agricultural scientist, **George Washington Carver** (1860–1943) from Missouri. A Russian plant geneticist, **Nikolai Ivanovitch Vavilov** (1887–1943), brought over 50 000 varieties of plants from all over the world to his country and tested their suitability for crop rotation. He published *Centers of Origin of Cultivated Plants* in 1920. *See agriculture.*

Ahmes Papyrus The oldest existing mathematical manuscript copied from an earlier manuscript (1825 BC) by Ahmes of Egypt during the reign of Auserre Apopi I (1607–1566 BC). The Ahmes papyrus was bought by a Scottish Egyptologist, **Alexander Henry Rhind** (1833– 1863) in Cairo in 1858 and was brought to London. The papyrus, which is also known as the Rhind papyrus, is now in the British Museum in London. *See mathematics.*

Aiken, Howard Hathaway (1900–1973) *See calculating machine, computers.*

Air A Greek philosopher, **Anaximenes** of Miletus (b 550 BC), who was a follower of **Thales** (640–546 BC), proposed that air is the essence of all things including life and named it *pneuma* to mean breath. **Empedocles of Agrigento** was the first to demonstrate that air has weight, in 450 BC. **Philo** of Byzantinium (*c.* AD 200) was probably the first to record the diminution of volume of air in a globe when a candle is burnt in it. The first study on the physical properties of air, including its compressibility, elasticity and weight was done by **Robert Boyle** (1627–1691) and his assistant, **Robert Hooke** (1635–1703), in 1660. The first experiments on the composition of air were done by **John Mayow** (1640–1679), an English physician, in 1674. He showed that when a substance was burnt in a closed vessel the volume of air diminished and that combustion ceased. **Stephen Hales** (1696–1761), an English vicar at Teddington, during his experiments in 1724 came to the conclusion that air had a certain amount of elasticity which was destroyed by a burning candle. Nitrogen was obtained from air by

Daniel Rutherford (1749–1819), a pupil of **Joseph Black** (1728–1799), in 1772. A Swedish apothecary and chemist, **Carl Wilhelm Scheele** (1742–1786) demonstrated the presence of oxygen in atmospheric air in 1773. **Henry Cavendish** (1731–1810) published his treatise on the composition of air in 1784. The French chemist **Joseph Louis Gay-Lussac** (1778–1850) took several samples of atmospheric air from a balloon at different altitudes; further studies led to the law of combination of gases. **Antoine Laurent Lavoisier** (1743–1794) published his work *Elementary Treatise on Chemistry,* describing the properties of hydrogen, nitrogen and oxygen in the air, in 1789.

Air Balloon   The idea of the air balloon was proposed by **Albert of Saxony** (*c.* 1316–1390), an Augustinian monk of the 14th century. **Roger Bacon** (*c.* 1214–*c.* 1298) of Oxford believed that a globe made of copper and filled with air might fly. The principle of the balloon was demonstrated before the King of Portugal by a Jesuit priest, **Laurenço de Guzmon** or **Bartolomeu de Gusmao** (1685–1724) in 1709. Two brothers and sons of a wealthy paper maker in France, **Joseph Michel Montgolfier** (1740–1810) and **Jacques Étienne Montgolfier** (1745–1799) demonstrated the flight of a 35 meter diameter balloon in 1783. In the same year a French physicist and professor of physics in Paris, **Jacques Alexandre César Charles** (1746–1823) became the first to use a hydrogen balloon, which he made from rubberized silk. The first flight carrying a live cargo – of a sheep, a cock and a duck – was performed before Louis XVI later in the same year. **Count Francesco Zambeccari** (1756–1812) of Bologna pioneered the navigation of air balloons with the use of oars and other methods, but died when his balloon became entangled in a tree and caught fire. The first crewed ascent in a balloon was made by **François Pilâtre de Rozier** (1757–1785), on 15 October 1783. The first balloon crossing of the English Channel was achieved by an American physician from Boston, **John Jeffries** (1744–1819), who emigrated to England. The first powered balloon or airship with a steerable rudder was built and flown over a distance of 17 miles by a French engineer, **Henri Giffard** (1825–1882), in 1852. A French pioneer, **Gaston Tissandier** (1835–1899), invented a navigable balloon propelled by electricity. The first scientific observations and physiological data in aviation were recorded during a balloon ascent by an English meteorologist, **James Glaisher** (1809–1903), and a surgeon, **Henry Tracy Coxwell** (1819–1900), at a height of *c.* 8800 m in 1862. A Swiss physicist, **Auguste Antoine Piccard** (1884–1962), made pioneering studies of the stratosphere by constructing a special balloon with which he reached a height of over

15 000 meters in 1931. His balloon was the first to be fitted with a pressurized cabin. *See airship.*

Air Brake   A compressed air brake for railways was invented by the English inventor **Samuel Cunliffe Lister** (1815–1906) of Bradford in 1848. An improved and safer form was devised by an American engineer, **George Westinghouse** (1846–1914) of New York, in 1869. His device allowed the driver of the locomotive to apply uniform and simultaneous braking to all the carriages. He founded the Westinghouse Electrical Company in 1886.

Air Conditioner   The first practical air conditioner was invented by **Willis Haviland Carrier** (1876–1950) of New York in 1902. In 1915 he founded the Carrier Engineering Corporation, which built an advanced air condition system for the skyscrapers of New York in 1939.

Air Cushion Vehicle (ACV)   *See hovercraft.*

Air Pump   Invented by **Otto von Guericke** (1602–1686), mayor of Magdeburg in Prussia, in 1656. His work was published by a Jesuit priest, **Kasper Schott** (1608–1666), in his *Mechanica Hydraulico-Pneumatica* in 1657. Schott's book was studied by **Robert Boyle** (1627–1691) and his assistant, **Robert Hooke** (1635–1703), who modified and improved the pump in 1659. Using this device Boyle was able to create a vacuum and demonstrate that air is essential to life. His experiments on air with the use of the air pump, entitled *New Experiments Physico-Mechanicall touching the spring of the Air*, was published in 1660.

Air Raid   *See warplanes.*

Air Thermometer   *See thermometer.*

Aircraft   *See airplane.*

Airlines   The German airship pioneer **Count von Ferdinand Zeppelin** (1838–1917) operated the world's first airline from 1910 to 1914, during which time 30 000 passengers were carried without any casualties. The world's first long distance passenger plane, the *Goliath,* was built in 1917 by two French brothers, **Henri Farman** (1874–1958) and **Maurice Farman** (1878–1964). The national airline of The Netherlands, *Koninklijki-Luchtvart-Maatschappiji NV* (KLM) conducted the world's first scheduled airplane flights, between Amsterdam and London, in 1920. The Handley-Page Transport Company, which later developed into British Airways, was established in 1919 and merged with Imperial Airways in 1924. One of the first commercial passenger airlines, Pan American Airways, was founded in 1927 by **Juan Terry Trippe** (1899–1981), a bomber pilot from New Jersey. The USSR state airline was founded in

1923 and was named *Aeroflot* in 1932. **Charles Thomas Phillipe Ulm** (1898–1934) of Melbourne founded the first Australian National Airways in 1929. It lasted for only 2 years. The airline now known as QANTAS was established in 1931 under the name Queensland and Northern Territory Aerial Services Limited by Australian aviator **Wilbot Hudson Fysh** (1895–1974). He was a historian of aviation and was knighted in 1953. **William Edward Boeing** (1881–1956), an American aircraft manufacturer, established the Boeing Air Transport Company in 1927 which became United Air Lines in 1934. The Boeing 747, known as the Jumbo Jet, first flew in 1969. The first supersonic passenger plane, *Aérospatiale Concorde,* with a speed of 1450 mph and designed for 100 passengers, was flown in 1969. It was launched as a regular passenger airliner through a joint French–British project in 1976. *See airplane, supersonic flight.*

Airplane [Latin: *aer*, air + *planus*, flat] The possibility of flight was explored by an Augustinian monk, **Albert of Saxony** (*c.* 1316–1390) in the 14th century. The first design for a flying machine, although impractical, was drawn by **Leonardo da Vinci** (1452–1519) around 1500. A Jesuit priest, Francesco de Lana de Terzi, designed an airship made of copper spheres in the 17th century. A practical design for an airplane was published by **Emanuel Swedenborg** (1688–1722) of Sweden in 1717. In 1847 an English mechanic, **John Stringfellow** (1799–1883), and William Henson built a steam-powered airplane with a 20-feet wing span. It was unsuccessful owing to the excessive weight of the engine. Later, in 1848, Stringfellow demonstrated a smaller model in London which was capable of flying up to 120 feet. The term *aeroplane* was coined by French pioneer of aviation, **Clement Ader** (1841–1926), who first succeeded in flying a plane heavier than air with a light-powered steam engine, for a distance of 50 meters in 1890. His flight was followed by that of the American brothers, **Orville Wright** (1871–1948) and **Wilbur Wright** (1861–1912) of Dayton, Ohio, who demonstrated their first glider at Kitty Hawk, North Carolina in 1901. In 1878 **Lawrence Hargrave** (1850–1915), an Australian pioneer, born in Greenwich, England, studied aeronautics and designed a box-kite with wings, which was translated into early aircraft. He used four of these kites to lift him 5 meters from the ground. In 1899 he designed a rotary engine used in most of the early aircraft. A German engineer and a pioneer in aeronautics, **Otto Lilienthal** (1848–1896), published *Bird Flight as a Basis of Aviation* in 1889. After his first successful glider was built in 1891 he was killed during a glide in 1896. The first motor-driven plane was demonstrated by G.

Whitehead in the same year. Orville Wright flew the first plane fitted with a combustion engine, the *Flyer I,* over a distance of 120 feet for 12 seconds in 1903. Later in 1905 he made a non-stop flight of 40 kilometers. **Alberto Santos Dumont** (1873–1932) of Brazil who was a pioneer in heavier-than-air flying demonstrated his first flight at Bagatelle, near Paris, in 1906. The first public one-kilometer airplane flight in America was achieved by **Glen Hammond Curtiss**, (1878–1930) of New York in his *June Bug* at a speed of 40 kilometers per hour in 1908. He also constructed the first practical sea plane which he patented in 1911. A British aircraft pioneer, **Alliot Verdon Roe** (1877–1958) from Manchester was the first Englishman to construct and fly his own aircraft, in 1908. He later developed the famous Avro series aircraft. An American pilot, **Samuel Franklin Cody** (1861–1913) made the first official flight in Great Britain at Farnborough, Hants in 1908. **John Theodore Cuthbert Moore-Brabazon** (1884–1964) made three short but sustained flights in Britain in 1909. A Frenchman, **Louis Blériot** (1872–1936), made the first cross-channel flight in his monoplane in the same year. **Frederick William Lanchester** (1868–1948) of Lewisham, London after an unsuccessful attempt in 1911 produced an aircraft that successfully flew in 1913. The aircraft that performed the historic round-the-world flight in 1924 was designed by **Donald Willis Douglas** (1892–1971), an aeronautical engineer from Brooklyn, New York. Douglas founded an aircraft company which started making a series of DC planes in 1920. He later joined with the American pioneer in space technology, **James Smith McDonnell** (1899–1980) from Denver, and floated the McDonnell Douglas Corporation for making aircraft in 1967. An English historian in the field, **Charles Harvard Gibbs-Smith** (1909–1981) of Teddington, published *Aviation – an Historical Survey from its Origins to the End of World War II* in 1960. *See aerodynamics, airlines, airship, supersonic flight, transatlantic flight, warplanes.*

Airships Also known as dirigibles. The term refers to semi-rigid or rigid air balloons, which became the first practical means of air travel. A Jesuit priest, Francesco de Lana de Terzi, designed an airship made of copper spheres and a mast in 1670. He believed that it might fly if the air was extracted from the spheres. The first steam-powered airship with a steerable rudder was built and flown by a French engineer, **Henri Giffard** (1825–1882) of Paris in 1852. The German airship pioneer **Count von Ferdinand Zeppelin** (1838–1917) flew his first airship, powered by two 16 horse-power engines, at a speed of 20 mph in 1900. His airships operated the world's first airline from 1910 to 1914, during which time 30 000 passengers were carried without any casualties. His airships were used against the Allies during the First World War. The first British airship was built by Stanley Spencer, who made his maiden flight from Crystal Palace, North London, in 1902. The first scheduled flights, using airships, were started by Delag (Deutsche Luftschiffahrt) at Frankfurt am Main in 1910. The largest British airship, made at the Royal Airship Works in Cardington, Bedfordshire, was first flown in 1929. It later crashed near Beauvais, France, in 1930, killing all 48 passengers. An English aeronautical engineer, **Sir Barnes Neville Wallis** (1887–1979) designed an airship for Vickers Company which, after its maiden flight in 1929, later made a successful Atlantic crossing. The ill-fated American airship *Hindenberg,* launched in 1936, made 54 flights until it caught fire over Lakehurst, New Jersey, killing 36 passengers. The US airship, *Akron,* launched in 1931, had room for 207 passengers.

Airy, Sir George Biddle (1801–1892) of Northumberland. The seventh Astronomer Royal, who modernized the observatory at Greenwich. He applied photography to astronomical research and founded the magnetic department of Greenwich Observatory in 1834. Airy did research on optics and corrected astigmatism with the use of a lens in 1824. He performed a series of pendulum experiments to determine the mean density of the earth at Harton Colliery, South Shields, near Newcastle and published over 500 papers. *See Greenwich Mean Time.*

Aitken, John (1839–1919) A Scottish physicist from Falkirk who did extensive studies on climatology, dealing with atmospheric dust, dew and cyclones. His collected works were published posthumously in 1923.

Aitken, Robert Grant (1864–1951) An American astronomer from California who, at the Lick Observatory, discovered more than 4000 new double stars and published *Binary Stars* in 1918.

Aki, Keiiti (b 1930) *See seismology.*

Al-Battani, Abu Abduallah (*c.* AD 1100) *See zij.*

Albert of Saxony (*c.* 1316–1390) *See airplane, air balloon, motion, vacuum.*

Alberti, Leone Battista (1404–1472) *See architecture, Italian.*

Albertus, Magnus (1192–1280) or Albrecht of Cologne. A Dominican priest, philosopher and scientist who also dealt in astrology and alchemy. His compilation of botanical plants in 1250, *De Vegetabilibus* (on plants), remained a popular work on the subject for many centuries. He was a faithful follower of Aristotle and wrote voluminous commentaries

on his works. He was one of the first to describe arsenic in detail. *See affinity, alchemy, arsenic, fossils, hybridization.*

Albin, Elezar (d 1759) *See entomology, ornithology.*

Albright, Arthur (1811–1900) *See matches.*

Albright, William Foxell (1891–1971) *See cave exploration.*

Albuzjani or Abdul Wafa (AD 940–998) *See trigonometry.*

Alchemy [Greek: *chemia*; Arabic: *al*, the + *kimiya*, the art of counterfeiting gold or silver] The fundamental aim of alchemy was to obtain the 'essence' which would change base metals into gold, cure all diseases and give eternal youth. The guardian or possessor of this essence or 'philosopher's stone' was a mythical personality, Hermes Trismegeastos. Its origin is difficult to trace but alchemy is supposed to have been practiced by the Chinese in 133 BC. The earliest documented literature on the subject was written in the 4th century in Alexandria by **Zosmismus of Papolis**. The pursuit of this goal contributed to the development of chemistry and metallurgy. Some of the works on alchemy are found in the writings of **Geberius** in the middle ages, **Albertus Magnus** (1192–1280), **Roger Bacon** (*c.* 1214 – *c.* 1298) of Oxford, and a Benedictine monk, **Basilus Valentinus** (*c.* AD 1500). The English alchemist **Robert of Chester** (*c.* 1200) wrote his *Book of the Composition of Alchemy* in 1144. **Paracelsus or Theophrastus Bombastus von Hohenheim** (1493–1541) proposed that the true aim of alchemy should be to cure diseases and the preparation and study of drugs should be the main object of the chemist. An English alchemist, **Thomas Norton** (*c.* 1480) of Bristol, wrote on the subject in the form of a verse entitled *The Ordinall of Alchimy* around 1477 which first appeared in print in English in 1652 in **Elias Ashmole's** (1617–1692) *Theatrum Chemicum.*

Alcmaeon (*c.* 500 BC) *See Empedocles.*

Alcock, John William (1892–1919) *See Transatlantic flight.*

Aldehyde [Arabic: *alkohl*, powder of antimony + Latin: *de,* away + Greek: *hydros,* water] The term was introduced into chemistry by **Johann Christian Poggendorf** (1796–1877) of Berlin while he was working with another German chemist, **Justus von Liebig** (1803–1873). An industrial organic chemist, **Ludwig Gatterman** (1860–1920), devised a synthesis of aromatic aldehydes by the reaction of a mixture of hydrogen chloride and hydrogen cyanide, in the presence of a catalyst, on reactive aromatic compounds such as phenols (the Gatterman reaction).

Alder, Kurt (1902–1958) *See Diels–Alder reaction.*

Aldrin, Edwin 'Buzz' (b 1930) *See astronauts.*

Aldrovandi, Ulysses (1522–1605) A professor at the papal university of Bologna and first director of the botanical gardens established there in 1567. He published a voluminous work on birds (1599) in three volumes and another on insects (1602). *See ornithology.*

Ale [Anglo-Saxon: *Alu, beer*] The Egyptians were supposed to be the first to have made liquor from corn by fermentation. Ale was known as a beverage as early as 404 BC. Ale-houses were mentioned in the laws of the king of Essex in AD 688 and they were regulated in 1551. In 1603, during the reign of James I of England, the price and the measure of ale were specified, and a duty on ale was introduced in 1643.

Aleksandrov, Pavel Sergeevich (1896–1982) *See topology.*

Alembert, Jean de Rond d' (1717–1783) *See calculus, d'Alembert principle.*

Alessi, Galeazzo (1512–1572) *See architecture, Italian.*

Alexander Polynomial Theorem If different polynomials are computed from two drawings, the two drawings represent different knots. Proposed independently by **James Waddell Alexander** and **Kurt Reidemeister** in the late 1920s. In 1984 **Vaughan Jones**, a mathematician at the University of California, Berkeley, invented a new rule for assigning a group of integers to each drawing.

Alexander Technique A system of mental and bodily control of self-cure for bad posture, muscular tension and other conditions, proposed by an Australian, Frederick Matthias Alexander (1869–1955). He initially developed the method to cure his throat and voice trouble, and published *Use of the Self* (1931).

Alexander the Great (355–323 BC) *See Alexandrian Museum and Library, Aristotle, diamonds.*

Alexander, Tilloch (1759–1829) *See printing.*

Alexanderson, Ernst Frederick Werner (1878–1975) *See color television.*

Alexandrian Museum and Library An ancient academic institution, which linked the culture and education from Egypt to Macedonia, which was established by Ptolemy I Soter around 284 BC following the death of **Alexander the Great** (355–323 BC). It became a great university where scholars from all over the world, such as **Euclid** (*c.* 300) the mathematician, **Archimedes** (287–212 BC) the physicist, **Herophilos of Chalcedon** (*c.* 250 BC) the anatomist,

Erasistratus (310–250 BC) the physiologist and scores of other important men came to study and participate. The museum consisted of four departments, literature, mathematics, astronomy and medicine, and its library was the largest and most famous in the world. It had over 400 000 volumes or scrolls, out of which about 200 000 rolls from Pergamnus were supposed to have been given by Marc Anthony to Cleopatra in 40 BC. The museum and library were destroyed during a civil war in AD 272.

Alfonsine Tables A set of astronomical tables mainly derived from **Ptolemy's** (*c.* AD 127–151) *Almagest*. They were compiled at Toledo by Hazen, a Jewish astronomer in around 1270, under the sponsorship of Alfonso X of Castille (*c.* 1221–1284). The tables were introduced into Paris around 1327 and **John of Saxony** (*c.* 1327–1355) provided the Latin instructions.

Algae [Latin: *alga*, seaweed] Primitive water plants with single or multiple cells containing chlorophyll. A German botanist and physician, **Johannes Hedwig** (1730–1799), was the first to observe and illustrate conjugation in algae. He published *Cryptogamia* and several other botanical works. His *Species Muscotum*, posthumously published in 1801, was a starting point in naming the algae. An Irish botanist and keeper of the herbarium collection at Trinity College, Cambridge, **William Henry Harvey** (1811–1866) published the *Manual of British Algae* in 1840. A German botanist, **Nathaniel Pringsheim** (1823–1894), introduced a uniform terminology for the reproductive structures of algae.

Algebra [Arabic: *al-jabr*] The study of structural or manipulative properties in mathematics. It represents a form of generalized arithmetic where variables or letters are used for numbers. The use of a letter for a number is found in the works of **Aristotle** (384–322 BC). The Alexandrian mathematician **Diophantus** (*c.* 250 BC) in his 13 books on arithmetic (*Arithmetica*) laid the foundation for the present system of algebra. An Arab, **Alkarismi** or **Abu Jafar Mohammed ibn Musa Al-Khowarimi** (*c.* 800–850) introduced letters, to represent numbers and measurement, in calculations for the first time, and this formed the basis for algebra. His treatise *al-jabr wa'l muqabalah'* [joining the parts to make a whole] gave origin to the term algebra. **Brahmagupta**, a Hindu mathematician from Ujjain around the 7th century, was the first to assign the rules for negative numbers in algebra. The first Latin treatise on algebra, *Liber Abaci*, was written by **Leonardo Fibonacci** (*c.* 1172–1250) of Pisa. In this book he introduced the Indian and Arabic numerals including the zero to the west. **Girolomo Cardan**

(1501–1576) published an advanced treatise on algebra, entitled *Ars Magna*, in 1545. It was the first printed book on algebra for solving equations. **Rafael Bombelli** (1526–1573) of Bologna published one of the most comprehensive accounts of the subject in the 16th century which, apart from some original work, revived the algebra of Diophantus. A German monk, **Michael Stifel** (1487–1567), used letters for unknown quantities. The use of symbols in algebra to designate known quantities was introduced into Europe by a French mathematician, **François Viète** (1540–1603). He published *In Artem Analyticam Isagoge* in 1591. Scientific classification of methods applied to cubic and biquadratic equations was proposed by the French mathematician **Jean Louis Lagrange** (1736–1813). He published *Théorie des Fonctions Analytiques* (1797), *Leçons sur le Calcul des Fonctions* (1806) and several other important works. The first treatise on algebra in English, *The whetstone of witte* (*c.* 1540–1542) was written by an English mathematician, **Robert Recorde** (*c.* 1510–1558). The equality sign was used for the first time in this book. The Oxford mathematician, **Thomas Harriot's** (1560–1621) treatise on algebra (*Artis analyticae praxis*) was published posthumously in 1631. Another important work, *De Algebra Tractatus; Historicus & Practicus* was published by one of the founders of the Royal Society and Savillian Professor at Oxford, **John Wallis** (1616–1703), in 1685. The concept of the group, the cornerstone of modern algebra, was proposed by the French mathematician **Evariste Galois** (1811–1832) around 1829.

Alhazen or **Abu Ali al-Hassan Ibn Al-Haitham** (965–1038) An Arab mathematician from Basra who was the first to study the properties of light and convex lenses. His work *Kitab Al-Manazir* (Book of Optics) on refraction, reflection and study of lenses, formed the basis for the invention of spectacles, the telescope and the microscope. Alhazen died in Cairo at the age of 73. The first Latin translation of Alhazen's mathematical works was written in 1210 by a clergyman from Sussex in England, **Robert Grosseteste** (1175–1253), who became bishop of Lincoln in 1235. Alhazen's treatise on astrology was printed in Latin at Basle in 1572.

Alizarin *See dyes.*

Al-Kashi, Ghiyath al-Din (*c.* 1400) A physician and astronomer from Iran who became the first director of Ulugh Beg's observatory at Samarkand, in 1424. He calculated the value of π to 16 decimal places.

Al-Khowarimi, Alkarismior Abu Jafar Mohammed ibn Musa (*c.* 800–850) *See algebra, irrational numbers, quadratic equation, zij.*

Allen, James Alfred van (b 1914) *See magnetosphere, Van Allen belts.*

Alloy [Latin: *ad*, to + *ligo*, bind] A blend of two or more metals. *See amalgam, brass, bronze, invar, pewter, soldering.*

Almagest [Arabic: *Al magiste*, the greatest] One of the greatest works on astronomy, entitled *Megale tes astronomias*, written by **Ptolemy of Alexandria** (AD 127–145). It was named *Al magiste* by the Arabs to mean the greatest. It contains illustrations of ancient astronomical instruments and elaborate astronomical tables and was translated into Latin in the 12th century. The first printed version appeared in Basle in 1538.

Al-Masudi, Abul Hassan (*c.* 900–956) An Arabian geographer from Baghdad who traveled widely in India, Africa and Islamic countries. He realized the influence of the geographical environment on animal and plant life, and wrote history based on science. He is regarded by some historians as the Pliny of the Islamic world.

Alpha First letter [α] of the Greek alphabet, sometimes used to denote the first member of a series or group. It is derived from the Phoenician word *aleph* for ox.

Alpha Decay Type of radioactive disintegration in which alpha particles are emitted by the nucleus of a radioactive element. *See alpha particles.*

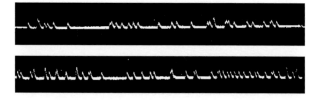

Figure 4 Photographic recording of alpha particles with a string galvanometer by Ernest Rutherford. Rutherford, Ernest. *Radioactive Substances and their Radiation*. Cambridge: Cambridge University Press, 1913

Alpha Particles Two English physicists, New Zealand-born **Lord Ernest Rutherford** (1871–1937), and **Frederick Soddy** (1877–1965) in 1902 proposed that radioactive elements underwent spontaneous changes or disintegration with the emission of high velocity negatively charged electrons or beta rays, and positively charged particles or alpha rays. The term alpha rays was first used by Rutherford to refer to less penetrating rays from radium, which were unable to pass through an aluminum foil of greater than a fiftieth of a millimeter thickness. The behavior of alpha particles was studied in detail by **Charles**

Thompson Rees Wilson (1869–1959), professor of natural philosophy at the University of Cambridge. An explanation for alpha decay on the basis of quantum mechanical tunneling was given by an American physicist, **Edward Uhler Condon** (1902–1974) from Almogorda, New Mexico. A Russian-born American physicist, **George Gamow** (1904–1968) independently gave a similar explanation in 1928. The term alpha ray has been superseded, as the so-called rays are now known to consist of a stream of particles – alpha particles or the nuclei of helium atoms.

Alpha Radiation   *See alpha particles.*

Alphabet [Greek: *alpha,* the first letter of the Greek alphabet + *beta,* the second letter of the Greek alphabet]   *See writing.*

Alpher, Ralph Asher (b 1921)   *See Big Bang theory.*

Alpine Flora   Plants suited to mountain districts. An Irish botanist, **John Ball** (1818–1889), was a pioneer in the field and the first president of the Alpine Club in 1857. He published the *Alpine Guide* (1863–1868) and proposed an ecological theory for Alpine plants of South America.

Alpini, Prospero (1533–1617)   *See botany, coffee plant.*

Al-Qibaji, Baylak (*c.* 1350)   *See compass (1).*

Alter, David (1807–1881)   *See spectroscopy.*

Alternating Current [AC]   The theory was first proposed by a Polish-born electrical engineer, **Charles Proteus Steinmetz** (1865–1923), who emigrated to the USA in 1888. An American engineer, **Arthur Edwin Kennelly** (1861–1939), professor of electrical engineering at Harvard (1902–1930), contributed to the theory and defined the term inductance speed. The first successful commercial generator for producing alternating current was built by a Belgian electrical engineer, **Zenobe Theophile Gramme** (1826–1901), in 1867. A Croatian-born US electrical engineer, **Nikola Tesla** (1856–1943), built an AC motor in 1888. An electricity generator that produces an alternating current was invented by the English electrical engineer **Sir John Ambrose Fleming** (1849–1945), of Lancaster, in 1904. An American engineer, **George Westinghouse** (1846–1914) of New York, was a pioneer in the use of alternating current for distributing electric power and he founded the Westinghouse Electric Company in 1886. **William Stanley** (1858–1916) of Brooklyn, New York, developed a long-range transmission system for alternating current. An English-born US inventor, **Elihu Thomson** (1853–1937) developed the three-phase alternating current generator.

Alternation of Generations [Latin: *alter,* the other, Greek: *genos,* offspring]   The resemblance of the offspring of certain animals to their grandparents or remote ancestors but not to their parents. A Danish zoologist, **Johann Lapetus Steenstrup** (1813–1897), first described this in his treatise *Propagation and Development of Animals through Alternate Generations* in 1892. He was appointed professor of zoology and director of the Zoological Museum at the University of Copenhagen in 1848.

Alternator [Latin: *alter,* the other]   An electricity generator that produces an alternating current, invented by an English electrical engineer **Sir John Ambrose Fleming** (1849–1945) of Lancaster in 1904. *See alternating current.*

Altman, Richard (1852–1900)   *See freeze drying.*

Altman, Sidney (b 1939)   *See ribonucleic acid.*

Altum, Bernard (1824–1900)   *See ecology.*

Al-Tusi, Sharaf al-Din (*c.* 1150)   *See astrolabe.*

Alum [Latin: *alumen*]   A compound used in ancient times to treat hide stripped from animals to prepare leather. Preparation of leather by a similar method is mentioned in Homer's (*c.* 800 BC) *Iliad.* The first mention of alum is found in the Ebers papyrus, suggesting that it was in use around 2000 BC. The first alum sources found in Britain were in the Isle of Wight and Yorkshire. Sir Thomas Chaloner of Longhull Manor, Yorkshire, was the first to start manufacturing alum in England, in 1600. An economic way of producing alum on a large scale by using sulfuric acid was invented by a Scottish chemist, Peter Spence, in 1845.

Aluminum [Latin: *alumen,* alum]   The element with atomic number 13. The term *alumen* was used by the Romans to denote general substances with astringent properties. The presence of aluminum in the earth's clay was demonstrated by a German chemist, **Andreas Sigismond Marggrafe** (1709–1782), in 1754, and **Hans Christian Oerstedt** (1777–1851) of Copenhagen obtained the chloride of aluminum in 1826. The pure metal was extracted by **Friedreich Wöhler** (1800–1882) in 1827 and his method was simplified by **Robert Bunsen** (1811–1899). The first production of aluminum in commercial quantities was achieved in 1855 by **Henri Étienne Saint-Claire Deville** (1818–1881), a French chemist of West Indian origin. The world's first aluminum factory was set up by **James Fern Webster** at Solihull Lodge near Birmingham in 1881. An economic electrolytic method of producing aluminum was invented by an American industrial chemist, **Charles Martin Hall** (1863–1914), of Ohio, in 1886. A French metallurgist, **Paul Louis Toussaint Héroult** (1863–1914), invented an electrolytic method for extracting aluminum from cryolite.

Alvarez, Louis Walter (1911–1989) *See bubble chamber, radar.*

Alfvén, Hannes Olof Gösta (1908–1995) *See magnetic recording, plasma physics.*

Al-Zalqali, Abu Ishaq (*c.* 1100) *See waterclock, zij.*

Amagat, Emile Hilaire (1841–1915) *See gas laws.*

Amalgam [Greek: *a,* without + *malakos,* soft] The term was introduced by **Thomas Aquinas** (1225–1274) of Naples to denote alloys of various metals. It is now used to denote an alloy of mercury with one or more metals.

Amber A term for fossilized resin. *See Gilbert, William, electricity, physics.*

Ambrotypes *See photography.*

America Named after **Amerigo Vespucci** (1451–1512), a son of a notary from Florence, who helped to fit the ships for Columbus before his second expedition. In his own inaccurate description of his travels Vespucci claimed to have set sail and reached Florida via the Gulf of Mexico in 1497. He published a pamphlet in 1503 in which he recommended that his newly discovered land be called the 'New World'. The first printed map with the name America for the New World was produced by a German cartographer, **Martin Waldseemuller** (*c.* 1480–1521), in 1507. **Christopher Columbus** (1451–1506) reached the Bahamas in 1492 and the South American mainland in 1498. **Peter Apian** (1495–1552), a professor of mathematics at Ingolstadt and a physician, used the name America on his map in 1520. The first map of the United States as a new nation was published by Abel Buell in 1783.

American Academy of Arts and Sciences Founded in 1780 in Boston.

American Association for the Advancement of Science Founded in 1847 with **William Redfield** (1789–1857) of Connecticut as its first president.

American Institute of Electrical Engineers Founded in 1884 and held its first American electrical exhibition in the same year in Philadelphia.

American Journal of Mathematics The first US research journal in mathematics, founded in 1878 by **James Joseph Sylvester** (1814–1897), a mathematician from London,

while he was professor of mathematics at the Johns Hopkins University, Baltimore.

American Journal of Science Founded in 1818 under the elaborate title *American Journal of Science, more especially of Mineralogy, Geology, and the Branches of Natural History including also agriculture and the ornamental as well as useful arts* by an American chemist, **Benjamin Silliman** (1779–1864), of Connecticut. He was the father of **Benjamin Silliman** (1816–1885), a professor of chemistry at Yale, who first showed that petroleum was a mixture of hydrocarbons.

American Mathematical Society Founded under the name New York Mathematical Society in 1888. It changed to its present name in 1894.

American Philosophical Society First proposed by **Benjamin Franklin** (1706–1790) in 1743, held its first meeting in Philadelphia in 1769. It was the first society to be formed in America for the promotion of science. The first issue of its *Transactions* appeared in 1771.

American Scientific Journals The *American Journal of Science, more especially of Mineralogy, Geology, and the Branches of Natural History including also agriculture and the ornamental as well as useful arts* was founded by a chemist, **Benjamin Silliman** (1779–1864), of Connecticut, in 1818. Its title was shortened to *American Journal of Science and Arts* a year later, and it eventually became the *American Journal of Science*. The *Astronomical Journal,* which was the first American periodical on astronomy, was founded by **Benjamin Apthorp Gould** (1824–1896), an astronomer at Boston, Massachusetts, in 1849, and it continued until 1861. The *Scientific American,* the first American scientific magazine for the general reader, was founded by a New York inventor, Rufus Porter, in 1845. He published a list of his inventions weekly in his newspaper, until he sold it to another inventor, Beach (1826–1896) in 1846. The first US research journal in mathematics, the *American Journal of Mathematics,* was founded by **James Joseph Sylvester** (1814–1897), an eminent mathematician from London, in 1883. An American agriculturalist, **Henry Wallace** (1836–1916), of West Newton, Pennsylvania, founded the periodical *Wallace's Farmer* in 1895. *See scientific journals.*

Americium The element with atomic number 95 was synthesized in 1944 by an American physicist, **Glenn Theodore Seaborg** (b 1912) and his team at Berkeley. He shared the Nobel Prize for Chemistry in 1951 with another American atomic scientist, **Erward Mattison McMillan** (1907–1991) of Redondo Beach, California. Ten isotopes of Americium are known, all radioactive.

Ames Test Used for identifying chemicals that damage DNA. Devised by Bruce Ames in 1973.

Amici, Giovanni Battista (1786–1863) of Modena. An Italian physicist who constructed the reflecting microscope and improved the achromatic objective of the microscope in 1812. He invented the water immersion objective for the microscope in 1840, and produced the first high-power objectives by using meniscus lenses in 1844. Amici was appointed professor of astronomy at the University of Pisa in 1835. *See achromatic lens, microscope, pollination.*

Amines A German organic chemist, **August Wilhelm von Hofmann** (1818–1892), classified amines as formal derivatives of ammonia in which one or more hydrogen atoms were replaced by compound radicals. His theory was further developed by **Charles Frederic Gerhardt** (1816–1856), an eminent chemist of Strasbourg.

Amman, Othmar Hermann (1879–1965) *See suspension bridges.*

Ammeter A device for measuring the flow of electric current in a circuit in amperes, invented by a London physicist, **William Edward Ayrton** (1847–1908), around 1884.

Ammonia Named by a Swedish chemist, **Torbern Olof Bergman** (1735–1784), in 1782, owing to the belief that it was first obtained by burning camel dung in the temple of Ammon in Libya. It was suggested to be a mixture of nitrogen and hydrogen in 1774 by **Joseph Priestley** (1733–1804), a clergyman and chemist from Leeds. His theory was experimentally demonstrated by a French chemist, **Claude Louis Compte de Berthollet** (1748–1822). **Joseph Louis Proust** (1754–1826) demonstrated the proportions of nitrogen and hydrogen in ammonia. A method of synthesis of ammonia was invented by a German chemist, **Karl Bosch** (1874–1940). He shared the Nobel Prize for Chemistry with **Friedrich Karl Rudolf Bergius** (1884–1949) for developing high-pressure chemical methods. *See Haber process, refrigeration.*

Amontons, Guillaume (1663–1705) A French mathematician from Normandy who became an instrument maker in Paris, and invented various instruments including an air thermometer (1702), conical nautical barometer (1695), hygrometer (1687) and a folded barometer (1688). He was one of the first to propose the relationship of air pressure to temperature, in 1669.

Ampere An SI unit (Système International d'Unités) of electric current, named after the French physicist, **André**

Marie Ampère (1775–1836), by **William Thomson, Lord Kelvin** (1824–1907), in 1880.

Ampère, André Marie (1775–1836) A French physicist from Lyon during the time of the French revolution, when his father was guillotined. He deduced the formula for measuring electricity while he was a professor at the École Polytechnique of Paris in 1827. The SI unit (Système International d'Unités) of current, ampere, is named in his honor. *See ampere, electricity, electromagnetic theory, galvanometer.*

Amphora [Latin: *amphora*, vessel] A double-handled vessel used to measure liquids in ancient times which remained a standard measure in Europe until the 17th century.

Amplifier Invented by an American physicist and pioneer in radio and wireless telegraphy, **Lee De Forest** (1873–1961) of Iowa. It consisted of a thermionic valve to enable a weak radio signal to control a stronger electric current which fluctuated in the same way as the signal. *See thermionic valve.*

Amplitude Modulation [AM] Modulation of radio waves by superimposing on a carrier so as to vary its amplitude. *See broadcasting, radio.*

Amsler-Laffon, Jakob (1823–1912) *See polar planimeter.*

Amundsen, Roald Engelbrecht Gravning (1872–1928) *See magnetic poles, South Pole.*

Amyl Alcohol An aliphatic alcohol discovered by a French professor of chemistry in Paris, **Auguste Cahours** (1813–1891).

Amylase [Greek: *amygdale*, almond + *lysis*, loosening] A French chemist **Anselme Payen** (1795–1871) extracted the substance that was capable of breaking down starch to sugar from germinated barley seeds in 1833, and named it amylase. The term is now applied to any of a group of closely related enzymes.

Anacharasis of Scythia (*c.* 569 BC) *See bellows, smelting.*

Analytical Chemistry [Greek: *analusis*, loosening] Pioneer work in the field was done by the Swedish chemist **Torbern Olof Bergman** (1735–1784). He compiled extensive affinity tables for acids and bases. A German chemist, **Karl Remigius Fresenius** (1818–1897), was a pioneer in analytical chemistry. He designed a systematic way of identifying compounds by precipitating various radicles through precipitation reactions. The English translation of his work, entitled *Elementary Instruction in Qualitative Analysis,* appeared in 1841.

Analytical Geometry [Greek: *analusis*, loosening] Also known as coordinate geometry. A system of geometry in which points, lines, shapes and surfaces are represented by algebraic expressions. Application of analytical methods to geometrical problems was known to the ancient Greeks including **Menaechmus** (375–325 BC) and **Apollonius of Perga** (260–200 BC). **Pappus of Alexandria** (AD 300–350) was one of the first to write on the subject. **René Descartes** (1596–1650) in the 17th century revived the Greek method of analytical geometry. He introduced variables and constants into conventional geometry so as to express curves in the form of algebraic equations. The important concept of applying motion into a geometric field was proposed by Descartes in his work *La Géométrie* in 1637. The credit for the invention of modern analytical geometry belongs to the French mathematician **Pierre de Fermat** (1601–1665), who published an important work on the subject entitled *Ad locos planos et solidos isagoge*. A German physicist and mathematician, **Julius Plücker** (1801–1868), made important contributions and published *Theorie der algebraischen Curven* (1839) and *System der Geometrie des Raumes in neur analytischer Behandlungweise* (1846).

Anaphase [Greek: *ana*, upon + *phasis,* appearance] A stage in mitotic cell division, described and named by a German botanist and professor at Bonn, **Eduard Adolf Strasburger** (1844–1912), in 1884.

Anatomy [Greek: *ana*, upon + *temnein*, to cut] **Herophilos of Chalcedon** and **Erasistratus** (310–250 BC) of the University of Alexandria, were the first to do public dissections for teaching human anatomy, around 250 BC.

Anaxagorus (*c.* 500–428 BC) *See circle, cosmology, earthquake, eclipse, element, physics, rainbow.*

Anaximander (611–547 BC) A Greek philosopher and astronomer born in Miletus (now Turkey). He was the first Greek to draw a map of the earth giving details of its surface, and speculate on the size and distances of the heavenly bodies or stars. His proposal that imperfectly organized beings developed from the action of the sun's heat on the cold earth and these beings evolved into animals, was probably the first idea of evolution. *See astronomy, cartography, earth, evolution, geogeny, gnomon.*

Anaximenes (b 550 BC), **of Miletus** *See air, astronomy.*

Anchor [Greek: *ancho*, press tight] Used for mooring ships. It is believed to have been invented by Anarcharis the Scythian, around 600 BC.

Andel, Tjeerd Hendrik Van (b 1923) *See oceanography.*

Anderson, Carl David (1905–1991) *See antimatter, cloud chamber, cosmic rays, positron.*

Anderson, Herbert L. (b 1914) *See atomic pile.*

Anderson, James (1739–1808) *See agricultural instruments.*

Anderson, John (1726–1796) A professor of oriental languages at Glasgow University in 1755. He was a mechanical genius and invented a gun with an air chamber to absorb the recoil in 1791. In his frustrated attempts to reform the university he conceived the idea of establishing a rival university. The Andersonian College of Glasgow was founded with the wealth he left when he died. He published *Institutes of physics* in 1786.

Anderson, John Stuart (1908–1990) *See crystallography.*

Anderson, Phillip Warren (1923–1994) An American physicist born in Indianapolis. He became professor of physics at Princeton University in 1975, and he shared the Nobel Prize for Physics in 1977, for his work on the electric and magnetic disordered system, with an English physicist, **Nevill Francis Mott** (1905–1996), and another American physicist, **John Hasbrouck van Vleck** (1899–1980).

Anderson, Tempest (1846–1913) *See volcanoes.*

Anderson, Thomas (1819–1874) *See pyridine, pyrrole.*

Anderson, Thomas Foxen (b 1911) *See electron microscope.*

Andersson, Johan Gunner (1874–1960) *See Peking man, prehistory.*

Andrews, Roy Chapman (1870–1948) *See dinosaurs, fossils.*

Andrews, Thomas (1813–1885) *See liquefaction of gases, critical temperature, ozone.*

Andromeda Nebula Named after the Greek goddess Andromeda. One of the four large galaxies visible from the earth with the naked eye. With a diameter of 200 000 light years, it contains 300 globular clusters and is one and a half times bigger than our own. It was first observed through a telescope by **Simon Marius** (1573–1624) of Germany in 1612. Detailed study of the stars in the galaxy was carried out independently by two American astronomers, **Edwin Powell Hubble** (1889–1953) from Missouri, and German-born **Walter Baade** (1893–1960). Hubble also determined the distance to the Andromeda nebula in 1923. The large space telescope placed in orbit in 1990 is named after him. The first radiomap of Andromeda nebula was obtained by a British radio astronomer, **Robert Hanbury-Brown** (b 1916), and Cyril Hazard in 1951. **Caroline Lucretia Herschel** (1750–1848), a German-born British astronomer and sister of **Sir Fredrick William Herschel** (1738–1822), discovered the companion of the nebula in 1783.

Andronicus of Cyrrus (*c.* 100 BC)   *See architecture, observatories, ancient.*

Andronicus of Rhodes (*c.* 70–50 BC)   *See metaphysics.*

Anemometer [Greek: *anemos,* wind + *metron,* measure] A device for measuring wind speed. The most basic form, the cup-type anemometer, consists of cups at the ends of arms, speed of rotation of which indicates the wind speed. Vane-type anemometers have vanes, like a small windmill or propeller, which rotate when the wind blows. An Irish astronomer, **John Thomas Romney Robinson** (1792–1882) of Dublin, designed a vane-type in 1846. Modern pressure-tube anemometers use the pressure generated by the wind to indicate speed. Hot-wire anemometers work on the principle that the rate at which heat is transferred from a hot wire to the surrounding air is a measure of the air speed.

Aneroid Barometer [Greek: *a,* without + *neroid,* moisture] The first suggestion that the fluid column can be dispensed with altogether in a barometer was made by **Gottfried Wilhelm Leibniz** (1646–1716) in 1700. The first aneroid barometer was constructed by **Jacques Nicholas Conte** (1755–1805) in 1798 and improved by Vidi in 1848.

Anfinsen, Boehmer Christian (1916–1995)   *See chromatography, ribonucleic acid.*

Angstrom Unit   Unit of length equal to 10^{-10} meter. Formerly used to measure wavelengths and intermolecular distances, but has now been replaced by the nanometer, 10^{-9} meter; 1 Å = 0.1 nm. It was defined and proposed by a French physicist, **Jacques Babinet** (1794–1872), and it was officially adopted in 1907. It is named in honor of the Swedish physicist **Anders Jonas Ångström** (1814–1874), and is used for atomic measurements and the wavelengths of electromagnetic radiation.

Ångström, Anders Jonas (1814–1874)   A Swedish physicist from Lodgo who introduced a unit of a ten millionth of a millimeter for measuring the wavelength of light. It was first called the tenth-meter and was later renamed the Ångström unit. Ångström was awarded the Rumford medal of the Royal Society in England in 1872. He discovered hydrogen in the solar atmosphere, and published a map of the solar spectrum in 1868. His *Researches in the Solar Spectrum* appeared in 1869. *See absorption spectra, aurora borealis, thermal conductivity.*

Aniline [Sanskrit: *nila,* dark blue] A primary aromatic amine, first observed in 1826 to be a product of the dry distillation of indigo, by an organic chemist from Potsdam, **Otto Unverdorben** (1806–1873). A German physician who later became an industrial chemist, **Friedlib Ferdinand Runge** (1795–1867), identified it in coal tar in 1834. Coal tar was an unwanted waste product of the coal gas industry until **August Wilhelm von Hofmann** (1818–1892) of Giessen in 1843 extracted aniline from it, thereby laying the foundations of the synthetic-dye industry. The first aniline dye, mauve, was prepared by London chemist **Sir William Henry Perkin** (1838–1907), who worked with August Hofmann at the age of 17, in 1856. A year after his discovery Perkin built his own dye factory near Sudbury, and received a knighthood in 1906.

Animal Behavior   *See ethology.*

Animal Breeding   *See animal husbandry.*

Animal Husbandry [Anglo-Saxon: *husbonda,* master of the house] The first animal to be domesticated, around 10 000 BC, was the dog. It was used to herd other animals that were in turn domesticated. The first known domesticated dog was kept in Idaho Valley in 8400 BC. Carbon dating indicates that pigs and chickens were domesticated in eastern Asia and China around 7000 BC. Goats and sheep were domesticated in Asiah, Persia, in 9000 BC and in Anatolia (now Turkey) in 7000 BC. Horses were tamed for their flesh and milk at Dereisk, Ukraine, around 4000 BC. English inventor and pioneer in new farming methods, **Jethro Tull** (1674–1741) of Basildon, Essex published *The Horse-Hoeing Husbandry* in 1733. Selection and modern inbreeding of sheep, cattle and horses in England was initiated by an agriculturist, **Robert Bakewell** (1725–1795) of Leicestershire. He established the Leicester breed of sheep and Dishley breed of Longhorn cattle. **Thomas William Coke, Earl of Leicester** (1752–1842) of Holkham was one of the first in England to promote better breeds of sheep, pigs and cattle. **John Ellman** (1753–1832) of Glynde used methods similar to Bakewell's and improved the Southdown sheep. A French zoologist in Paris, **Isidore Geoffrey Saint-Hilaire** (1805–1861), studied the domestication of animals and published *Domestication et naturalisation des animaux utiles* in 1854. An American agricultural chemist and dairy farmer, **Stephen Moulton Babcock** (1843–1931), started studying the effect of a selective diet on cattle. A Scottish biologist, **Lord John Boyd Orr** (1880–1971) was a pioneer in animal nutrition and fat stock. He was director general of the United Nations Food and Agricultural Organization and was awarded the Nobel Prize for Peace in 1949. A Scottish zoologist, **James Cossar Ewart** (1851–1933) of Penicuik, was another pioneer of animal breeding in Britain. L. M. Winters published an important work *Animal Breeding* in 1925. An American geneticist, **Sewall Wright** (1889–1988) of Massachusetts, developed breeding methods to improve livestock while he was with the US Department of Agriculture. **Charles Robert Darwin** (1809–1882) published *Animals and Plants under Domestication* in 1868.

Animals [Latin: *animal,* life or breath] *See animal husbandry, ethology, zoo, zoology.*

Anion [Greek: *ana,* upon + *ienai,* to go] A negatively charged particle which moves towards the anode or positive pole. **Johann Wilhelm Hittorf** (1824–1914), a professor at the academy of Münster in Westphalia, studied the rate of movement of anions and cations during electrolysis. *See electrolysis.*

Anning, Mary (1799–1847) *See ichthyosaurus, plesiosaurus.*

Anode A term derived from the Greek term meaning the 'upward way in which the sun rises'. **Michael Faraday** (1791–1867) first used the term to refer to a positive electrode in electrolysis in 1833. *See cathode.*

Antarctic Region The area of the planet south of the Antarctic Circle, *c.* 66° 30′ South. Evidence suggests that the land surface of the earth was once a single primeval continent, now called *Pangaea.* The area of land now at the South Pole was apparently in the region of the Sahara during the Ordovician period, about 450 million years ago. *See South Pole.*

Anthracene An organic compound discovered in 1832 by a French chemist, **Auguste Laurent** (1807–1853).

Antimatter [Greek: *anti,* against + *materia,* thing] The fundamental theory of antimatter was proposed by an English mathematician, **Paul Adrien Maurice Dirac** (1902–1984) from Bristol, in 1930. He was made professor of mathematics at Cambridge in the same year and shared the Nobel Prize for Physics with **Erwin Schrödinger** (1887–1961) in 1933. The first type of antimatter to be found, the positive electron or positron, was discovered by an American physicist, **Carl David Anderson** (1905–1991) of New York, in 1932. He was awarded the Nobel Prize for Physics for his work on cosmic rays, jointly with the Austrian-born US physicist **Victor Francis Hess** (1883–1964) in 1936. Important studies on antimatter outside our galaxy were carried out by an American physicist, **Val Lodgson Fitch** (b 1923) from Nebraska. He shared the Nobel Prize for Physics for his work on particle physics with **James Watson Cronin** (b 1931) from Chicago, Illinois, in 1980.

Antimony The metallic element with atomic number 51. It was used in its metallic form for making vases and drinking cups by the ancients including the Fifth and Sixth Dynasty of Egypt. **Pliny the Elder** (AD 28–79) mentioned two forms of antimony. The French chemist **Pierre Eugène Marcellin Berthelot** (1827–1907) analyzed a vase of the Chaldeans in 1888 and found it be composed of almost pure antimony. It was widely used as a medicine during the middle ages.

Antiphon (*c.* 430 BC) *See exhaustion.*

Antiproton [Greek: *anti,* against + *protos,* first] A subatomic particle consisting of a proton carrying a negative charge of electricity instead of the usual positive charge. When it meets a proton mutual annihilation takes place. It was discovered by Italian-born US physicist **Emilio Segre** (1905–1989) and **Owen Chamberlain** (b 1920) of San Francisco, for which they shared the Nobel Prize for Physics in 1959. An Italian-born American physicist, **Carlo Rubbia** (b 1934), discovered that antiprotons and protons, because they have the same mass but opposite charges, could be predicted to have the same orbit though in opposite directions, in a magnetic field. This finding led to the development of the Super Proton Synchrotron (SPS) accelerator for colliding protons and antiprotons. He became the professor of physics at Harvard in 1971 and shared the Nobel Prize for Physics, for the above work, with a Dutch physicist, **Simon van der Meer** (b 1925), in 1984.

Antoniadi, Eugène Marie (1870–1944) A Turkish-born French astronomer who proposed that the intricate pattern of canals on the surface of Mars previously pointed out in 1877 by Italian astronomer Giovanni Schiaparelli, were really an optical illusion. Antoniadi was also a historian of ancient Greek and Egyptian astronomy.

Apian, Peter or **Petrius Apianus** (1495–1552) *See America, cartography, comet, Pascal triangle.*

Apollonius of Perga (260–200 BC) *See analytical geometry, conics, geometry.*

Apollo Space Program *See space travel.*

Appert, Nicolas François (1749–1841) *See canned food, food industry.*

Apple Computer Company *See computers.*

Applegarth, Augustus (1788–1871) *See printing.*

Appleton Layer *See Appleton, Sir Edward Victor.*

Appleton, Sir Edward Victor (1892–1965) An English physicist from Bradford, who served as professor of experimental physics at King's College, London (1924–1936), and later as Jacksonian professor of natural philosophy (1936–1939) at Cambridge. He was appointed secretary to the Department of Scientific and Industrial Research in 1939 and was knighted in 1941. He is well known for his discovery of the Appleton layer, the next part of the earth's atmosphere above the Heaviside layer, which contains a relatively high concentration of electrons. This layer was later found to play an essential role in wireless communication between distant stations, and in the development of radar. *See ionosphere.*

Aqualung [Latin: *aqua,* water + Anglo-Saxon: *lungen,* lung] or self-contained underwater breathing apparatus (scuba). The first diving helmet was invented by Augustus Siebie in 1837. The aqualung, the first apparatus which allowed a diver to descend more than 30 meters without being attached to the boat for his supply of air, was invented by **Jacques-Yves Cousteau** (1910–1997) and Emile Gagnon of France in 1943. They used compressed air contained in tanks or bottles fitted with valves to control the delivery. The use of a mixture of helium and oxygen for deep-sea diving was introduced by a chemist from New Jersey, **Joel Henry Hildebrand** (1881–1983) who was professor of chemistry at the University of California, Berkeley.

Aquarium [Latin: *aqua,* water] The term was coined by **Phillip Henry Gosse** (1810–1888), a naturalist from Worcester whose special interest was coastal marine biology in Jamaica. He published *History of Sea-anemones and Corals* (1860) and several other books on natural history.

Aqueduct [Latin: *aqua,* water + *ducere,* to lead] A channel raised above the ground to convey water. *See water supply.*

Aquinas, Thomas (1225–1274) A Dominican monk and philosopher, born in Monte Cassino and educated at the University of Naples. He sought to reconcile Aristotelian science and Christian orthodoxy.

Arago, Dominique François (1786–1853) *See electromagnetic theory, polarization, quartz.*

Aramatus, Savinus of Pisa (*c.* 1300) *See optics.*

Arber, Agnes (1879–1960) *See monocotyledons.*

Arc Light [Latin: *arcus,* bow] The first electric lamp, produced by passing electricity between two carbon electrodes. It was invented by **Sir Humphry Davy** (1778–1829) in 1803. Although his device produced a brilliant light, it had the disadvantage of releasing large amounts of smoke and heat. Despite these disadvantages it was used to light up Paris and London in the 19th century. The lighthouse in Foreland, Kent, was the first in England to be equipped with electric arc light, in 1858. In 1876 a Russian inventor in Paris, **Pavel Nikolaivitch Jablochkoff** (1847–1894), invented a low-current arc lamp known as the electric candle (Jablochkoff candle). **Edwin James Houston** (1847–1914) of Alexandria, Virginia, and **Elihu Thomson** (1853–1937) from Manchester, who emigrated to the US, patented an arc light in 1881. *See electric lighting.*

Archaeopteryx Archaeopteryx is the oldest fossil bird known, and dates from 160 million years ago. Although it had a fully-feathered body and wings, it is now thought likely that it was incapable of proper flight, but could glide; some maintain that it was a sort of feathered dinosaur which evolved into modern birds. It was first described by **Richard Owen** (1804–1892).

Archer, Frederick Scott (1813–1857) *See photography.*

Archimedes (287–212 BC) Father of hydrodynamics, born at Syracuse in Sicily. He discovered the principles of flotation while he was contemplating an experiment to determine the content of gold in King Hiero's crown at a royal request. He announced his discovery with a joyous expression *heureka* (I have found it) and it formed the basic concept of specific gravity. The story of his discovery was recounted by the Roman architect, **Marcus Vitruvius** in 100 BC. Archimedes also enunciated the principle of moments on which the working of a lever depends, and invented the Archimedian Screw. He was killed by a Roman soldier during the capture of Syracuse. The tomb of Archimedes, with a cylinder inscribed on it, was located by Cicero in 80 BC but it was subsequently lost. *See Alexandrian Museum and Library, burning glass, calculus, diopter, geometry, hydrodynamics, hydrometer, hydrostatics, lever, mathematics, mechanical engineering, mensuration, military engineering, physics, pi.*

Archimedes Name given to a home computer produced in 1987 by the British computer firm *Acorn,* as a successor to its BBC microcomputer. Despite its advanced design it was not successful.

Archimedian Screw A mechanical device for raising water which was invented by **Archimedes** (287–212 BC) during his visit to Egypt around 250 BC. His device has been in continual use in Egypt up to the present times.

Architecture [Greek: *architekron,* master builder] *See architecture, ancient, architecture, American, architecture, British, architecture, European, building.*

Architecture, American An English architect, **Benjamin Henry Latrobe** (1764–1820) from Yorkshire emigrated to America in 1796 and introduced the Greek revival there. **Louis Henri Sullivan** (1856–1924) of Boston was one of the first to design skyscrapers. After studying in Paris he designed the Wainwright Building in St Louis (1890–1891) and the Carson Store in Chicago (1899–1904). **Frank Lloyd Wright** (1867–1959) studied civil engineering in his local Wisconsin University and modernized American architecture with the application of engineering principles. He planned several homes, including his own in Wisconsin. He is best known for his earthquake-proof Imperial Hotel of 1916–1920. His American buildings include Florida Southern College (1940) and the Guggenheim Museum of Art in New York (1959). The world's first substantial skyscraper and the tallest structure after the Eiffel Tower at that time (1912), the 66-storey Woolworth Building in New York, was built by an American architect, **Cass Gilbert** (1859–1934) of Ohio. He also designed many other important buildings in America. Further skyscrapers in America, including the American Radiator Building, New York (1924) and the Rockefeller Center (1940), were designed by **Raymond Mathewson Hood** (1881–1934) of Rhode Island. A Chinese-born US architect, **Ieoh Meng Pei** (b 1917) designed the John Hancock Tower at Boston and numerous other skyscrapers worldwide.

Architecture, Ancient The Egyptian demi-God **Imhotep** who designed the stepped pyramid at Saqqara in Egypt in 2750 BC is regarded as the first architect of whom we have record. He was the principal officer of King Djoser of the Third dynasty. The well-planned towns of Harrapa and Mohanjadaro in the Indus Valley, dating from 2500 BC, indicate the advanced knowledge of architecture in the east. **Dinokrates**, a celebrated ancient architect, in 330 BC rebuilt the temple of Diana and was commissioned by **Alexander the Great** (355–323 BC) to plan the city of Alexandria. His attention to fine detail led to the magnificent city of Alexandria. Another ancient architect of importance, **Scopas of Ephesus,** who lived around 430 BC, constructed the mausoleum for Artemisia's husband. The lighthouse of Alexandria was built by Sostratus, an eminent architect of the pre-Christian era, during the reign of Philadelphus, the King of Egypt (300 BC). A Greek architect, **Andronicus of Cyrrus** (*c.* 100 BC) built the Tower of the Winds at Athens. The Roman architect **Marcus Pollio Vitruvius** in the 1st century wrote *De Architecture* (*c.* AD 25) which is the only extant Roman treatise. *See building.*

Architecture, Australian Most of the early colonial buildings in Australia were built by **Francis Howard Greenway** (1777–1837) from Gloucestershire who was a student of **John Nash** (1752–1835). He was sent to Sydney after being convicted for forgery and established his practice as an architect there. A Danish architect, **Jörn Utzon** (b 1918) designed the Sydney Opera House.

Architecture, British An eminent English architect, **Robert Smythson** (1534–1614), who started his career as a mason, designed Wollaton Hall at Nottingham (1580–1588) and Hardwick Hall, Derbyshire (1591–1597). He developed a vertical plan with the great hall set transversely, which influenced contemporary building in England. Classical architecture in England was revived by **Inigo Jones** (1572–1652), a celebrated London architect of the 17th century. He studied landscape painting and architecture in Italy before introducing the Palladian style into England. He rebuilt the Banqueting Hall at Whitehall and designed Covent Garden and Lincoln's Inn Fields. **William Kent** (1684–1748) of Yorkshire further promoted the Palladian style in Britain. He designed several important buildings in London, including the Royal Mews at Trafalgar Square. A Scottish architect, **Colen Campbell** (1679– 1726), of Argyll, published an important work *Vitruvius Britannicus* (1712). **Thomas Sandby** (1729–1809), an English architect from Nottingham, became the first professor of architecture to the Royal Academy, in 1770. He developed Lincoln's Inn Fields in London in 1776. **James Wyatt** (1746–1813) of Staffordshire did the neo-classical design for the London Pantheon (1772) and carried out restorations of several medieval cathedrals. His son **Benjamin Dean Wyatt** (1775–1850) designed Drury Lane Theatre in 1811. Many important parts of London, including Trafalgar Square, St James's Park and Marble Arch, were designed by an English architect, **John Nash** (1752–1835). In 1825 he laid out Regent Street to link Regent's Park with Westminster. **Sir Robert Smirke** (1781–1867) built the Covent Garden Theatre (1809), the British Museum (1823–1847) and several other important buildings in London. His brother **Sydney Smirke** (1799–1877) completed the west wing of the museum. A German architect, **Gottfried Semper** (1803–1873) from Hamburg, designed the Victoria and Albert Museum in London. A Scottish architect, **Sir William Chambers** (1726–1796), published a *Treatise of Civil Architecture* in 1759. A London architect, **Decimus Burton** (1800–1881), designed the new layout for Hyde Park and the triumphal arch at Hyde Park Corner. **Sir George Gilbert Scott** (1811–1878) designed St Pancras Station and Hotel in London (1865), Glasgow University (1865) and the Albert Memorial (1862) before he became professor of architecture at the Royal Academy in 1868. His grandson **Sir Giles Gilbert Scott** (1880–1960) designed the new Cambridge University Library (1931–1934) and helped to redesign the House of Commons after the Second World War. **Sir John Soane** (1753–1837) designed his own home at Lincoln's Inn Fields, which he bequeathed to the nation as the Sir John Soane Museum. Another English architect, **Benjamin Henry Latrobe** (1764–1820) from Yorkshire, who emigrated to America in 1796, introduced the Greek revival there. A London architect, **August Welby Northmore Pugin** (1812–1852) revived Gothic architecture and published *Contrast between the Architecture of the 15th and 19th Centuries* (1836). **Alfred Waterhouse** (1830–1905) of Liverpool revived Gothic architecture in England and designed the Natural History Museum in Kensington, London (1873–1881).

Architecture, European   Classical architecture in Holland was revived by **Jacob van Campen** (1595–1657). **Hendrik de Keyser** (1565–1621) designed three important churches and other well-known structures in Amsterdam. **Michael Beer** (1605–1666) of Germany in 1657 established *Auer Zunft* (Guild of Au) in his home town Au for theoretical training in architecture through workshops. Another German, **Balthaser Neumann** (1687–1753), revived the Baroque style in Germany. **Pierre Lescot** (1510–1578) of Paris, a leading French Renaissance architect, designed and rebuilt one wing of the Louvre. A French physician and architect, **Claude Perrault** (1613–1688), was also a Latin scholar and he produced a translation of **Marcus Pollio Vitruvius's** (*c.* 100 BC) work on architecture, including its elaborate drawings and engravings. His work was accepted for the façade of the Louvre in 1666 and he also designed the Paris Observatory. **Jacques Ange Gabriel** (1698–1782) of Paris designed the Place de la Concorde in 1753. **Charles Percer** (1764–1838) of Paris was the first to construct buildings in the Empire style. **Jacques Germain Soufflot** (1713–1780), an eminent French architect in Paris, rebuilt the Church of St Genevieve which became the Panthéon. He also designed several other important buildings in Paris. An influential book on the subject during the 18th and 19th centuries, *Architecture hydraulique* (1737–1739), was published by a Spanish-born French engineer, **Bernard Forest de Bélidor** (1698–1761). **Eugene Emmanuel Viollet-le-Duc** (1814–1879) of Paris restored many ancient buildings in France and published an important work, *Dictionnaire raisonné de l'architecture français du XIe au XVe siècle* (1854–1886). A Swedish architect, **Nicodemus Tessin** (1615–1681) of Stralsund, went to Stockholm in 1636 and designed several important buildings there, including Kalmar Cathedral, the present Supreme Court, and the

Bank of Sweden. His son **Nicodemus Tessin** (1654–1728) succeeded his father as the royal architect in 1676 and built the Royal Palace at Stockholm. **Johann Bernard von Erlach Fischer** (1656–1723) introduced the Austrian Baroque style and built several palaces in Vienna. **Otto Wagner** (1835–1917) modernized Austrian architecture with his art nouveau style and application of modern materials and technology. A Finnish architect, **Johann Carl Ludwig Engel** (1778–1840) planned the layout of Helsinki as the capital of his country. *See architecture, British, architecture Italian.*

Architecture, Italian   The pioneers of modern and decorative architecture in Europe were mostly Italians. **Giotto** (*c.* 1266–1337) of Florence is regarded as the initiator of Renaissance architecture and art. In 1334 he was appointed master of works for the city of Florence and its cathedral. His earliest work was on mosaics for the Florence Baptistery. **Fillipo Brunelleschi** (1377–1446), a pioneer of Renaissance architecture in Italy, designed the dome of Florence Cathedral. Another Italian architect of Venice, **Leone Battista Alberti** (1404–1472) revived Roman classical architecture and the Roman methods of construction in his *De Re Aedificatoria,* published in 1485. **Baldassare Tommaso Peruzzi** (1481–1536) designed several buildings in Rome, including the Pallazzo Massiomo in 1535. His contemporary, **Sebastiano Serlio** (1475–1554) of Bologna, wrote an important work *Regole generali di architettura* (1537–1551). Another influential book on architecture during the Renaissance, the *Quattro Libri dell Architettura,* was published by **Andrea Palladio** (1518–1590) of Italy in 1580. **Giovanni da Udine** (1487–1564) became known for his decorative style labeled the 'grotesque'. His style later spread rapidly throughout Europe. He was responsible for most of the public buildings in his home town, Udine. **Giacomo Barozzi da Vignola's** (1507–1573) cruciform plans and side chapels became the standard for church building in France and Italy. **Vincenzo Scamozzi** (1552–1616) was another eminent Italian architect, whose principal works, including the Citadel of Palma, are in Venice. **Galeazzo Alessi** (1512–1572) of Perugia, Italy, designed palaces and churches in Genoa. Several important buildings in Rome were designed by an Italian baroque architect, **Francesco Borronomi** (1599–1667). A Flemish sculptor and architect, **Giovanni Bologna** (1524–1608), designed most of the important fountains in Florence. **Juvara Filipo** (1678–1736) of Sicily was an exponent of Rococo design in Italy. The *Arco della pace* of white marble in Milan was designed by **Luigi Marchese Cagnola** (1762–1833).

Archytas of Tarentum (428–347 BC) *See acoustics, automation, musical theory, pulley, sound, wheel.*

Arctic Regions The area north of the Arctic Circle, *c.* 66° 30′ north of the equator. The first scientific treatise on the subject, *An Account of Arctic Regions* (1820), was published by an English Arctic Explorer, **William Scoresby** (1789–1857) of Whitby. *See Magnetic Pole, North Pole.*

Arfwedson, Johan August (1792–1841) *See lithium.*

Argand, Aimé (1755–1803) *See Argand lamp.*

Argand, Jean Robert (1768–1822) *See Argand diagram.*

Argand Diagram A method used for representing complex numbers in algebraic equations or Cartesian coordinate in mathematics. Along its horizontal axis the real numbers are plotted, while the vertical axis has non-real, or imaginary, numbers. It was devised in 1806 in Paris by a Swiss mathematician, **Jean Robert Argand** (1768–1822).

Argand Lamp The first oil lamp with a glass chimney and wick in the form of a ring, invented in 1782 by a Swiss chemist, **Aimé Argand** (1755–1803). It had a circular burner that passed an air current up its center.

Argelander, Friedrich Wilhelm August (1799–1875) *See astronomy.*

Argon [Greek: *argon,* inactive] The first inert gas to be discovered – the element with atomic number 18. An English physicist, **Lord John William Strutt Rayleigh** (1842–1919), repeatedly noticed during his experiments that the nitrogen from the air was more dense than nitrogen obtained otherwise. He was at a loss to explain this phenomenon until the Scottish chemist **Sir William Ramsay** (1852–1916) pointed out to him at a Royal Society meeting in 1894 that **Henry Cavendish** (1731–1810) had also noted this finding a hundred years earlier. Cavendish, in his conclusions, stated that nitrogen in the air was inhomogeneous, implying that there was an impurity in air. Ramsay and Rayleigh carried out their investigations along this line and announced their discovery of argon, which had previously escaped detection owing to its inertness, at the British Scientific Research Workers meeting on 13 August 1894.

Aristarchos (*c.* 320–250 BC) A Greek philosopher from the island of Samos, who proposed the theory of rotatory movement of the earth. He initiated the heliocentric theory that the sun is the center of the solar system and the planets revolve around it.

Aristotle (384–322 BC) Greek philosopher and father of biology, born in a small town, Stagira, in the province of Chalcidice near Macedonia. His father was court physician to the king of Macedonia, Amyntas II, the grandfather of Alexander the Great (355–323 BC). At the age of 18 Aristotle traveled to Athens to study under **Plato** (428–348 BC) and remained his pupil for 20 years. At 41 he was appointed teacher to Alexander the Great, who was 13 years old. When Alexander's father, King Philip, was assassinated in 336 BC Alexander became king and Aristotle returned to Athens. His earliest treatise on biology, *Historia Animalorum* (History of Living Creatures), was written after his return to Athens. Some of his other works include *De Anima* on the psyche, *De Generatione Animalorum* and *De Partibus Animalorum.* Aristotle formed his University Lyceum in Athens during the year 336 BC and died at the age of 62. The first modern Latin translation of his three great biological treatises was published by **Theodore Gaza** (1400–1478) in Venice in 1476. Most of Aristotle's teachings remained valid for the 2000 years following his death. *See algebra, biology, embryology, ether, invertebrates, Lyceum, metaphysics, meteorology, motion, ornithology, physics, rainbow, vacuum, vertebrates.*

Arithmetic [Greek: *arithmos,* number] Science of numbers and art of computation. The origin of arithmetic is difficult to trace as it began when man first started counting. The earliest documentation on the subject is found in the papyrus written by a priest named Ahmose or Ahmes in 1650 BC. The information originates from 2200 BC during the time of the XII dynasty. This papyrus, containing some common arithmetic operations and multiplications, was given as a part of **Alexander Henry Rhind's** (1833–1863) collection to the British Museum. The ancient Babylonian numerals had bases of 10 and 60 in their calculations, and the Egyptian numerals were based on symbols for 1 and multiples of ten. Hieroglyphic symbols were allocated earlier for numbers by the Egyptians. The oldest Greek numbering system consisted of numbers assigned to twenty-four letters of the Greek alphabet. The ancient Roman numbers had symbols for multiples of five as well as for powers of ten. The chief sources of our knowledge of Greek arithmetic are **Euclid's** (*c.* 300 BC) *Elements,* the *Introduction to Arithmetic* by **Nicomachus** (*c.* AD 100), and the *Arithmetic* of **Diophantus** (*c.* AD 250). The first printed book on arithmetic in England, *De Arte Supputandi,* was published by **Cuthbert Tonstall** (1474–1559) in 1522. An important work, *Arithmetica Infinitorum* (Arithmetic of Infinites), was published by one of the founders of the Royal Society and the Savillian Professor at Oxford, **John Wallis** (1616–1703), in 1655. *See accountancy, mathematics, numbers.*

Arkwright, Sir Richard (1732–1792) *See spinning mule.*

Armature Any moving part in an electrical machine in which a voltage is induced by a magnetic field; particularly applied to the coils of an electric motor or generator. *See dynamo.*

Armour, Phillip Danworth (1832–1901)　*See food industry.*

Armstrong, Edwin Howard (1890–1954)　*See radio.*

Armstrong, Henry Edward (1848–1937)　*See affinity.*

Armstrong, Neil (b 1930)　*See astronauts, space travel.*

Armstrong, William George (1810–1900)　*See crane, electricity.*

Arnold, John (1736–1799)　*See escapement.*

Arnott, Neil (1788–1874)　*See heating.*

Aromatic Compounds [Greek: *aromatos,* spice] Organic compounds which have one or more closed rings of atoms which are partly unsaturated but which are, nevertheless, much more stable than would be expected from any simple structural formula, involving double and triple bonds, that could be devised. Many such compounds smell strongly – hence the name. Aniline, a primary aromatic amine, was first observed to be a product of the dry distillation of indigo by an organic chemist from Potsdam, **Otto Unverdorben** (1806–1873), in 1826. The French chemist **Pierre Eugène Marcellin Berthelot** (1827–1907), professor of organic chemistry at the École de Pharmacie, investigated aromatic compounds and isolated benzene and naphthalene in 1851. The Friedel–Crafts reaction, in which aluminum chloride or other acidic catalyst is used to promote the alkylation or acylation of aromatic hydrocarbons, was discovered by a French organic chemist, **Charles Friedel** (1832–1899), and an American chemist, **James Mason Crafts** (1839–1917) of Boston, Massachusetts. Assigning a structure to the archetypal aromatic hydrocarbon, benzene, proved to be a severe problem; the first step towards its solution came in 1865 when Kekulé deduced that instead of a chain of six carbon atoms it contains a highly symmetric ring of carbons, to each of which is attached a hydrogen atom. Modern spectroscopic methods and quantum mechanical calculations have confirmed his inspired guess. In 1890 a German chemist, **E. Bamberger** (1857–1932), suggested that the aromatic character of compounds may be related to unused valencies. Another German chemist, **Karl Graebe** (1841–1927) of Frankfurt am Main, introduced the terms ortho, meta and para for the spatial positions of substituents in aromatic compounds. In 1931 a German chemist, **Erich Hückel** (1896–1980) formulated the criterion (the Hückel rule) for aromaticity of cyclic unsaturated compounds. A

London chemist, **Sir Christopher Kelk Ingold** (1893–1970) studied the mechanism of aromatic nitration in detail. His monumental work *Structure and Mechanism in Organic Chemistry* was published in 1953.

Arrhenius, Svante August (1859–1927) A Swedish chemist, born in Wijk near Uppsala. After studying for 5 years at Uppsala University he moved to Stockholm in 1881 and became a student of **Jacobius Henricus van't Hoff** (1852–1911). He advanced the theory of electrolyte dissociation or the ionic theory, previously proposed by Henricus van't Hoff, and established the concept of the dissociation constant in 1883. He formulated the effect of temperature on the rate of chemical reactions in 1889 and was awarded the Nobel Prize for Physics in 1903.

Arrol, William (1839–1913) *See bridges.*

Arrow [Anglo-Saxon: *arewe*] The bow and arrow, according to evidence from sites at Parpallo (Spain) and in the Sahara, were invented around 25 000 BC. Evidence remains for the arrow's use in the Mississippi Valley in the Americas around 800 BC. Although stone arrow heads belonging to the Neolithic period were observed and described by **George Agricola** (1494–1555) and **Conrad Gesner** (1516–1565), no adequate explanation for their origin was given until a Danish archaeologist, **Christian Jörgensen Thomsen** (1788–1865), and **Jacques de Perthes** (1788–1868), a French archaeologist, identified them as instruments of the Stone Age. *See prehistory.*

Arrowsmith, Aaron (1750–1823)　*See cartography.*

Arrowsmith, John (1790–1873)　*See cartography.*

Arsenic [Greek: *arsenikon*] The element of atomic number 33, one of whose sulfide compounds was known to **Aristotle** (384–322 BC). The Greek herbalist **Dioscorides** (AD 40–90) used the term *arsenikon* in AD 60. **Albertus Magnus** (*c.* 1192–1280) is supposed to have been the first to obtain it in its elementary form and describe it. White arsenic was known as ratsbane in England during the 15th century owing to its use as a rat poison.

Artachaies (*c.* 500 BC)　*See canals.*

Artedi, Peter (1705–1735)　*See ichthyology.*

Artesian Wells A well in which water is forced up to the surface by hydrostatic pressure. The necessary conditions for an artesian well are a basin in the earth's crust in which an aquifer, or zone of water-bearing rock, is confined between impermeable beds in such a way that water can only enter it where it outcrops on the surface at a point (or points) that are higher than the area within the basin. As a result, if a hole is bored into the aquifer, the hydrostatic pressure above will force water to the surface without the need for pumping. It derives its name from the province of Artois, in France, where the phenomenon was first observed.

Artificial Diamond The first attempt to produce artificial diamonds was made by a Scotsman, James Ballantyne Hannay, in 1878. Two years later he sent a few tiny crystals which he claimed were produced in his laboratory to a mineralogist who declared them to be real diamonds. The mystery of these diamonds has not been solved up to date. A French chemist, **Ferdinand Frederic Henri Moissan** (1852–1907), the inventor of the electric oven and discoverer of carborundum, made further attempts to produce artificial diamonds in 1896. After several trials other workers at the General Electric Company produced an artificial diamond of high quality in 1970. However, the cost of the production of such a high-quality diamond was found to exceed the production costs of real diamonds by several times. A new method of synthesizing artificial diamonds was developed by an American physicist, **Percy Williams Bridgman** (1882–1961) of Cambridge, Massachusetts in 1955. *See diamonds.*

Artificial Gene The first artificial gene to function naturally when inserted into a bacterial cell was constructed by an Indian-born US chemist, **Har Gobind Khorana** (b 1922) from Raipur, Punjab, and his co-workers in 1976. Khorana was awarded the Nobel Prize for Physiology or Medicine for his work on the genetic code and its role in protein synthesis, in 1968.

Artificial Ice *See refrigeration.*

Artificial Intelligence A branch of computing science which seeks to match human intelligence via machines or computers. The study of machine intelligence was developed in England by a British physicist, **Donald Michie** (b 1923), who was born in Rangoon, Burma. He became the director of intelligence programming at Edinburgh in 1963, and was made professor of machine intelligence in 1967. He proposed that computers are able to generate new knowledge, and founded the Turing Institute in Glasgow in 1984. His work *On Machine Intelligence* was published in 1974.

Artificial Magnet First produced by an English physicist, **John Canton** (1718–1772), of Stroud, Gloucestershire.

Artificial Rain An American physicist, **Vincent Joseph Schaefer** (1906–1993) of Schenectady, New York, during his experiments on the problem of icing on airplanes, dis-covered that dry ice or solid carbon dioxide when introduced into a cold box containing water vapor resulted in a small snow storm. In 1946 he used his discovery to demonstrate the possibility of inducing rainfall by dropping dry ice from an airplane on to clouds. **Bernard Vonnegut** (b 1914) of Indianapolis, professor of atmospheric physics at New York State University, used silver iodide as a cloud-seeding agent for artificial rain in 1947.

Artificial Rubber A Belgian-born US chemist, **Julius Arthur Nieuwland** (1878–1936) in 1920 discovered that acetylene could be polymerized in the presence of a catalyst. He investigated this reaction in 1925 and synthesized the first artificial rubber, neoprene, in 1929. **Sir William Augustus Tilden** (1842–1926), a chemist at St Pancras, in London, and professor at the Royal College of Science, manufactured artificial rubber from a synthetic preparation of isoprene. Butyl rubber was invented by two Americans, Robert Thomas and William Sparks, of Exon Company, in 1937.

Artificial Silk As early as 1664 **Robert Hooke** (1635–1703) in his *Micrographia* suggested the possibility of making an artificial glutinous compound resembling silk. In 1883 **Sir Joseph Wilson Swan** (1828–1914) of Sunderland first produced such filaments by squirting solutions of nitrocellulose. His method was adopted commercially by a French chemist, **Hilaire Bernigaud Comte de Chardonnet** (1839–1924), who exhibited his material, which had a remarkable resemblance to the fibers spun by the silkworm, in 1889. An improved way of producing this substance – rayon – was invented by two English chemists, **Frederick Charles Cross** (1855–1935) of Brentford, Middlesex and **Edward John Bevan** (1856–1921) of Birkenhead.

Artificial Transmutation The Greek philosopher **Plato** (428–348 BC) and others during his period believed that metals could undergo transmutation with age. Artificial transmutation was first attempted by the alchemists of the middle ages when they tried to convert other metals into gold. The radioactive decay of elements observed in the early 20th century by several workers, including **Lord Ernest Rutherford** (1871–1937) and **Frederick Soddy** (1877–1965) is an example of natural transmutation. **Bertram Borden Boltwood** (1870–1927), an American chemist from Amhurst, Massachusetts, in 1905 showed that when uranium decays it produces radium and the end product of further decay is lead. Artificial transmutation of boron into helium by bombarding it with neutrons was demonstrated by an Austrian chemist, **Frederick Adolf Paneth** (1887–1958) in the 1930s. Several other artificial transmutations were demonstrated around the same time by a number of workers including Rutherford.

Artillery Science *See military engineering.*

Aryabhata (AD 475–550) *See astronomy, mathematics, sines, trigonometry.*

Ashmole, Elias (1617–1692) An eminent antiquary from Litchfield who initially was an attorney in London before he moved to Oxford. He was a member of the Society of Astrologers and a great collector of curiosities and coins. He presented his collection of books and manuscripts to Oxford University in 1677 and it formed the basis of the Ashmolean Museum in 1682. *See alchemy, museum.*

Ashmolean Museum *See Ashmole, Elias.*

Asparagine The first amino acid to be discovered by a French chemist, **Louis Nicolas Vauquelin** (1763–1829), in 1806.

Aspdin, Joseph (1779–1855) *See cement.*

Astatine The element with atomic number 85; all its isotopes are radioactive. D.R. Corson and K.R. Mackenzie obtained it by bombarding bismuth-200 with alpha particles in 1940.

Astbury, John (1688–1743) A potter, born in Staffordshire, England who developed a distinctive type of earthenware pottery known as Astbury ware.

Astbury, William Thomas (1898–1961) *See polymer, textile chemistry.*

Asteroids [Greek: *asteroid*, small star] Minor planets too small to be measured. About 40 000 minor planets or asteroids orbit the sun between Mars and Jupiter. The first one, *Ceres,* was discovered by an Italian monk, **Giuseppe Piazzi** (1749–1826) at Palermo, Italy in 1801. He served as director of Palermo Observatory from its establishment in 1790 until his death. The first one visible to the naked eye, *Vesta,* was discovered by a German physician and astronomer, **Heinrich Wilhelm Matthaus Olbers** (1758–1840), in 1807. Bifurcated asteroids, first discovered in 1990, are in fact two chunks of rock that touch each other, and it is estimated that about 10% of asteroids approaching the Earth are bifurcated.

Aston, Francis William (1877–1945) *See mass spectrograph.*

Aston, John G. (1902–1990) *See absolute zero.*

Astrolabe [Greek: *aster,* star + *lambanein,* to take] An instrument used by ancient Greek and Babylonian astronomers to

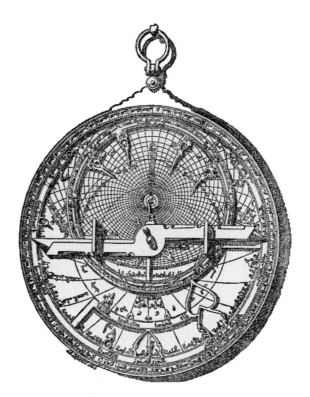

Figure 5 Arabic astrolabe. Rolt-Wheeler, Francis. *The Science-History of the Universe, Mathematics*. London: The Waverley Book Company Limited, 1911

map the stars. An Assyrian astrolabe dating back to 700 BC found at Nineveh is now located in the British Museum. **Hipparchus of Bithynia** (190–120 BC) used the astrolabe for locating celestial bodies around 130 BC. Arab sailors used the instrument around AD 600 to plot their position at sea. An Arabian mathematician, **Alkarismi** or **Abu Jafar Mohammed ibn Musa Al-Khowarimi** in the 9th century wrote on the Greek astrolabe, an instrument which the Arabs developed to a great extent. **Gerbert** (d 1003), who became Pope Sylvester II, wrote a Latin translation of an earlier Arabic work on the astrolabe in 970. The first original account of the plane-astrolabe in Latin was given by **Herman the Cripple** (1013–1054), a Benedictine monk from Switzerland. Another early treatise on the astrolabe was written by a Hebrew writer, Rabbi Ben Ezra, in the 12th century. A mathematician and astronomer in Damascus, **Sharaf al-Din al-Tusi** (*c.* 1150) invented a linear astrolabe consisting of a graduated wooden rod with a plumb line and a double cord, which he used for making angular measurements. Large and cumbersome astrolabes made of iron were in use in Europe during the 13th century. The instrument was introduced into England in the 14th century. The English poet **Geoffrey Chaucer** (1340–1400) gave an astrolabe to his 10-year-old son and wrote a treatise on the subject entitled *Tractus de Conclusonibus Astralabi* which is considered to be the earliest treatise on science in England. A comprehensive treatise on the astrolabe *Elucidatio Fabricae Vsuque Astralabii* (Elucidation on the manufacture and use of astrolabe) was written by Johann Stoeffler in 1564. James Bassantin, a Scottish astronomer, published *A Treatise on Astrolabe* in 1555. A modern telescope currently used in astronomy for making accurate determinations of the positions of stars and planets is known as a prismatic astrolabe. This modern version has a small pool of mercury and a refracting prism, with a small aperture.

Astronautics [Greek: *aster,* star + *nautes,* sailor] A science which deals with space flights. *See astronauts, space travel.*

Astronauts [Greek: *aster,* star + *nautes,* sailor] The first man to travel in space was a Russian, **Yuri Alekseyevich Gagarin** (1934–1968). He completed a circuit of the earth in the Russian space satellite *Vostok I* in 1961. Gagarin later died in a plane accident during training. **Alan Bartlett Shepard** (1923–1998) from East Derry, New Hampshire, was the first American to travel in space. He was launched 116 miles into space in *Freedom 7,* 23 days after Yuri Gagarin's historic orbit around the earth. The first American to orbit the earth was **John Herschel Glenn** (b 1921) from Cambridge, Ohio. He made a three-orbit flight in the *Friendship* 7 space capsule in 1962. **Valentina Vladimirovna Tereshkova** (b 1937) became the first woman astronaut in *Vostok 6,* launched from Tyuratum, USSR, in 1963. The first man to walk in space was a Russian astronaut, **Aleksey Arkhipovich Leonov** (b 1934) from Listvyanka. He stepped out of the spacecraft *Voskhod 2* during its orbit around the earth and walked in space for ten minutes in 1965. Edward White was the first American to walk in space from his spacecraft, *Gemini 4,* in the same year. The historical landing on the moon was achieved by the American astronauts, **Neil Armstrong** (b 1930) **Edwin 'Buzz' Aldrin** (b 1930) and **Michael Collins** (b 1930) in their *Apollo 11,* on 20 July 1969. The first woman American astronaut, **Sally Kristen Ride** (b 1951) of Los Angeles was selected by NASA in 1978 and served on a six-day flight of the *Challenger* in 1983. The record for the longest time spent in space – 326 days – was achieved by the Soviet astronaut, Yuri V. Romanenko in 1987. **Helen Sharman** (b 1963) became the first British woman in space, in 1991. *See space travel.*

Astronomical Clock A device for keeping time and showing the movements of planetary bodies. **Richard of Wallingford** (*c.* 1292–1336), an English Benedictine monk and engineer from Wallingford in Berkshire, constructed

one of the first mechanical astronomical clocks in England. A professor of astronomy at Padua and a physician, **Giovanni de Dondi** (1318–1389) took 18 years to construct an astronomical clock at the library of Pavia. In addition to hours and days it showed the movements of the sun, moon and planets. The world's largest – at the Cathedral of St Pierre, Beauvais, in France, containing 90 000 parts – was constructed around 1865.

Astronomical Instruments *See astrolabe, astronomical clock, coronograph, diopter, heliometer, heliostat, reflecting telescope, siderostat, spectroscope, telescope.*

Astronomical Journal First American periodical on astronomy, founded by an astronomer from Boston, Massachusetts, **Benjamin Apthorp Gould** (1824–1896) in 1849; it continued until 1861.

Astronomical Paintings Representations or paintings of space, planets and the outer universe before space exploration became established. A French artist and amateur astronomer, **Lucien Rudaux** (1874–1947) used the telescope and interpreted his findings before he painted lunar and Martian landscapes. His *Sur les autres mondes* (On the other worlds) in 1937 contained masterly illustrations of a variety of space phenomena. In 1865 a French novelist, **Jules Verne** (1828–1905), of Nantes published *De la Terre à la Lune* (From the Earth to the Moon), the first fiction on space travel to contain scientific illustrations beyond the earth. **Chesley Bonestell's** (1888–1986) color-illustrated book *The Conquest of Space* (1949) is a major work on illustrative space art.

Astronomical Photography *See celestial photography.*

Astronomical Society of England Founded at the premises of Freemason's Tavern, London, in 1820. An English astronomer, **Francis Bailey** (1774–1844) from Newbury, Berkshire, who was one of its founder members, framed its constitution while he was secretary to the society.

Astronomical Tables *See Alfonsine tables, Almagest, Zij.*

Astronomy [Greek: *astro,* star + *nomy,* to classify] One of the earliest of the sciences, practiced by the ancients including the Babylonians, the Chinese and the Greeks. In China the planets were studied and their positions were recorded as early as 2513 BC, during the time of Emperor Cheuni. Around 400 BC three Chinese astronomers, Shih Shen, Gan De and Wu Hsien, compiled a catalogue of stars which was in use for nearly a thousand years. Some of the notable Greek philosophers who studied astronomy include **Thales** (640–546 BC) of Miletus, **Anaximander** (611–547 BC) of Miletus, **Anaximenes** (*c.* 550 BC), and **Pythagorus**

(*c.* 580–500 BC). **Hipparchus of Bithynia** (190–120 BC), who came to be regarded as the father of observational astronomy, measured the motion of the sun and the moon. **Ptolemy** (*c.* AD 127–145) wrote a cyclopedia of astronomy, the *Almagest* [Greek: *megiste,* the greatest] and explained the unequal movements of the sun and the moon around AD 130. A Hindu mathematician, **Aryabhata** (475–550) of Patna, attempted to determine the distances of the moon and the sun by mathematical methods similar to those of Hipparchus. An English mathematician, **John of Halifax** or **Johannes de Sacrobosco** (*c.* 1250) wrote one of the few important works in astronomy during the middle ages, entitled *De Sphaera Mundi.* It was based on Ptolemaic and previous Arabic writings. The greatest astronomer of early Renaissance times was **Nicolas Copernicus** (1473–1543), a priest born in Prussia. He devised methods of accurately predicting the positions of the sun, moon, and planets and increased the accuracy of calculations and tables. He was followed by **Tycho Brahe** (1546–1601), a Danish astronomer who catalogued over a thousand stars and studied the motion of the planet Mars. The progress of astronomy continued with **Johannes Kepler** (1571–1630) of Wurtemberg who discovered in 1609 three laws of planetary motion. They state that: (1) the orbits of the planets are elliptical, with the sun at one focus of the ellipse; (2) an imaginary line (*radius vector*) connecting the sun to a planet sweeps across equal areas in equal times; (3) the ratio of the square of each planet's sidereal period to the cube of its distance from the sun is constant for all the planets. His above three discoveries later proved to be the precursors to Newton's Law of Gravitation. Kepler's book *Astronomia Nova* was published in 1609. Around the same time as Kepler's *Astronomia,* **Galilei Galileo** (1564–1642) made one of the first telescopes to be used in astronomy. With his telescope he discovered the black spots on the sun, and the hills and valleys of the moon. He also demonstrated that the Milky Way was composed of a multitude of stars. **Sir Isaac Newton** (1642–1727), while meditating on the logic of the movements of the planets, moon and sun, saw the apple fall and realized its relevance. Newton's Law of Gravitation, published in 1687, gave a physical meaning to Kepler's three laws. **Edmund Halley** (1656–1742), another great astronomer, among his other contributions accurately predicted the reappearance of a comet, which had been observed to occur at intervals of 75 years since 1380. This comet, later known as Halley's comet, contributed to the development of Newton's theory of gravitation. The development of the spectroscope through the efforts of **Gustav Robert Kirchhoff** (1824–1887) in 1859 contributed to the analysis of atmospheric materials surrounding the planets and stars. The first international organization of astronomers, *Astronomische Gesellschaft* was founded by a German astronomer, **Friedrich Wilhelm August Argelander** (1799–1875), in 1863. *See astrophysics, celestial photography, eclipse, observatories, radioastronomy, X-ray astronomy.*

Astrophysics [Greek: *astro*, star + *phusis*, nature] The application of mechanics to the investigation of the motion and nature of stellar and planetary bodies. The modern study of astrophysics began with the examination of the solar spectrum by an English physician and chemist, **William Hyde Wollaston** (1766–1822) in 1802. His work was followed by that of a Bavarian instrument maker, **Joseph von Fraunhofer** (1787–1826), who attached a telescope to a prism and examined the solar spectrum in 1816. He noticed that the spectra of the stars were slightly different from those of the sun. The significance of this finding was realized in 1859 by **Gustav Robert Kirchhoff** (1824–1887), whose work made it possible to determine the chemical composition of the sun from the earth. Among the earliest contributors to the subject was **Sir William Huggins** (1824–1910), who had his own small observatory in London in 1855. He confirmed that the stars were made of the same elements as those found on the earth. A Jesuit priest, **Pieto Angelo Secchi** (1818–1878), began his observations on the stellar spectra around the same time, at the Vatican Observatory in Rome, and classified the stars according to their spectral type for the first time, in 1867. **Sir Norman Joseph Lockyer** (1836–1920) around the 1870s did work on astrophysics as a professor at the Norman School of Science Observatory at Exhibition Road, Kensington, which later became the Royal College of Science. He was also instrumental in founding the Science Museum in London. The first Astrophysical Observatory in Europe was founded at Potsdam in Germany in 1874. The problem of determining the huge distances to the stars was first tackled by the German astronomer **Friedrich Bessel**, who used the method of parallax. This method works well for distances of a few hundreds of light years, but cannot be used for very distant stars and galaxies. In 1912 **Henrietta Swan Leavitt** (1868–1921) established that variable stars have a simple relationship between period of variation and luminosity; assuming that Cepheid variables in distant galaxies obey the same law enabled comparison to be made between the observed and actual luminosity, hence establishing the distances to these galaxies. The distances to still more remote galaxies are estimated from their *redshift* – the change in wavelength of the light they emit – which is proportional to their recessional velocity, in turn proportional to their distance; relativistic and, possibly, gravitational redshift complicate this simple idea. Quantum theory was applied to the study of cosmic radiation by a Russian astrophysicist, **Vitalii Lazarevich Ginzberg** (b 1916). *See cosmic radiation, X-ray astronomy.*

Atanasoff, John Vincent (1903–1995) *See calculating machine.*

Atherstone, W. Guybon (1813–1898) *See diamond.*

Atkinson, Robert D'escourt (1898–1982) A Welsh astrophysicist who worked out a theoretical model for a way in which matter could be annihilated. He worked with Arthur Eddington (1882–1944) at the Greenwich Observatory and determined the amount of energy released from atomic reactions within stars.

Atlantic *See transatlantic communication, transatlantic flight, transatlantic voyage.*

Atlantis A large island in the Atlantic Ocean supposed to have been located west of the Strait of Gibraltar. According to **Plato** (428–348 BC) 'in a single day and night of misfortune, it sank into the sea'. Its disappearance was probably due to the eruption of the volcano Santorini around 1645 BC.

Atlas [Greek: *atlao,* I endure or sustain] The word was used for the first time to describe a book of maps by a Flemish geographer, **Gerardus Mercator** (1512–1594) in 1585. His book, which had a cover with a drawing of the Greek god Atlas, was completed by his son in 1595. *See cartography.*

Atmosphere [Greek: *atmos,* vapor + *sphaira,* globe] Atmospheric air was regarded as a single substance until 1674 when an English physician, **John Mayhow** (1640–1679) demonstrated that if a substance is burnt in an enclosed vessel, the volume of air diminished until combustion no longer took place. Further knowledge on the composition of the atmosphere was gained by a Swedish apothecary and chemist, **Carl Wilhelm Scheele** (1742–1786). In the latter half of the 19th century, experiments from balloons contributed significantly to the study of the atmosphere and the discovery of the stratosphere, a region of uniform temperature above an altitude of 10 kilometers, was made around 1898. The region below it, which exhibited a non-uniform temperature, was called the troposphere. The radio-sonde, a device to transmit atmospheric changes from high altitude to the ground, a forerunner of the modern weather satellite, was introduced in 1930. *See air.*

Atmospheric Electricity *See lightning.*

Atmospheric Engine An engine in which cooling of steam and its condensation allowed the atmosphere to push a piston. Developed by **Thomas Newcomen** (1663–1729) of Dartmouth in Devon. The first one was built in 1712 at Dudley Castle, near Staffordshire, and only an engraving of it remains. *See steam engine.*

Atmospheric Pressure The mayor or burgomaster of Magdeburg in Prussia, **Otto von Guericke** (1602–1686), who invented the air pump, demonstrated the effects of atmospheric pressure for the first time at the royal court of the emperor and devised a method of measuring it in 1657. *See barometer.*

Atom [Greek: *a,* without + *tomy,* cut] The smallest part of an element that still retains all the properties of that element. *See atomic bomb, atomic disintegration, atomic structure, atomic theory, atomic volume.*

Atomic Bomb The possibility of obtaining energy from the spontaneous disintegration of an atom was first suggested by the English physicist, **Ernest Rutherford** (1871–1937). In 1938 a group of Germans, **Otto Hahn** (1879–1968), **Lise Meitner** (1878–1968), **Otto Robert Frisch** (1904–1979) and **Fritz Strassmann** at the Kaiser Wilhelm Institute for Chemistry, discovered by chance that uranium-235 when bombarded with neutrons was capable of breaking down into two other elements, barium and krypton, with the release of a large amount of energy. This process – named fission by Frisch and Meitner – opened the doors to the making of the first atom bomb. Meitner, after escaping from the Nazis and going to Sweden, became concerned about the possibility of the Germans making such a bomb. The Danish physicist **Niels Henrich David Bohr** (1885–1962) realized this danger through Meitner and traveled to America to caution the Americans of this possibility. In America Bohr worked with **John Archibald Wheeler** (b 1911), an American physicist at the Princeton laboratory, on the project and established that an atomic bomb could be produced with the use of uranium-235. Their findings led to the first nuclear reactor, built by an Italian, **Enrico Fermi** (1901–1954) and a Hungarian biochemist, **Leo Szilard** (1898–1964) at the University of Chicago, the United States, in 1942. The technique of bringing together several small, sub-critical, pieces of fissile material to make one piece above the critical mass, which would then explode, was devised by an American, Seth Neddemeyer, in 1943. The development of the atomic bomb was carried out at the Los Alamos Scientific Laboratories in New Mexico headed by its director, **Julius Robert Oppenheimer** (1904–1967) from New York. The first trial of an atomic bomb, code-named Trinity, was carried out on

16th July 1945 in New Mexico, 20 days before the atomic drop on Hiroshima. The energy released during this trial turned out to be nearly 10 times more than the expected amount. The atomic bomb code named fat boy, and made of uranium-235, was dropped over Hiroshima on 6th August 1945. The second bomb, dropped on Nagasaki on August 9th, was made of plutonium-239. The photographs of the immediate effects of the bomb on Hiroshima and Nagasaki were first released by the US Government in December 1960. A London physicist, **Baron William George Penney** (1909–1991), who was an observer when the atomic bomb was dropped on Nagasaki, became instrumental in the British developing their own atomic bomb in 1952. He was the chairman of the UK Atomic Energy Authority from 1964 to 1967.

Atomic Clock   The ammonia clock makes use of the oscillations of the nitrogen atom in ammonia which occur at a regularity of approximately 24×10^9 times a second. It was invented by an American scientist, Harold Lyons, in 1948 and was unveiled at the National Bureau of Standards, USA, in January 1949. Its accuracy is within one second in 1000 years. Two American physicists, **Norman Foster Ramsey** (b 1915) of Washington DC and German-born **Hans Georg Dehmelt** (b 1922) developed methods to accurately measure the energy of atomic transitions. Their work led to a more accurate atomic clock based on cesium, with an accuracy of one second in several thousand years, which has been in use for international time standards since 1972. Twin atomic hydrogen masers based on the frequency transition period for reading time were installed at the US Naval Research Laboratory in Washington DC.

Atomic Disintegration   A hypothesis stating that radioactive elements, made of complex particles, undergo spontaneous changes or disintegration and discharge high velocity negatively charged electrons or beta rays, or positively charged particles or alpha rays, was put forward by **Lord Ernest Rutherford** (1871–1937) and **Frederick Soddy** (1877–1965) in 1902. An English physicist, **Patrick Maynard Stuart Blackett** (1897–1974) was the first to observe nuclear disintegration by cosmic rays. He was awarded the Nobel Prize for Physics for his work on atoms in 1948. *See isotopes, radioactivity.*

Atomic Energy   The possibility of using atomic energy first became apparent with **Albert Einstein's** (1879–1955) equation on energy and matter in 1907. In 1938 a group of Germans, **Otto Hahn** (1879–1968), **Lise Meitner** (1878–1968) and **Fritz Strassmann** discovered by chance that uranium-235, when bombarded with neutrons, was

capable of breaking down into two other elements (barium and krypton), with the release of a large amount of energy. The first nuclear reactor, which produced electricity – the thermal fast nuclear reactor – was built at the Argonne National Laboratory in 1951. *See atomic power, nuclear fission, nuclear fusion.*

Atomic Heat   Refers to the product of relative atomic mass and specific heat. The law (Dulong and Petit Law), stating that the product of specific heat and relative atomic mass is constant for solid elements, was proposed by a French physician, **Alexis Thérèse Petit** (1791–1820) and a Parisian chemist, **Pierre Louis Dulong** (1785–1838) in 1818. Although only approximate, the law applies reasonably well at normal temperatures to elements with a simple crystal structure.

Atomic Nucleus   The atomic nucleus is the central core of an atom, that contains most of its mass. Except for hydrogen, whose nucleus comprises a single proton, it consists of a mixture of protons and neutrons, the former conferring on it a positive electrical charge, while the neutrons contribute to the nuclear mass (but are themselves uncharged). It was discovered and named by **Lord Ernest Rutherford** (1871–1937) in 1911. The shell model for nuclear structure was proposed independently by two German-born US physicists, **Maria Goeppert-Mayer** (1906–1972) and **Johannes Hans Daniel Jensen** (1907–1973) who shared the Nobel Prize for Physics with a Hungarian-born US physicist, **Eugene Paul Wigner** (1902–1995) in 1963.

Atomic Number   The number of protons in the nucleus of an atom. A professor of physics at King's College, London, **Charles Glover Barkla** (1877–1944), was one of the first to correlate the position of an element in the periodic table with the number of electrons it contained. This was the first step towards the determination of atomic numbers of elements. An English physicist, **Henry Gwyn Jeffreys Moseley** (1887–1915), of Weymouth, demonstrated that the number of positive charges in the nucleus is equal to its atomic number in 1913.

Atomic Pile   The first nuclear reactor or atomic pile was demonstrated in   December 1942 at the University of Chicago by **Enrico Fermi** (1901–1954), **Herbert Anderson** (b 1914) and **Walter Henry Zinn** (b 1906). *See atomic bomb, chain reaction.*

Atomic Power   The term usually refers to the use of atomic energy for peaceful purposes. The world's first atomic power station producing electricity, the ERR-1, was installed in the USA in 1951. The United Kingdom Atomic Energy

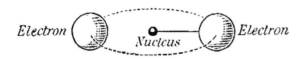

Figure 6   Structure of neutral helium atom, according to Nils Henrick David Bohr. Graetz, Leo. *Recent Developments in Atomic Theory*. London: Methuen & Co, 1923

Authority, responsible for the development of atomic energy in the UK, was established by an act of parliament in 1954. It operates under five groups: research, weapons, production, reactor and engineering. The world's first large-scale atomic power station, with four nuclear reactors, at Calder Hall in Cumbria, was built by **Christopher Hinton** (1901–1983) of Tisbury, Wiltshire, and it officially opened on 17 October 1956. The heat from its reactors was harnessed to drive turbo-alternators which generated electric power for the national electricity supply. Another nuclear power station was opened at Dounray, near Thurso, in Scotland, by the United Kingdom Atomic Energy Authority. The nuclear station at Harwell, Berkshire, was established around 1955. An English nuclear physicist, **William Frederick Fenning** (1919–1988) was mostly responsible for the development of nuclear reactors there. A Soviet physicist, **Igor Vasilevich Kurchatov** (1903–1963) was instrumental in establishing Russia's first industrial nuclear power plant in 1954. A nuclear reactor for power production at Shippingport in the USA became operative in 1957. The Chapplecross Power Station at Chapplecross, Annan, Dumfrieshire, Scotland, first opened in 1958. The Centrale de Chinon power station at Avoine, near Chinon in France, became operative in 1959. The Dresden Nuclear Power Station at Grundy County, Illinois, in the USA, started operating in the same year. The Elk River Reactor for power production at Elk River, Minnesota, followed in 1960.

Atomic Ships   The world's first atomic-powered submarine, *Nautilus,* was engineered and built by a Russian-born US naval engineer, **Hyman George Rickover** (1900–1986), and was launched at Groton, Connecticut in 1954. It was the first submarine to make a North Pole crossing under the ice. The world's first atomic or nuclear-powered merchant ship, the *Savannah,* was launched at Camden, New Jersey, in the USA, in 1959. The Soviets launched the first nuclear-powered icebreaker, *Lenin,* in the same year. The first British nuclear submarine, HMS *Dreadnought,* was launched at Barrow-on-Furness in 1960.

Atomic Structure   Two Greek philosophers, **Democritus** (460–370 BC) and his master **Leucippus** at the school of

Abdera (*c.* 500 BC) were the first to state that all things in nature were made of small particles. These particles were named atoms [Greek: α, without + *tomy*, cut] by Leucippus. The Roman poet and philosopher, **Lucretius** (98–55 BC), in his first two books of the *De Rerum Natura* considers matter as consisting of atoms of various sizes and shapes, and discusses their combinations. Ancient Hindu Sanskrit writings also describe an atom as a particle of indivisible matter. A French analytical chemist, **Joseph Louis Proust** (1754–1826), from Angers, France, proposed the Law of Multiple Proportions, which is related to the combining properties of atoms. **John Dalton** (1766–1844), who is regarded as the father of atomic theory, determined the atomic weight of various elements in 1808. J. W. Nicholson, professor of Mathematics at King's College, London, was the first to make successful calculations of the wavelengths of spectral lines from a model of an emitting atom in 1911. The first constructive hypothesis that led to the modern theory of atomic structure was proposed by the English physicist, **Lord Ernest Rutherford** (1871–1937) at the Manchester Literary and Philosophical Society on May 7 1911. Earlier, in 1909, he had conceived the idea of an atom as a miniature replica of our solar system with the positively charged central nucleus as the sun, and the electrons as the planets. **Henry Gwyn-Jefreys Moseley** (1887–1915) of Weymouth, a student of Ernest Rutherford, demonstrated that the number of positive charges on the nucleus is equal to its atomic number, in 1913. **Niels Henrick David Bohr** (1885–1962), a Danish physicist, was the first to propose the dynamic theory for the structure of the atom in 1913. He proposed that the electrons rotate in orbits with quantized energy, and used his theory to explain the spectral lines emitted by the hydrogen atom and simple ions such as He^+. The theory has been superseded by more modern ones based on the idea of electrons occupying atomic orbitals. Two theories existed up to 1950 to explain the atomic nucleus: one stated that nuclear particles were arranged in concentric shells, and the other described the nucleus as analogous to a liquid drop. Both these theories were explained through the same idea by one model by an American physicist, **James Leo Rainwater** (1917–1986) of Idaho, in the early 1950s. **Aage Niels Bohr** (b 1922) and **Benjamin Roy Mottelson** (b 1926) used Rainwater's theory to develop a more acceptable one which explained the shape of the nucleus. Rainwater, Bohr and Mottelson shared the Nobel Prize for Physics in 1975, for this work. In 1928 two Austrian physicists, **Wolfgang Pauli** (1900–1958) and **Erwin Schrödinger** (1887–1961), described the atom on the basis of quantum mechanical principles.

Atomic Theory The Greek philosopher and scientist **Democritus** around 450 BC proposed that the world consisted of atoms. His theory was advocated by **Epicurus** (342–271 BC) of Samos. A Hindu philosopher, **Kanada** (*c.* 300 BC) in his *Vaiseshika Sūtra* held the view that things are made of invisible, eternal atoms of earth, water, light and air. A French astronomer and philosopher, **Pierre Gassendi** (1592–1655), revived the atomic theory of Democritus and Epicurus. The proof for it was given nearly 200 years later by English schoolmaster and chemist **John Dalton** (1766–1844) in 1803. The theory of atomic structure was proposed by **Lord Ernest Rutherford** (1871–1937). *See atomic structure.*

Atomic Volume The volume of one gram-atom of an element. The relationship of relative atomic volume to relative atomic mass was demonstrated by a German chemist, **Julius Lothar von Meyer** (1830–1895), in 1870. He was professor of chemistry at Zurich (1872), Göttingen (1885) and Heidelberg (1889). He suffered from depression and committed suicide.

Atomic Weight The old name for relative atomic mass. The English chemist **John Dalton** (1766–1844) was one of the first to suggest, in 1803, that the atoms of different elements had different characteristic masses. **Johann Wolfgang Dobereiner** (1780–1849), a German professor of chemistry in Jenna, demonstrated the relationship of relative atomic masses between the elements calcium, barium and strontium. **Jons Jacob Berzelius** (1779–1848) determined the relative atomic mass of many elements in 1826 and prepared the first accurate list. The Dulong and Petit Law (the product of specific heat and relative atomic mass is constant for solid elements) was proposed by a French physician, **Alexis Thérèse Petit** (1791–1820) and a Parisian chemist, **Pierre Louis Dulong** (1785–1838) in 1818. **Stanislao Cannizaro** (1826–1910), an Italian organic chemist, distinguished between relative atomic mass and relative molecular mass **John Alexander Reina Newlands** (1837–1898), a London chemist, was the first to arrange the elements in order of their atomic weights and recognize the similarity between every eighth element. His law of octaves became a forerunner of the periodic table. A theory of relative atomic masses, suggesting a periodic system, was proposed by a Boston chemist and a professor of chemistry and mineralogy at Harvard, **Josiah Parsons Cooke** (1827–1894). A periodic table of the elements, arranged in the order of relative atomic masses was designed by **Dmitri Ivanowitsch Mendeleeff** (1834–1907) in 1869. A more accurate method for determining relative atomic mass was devised by an American chemist and Harvard graduate, **Theodore William Richards** (1868–1928) of Pennsylvania, around 1900. He calculated the relative atomic masses of over 25 elements and was awarded the Nobel Prize for Chemistry for his work in 1914.

Atwood, George (1746–1807) *See acceleration, motion.*

Aublet, Jean Baptiste Christophe (1723–1788) *See forestry.*

Audiocassette *See magnetic recording.*

Audion *See thermionic valve.*

Audubon, John James (1785–1851) *See ornithology.*

Auerbach, Charlotte (1899–1994) *See mutation.*

Auger Electrons Particles emitted instead of photons when an electron drops from a higher to a lower energy level in an atom. They were discovered by a French physicist, **Pierre Victor Auger** (1899–1994) in 1925.

Auger Showers Cascades of large numbers of particles produced by the interaction of cosmic rays with the earth's upper atmosphere. Discovered by a French physicist, **Pierre Victor Auger** (1899–1994) who was a professor at the University of Paris.

Auger, Pierre Victor (1899–1994) *See Auger electrons, Auger showers.*

Aurora Australis A similar phenomenon to the aurora borealis found first in 1773 in the southern skies. *See aurora borealis.*

Aurora Borealis or northern lights [*Aurora*, Greek goddess of dawn] A luminous phenomenon in the northern sky. When observed in London in 1560 it was referred to as *burning spears* and was considered as an omen for an impending disaster. It was described by professor Cornelius Genune in 1575, and by Michael Mestin, who was a pupil of the German astronomer **Johannes Kepler** (1571–1630). **Edmund Halley** (1656–1742) suggested a terrestrial magnetic cause for it in 1714. The phenomenon was thought to be due to a disturbance of terrestrial magnetism and electricity by **Anders Celsius** (1704–1744), a Swedish astronomer, in 1733. A French scientific commission was appointed to investigate the phenomenon in 1838, and most of its members confirmed the phenomenon to be electrical in origin. A London meteorologist, **James Glaisher** (1809–1903), studied it with the help of a compass in 1847. The first spectroscopic analysis was performed by a Swedish physicist, **Anders Jonas Ångström** (1814–1874). The electromagnetic nature of the aurora borealis was demonstrated by a Norwegian physicist, **Kristian Olaf Bernhard**

Birkeland (1867–1917), in 1900. A Hungarian-born physicist, **Joseph Kaplan** (b 1902), first reproduced its spectrum in the laboratory, in 1931. It is now known to be caused by the interaction of the atoms and molecules in the upper atmosphere (mainly atomic oxygen) with charged particles streaming from the sun.

Australopithecus africanus A fossil primate discovered in the west of the Rift Valley in South Africa in 1925 by **Raymond Arthur Dart** (1893–1988) from Brisbane. Originally thought to be a primitive human, it was nicknamed *Abel*. Since this finding eight other *Australopithecus* remains, believed to be 1.2 to 2.5 million years old, have been found. *See hominids.*

Autogyro [Latin: Greek: *autos,* self + *gyro,* turn around] The forerunner of the helicopter, a rotating-wing aircraft, invented by a Spanish aeronautical engineer, **Juan de la Cierva** (1895–1936) in 1923. *See helicopter.*

Automatic Musical Instruments The mechanical scientist, **Hero of Alexandria** (*c.* AD 100) constructed a hydraulic organ. Barrel organs, the first mechanical recording devices that could reproduce music, came into use around AD 1200. Musical boxes were introduced in early 1800, following the invention of a metal comb with vibrating teeth by a clockmaker, Antoine Favre of Geneva. David Lecoultre was the pioneer manufacturer of musical boxes, in Geneva, around 1815. Automatic organs were first built around 1870, mainly for use in fairgrounds. The earliest of these, the trumpet barrel organ, was operated by a steam engine. A pioneer manufacturer of organs, Gavioli and his brother invented a book-organ operated by electricity around 1892. The pianola, which operated pneumatically, was invented in 1904. It consisted of a piano with a punching system which operated the keys through compressed air. *See barrel organ, gramophone, musical synthesizer.*

Automation [Latin: Greek: *autos,* self] A term coined in 1946 for a process that is taken to a point where human intervention is not required. **Archytas of Tarentum** (428–347 BC) constructed a wooden model of a dove which could fly, based on pneumatic principles. In AD 100 **Hero of Alexandria** designed a device for automatically opening and closing temple doors. He heated the air which caused it to expand and move a fluid column which controlled the pillars of the temple doors. **René Descartes** (1596–1650), a French philosopher and scientist, was the first to compare the automaticity in animals with the automatic activity of machines such as hydraulically animated toys, in the 17th century. The governor, an automatic controlling device used in the steam engine, was invented by **James Watt**

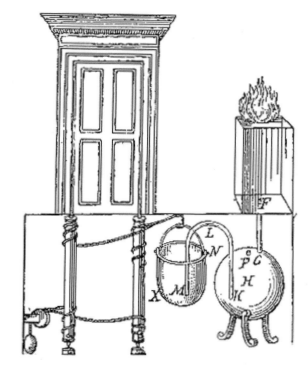

Figure 7 Hero's device for automatically opening a temple door. Findlay, Alexander. *The Spirit of Chemistry.* London: Longmans, Green and Co, 1930

(1736–1819). The self-governed steam engine is one of the early examples of a feed-back mechanism. The earliest automatic machine for industrial use was invented in 1773 by **Jesse Ramsden** (1735–1800), an English mathematical instrument maker from Halifax. It was used to divide a graduated circle. Self-regulating devices for windmills were starting to be used in 1830. Another automation mechanism, the servo, was developed in the 1920s. An American, **Nobert Wiener** (1894–1964), of Columbia, Missouri, in 1948 made a study of communication and control in animal and machine and named the science cybernetics. His concept has important relevance to many fields, such as computers, physiology, mathematics and engineering. He served as professor of mathematics at the Massachusetts Institute of Technology from 1932 to 1960. Many common terms, such as feedback, input and output originate from his work. Electronic automation and miniaturization were pioneered in 1948 by an American electrical engineer, **Jack Saint Clair Kilby** (b 1923) and he patented over 50 inventions related to integrated circuits.

Automobile [Latin: Greek: *autos,* self + *mobilis,* movable] The earliest automobile, a two-feet long steam model, was constructed in 1668 by a Belgian Jesuit priest, **Ferdinand Verbiest** (1623–1687). A full scale three-wheeled steam-powered road tractor capable of carrying passengers at a speed of 6 kilometers per hour was built in 1770 by a French army engineer, **Nicholas Joseph Cugnot** (1725–1804). A Cornish engineer, **George Trevithick** (1771–1833), built a practical passenger road vehicle powered by steam in 1801. Amedée Bollée from Le Mans was a pioneer of steam-powered road vehicles in France and his model in 1881 had a two cylinder front-mounted engine with camshaft and differential gear for transmission. Pierre Alexandre Darracq (1855–1931) of Bordeaux, France was one of the first to produce motor vehicles on a mass scale. *See car.*

Automobile Industry *See automobile, car, Chrysler, Walter Percy, Citroën, André Gustav, Daimler, Gottlib, Ford, Henry, Farina, Battista, Ferrari, Enzo, Rolls, Charles Stewart, Royce, Sir Henry, Holden, Sir Edward Wheewall.*

Auxin *See plant growth.*

Auzont, Adrian (1622–1691) *See micrometer, photometry.*

Avery, Theodore Oswald (1877–1955) *See deoxyribonucleic acid.*

Aviation *See aerodynamics, airlines, airplane, air balloon, airships, ejection seat, jet engine, supersonic flight, transatlantic flight, warplanes.*

Avicenna (980–1037) *See fossils.*

Avogadro, Amedeo (1776–1856) An Italian physicist at the University of Turin who proposed Avogadro's Law – sometimes called Avogadro's Hypothesis – in 1811. He was the first to use the term molecule to denote the smallest possible quantity of water. *See Avogadro's Law.*

Avogadro's Law Equal volumes of gases at the same temperature and pressure contain an equal number of molecules. Proposed by an Italian physicist, **Amedeo Avogadro** (1776–1856) of Turin in 1811. He was made the first professor in mathematical physics, in Italy, at Turin in 1820. According to **M.A.A. Gaudin** (1804–1880) the French physicist, **André Marie Ampère** (1775–1836) suggested a similar theory in 1814.

Axel, Richard (b 1946) *See genetic engineering.*

Ayrton, Hertha (1854–1923) A woman pioneer in British engineering who became the first woman member of the Institution of British Electrical Engineers. She did extensive research on arc lamps and took out several patents and published *The Electric Arc* in 1902.

Ayrton, William Edward (1847–1908) A London electrical engineer who founded the first laboratory in the world for teaching applied electricity, at Tokyo in 1873. He was the first to advocate power transmission at high voltage. *See ammeter, telpherage, tricycle.*

Azimuth [Arabic: *as-samut*, points of the horizon] A specific unit of distance through a defined meridian in astronomy. The instrument designed to measure this distance and direction called the Azimuth compass was built by a German astronomer, **Johannes Hevelius** (1611–1687) in 1641.

Azo Dye A class of dye discovered by a German industrial chemist, **Peter Johann Griess** (1829–1888), during his study of reactions of amines and phenols in 1861.

Azote [Greek: *a*, without + *zoe*, life] *See nitrogen.*

B

Baade, Walter (1893–1960)   *See Andromeda nebula, radioastronomy.*

Babbage, Charles (1792–1871)   A British mathematician from Teignmouth, Devon, who founded the Analytical Society in 1812. He is mostly known for his construction (1842) of the calculating machine, which he could not complete owing to the enormous additional funds that were needed despite an initial sum of 6000 GBP of his own money and a public sum of 17 000 GBP. However, the prototype of the machine which he described to the Royal Astronomical Society in 1822 earned him the first Gold Medal of the society. His unfinished calculating machine is now exhibited at the Science Museum in London.

Babcock, George Herman (1832–1893)   *See Babcock–Wilson steam boiler.*

Babcock, Harold Delos (1882–1968)   An American physicist from Edgerton, Wisconsin, who worked at the Mount Wilson Observatory. He measured the magnetic field of the stars, which provided a link between the theories of electromagnetism and relativity. *See solar magnetograph.*

Babcock, Stephen Moulton (1843–1931)   *See animal husbandry, dairy industry.*

Babcock–Wilson Steam Boiler   Made of cast iron to withstand high pressures with protection against explosion. Developed by two American engineers, **George Herman Babcock** (1832–1893) of Otego, New York and Stephen Wilson, in 1867.

Babinet, Jacques (1794–1872)   *See Ängström unit.*

Babo, Clemens Heinrich Lambert von (1818–1899)   *See Babo tube.*

Babo Tube   An apparatus for making ozone, invented by a German chemist, **Clemens Heinrich Lambert von Babo** (1818–1899). It was the first laboratory apparatus to incorporate a centrifuge.

Babylon   Capital of the Assyrian empire and one of the most ancient cities, it is regarded as the seat of the first civilization. It is said to have been founded by Belus, the Nimrod of the sacred scriptures, around 2300 BC. As early as 2200 BC

Babylonians defined the units of physical measurement for length, weight, and time. The Babylonian year consisted of twelve months or 360 days, and length was measured in units of fingers, feet and poles. Clay tablets dating back to 2000 BC discovered in the 19th century have revealed an advanced system of astronomy practiced by the Babylonians. By their methods they were able to predict eclipses and the positions of the moon and the sun. Babylon was taken control by the Amorite king Nebuchadnezzar in 1124 BC and it became the largest city on earth, with 25 000 acres, under Nebuchadnezzar II in 601 BC. Knowledge of astrology reached its zenith in Babylon around 540 BC when the Chaldeans conquered Babylon. The remains of this ancient city were discovered by Paris-born Anglo-Spanish archaeologist, **Henry Austen Layard** (1817–1894) in 1849.

Bache, Alexander Dallas (1806–1867)   *See academy, geological map.*

Bachman, John (1790–1874)   *See zoology.*

Back, Ernst (1881–1959)   *See Pauli's exclusion principle.*

Background Radiation   Residual microwave radiation in space. Its existence was predicted by **Ralph Asher Alpher** (b 1921) in 1948. Its presence as a result of the Big Bang was confirmed by **Arno Allan Penzias** (b 1933) and **Robert Woodrow Wilson** (b 1936) in 1964.

Backhouse, William (1593–1662)   An English alchemist and astrologer from Berkshire who wrote *The Complaint of Nature,* and translated *The Pleasant Fountain of Knowledge* from the French. He invented an instrument called waywiser, an early form of odometer.

Backus, John (b 1924)   *See Fortran.*

Bacon, Francis (1561–1626)   The lord chancellor of England, who was a philosopher as well as a scientist. He introduced the science of experimental or inductive method of reasoning for interpreting nature in his great work *Novum Organum* published in 1620. *See tectonic theory, thermometer.*

Bacon, Richard (1775–1844)   *See printing.*

Bacon, Roger (*c.* 1214–1298) of Ilchester, an English monk of the Franciscan order, a scientist and an alchemist. His work on alchemy in search of the philosopher's stone enhanced the science of experimentation. He investigated the phenomena of raindrops and refraction, and suggested many futuristic ideas such as flying machines, the camera obscura and mechanized ships. He is also considered by some historians to be the inventor of gunpowder, though it seems more likely that gunpowder was invented by the

Chinese, probably in the tenth century. His *Opus Majus,* containing his views, led to his imprisonment in 1277 by Pope Nicholas IV for over 10 years. *See air balloon, alchemy, camera, compass (1), gunpowder, rainbow, spectacles, telescope, vision.*

Bacteriophage [Greek: *bakterion,* rod + *phagein,* to devour] Viruses that infect and lyse bacteria. Discovered in 1915 by an English bacteriologist, **Frederick William Twort** (1877–1950) of Camberley, Surrey, and by **Felix Hubert D'herelle** (1873–1949) in 1917. In 1955 a German-born US biochemist, **Heinz Fraenkel-Conrat** (b 1910) showed that it was the nuclear component that was responsible for its infectivity and not the outer protein case.

Badarayana A Hindu philosopher who wrote *Vedante Sutra,* one of the six classic systems of Hindu philosophy, in the 5th century. He is also credited with the compilation of the Hindu epic *Mahabarata.*

Baekeland, Leo Hendrick (1863–1944) An American chemist of Belgian origin who is regarded as the founder of the plastics industry owing to his discovery of the first synthetic phenolic resin, which is now known as Bakelite. Baekeland invented the photographic paper that could be used with artificial light in 1893 and made several other important contributions to the fields of organic chemistry and electrochemistry.

Baer, Karl Ernst Ritter von (1792–1876) *See embyology.*

Baeyer, Johann Friedrich Wilhelm Adolf von (1835–1917) An organic chemist from Berlin who was a student of **Robert Bunsen** (1811–1899) and **Friedrich August Kekulé** (1829–1896). His research included the mechanism of photosynthesis, and condensation of phenols and aldehydes. His work on the synthesis and study of the dye indigo in 1882 led to the recognition of the phenomenon currently known as tautomerism. Baeyer was awarded the Nobel Prize for chemistry in 1905.

Baffin, William (1584–1622) An explorer from London during the time of Shakespeare and the reign of Queen Elizabeth I. He served as a member of the polar expedition on the ship *Discovery,* organized by Sir Thomas Smith in 1615. He was the first person to determine a degree of longitude at sea by lunar observation. The largest island in the Canadian Arctic, Baffin Island, is named after him.

Bagnold, Ralph Alger (1896–1990) *See sand dunes.*

Bailey, Liberty Hyde (1858–1954) *See horticulture.*

Bailly, Jean Sylvain (1736–1793) A French astronomer and politician who wrote *Histoire de l'Astronomie* (1775–1787). He was guillotined during the revolution.

Baily, Francis (1774–1844) *See Astronomical Society, solar eclipse.*

Bain, Andrew G. (1797–1864) *See geological map.*

Bainbridge, Kenneth Tompkins (1904–1996) *See mass spectrograph.*

Baird, John Logie (1888–1946) *See broadcasting, television.*

Baird, Spencer Fullerton (1823–1887) An American zoologist from Reading, Pennsylvania, and secretary to the Smithsonian Institution. His most important work *Mammals of North America* was published in 1859.

Bakelite Trade name of a synthetic material used for insulating and other purposes. **Leo Hendrick Baekeland** (1863–1944), an American chemist of Belgian origin, first produced it by condensing phenol with formaldehyde.

Baker, Sir Benjamin (1840–1907) *See bridges, tunnel.*

Baker, Herbert Brereton (1862–1935) An English physical chemist from Blackburn who became professor of chemistry at Imperial College, London in 1912. His main research was on the effect of intensive drying on chemical systems.

Baker, Samuel (d 1778) *See bookshops.*

Baker, Sir Samuel (1821–1893) An African explorer from London who was the first European to see Lake Albert Nyanza, in 1864. He also traveled widely to other parts of the world and he published *The Rifle and the Hound in Ceylon* (1853) and *Eight Years Wanderings in Ceylon* (1855).

Bakewell, Robert (1725–1795) *See animal husbandry, geology.*

Balard, Antoine Jerome (1802–1876) *See bromine, starch.*

Baldwin, Matthias William (1795–1866) *See locomotive.*

Balfour, Francis Maitland (1851–1882) *See chordata, genetics.*

Balfour, George (1872–1941) A construction engineer of Scottish origin from Portsmouth, who founded the Balfour Beatty construction firm and installed the first major hydroelectric scheme in Scotland.

Balfour, John Hutton (1808–1884) A Scottish botanist of Edinburgh who became professor of botany there in 1845. He was instrumental in establishing the Botanical Society of Edinburgh which later became the Botanical Society of

Scotland. His son Sir Isaac Bayley Balfour (1853–1922) founded the journal *Annals of Botany*.

Baliani, Giovanni (1582–1666) *See barometer.*

Ball, John (1818–1889) *See alpine flora.*

Ball-Point Pen *See pen.*

Ball, Sir Robert Staywell (1840–1913) An eminent astronomer, born in Dublin and educated at Trinity College. He was appointed Andrew's professor of astronomy at Dublin University and Astronomer Royal for Ireland in 1874. He made valuable studies on nebulae and stellar parallax, and published *The Story of the Heavens* (1885) and *Popular Guide to the Heavens* (1892).

Ballantyne, James (1772–1833) *See bookshops.*

Ballantyne, John (1774–1821) *See bookshops.*

Ballistics Study of the properties and behavior of projectiles. The mechanisms of projectile motion were discussed and explained by **John Buridan** (*c.* 1300–1358) from Béthune, in the North of France, who was rector at the University of Paris. The first scientific work on the subject was presented by **Niccolò Fontana Tartaglia** (1499–1557) in his *Della Nova Scienza* (of the new science) published in 1537. His theorem, relating the projectile to its speed and elevation, is named after him. Pierre Varignon's French *Treatise on bomb propulsion and in General on Propelling Bodies* (1704–1707) was an important landmark. An English physicist, **Benjamin Robin** (1707–1751), used the pendulum for experimental studies on ballistics.

Ballot, Christoph Hendrik Diederik Buys (1817–1890) *See meteorology, weather forecast.*

Balmer Series *See Balmer, Johan Jacob.*

Balmer, Johan Jacob (1825–1898) A Swiss physicist from Lausanne. He discovered the visible atomic spectrum of hydrogen, consisting of a convergent series of lines seen near the ultraviolet region of the spectrum (Balmer series) in 1885. He deduced the mathematical formula for the wavenumber of these spectral lines, $1/\lambda = R\left(1/n_1^2 - 1/n_2^2\right)$ where λ is the wavelength, R the Rydberg constant, and n_1 and n_2 are integers.

Baltimore, David (b 1938) *See deoxyribonucleic acid.*

Bamberger, E. (1857–1932) *See aromatic compounds.*

Bampton Theological Lectures Established at Oxford with the proceeds of the estate left by a clergyman, **John Bampton** (1690–1751). The first lecture was given by James Bandinel in 1780.

Bampton, John (1690–1751) *See Bampton Theological Lectures.*

Banach, Stefan (1892–1945) A Polish mathematician from Krakow who is regarded as one of the founders of functional analysis. He published *Théorie des opérations linéaires* (1932) which is regarded as a classic on functional analysis.

Bancroft, Sir Joseph (1836–1894) *See parasitism.*

Banks, Sir Joseph (1743–1820) A London naturalist and botanist who accompanied Captain **James Cook** (1728–1779) on his voyage around the world in the ship *Endeavour*. He bequeathed his botanical collection and books to the British Museum to which **Robert Brown** (1773–1858) was appointed as the first curator.

Banting, Frederick (1891–1941) *See insulin.*

Barbaro, Daniello (d 1570) A Venetian who was the first to use the lens for construction of a pinhole camera, in 1568. *See camera.*

Barbed Wire A device for confining cattle to the farmyard. The initial device used was a length of wire with strips of wood for holding the spikes. An American farmer, Joseph Glidden of De Kalb, Illinois, constructed the first barbed wire by hand, and patented it in 1873. He twisted two strands of fencing wire together, with knots containing spikes at regular intervals. Another American, Lucien B. Smith, invented a primitive form of barbed wire in 1867.

Barbon, Nicholas (1637–1698) *See insurance.*

Bardeen, John (1908–1991) An American physicist from Madison, Wisconsin, who had the singular honor of receiving the Nobel Prize for physics twice. He invented the transistor in 1947 and proposed (with **Leon Niels Cooper** and **John Robert Schrieffer**) the Bardeen–Cooper–Shrieffer theory of superconductivity. *See Bardeen–Cooper–Schrieffer Theory, superconductivity, transistor.*

Bardeen–Cooper–Schrieffer Theory Accounts for the zero electrical resistance of superconductors. Developed by three American physicists, **John Bardeen** (1908–1991) of Madison, Wisconsin, **Leon Niels Cooper** (b 1930) of New York, and **John Robert Schrieffer** (b 1931) of Oak Park, Illinois, who jointly shared the Nobel Prize for physics in 1972.

Barium [Greek: *barytes*, heavy] An element with atomic number 56. Its presence in the earth was demonstrated by a

Swedish apothecary and chemist, **Carl Wilhelm Scheele** (1742–1786) in 1774, and a process for obtaining it was suggested by **Jons Jacob Berzelius** (1779–1848). **Sir Humphry Davy** (1778–1829) first used the method to obtain the element, in 1808.

Barkhausen Effect Magnetization of iron proceeding in discrete steps, discovered in 1919 by a German physicist, **Heinreich Georg Barkhausen** (1881–1956) of Bremen. He also devised a loud speaker system to demonstrate these steps.

Barkhausen, Heinreich Georg (1881–1956) *See Barkhausen effect.*

Barkla, Charles Glover (1877–1944) A professor of physics at King's College, London, from Lancashire, who studied X-rays and established them to be of the same nature as light, but of a shorter wavelength. He was one of the first to correlate the position of an element in the periodic table to the number of electrons it contained, which was the first step towards the determination of atomic number of elements. He became professor of natural philosophy at the University of Edinburgh in 1913, and was awarded the Nobel Prize for physics in 1917.

Barlow, Peter (1776–1862) A physicist from Norwich whose main research was on marine engineering. He published *New Mathematical Tables* (1814) which was reprinted under the title *Barlow's Tables* in 1947.

Barlow's Tables *See Barlow, Peter.*

Barnard, Edward Emerson (1857–1923) An American astronomer born in Nashville, Tennessee. In 1895 he was appointed professor at the Yerkes Observatory, University of Chicago, and was instrumental in constructing two of the largest telescopes in the world. In 1892 he discovered the fifth satellite of Jupiter, Amalthea.

Barnard, Joseph Edwin (1870–1949) *See ultraviolet microscope.*

Barnard's Star A small star, the second-nearest star to the sun. It was discovered in 1916 by **Edward Emerson Barnard** (1857–1923), an American astronomer of Nashville, Tennessee.

Barometer [Greek: *baros*, heavy + *metron*, measure] **Galilei Galileo** (1564–1642) observed that water would rise only to a height of *c.* 10 meters in a suction pump, implying the existence of atmospheric pressure. **Giovanni Baliani** (1582–1666) of Italy suggested that the weight of the external air balanced that of the column of water. Another Italian,

Evangelista Torricelli (1608–1647), of Faenza, a contemporary of Galileo, developed the theory of atmospheric pressure and set out to prove it. During his researches Torricelli discovered that the height of a column of water or mercury that can be supported by the air is a measure of the pressure exerted by the atmosphere; an important point is that the height of the column is independent of the cross-sectional area of the tube containing the liquid. Based on this finding he worked with **Vincenzo Vivianni** (1622–1703) and constructed the first barometer in 1643. An important principle in barometry, that the height of fluid in the barometer depends on the external pressure, was proved by **Robert Boyle** (1627–1691) in 1659. In 1665 he suggested a form of barometer with narrowing towards the closed end suitable for use at sea. **Otto von Guericke** (1602–1686) constructed a water barometer in 1672. Wheel barometers were introduced in 1668 and pendent barometers came into use in 1695. The heights of mountains were recorded accurately for the first time with the use of the barometer by a Swiss geologist, **Jean André de Deluc** (1727–1817) from Geneva, who settled in England in 1774 and became the reader to Queen Charlotte Sophia at Windsor Castle. The mercury barometer (or cistern barometer) has been replaced in many applications by the aneroid barometer, in which air pressure is measured through its effect on the thin corrugated metal lid of a box; this, although not as accurate as the mercury barometer, is much more robust and convenient.

Barr Stroud Ltd A British firm of scientific instruments makers and pioneers of naval range finding and anti-aircraft guns, founded in 1931 by **William Stroud** (1860–1938) of Bristol, and **Archibald Barr** (1855–1931) of Paisley, Glasgow.

Barr, Archibald (1855–1931) A Scottish engineer from Paisley who graduated from Glasgow University where he became regius chair of civil engineering in 1889. He was instrumental in establishing the James Watt research laboratories in 1900. *See Barr Stroud Ltd.*

Barrel Organ A mechanism in which music is preserved as a mechanical recording and could be reproduced. The first mechanical recording devices or barrel organs that could reproduce music came into use around AD 1100. A historian, William of Malmesbury (b 1142) described a barrel organ built by **Gerbert** or **Pope Sylvester** II (d 1003). Queen Elizabeth in 1597 presented a barrel organ to the sultan of Turkey. It was designed and built by an English organ-maker, **Thomas Dallam** (*c.* 1599–1630). His son **Robert Dallam** (1602–1665) built the organs at St Paul's

Cathedral, Jesus College, Cambridge, and Canterbury Cathedral.

Barrett, Alan H. (1927–1991) *See radioastronomy.*

Barrow, Isaac (1630–1677) A teacher of **Sir Isaac Newton** (1642–1727) at Cambridge who wrote several treatises on geometry including *Elements* (1655) and *Data* (1657). The method of drawing a tangent on a given point on a curve, first described by him in his book *Lectiones opticae et geometricae* (1669) is supposed to have aided the discovery of fluxions by Newton.

Barry, Martin (1802–1855) *See embryology.*

Bartholinus, Erasmus (1625–1698) *See crystallography.*

Bartholomew, John George (1860–1920) *See cartography.*

Bartlett, John (1820–1905) *See bookshops.*

Bartlett, Neil (b 1932) *See xenon.*

Barton, Sir Derek Harold Richard (1918–1998) *See stereochemistry.*

Bartram, John (1699–1777) A self-taught botanist and farmer from Pennsylvania who had one of the greatest collections of North American plants in his garden. **Karl Linnaeus** (1707–1778) considered him as the greatest natural botanist in the world.

Bary, Heinrich Anton De (1831–1888) *See plant anatomy, symbiosis.*

Barycentric Calculus [Greek: *barys,* heavy] A system of calculatory procedures useful in geometrical problems. Invented by a German mathematician, **August Ferdinand Möbius** (1790–1868).

BASIC [**B**eginners **A**ll-purpose **S**ymbolic **I**nstruction **C**ode] *See computers.*

Baskerville, John (1706–1775) *See typography.*

Basov, Nikolay Gennadiyevich (b 1922) *See laser, maser.*

Bassi, Agostino (1773–1856) *See silkworms.*

Bates, Henry Walter (1825–1892) *See mimicry.*

Bateson, William (1861–1926) An English geneticist from Whitby, Yorkshire, who is regarded as the father of genetics in Britain. He became the first professor of genetics at Cambridge, in 1908, and was appointed director of John Innes Horticultural Institution in 1910. Some of his published works on genetics include *Materials for Study of Variation* (1894), *Mendel's Principles of Heredity* (1902) and *Problems of Genetics* (1913). *See genetics.*

Bathyscaphe *See bathysphere.*

Bathysphere [Greek: *bathos*, depth + *sphaira,* a ball] A term coined by an American explorer, **Charles William Beebe** (1877–1962) of Brooklyn, New York, for his 1.45 meter ocean diving device for studying deep sea marine forms. He reached a new record of 923 meters for diving with his invention in 1934. A Swiss physicist, **Auguste Antoine Piccard** (1884–1962) constructed another device (bathyscaphe) in 1948, and explored the sea below a depth of 3000 m in 1953.

Battery An assembly of electrochemical cells for the production of electricity. The first primitive form of battery, consisting of zinc, silver and a moistened card, was devised by **Alessandro Volta** (1745–1827), in 1797. An English physicist, **William Sturgeon** (1783–1850), of Lancashire, improved it by using zinc and mercury amalgam. The first dry cell battery was constructed by a German physicist, **Johann Wilhelm Ritter** (1776–1810), in 1802. The first reliable source of direct current electricity (Daniell cell), with a zinc cathode and copper anode in copper sulfate solution, was invented in 1836 by **John Frederick Daniell** (1790–1845), professor of chemistry at King's College, London. **Robert Bunsen** (1811–1899) of Göttingen invented the carbon–zinc electric battery, which became known as the Bunsen battery, in 1841. The first practical storage battery with a secondary cell that could be recharged several times was constructed by a French physicist, **Gaston Plante** (1834–1889) in 1860. A Guernsey-born British scientist and astronomer, **Warren de la Rue** (1815–1889) invented the silver chloride battery. *See Grove cell, zinc–carbon cell.*

Bauhin, Casper (1560–1624) *See botany.*

Baume, Antoine (1728–1804) *See Baume's scale.*

Baume's Scale Used in hydrometers for the measurement of the specific gravity of liquids. Proposed by a French chemist, **Antoine Baume** (1728–1804), in 1768. Baume was appointed professor at the School of Pharmacy in 1752 where he invented the hydrometer which is named after him.

Baxter, John (1781–1858) The first English printer to use an ink roller. He published a bible and the first book on cricket rules.

Bayer, Johann (1572–1625) A Bavarian astronomer who first used the letters of the Greek alphabet to represent the brighter stars. He published *Uranometria* (1603) which gave positions of nearly 1000 more stars, in addition to those described by the Swedish astronomer **Tycho Brahe** (1546–1601).

Bayes, Thomas (1702–1761) *See statistics.*

Bayliss, Sir Willam Maddock (1860–1924) *See digestion, hormones.*

Bazalgette, Sir Joseph William (1819–1891) A London civil engineer who installed a complete drainage system for the city of London. He was knighted in 1874 for his contribution to public health, and became president of the Institute of Civil Engineers in 1884.

Beach, Frank Ambrose (b 1911) *See ethology.*

Beadle, George Wells (1903–1989) An American geneticist from Wahoo, Nebraska who worked with **Edward Lawrie Tatum** (1909–1975) at Stanford University to develop the concept that specific genes controlled specific enzymes. He shared the Nobel Prize for Medicine or Physiology for his work on biochemical genetics with Tatum and **Joshua Lederberg** (b 1925) in 1958.

Beagle, HMS The English naval ship with **Charles Robert Darwin** (1809–1882) as its naturalist during its voyage to complete the unfinished survey of Patagonia and Tierra del Fuego, to map out the shores of Chile and Peru, to visit Pacific Archipelagos, and to carry out chronometrical measurements around the world. Captained by a meteorologist, **Robert Fitzroy** (1805–1865), from Suffolk, it set sail from Devonport in 1831 and returned to Falmouth in 1836. Darwin spent 4 years on the ship during this voyage without pay, studying the flora and fauna of South America and the Galapagos Islands. On his return, he worked on his theory of evolution for the next 20 years and published his monumental work *On the Origin of Species by Means of Natural Selection* in 1859. *See evolution theory, Darwin, Charles.*

Beale, Dorothea (1831–1906) A pioneer of women's education from London; she founded the first training college for women teachers in England, the St Hilda's College, at Cheltenham, in 1885.

Beauchamps, Joseph (1752–1801) An eminent French astronomer and scientist who was recruited by Napoleon Bonaparte as a spy. He was captured by the English and was handed over to Turks who imprisoned him until the last year of his life.

Beaufort Scale The scale used for classification and description of wind force, first proposed by **Sir Francis Beaufort** (1774–1857) in 1805. It was revised and improved in 1921 by an English meteorologist from Derby, **Sir George Clark Simpson** (1878–1965).

Beaufort, Sir Francis (1774–1857) A naval officer from Lebanon, Connecticut, who did research on hydrography. The tabulated system of weather registration was developed by him around 1829. *See Beaufort scale.*

Beaumont, William (1785–1853) *See digestion.*

Beccaria, Giambatista (1716–1781) *See lightning.*

Beche, Sir Henry Thomas de la (1796–1855) A London geologist and founder of the Geological Museum, Geological Survey of Britain, and the Royal School of Mines. In 1832, he was appointed as the first director of geological survey of Great Britain, and published *Manual of Geology* (1831), *Researches in Theoretical Geology* (1834), *Geological Observer* (1853) and several other books. He was knighted in 1842.

Becher, Johann Joachim (1635–1682) *See mineralogy, physical chemistry.*

Becker, Heinrich (1911–1942) *See beryllium.*

Becker, Wilhelm (b 1907) *See celestial photography.*

Beckmann Thermometer A sensitive thermometer used in the cryoscopic method for determination of relative molecular masses in solutions. It is named after its inventor, a German chemist, **Ernst Beckmann** (1853–1923), who was professor of chemistry at Erlangen and Leipzig.

Beckmann, Ernst (1853–1923) *See Beckmann thermometer.*

Becquerel, Alexandre-Edmond (1820–1891) A French physicist and assistant to his father **Antoine-César Becquerel** (1788–1878). He succeeded his father as director of the National History Museum in Paris in 1878, and made important contributions to the study of electricity and magnetic properties of solar radiation. He devised an actinometer to measure the intensity of sunlight.

Becquerel, Antoine Henri (1852–1908) A French physicist who discovered in 1895 that certain substances like uranium emit radiation similar to X-rays. This was the first recognition of radioactive substances and he named the phenomenon radioactivity. He shared the Nobel Prize for physics for his work on radioactivity with **Marie Curie** (1867–1934) and **Pierre Curie** (1859–1906), in 1903.

Becquerel, Antoine-César (1788–1878) A French chemist from Châtillon-sur-Loire who did research on electricity. He improved the electric magnet, invented several instruments for precise measurements of electromagnetic forces

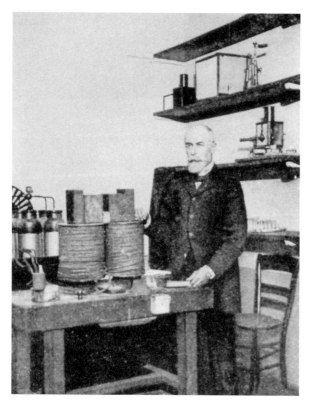

Figure 8 Antoine Henri Becquerel (1852–1908) in his laboratory in Paris. Courtesy of the National Library of Medicine

and published *Traité Expérimental de l'electricité et du Magnétisme* (1834–1840). He was the first to use electrolysis as a means of isolating metals from their ores.

Beddoes, Thomas (1760–1808) A physician from Shiffnal, in Shropshire, who graduated in medicine from Edinburgh in 1786. He was appointed to the chair of chemistry at Oxford which he gave up in 1792 to practice medicine in Bristol. He published *Translations of Schlee's Chemical Essays* in 1786 and *Chemical Experiments and Opinion*. In 1799 he founded the Medical Pneumatic Institution to study the role of inhalation of gases in the treatment of diseases.

Bede, Venerable (*c.* 673–735) *See Christian era, tides.*

Bednorz, Johannes Georg (b 1950) *See superconductivity.*

Beebe, Charles William (1877–1962) *See bathysphere.*

Beer, Sir Gavin Rylands de (1899–1972) *See recapitulation theory.*

Beer [Anglo-Saxon: *beor*] An alcoholic beverage known in Mesopotamia around 4000 BC. Bone inscriptions on beer making, dating back to 1500 BC, have been found in China.

The oldest brewery in the world, Weihenstephan, at Freising, near Munich, was established in AD 1040. Beer became popular in Europe through Germany around AD 1600. Beer cans were first introduced in New Jersey, United States, in 1935. The push-through tabs on beer cans were introduced in 1973.

Beer, Michael (1605–1666) *See architecture, European.*

Bees The habits of bees, including the fertilization of the queen bee and the expulsion of the drones, were discovered by a Swiss naturalist, **François Huber** (1750–1831). Detailed accounts of the behavior of wasps and bees, and life cycles of beetles, were given by a French entomologist, **Jean Henri Fabre** (1823–1915).

Beet Sugar First extracted from beet root by a German chemist, **Andreas Sigismond Marggrafe** (1709–1782) in 1747. He used the microscope to demonstrate that the crystals found in beet sugar were identical to those of sucrose. This was probably the first instance of the use of the microscope in chemistry. A German agricultural chemist, **Franz Karl Achard** (1753–1821) of Berlin, who in 1799 succeeded Marggrafe as director of the Royal Prussian Academy, established the first beet sugar factory in Silesia, in 1801.

Béguyer, Alexandre Emile De (1819–1886) *See periodic law.*

Behaim, Martin (1440–1506) *See globe.*

Behr, Fritz Bernhard (b 1842) *See monorail.*

Beijerinck, Wilhelm Martinus (1851–1931) *See virus.*

Beilby, Sir George Thomas (1850–1924) A Scottish industrial chemist and father-in-law of the English physicist **Frederick Soddy** (1877–1965). He is known for his invention of several industrial chemical processes.

Beilstein, Friedrich Konrad (1836–1906) *See organic chemistry.*

Bélidor, Bernard Forest De (1698–1761) A French pioneer in engineering, born in Spain. He described various hydraulic mechanisms of water supply for dams in Europe in his *Architecture Hydraulique* (1737–1753). *See architecture, European, military architecture.*

Bell [Anglo-Saxon: *belle*] A tower bell dating back to 1106 is at Pisa, Italy. Another bell, found in 1849 in the Babylonian palace of Nimrod by **Austen Henry Layard** (1817–1894) has been dated 1100 BC. The oldest tower bell (AD 1010) in Britain, at St Botolph, Hardham, Sussex, is still in use.

Bell, Alexander Graham (1847–1922) The inventor of the telephone; born in Edinburgh and educated at London University. He moved to Canada in 1870 and was appointed professor of vocal physiology at Boston University in 1873. He invented an electrical device by the aid of which speech could by represented in a visible form in 1876. His work in this field led to the invention of the telephone, which he patented on 4 February 1876.

Bell, Chester Gordon (b 1934) *See computers, pulsar.*

Bell, Henry (1737–1830) A Scottish pioneer in steam navigation from Linlithgow. He constructed the first practical passenger steam vessel *Comet* which operated regularly between Greenock and Glasgow.

Bell, Lawrence Dale (1895–1956) An aircraft designer from Indiana who founded the Bell Aircraft Corporation in 1935. The company produced its first jet propelled aircraft in 1942, followed by the first manned aircraft to exceed the speed of sound, in 1947.

Bell, Patrick (1799–1869) *See agricultural instruments.*

Bellinghausen, Fabian Gottlieb Benjamin von (1778–1852) *See South Pole.*

Bellows [Anglo-Saxon: *belg,* bag] First invented for the purpose of smelting metals and to keep the fire continuously burning. **Anacharasis of Scythia**, who lived around 569 BC, has been credited with its invention although evidence suggests that the device existed for the purpose of manufacturing glass and smelting in 1600 BC in Mesopotamia. In 310 BC the Chinese introduced a form of double acting piston bellows to produce a continuous stream of air. Water powered bellows for making cast iron were invented by **Tu Shih** of China in AD 31. Wooden bellows were invented in 1669 by two brothers, Martin Schelhorn and Nicholas Schelhorn, from Schmalebuch, a small German village in Coburg. Before their invention bellows were usually made of leather. Bellows were also used for raising water.

Belon, Pierre (1517–1574) *See comparative anatomy, ornithology.*

Benda, Carl (1857–1933) *See mitochondrion.*

Beneden, Edouard Joseph Louis-Marie Van (1846–1910) *See fertilization, genetics, meiosis.*

Benedetti, Giovanni (1530–1590) *See acoustics.*

Benioff, Victor Hugo (1899–1968) *See seismology, Wadati–Benioff zones.*

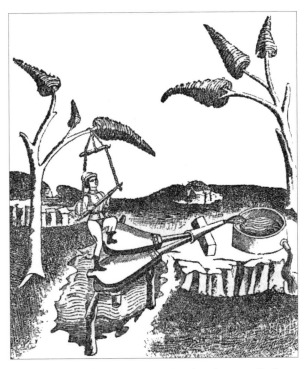

Figure 9 A 15th century print showing the use of bellows for raising water. Rolt-Wheeler, Francis. *The Science-History of the Universe, Mathematics.* London: The Waverley Book Company Limited, 1911

Bennet, Ethelred (1776–1845) The first prominent woman geologist in Britain, who published *A Catalogue of Organic Remains of the County of Wilts* in 1831.

Bennett, Abraham (1750–1799) *See gold leaf electroscope.*

Bennett, Floyd (1890–1928) *See North Pole.*

Benson, Sidney William (b 1918) An eminent New York physical chemist who contributed to photochemistry, kinetics, thermochemistry and laser chemistry. He was chief editor (1967–1983) of the *International Journal of Chemical Kinetics* and published *Thermochemical Kinetics* in 1968.

Bentham, Sir Samuel (1757–1831) *See military architecture.*

Bentham, George (1800–1884) A British botanist from Devon, who served as the president of the Linnean Society from 1863 to 1874. He published *Genera Plantarum* which took over 20 years to write and became a standard work on plant classification.

Bentham, Jeremy (1757–1831) One of the first engineers in England to start making machine tools. **Henry Maudslay** (1771–1831) was one of his pupils.

Bentley, Charles Raymond (b 1929) *See glaciology.*

Benz, Carl Friedrich (1844–1929) Son of a railway mechanic from Karlsruhe, Germany, who became a pioneer in automobile engineering. In 1879 he developed a two-stroke engine and exhibited his first practical car at the Paris Fair of 1889. *See car.*

Benzene [Latin: *benzoin,* aromatic resin] First observed in 1825 by **Michael Faraday** (1791–1867) in the whale gas prepared by the *Portable Gas Company.* A German chemist, **Eilhardt Mitscherlich** (1794–1863) synthesized it, in 1834, and named it benzin. **August Wilhelm von Hofmann** (1818–1892) discovered it in coal tar around 1840. **Friedrich August Kekulé, von Stradonitz** (1829–1896) deduced the cyclic six carbon ring structure of the compound in 1865. A Scottish chemist, **Alexander Crum Brown** (1838–1922), of Edinburgh, proposed the Crum Brown rule, related to substitution in benzene derivatives and proposed a modern structure for benzene in 1864.

Berard, Jacques Etienne (1789–1869) *See radiation of heat.*

Berg, Paul (b 1926) *See cytogenetics, genetic engineering.*

Bergeron, Harold Percival (1891–1977) *See clouds.*

Bergius, Friedrich Karl Rudolf (1884–1949) *See ammonia, Bosch, Carl, petroleum.*

Bergman, Torbern Olof (1735–1784) *See affinity, ammonia, analytical chemistry.*

Berkeley, George (1685–1753) *See perception.*

Berkelium The element with atomic number 97, synthesized in 1949 by three American physicists, **Glenn Theodore Seaborg** (1912–1999), S.G. Thompson and A. Ghiorso, at Berkeley, California by bombarding americium-241 with alpha particles; all its isotopes are radioactive.

Berliner, Emile (1851–1929) *See gramophone.*

Bernal, John Desmond (1901–1971) *See crystallography.*

Bernoulli, Daniel (1700–1782) Second son of **Jean Bernoulli** (1667–1748) from Groningen, The Netherlands. He was educated in Basle, Switzerland, and graduated as a physician in 1721. His main interest was mathematics and he published *Excitationes Mathematicae* in 1724. After becoming professor of mathematics at St Petersburg in 1725, he returned to Basle as professor of anatomy in 1732. He wrote several treatises on science, astronomy and differential equations. His *Hydrodynamica* (1738) explored the relationship between pressure, velocity and density in flowing fluids. In the above work he formulated the laws for the flow of liquids through pipes of various diameters, and explained

Boyle's law of gases. He deduced Bernoulli's equation which helped to solve the differential equation proposed by **Count Jacopo Francesco Riccati** (1676–1754).

Bernoulli, Jacques (1654–1705) *See Bernoulli numbers, Bernoulli theorem.*

Bernoulli, Jean (1667–1748) *See Bernoulli numbers.*

Bernoulli Numbers A sequence of rational numbers that represent a definite symbolic form. It was proposed by a Swiss mathematician, **Jacques Bernoulli** (1654–1705) in his *Ars Conjectandi* published posthumously in 1713. He was a brother of another eminent mathematician, **Jean Bernoulli** (1667–1748).

Bernoulli Theorem At any point in a pipe through which a fluid is flowing, the sum of the pressure energy, potential energy and kinetic energy of a given mass of the fluid is constant. This is in effect a statement of the law of conservation of energy. It is named after a Swiss mathematician, **Daniel Bernoulli** (1700–1782).

Bernoulli's Equation *See Bernoulli, Daniel.*

Bernstein, Richard Barry (1923–1990) *See femtochemistry.*

Berthelot, Pierre-Eugène Marcellin (1827–1907) A French chemist, born and educated in Paris where he was appointed to the chair of organic chemistry at the École Supérieure de Pharmacie in 1859. He investigated the aromatic compounds and produced benzene and naphthalene in 1851 and demonstrated acetylene in 1860. As a politician, he held several ministerial posts. *See antimomy, aromatic compounds, chemistry, nitrogen fixing bacteria, organic chemistry.*

Berthhold, Arnold (1801–1863) *See hormones.*

Berthholdus or Bertholet, Michael Schwartz (c. 1320) *See firearms, gunpowder, military engineering.*

Berthollet, Claude Louis Compte de (1748–1822) An eminent French chemist and physician from Talloires, Savoy. He discovered a relationship between the masses of the reagents involved in a chemical reaction, which led to the discovery of the law of definite proportions by **Joseph Louis Proust** (1754–1826). He demonstrated the proportions of nitrogen and hydrogen in ammonia. His *Essai de Statique Chimique* explaining the forces of chemical affinity was published in 1803. *See affinity, ammonia, bleaching powder, chlorine, law of constant composition, metric system, potassium chlorate.*

Berthoud, Ferdinand (1727–1807) *See marine chronometer.*

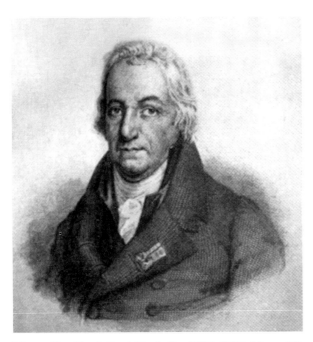

Figure 10   Claude Louis Berthollet (1748–1822). Moore, F.J. *A History of Chemistry*, International Chemical Series. New York: McGraw-Hill Book Inc, 1918

Beryllium [Greek: *beryllion*, dim]   The element with atomic number of 4. It was discovered in 1798 by a French Chemist, **Louis Nicolas Vauquelin** (1763–1829), from Normandy, who first named it Glucine, owing to the sweet taste of its salts. Beryllium in a pure state was isolated in 1828 by a German chemist, **Friedrich Wöhler** (1800–1882). A French chemist, **Antoine Alexandre Brutus Bussy** (1794–1882), of Marseilles, independently obtained it in the same year. In 1930 two German physicists, **Heinrich Becker** (1911–1942) and **Walter Wilhelm Georg Bothe** (1891–1957) during their nuclear research discovered that by bombarding beryllium with alpha rays a penetrating radiation could be produced.

Berzelius, Jons Jakob (1779–1848)   A Swedish chemist and physician who determined the relative atomic mass of many metals in 1826. He proposed the system of representing elements by the first Latin letter of their name. He was the first to use the term organic chemistry in his *Lectures in Animal Chemistry* (1806), and defined it as 'the part of physiology which describes the composition of living bodies, and the chemical processes which occur in them'. He also coined the term protein. *See atomic weight, barium, catalysis, cerium, chemistry, chemical symbols, halogens, iron, isomerism, selenium, silicon, sodium, thorium, titanium, zirconium.*

Bessel Equation   Relates to the calculation of statistical bias in astronomical observations. It was proposed by a German astronomer, **Friedrich Wilhelm Bessel** (1784–1846). He became the director of Königsberg Observatory in 1810.

Bessel, Friedrich Wilhelm (1784–1846)   *See Bessel equation, Sirius.*

Bessemer Process   Manufacture of iron and steel by passing compressed cold air through fused molten metal. Invented in 1856 by a British engineer of Huguenot origin, **Sir Henry Bessemer** (1813–1898) of Hitchin, Hertfordshire. A similar method was invented around the same time by an American metallurgist, **William Kelly** (1811–1888) of Pittsburgh, Pennsylvania, who patented it in 1857. An English metallurgist, **Robert Forester Mushet** (1811–1891), of Gloucestershire, improved the Bessemer process and made it a commercial success in the same year. A Swedish industrialist, **Göran Frederik Göransson** (1819–1900), further improved the process in 1858. In 1878 another English metallurgist, **Sidney Gilchrist Thomas** (1850–1885) of Canonbury, North London, added refinements for obtaining a pure yield. His improved method provided an inexpensive way of making steel. The Bessemer process has since been superseded by more efficient steelmaking methods.

Bessemer, Sir Henry (1813–1898)   An inventor and engineer from Charlton, Hertfordshire. He studied metallurgy at his father's foundry and invented the Bessemer converter, which enabled the economic production of steel. He established a steelworks at Sheffield in 1859.

Besson, Jacques (1535–1575)   A French mathematician and inventor. He anticipated some modern inventions in his illustrated work entitled *Théâtre des Instruments Mathématiques et Mécaniques* published posthumously in 1578.

Best, Charles Herbert (1899–1978)   *See insulin.*

Beta   The second letter (β) of the Greek alphabet. It is derived from the Phoenician word *beth* for house. The term beta is sometimes used to denote the second member of a series or group, especially a group of stars in a constellation, where the name is normally given to the constellation's second brightest star, e.g. Beta Centauri.

Beta Rays   *See radioactivity.*

Bethe, Hans Albrecht (b 1906)   *See carbon cycle, thermonuclear fusion.*

Betti, Enrico (1823–1892)   An Italian mathematician from Pistoria, who was the first to resolve integral functions of a complex variable into their primary factors. He gave explanations for many of **Evariste Galois's** (1811–1832) theorems.

Bevan, Edward John (1856–1921) *See textile chemistry.*

Beverton, Raymond John Heaphy (b 1922) *See marine biology.*

Bhabha Atomic Research Centre Named after the Indian physicist, **Homi Jehangir Bhabha** (1909–1966), who served as its director when it was originally known as the Atomic Energy Research Centre. He derived a correct expression for the cross-section of scattering positrons by electrons (Bhabha scattering). Bhabha was a student of **Paul Adrien Maurice Dirac** (1902–1984).

Bhabha Scattering A scattering process involving positrons and electrons, discovered by an Indian physicist, **Homi Jehangir Bhabha** (1909–1966) from Bombay.

Bhabha, Homi Jehangir (1909–1966) *See Bhabha Atomic Research Center, Bhabha scattering.*

Bhaskara (AD 1114–1185) A Hindu mathematician and astrologer from Ujjain. He named his treatise on arithmetic after his daughter, *Lilavathi. See mathematics, permutation.*

Bichat. Marie François Xavier (1771–1802) *See tissue.*

Bickford, William (1774–1834) *See metallurgy.*

Bicycle [Latin: *bis,* twice + Greek: *kyclos,* cycle] **Leonardo da Vinci** (1452–1519) made the first drawing of a two-wheeled machine propelled by cranks and pedals. The forerunner of the bicycle, the pedestrian hobby-horse, which consisted of a wooden bar joining the two wheels, was invented in France around 1770. Known as the *céléfère,* it had no steering or pedals and the rider had to roll it along while seated on its bar. Similar models were known in ancient Babylon and Rome. In 1817 a farmer and engineer in Baden, Baron **Karl Draise von Sauerbon** (d 1851), added a steering mechanism and it came to be known as the *Draisienne.* The first primitive bicycle was built in 1840 by a Scottish inventor and son of a village blacksmith, **Kirkpatrick Macmillan** (1813–1878), of Thornhill in Dumfriesshire. His model had two long levers attached to the rear wheel, which had to be moved back and forth with the feet to propel the vehicle. Kirkpatrick was also the first to add pedals to a tricycle, in 1838. He demonstrated his bicycle by riding it for 70 miles from Dumfriesshire to Glasgow in 1840. In 1855 a locksmith in Paris, Ernest Michaux, independently developed the idea of fitting pedals to the hub of the front wheel. **James Starley** (1831–1881) from Albourne in Sussex invented the prototype of the present bicycle which,

although greatly advanced, was still perilous to ride owing to its large front wheel. It was called the 'ordinary' bicycle, but colloquially referred to as the 'penny farthing' because of the relative sizes of the front and rear wheel (analogous of the British coinage). Starley also created the modern type of wheels with rim and hub connected by wire spokes, and the first practical tricycle. J. F. Tretz used a chain drive for the first time to propel the bicycle, in 1869. The modern safety bicycle, built by H. J. Lawson in 1876, started to be marketed in 1885. The pneumatic tire was adopted in 1891 and the free-wheel mechanism appeared in 1894. Variable gears were introduced in 1899.

Biela Comet Named after an Austrian army officer, **Wilhelm von Biela** (1782–1856), who observed it in 1826. The comet was discovered by Jacques L. Montaigne in 1772.

Biela, Wilhelm von (1782–1856) *See Biela comet.*

Bierman, Ludwig (1907–1986) *See comet, solar wind.*

Biffen, Sir Rowland Harry (1874–1949) *See hybridization.*

Bifilar Magnetometer A device made of bar magnet suspended by two vertical wires, first constructed by Sir W. Snow Harris in 1836. It was improved by two German physicists, **Wilhelm Eduard Weber** (1804–1891) and **Carl Friedrich Gauss** (1777–1855).

Bifocal Lens *See Franklin, Benjamin.*

Big Bang Theory A theory for the origin of the universe, based on an enormous explosion, was proposed in 1927 by a Belgian priest and astrophysicist, **Henri George Lemaître** (1894–1966). The theory maintains that about 10 000 million years ago all the matter in the Universe was packed into one superdense sphere, the primeval atom which exploded at a finite time. Lemaître's work *Discussion on the Evolution of the Universe* was published in 1933. His theory was developed by a Russian-born American physicist, **George Gamow** (1904–1968), Robert Hermann, and **Ralph Asher Alpher** (b 1921) of Washington DC, in 1948. These workers in their alpha, beta, gamma theory proposed that the abundance of chemical elements arose as a result of thermonuclear processes in the early stages of a hot evolving universe. In 1964 an American professor of physics at Princeton University, **Robert Henry Dicke** (1916–1997), and a Canadian-born cosmologist, **Phillips James Edwin Peebles** (b 1935) also predicted the existence of remnant background microwave radiation due to the Big Bang. An American astronomer, **Edwin Powell Hubble** (1889–1953) from Missouri found the first evidence for the expansion of the universe based on the theory of Lemaître.

His work set the date of creation at 15 000 million years. The existence of background radiation as a result of the Big Bang, predicted by Alpher and others, was confirmed by two American radioastronomers, **Arno Allan Penzias** (b 1933) of German origin, and **Robert Woodrow Wilson** (b 1936) in 1964. Microscopic black holes may have been formed in the chaotic conditions of the Big Bang. The English physicist **Stephen Hawking** has shown that such tiny black holes could 'evaporate' and explode in a flash of energy. *See Oscillating theory, Steady State theory.*

Bigelow, Erastus Bigham (1814–1879) An American engineer from West Boylston, Massachusetts, who invented various kinds of loom for the textile industry, including the first powered one for weaving ingrain carpets. He founded the Massachusetts Institute of Technology (MIT) in 1861.

Binary Stars A pair of stars revolving about a common center of mass. A German astronomer, **Hermann Carl Vogel** (1842–1907), of Leipzig discovered the spectroscopic binary stars which cannot usually be resolved by telescope, but can be detected by their spectra. An American astronomer, **Robert Grant Aitken** (1864–1951), from Jackson, California, identified more than 4000 new double stars at the Lick Observatory and published *Binary Stars* (1918) and *New General Catalogue of Double Stars* (1932). *See Plaskett Twins.*

Binary System The basis of modern computer language, with a system of numbers to base two, using combinations of the digits 1 and 0. Developed from a system of two-valued or binary algebra proposed by the English mathematician **George Boole** (1816–1864). *See Boole, George, Boolean algebra.*

Bingham, Eugene Cook (b 1878) *See viscosity.*

Binnig, Gerd Karl (b 1947) *See electron microscope.*

Binomial Nomenclature [Latin: *bi*, twice + Greek: *nomia*, to arrange or classify] A system of classification of organisms with the use of two terms, the genus and species. *See Linnaeus, Karl, Tournefort, Joseph Pitton de.*

Binomial Theorem [Latin: *bi*, twice + Greek: *nomia*, to arrange or classify] Began with **Euclid's** (*c.* 300 BC) formula for $(a + b)^2$ and culminated with **Niels Henrik Abel's** (1802–1829) proof of the theorem for any value of the exponent *n* in the expression $(a + b)^n$. In 1676, **Sir Isaac Newton** (1642–1727) deduced the theorem for negative and fractional exponents through the problem of finding the area under a curve.

Biochemistry [Greek: *bios*, life + *khemia*, alchemy] The application of chemistry to life was initiated by a Swiss alchemist and physician, **Theophrastus Bombastus von Hohenheim** (1493–1541), also known as **Paracelsus**. **Antoine Laurent Lavoisier** (1743–1794) stated that life is a chemical function. Important works which contributed to early biochemistry include: *Chemistry in its Application to Agriculture and Physiology* (1840) and *Organic Chemistry in its Application to Physiology and Pathology* (1842), both written by **Justus von Liebig** (1803–1873), and *Chemical and Physiological Balance of Organic Nature* (1844) by **Jean Baptiste André Dumas** (1800–1884) and **Jean Baptiste Joseph Dieudonné Boussingault** (1802–1887). **William Dobinson Halliburton** (1860–1931), professor of physiology at King's College, London, and an English pioneer in biochemistry wrote *The Essentials of Chemical Physiology* in 1892. A turning point in the study of structural biochemistry came with a German chemist, **Emil Fischer's** (1852–1919) research on the principal components of living matter such as fats, proteins and sugars. F. Lebenís in his *Geschichte der Physiologischen Chemie* (1935) has given a valuable account of early development of biochemistry. *See organic chemistry.*

Biology [Greek: *bios*, life + *logos*, a discourse] A term first introduced in 1802 by **Gottfried Reinhold Treviranus** (1776–1837) of Bremen to denote the science of life. Earlier, in 1800, a German naturalist, **Karl Friedrich Burdach** (1776–1847), used the term as synonymous with anthropology or the study of man. **Jean Baptiste De Monet Lamarck** (1744–1829) independently used the term biology in the same year. The first use of the word in the English scientific literature is found in the *Lectures on Physiology* published by **Sir William Lawrence** (1783–1867) in 1818. **Aristotle** (384–322 BC), who is sometimes referred to as the father of biology, wrote some of the oldest surviving works on the subject. His first book, *De Anima,* dealing with the essence of life or psyche, distinguished living from non-living things. His second book, *Historia Animalium,* contained observations, investigations and descriptions of several forms of animal life. He used the term *historia* to mean the process of learning by inquiry in the book. *De Generatione Animalium* on the generation of animals, and *De Partibus Animalium* on the parts of animals are two of his other extant works on biology. **Theophrastus** (380–287 BC), the founder of botany, wrote two extant treatises on plants. The next important contribution to botany was made by **Dioscorides** in the first century. Some of the notable biologists of the last three centuries include **Augustin Pyrame De Candolle** (1778–1841), **Herbert Spencer** (1820–1903), **John Ray** (1627–1705), **Karl**

Linnaeus (1707–1778) and **Charles Darwin** (1809–1882).

Biot, Jean Baptiste (1774–1862) *See polarization, Savart–Biot Law.*

Birch, Albert Francis (1903–1992) *See earth.*

Birds *See ornithology.*

Birdseye, Clarence (1886–1956) *See food industry.*

Biringuccio, Vanocchio (1460–1538) *See bronze, industrial chemistry, metallurgy.*

Birkeland, Kristian Olaf Bernhard (1867–1917) *See aurora borealis, nitric acid.*

Birkhoff, George David (1884–1944) *See Poincaré, Jules Henri.*

Biro or ball-point pen. *See pen.*

Bishop, John Michael (b 1936) *See oncogenes.*

Bismuth [German: *weisse masse,* white mass] An element discovered in 1520 by the German physician and metallurgist, **Georgius Agricola** (1494–1555); atomic number 83. A Spanish priest, Alvarez Alonso Barba, in his treatise on metallurgy in 1640, mentioned Bohemia as one of its major sources.

Bit Abbreviation for binary digit in computer language. A bit is the smallest unit of data stored in a computer. All data to the computer is coded into a pattern of individual bits. The first microprocessor, the Intel 4004 (launched 1971) had a 4-bit device. Several different 8-bit computers were introduced in the later 1970s. The Intel 8088 processor, which combined a 16-bit processor with an 8-bit data bus was used for the IBM personal computers in the 1980s. The 32-bit processors such as the Intel 80386 and Motorola 68030 were introduced in the late 1980s. The first 64-bit microprocessor, was installed into the Intel Pentium in 1993. *See computers.*

Bitumen Tarry substance obtained from coal tar or petroleum. *See roads.*

Bjerknes, Jacob Aall Bonnevie (1897–1975) *See cyclone, weather forecasting.*

Bjerknes, Vilhelm Friman Koren (1862–1951) *See cyclone, Sporer's law.*

Bjerrum, Niels Janniksen (1879–1958) *See dissociation.*

Black Body A hypothetical body that would absorb all radiation that fell on it, with perfect absorptance and emissivity.

Black Body Radiation Electromagnetic radiation emitted by a black body. In 1879 an Austrian physicist, **Josef Stefan** (1835–1893), showed that the amount of energy radiated from a black body is proportional to the fourth power of the absolute temperature. The concept of a perfect black body that would absorb and emit radiation was proposed by a German physicist, **Gustav Robert Kirchhoff** (1824–1887). The nearest approach to the hypothetical black body – a small aperture in a hollow sphere – was constructed by German physicist **Otto Richard Lummer** (1860–1925) and **Wilhelm Carl Werner Otto Fritz Franz Wien** (1864–1928) of East Prussia, and their work on thermal radiation led to **Max Karl Ernst Ludwig Planck's** (1858–1947) radiation formula. Wien was awarded the Nobel Prize for physics in 1911 for his discovery of the law related to thermal radiation that bears his name, and which can be stated: for a black body $\lambda mT =$ constant, where λm is the wavelength corresponding to the maximum radiation of energy and T the temperature.

Black, Davidson (1884–1934) *See Peking Man.*

Black Hole An object in space, the gravity of which is so great that nothing can escape from it, not even light. The existence of black holes in the universe was predicted in 1798 by a French mathematician and astronomer, **Pierre Simon Marquis de Laplace** (1749–1827) of Beaumont-en-Auge, in Normandy. A German astronomer, **Karl Schwarzschild** (1873–1916), of Frankfurt-am-Main, explained the phenomenon on the basis that when a star contracts under gravity, there will be a point of such gravitational intensity that light could not leave it. The term black hole was coined by an American physicist, **John Archibald Wheeler** (b 1911) of Jacksonville, Florida, to describe the result of this enormous gravitational force. Some of the fundamental theorems relating to black holes were proposed by an English mathematician from Colchester, Essex, **Roger Penrose** (b 1931), and an English theoretical physicist from Oxford, **Stephen William Hawking** (b 1942). An expression which describes the properties of the black hole predicted by earlier physicists was formulated by a New Zealand mathematician, **Roy Patrick Kerr** (b 1934). Four likely black holes in our galaxy had been identified by 1994. Microscopic black holes may have been formed in the chaotic conditions of the Big Bang, and **Stephen Hawking** has shown that such tiny black holes could 'evaporate' and explode in a flash of energy.

Black, Joseph (1728–1799) An eminent Scottish chemist who was a son of a wine merchant in Bordeaux, France. He was educated at Belfast and studied medicine at Glasgow and Edinburgh before he succeeded William Cullen (1710–1790) as professor of chemistry and anatomy at Glasgow in 1756. He later became a lecturer in chemistry at Edinburgh in 1766. During his researches he developed the theory of latent heat and rediscovered carbon dioxide. His doctorate thesis in 1754 *De Humore acido a cibis orto, et Magnesia Alba* is regarded as a model for philosophical investigation. *See air, carbon dioxide, latent heat, nitrogen, quantitative chemistry, steam engine.*

Black, Max (1909–1988) US professor of philosophy at Cornell (1954–1977) and mathematician who described mathematics as the study of all structures whose form may be expressed in symbols, and divided it into logical, formalist, and intuitional. He published *The Nature of Mathematics* (1950) and *Problems of Analysis* (1954).

Blackburn, James (1803–1854) An English engineer and architect, who was convicted of forgery and transported to Tasmania in 1833 where he designed churches including the Gothic Revival Holy Trinity and St Mark's, Pontville (1839). He also designed the Yan Yean water-supply works in Victoria 1850–1851.

Blackburn, Robert (1885–1955) A British aircraft designer and founder, in 1914, of Blackburn Aircraft Company which built military biplanes. He designed his first plane in 1910.

Blackett, Patrick Maynard Stuart (1897–1974) *See atomic disintegration, positron.*

Blackman, Frederick Frost (1866–1947) *See plant physiology.*

Blaes, Gerard (1646–1682) *See comparative anatomy.*

Blagden, Sir Charles (1748–1820) *See Blagden's law.*

Blagden's Law The depression of the freezing point of a pure liquid when another substance is dissolved in it is proportional to the concentration of the solute. It was discovered by an English chemist, **Sir Charles Blagden** (1748–1820), of Gloucestershire, in 1788.

Blakeslee, Albert Francis (1874–1954) *See horticulture.*

Blanchard, Jean Pierre François (1753–1809) *See parachute.*

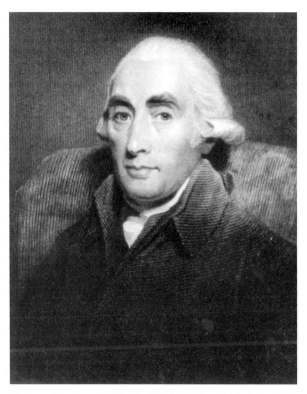

Figure 11 Joseph Black (1728–1799). Courtesy of the National Library of Medicine

Blast Furnace The first blast furnace in England was established at Bilston, by an English iron-master, **John Wilkinson** (1728–1808), of Clifton in Cumberland, in 1748.

Bleaching Powder A Scottish industrial chemist **Charles Tennant** (1768–1838) from Ochiltree, Ayrshire, patented the method of manufacture of bleaching powder from chlorine and slaked lime, in 1799. However the invention was probably that of his partner **Charles Macintosh** (1766–1843). **Louis Claude Comte de Berthollet** (1748–1822), a physician and chemist from Talloire, France, was one of the first to manufacture bleaching powder by the new method.

Blériot, Louis (1872–1936) *See airplane.*

Bloch, Felix (1905–1983) *See magnetic resonance imaging.*

Bloembergen, Nicolaas (b 1920) *See Electron Spectroscopy for Chemical Analysis (ESCA), laser, Rydberg constant.*

Blondel, Nicolaus François (1618–1686) *See military architecture.*

Blowpipe Analysis A method used in analytical chemistry, invented by a Swedish mineralogist, **Baron Axel Fredrik Cronstedt** (1722–1765) of Turinge. His *Essay towards a System of Mineralogy* was published in 1758.

Blume, Karel Lodewijk (1796–1862) *See horticulture.*

Blumenbach, Friedrich (1752–1840) *See dinosaurs.*

Boats Boats and paddles were some of man's earliest inventions, and the earliest sea-going devices were probably dugout canoes. Aborigines are believed to have crossed the Torres Strait from New Guinea to Australia on boats around 60 000 BC. A paddle found in North Yorkshire in 1948 which is now in the Cambridge Museum of Archaeology is estimated to be 7500 years old. A boat made of dug-out pine wood which is 6500 years old is now in the Provincial Museum at Assen. The oldest surviving boat is a wooden canoe discovered at Tybrind Vig on the Baltic Island of Fünen. It dates back to about 5000 BC. A cedarwood rowing boat belonging to King Cheops (d 2566 BC) was recovered near the Great Pyramid in 1954 by an Egyptian archaeologist, **Kamal el Malakh** (b 1918). *See sailing ships, shipping.*

Bode Law A mathematical formula for distances of planets, first proposed by **Johann Titius** (1729–1796) of Wittenberg. It was revived by a German astronomer, **Johann Elert Bode** (1749–1826) and became useful in the prediction and discovery of several planets including Uranus by **Sir William Herschel** (1738–1822), in 1781, and the large asteroid Ceres by **Giuseppe Piazzi** (1749–1826) in 1801. The rule was later partly discredited by other workers.

Bode, Johann Elert (1749–1826) *See Bode's law, Uranus.*

Bodenstein, Ernst August Max (1871–1942) *See halogens.*

Bodmer, Johann Georg (1786–1874) *See textile industry.*

Boehm, Theobold (1794–1881) *See flute.*

Boeing, William Edward (1881–1956) An American aircraft manufacturer, who established the Pacific Aero Products Co (1916) which became Boeing Airplane Company in 1917. His company subsequently became the world's largest producer of military and civilian aircraft. *See airlines.*

Boethius, Anicus Manlius Severinus (AD 480–524) *See musical theory, permutation, sound.*

Bogardus, James (1800–1874) *See engraving, postal service.*

Bogiliubov Transformation A mathematical technique for changing variables in quantum field theory, developed by a Russian mathematical physicist, Nikolai Nikolaevich Bogiliubov (b 1909). His above work contributed to research on particle physics.

Bohm, David Joseph (1917–1992) *See plasma physics, quantum mechanics.*

Bohr, Aage Niels (b 1922) Son of **Niels Henrik David Bohr** (1885–1962). He became a physicist at his father's Institute of Theoretical Physics at Copenhagen. He developed the collective model theory for the atomic nucleus and was awarded the Nobel Prize for physics in 1975.

Bohr, Harold August (1887–1951) Proposed the Bohr–Landau theorem, with Edmund Landau. *See Riemann zeta-function.*

Bohr, Niels Henrick David (1885–1962) A Danish physicist, who first proposed the dynamic theory of the structure of atom, in 1913. He realized the possibility of the Germans making the atomic bomb and traveled to America where he worked on the atomic project with **John Archibald Wheeler** (b 1911), an American physicist, at the Princeton laboratory. During their work they established that the atomic bomb could be produced using uranium-235. In his work on hydrogen, Bohr postulated a massive, charged central nucleus consisting, in the case of hydrogen, of a single proton, with an electron orbiting it in one of a number of well defined orbits with very specific – 'quantized' – energy. The theory has since been superseded, but marked a big advance in our understanding of atomic structure. Bohr also worked in England for a brief period with **Joseph John Thompson** (1856–1940) and **Lord Ernest Rutherford** (1871–1937). *See atomic bomb, atomic structure, hydrogen, quantum theory.*

Boisbaudran, Paul Emile Lecoq de (1838–1912) *See dysprosium, gallium, samarium.*

Boissier, Pierre Edmund (1810–1885) *See botany.*

Bok, Bart (1906–1992) *See Bok's globules.*

Bok's Globules Small circular dark spots seen in nebulae, supposed to be clouds of gas that are condensing into stars but are not yet hot enough to shine. Discovered by a Dutch astrophysicist, **Bart Bok** (1906–1992), who in 1966 became the director of the Stewart Observatory in Tucson Arizona, a post he held until his retirement in 1970.

Boksenberg, Alexander (b 1936) *See Image Photon Counting System, quasars.*

Bologna, Giovanni (1524–1608) *See architecture, Italian.*

Bolometer A sensitive instrument for measuring changes of as little as one millionth of a degree ($^{\circ}$C) in temperature, by registering the change in electrical resistance of a fine wire when it is exposed to heat or light. Built in 1880 by a professor of physics at the Western University of Pennsylvania, **Samuel Pierpont Langley** (1834–1906). He was a pioneer in aeronautics and secretary to the Smithsonian Institute in 1881. He used the bolometer for measuring radiation from stars.

Boltwood, Bertram Borden (1870–1927) An American chemist from Amhurst, Massachusetts, who was a pioneer in the study of isotopes. He discovered the element ionium, now known as thorium-203. He devised a method of dating rocks, based on their radioactivity, in 1907.

Boltzmann, Ludwig (1844–1906) An Austrian physicist from Vienna who served as professor of physics at several universities including Graz, Vienna, Munich and Leipzig. He proposed the law of equipartition of energy known as Boltzmann's Law. His two volumes of *Vorlessungen über Gastheorie* (1896, 1898) contain fundamental contributions to the kinetic theory of gases.

Boltzmann's Law *See Boltzmann, Ludwig.*

Bolyai, Wolfgang (1775–1856) *See Bolyai, Janos.*

Bolyai, Janos (1802–1860) A Hungarian mathematician and one of the founders of non-Euclidean geometry. His father, **Wolfgang Bolyai** (1775–1856), was an eminent mathematician.

Bolzano, Bernardus Placidus Johann Nepomule (1781–1848) Czech philosopher and mathematician who formulated a proof of the binomial theorem in his work, published in 1817. One of the most sigificant parts of this book was his definition of continuous functions. He proved the existence, and defined the properties, of infinite sets.

Bombay Natural History Society Established for the purpose of promoting the study of natural history in 1883. By 1913 it had expanded to include over 1700 members in India, Burma, Ceylon and Siam.

Bombelli, Rafael (1526–1573) *See algebra.*

Bond, George Phillips (1825–1865) A pioneer in celestial photography, from Dorchester, Massachusetts, and a son of **William Cranch Bond** (1789–1859). *See celestial photography.*

Bond, William Cranch (1789–1859) An American watch maker from Portland, who turned his attention to astronomy. He built one of the first private observatories in America at his home and was commissioned by Harvard University to design a new observatory. He worked with his son and made many discoveries, including 17 new comets. Bond was a pioneer in celestial photography.

Bondi, Sir Hermann (b 1919) *See steady-state theory.*

Bonds The concept of bonds in chemistry was introduced by a Scottish chemist, **Archibald Scott Couper** (1831–1892). He postulated the formation of links between atoms in his paper *On a New Chemical Theory* which was to have been presented to the French Academy in 1858 through his teacher **Charles Adolphe Wurtz** (1817–1884). Wurtz delayed the presentation of Couper's paper and the credit for the concept of bonds went to **Friedrich August Kekulé von Stradonitz** (1829–1896). The rules of electrovalence for chemical bonding were proposed by a Polish born US chemist, **Kasimir Fajans** (1887–1975), who became a professor at the University of Michigan, Ann Arbor. A French-born Swiss chemist and Nobel Prize winner in 1913, **Alfred Werner** (1866–1919), proposed the modern theory of coordination bonds between molecules, and published *Lehrbuch der Stereochemie* (1904). In 1931 **Linus Carl Pauling** (1901–1994), an American chemist from Portland, Oregon, used quantum mechanics to explain chemical bonding and the structure of molecules. He published *The Nature of the Chemical Bond* in 1939. In England, **Charles Alfred Coulson** (1910–1974), the first professor of theoretical chemistry at Oxford, studied the application of molecular orbital theory to chemical bonds and defined fractional bond order, and relation of this to bond-length. The first quadruple bond was discovered in 1963 by an American chemist, **Frank Albert Cotton** (b 1930) of Philadelphia. *See affinity, valency.*

Bonnet, Charles Étienne (1720–1793) *See catastrophism, evolution, plant nutrition.*

Bonnier, G. (1853–1922) *See parasitism.*

Bonrepos, Pierre Paul Riquet de (1604–1680) *See canals.*

Books [Anglo-Saxon: *boc,* book] The oldest extant hand written book, a Coptic Psalter, about 1600 years old, was found at Beni Suef, Egypt, in 1984. The Chinese discovered that wooden blocks could be used to print pages that could be bound together, and one such Chinese book dating to AD 868 is extant. Early books were hand written on papyrus or parchment. In AD 700 the monastery of Saint-Martin at Tours in France had around 200 monks writing books. They devised a script with rounded letters which made writing easier. The earliest mechanically printed book, the Gutenberg Bible, was printed at Mainz, Germany, around 1454. *See early printed books, libraries, printing.*

Booksellers *See bookshops.*

Bookshops An English bookseller, **John Dunton** (1659–1733) from Graffham, Huntingdonshire, was one of the first to establish the trade in London. The status of the book trade during his time is found in his *Life and Errors of John Dunton* published in 1705. Another early English book-seller, **George Thomason** (d 1666) had a valuable collection of pamphlets printed in England which were later acquired by George III, and presented to the British Museum in 1762. The London bookseller **Jacob Tonson** (1656–1736) published the works of several English poets. Another English bookseller in London, **John Newbery** (1713–1767), of Berkshire, was the first to publish little books for children in England. **Samuel Baker** (d 1778) established the first sale room for antiquarian books, manuscripts and prints, in 1744 at York Street, Covent Garden. The booksellers, W.H. Smith, was established by **William Henry Smith** (1792–1865) of London. He was joined by his son (1825–1891) of the same name in 1846, and his company first started selling newspapers at railway stations. Smith junior was also a leading politician and served as the first lord of the Admiralty (1877–1880) and the secretary of war (1880). The Blackwell's Oxford bookshop was founded in 1846. One of the first established bookselling firms in Scotland, Ballantyne & Co, was founded in 1808 by two brothers, **James Ballantyne** (1772–1833) and **John Ballantyne** (1774–1821), in partnership with the Scottish novelist, **Sir Walter Scott** (1771–1832). W. & G. Foyle Ltd, one of the largest book stores in London, began as a small shop in Islington in 1904. The English publisher **George Routledge** (1812–1888) started his profession as a book-seller in London in 1836. **John Bartlett** (1820–1905) of Plymouth, Massachusetts, was one of the early established booksellers in America and he owned the University Book Store at Harvard from 1849 to 1863. **Joshua Ballinger Lippincott** (1813–1886) of New York established a book-selling business in Philadelphia in 1834 and later founded the well known publishing firm named after him. The bookshop with the largest floor area in the world, Barnes & Noble Bookstore, is at 5th Avenue and 18th Street, New York.

Boole, George (1816–1864) A self-taught English mathematician, and son of a cobbler from Lincoln. He became professor of mathematics at Cork, and did important work on differential equations. He published several papers including *Mathematical Analysis of Logic* (1847) and *Laws of Thought* (1854). He invented the binary language or base-two number system, later used in computing.

Boolean Algebra A system of algebraic rules proposed by George Boole (1816–1864), in which true and false are equated to 0 and 1. It became the basis of computer logic because the true values can be directly associated with bits.

Boomerang A device discovered in Poland dating from about 25 000 years ago. They were made of mammoth tusk and preceded Australian boomerangs by 13 000 years. They were used to hunt animals for food.

Booth, Hubert Cecil (1871–1955) *See vacuum cleaner.*

Borax [Arabic: *booruk*] **Pliny the Elder** (AD 28–79) referred to the substance as *chrysocolla*. The main source of borax in the past was Tibet. The name chrysocolla [Greek: *krusos*, gold] was revived by a German physician, **Georgius Agricola** (1494–1555) in 1530, as it was used for soldering gold. **Wilhelm Homberg** (1652–1715) of Batavia prepared sal sedativum, a free acid of borax, in 1702. Borax – disodium tetraborate $10H_2O$ is an important substance in the glass and ceramics industries, and is a raw material for the manufacture of a variety of industrially important boron compounds.

Borda, Jean Charles (1733–1799) *See meridian, metric system.*

Bordeu, Théophile de (1722–1776) *See hormones.*

Borel, Emile Felix Edouard Justin (1871–1956) *See games theory.*

Borelli, Giovanni Alfonso (1608–1679) An Italian mathematician and biologist from Naples who founded the iatro-physical school of medicine. *See academy.*

Born, Max (1882–1970) A German physicist from Breslau who became professor of natural philosophy at Edinburgh in 1936. His research on quantum theory based on matrix mechanics led to a statistical approach to the subject. For this work, he was awarded the Nobel Prize for physics with another German physicist, **Walter Wilhelm Georg Bothe** (1891–1957) in 1954.

Bornmuller, Joseph Friedrich Nicolaus (1862–1948) *See botany.*

Boron [Arabic: *bauraq*] The element of atomic number 5. Its ore was known as *chrysocolla* [Greek: krusos, gold] to **Pliny the Elder** (AD 28–79), and the German physician and metallurgist **Georgius Agricola** (1494–1555) revived the term. In 1808 **Sir Humphry Davy** (1778–1829) produced small amounts of boron by passing an electric current through boracic acid. The non-metallic form was discovered independently by two French chemists **Joseph Louis Gay-Lussac** (1778–1850) and **Louis Jacques Thenard** (1777–1857), in 1808. In the 1950s an American organic chemist, **William Nunn Lipscomb** (b 1919) of Cleveland, Ohio, used X-ray diffraction crystallography to study a group of boron compounds and developed a theory to explain their chemical bonding. He was awarded the Nobel Prize for chemistry for this work in 1976. A London-born US chemist, **Herbert Charles Brown** (b 1912) studied the use of boron compounds in organic synthesis for which he was awarded the Nobel Prize for chemistry in 1979. *See borax.*

Borronomi, Francesco (1599–1667) *See architecture, Italian.*

Bosch Process *See Bosch, Carl.*

Bosch, Carl (1874–1940) A German chemist from Cologne, who invented the Bosch process, in which hydrogen is obtained from water gas and superheated steam through a high pressure method. His method of industrial synthesis of ammonia – a development of the Haber process devised by **Fritz Haber** (1886–1934) – enabled the cheap production of agricultural fertilizers and explosives. In 1931 he shared the Nobel Prize for chemistry, for his work on high-pressure methods, with another German industrial chemist, **Friedrich Karl Rudolf Bergius** (1884–1949).

Boscovich, Ruggiero Giusseppe (1711–1787) *See electrolysis.*

Bose, Satyendranath (1894–1974) *See Bose–Einstein Statistics.*

Bose, Sir Jagadis Chander (1858–1937) A physicist and botanist from Calcutta who did research on electric waves and growth of plants. He published *The Physiology of Photosynthesis* (1924) and *The Nervous Mechanisms of Plants* (1926). Bose was the first person to demonstrate the process of wireless telegraphy. In 1917 he founded the Bose Research Institute in Calcutta for the study of physical and biological sciences. He was knighted in the same year, and in 1920 became the first Indian physicist to be elected a fellow of the Royal Society.

Bose–Einstein Statistics A system of statistical quantum mechanics for integral-spin particles, developed by **Albert Einstein** (1879–1955). It originates from the work of an Indian physicist, **Satyendranath Bose** (1894–1974), who derived the black-body radiation law without reference to classical electrodynamics. **Paul Adrien Maurice** (1902–1984) named particles with integral spin bosons, in his honor.

Boson An elementary particle with integral spin named after an Indian physicist, **Satyendranath Bose** (1894–1974), by **Paul Adrien Maurice** (1902–1984). Independent researches by an Italian-born American physicist, **Carlo Rubbia** (b 1934) and a Dutch physicist, **Simon Van Der Meer** (b 1925) led to the development of the Super Proton Synchrotron (SPS) accelerator for colliding protons and antiprotons. This led to the first production of W and Z bosons. Van Der Meer and Rubbia shared the Nobel Prize for physics for this work, in 1984. *See fermion.*

Botanical Classification In his treatise *History of Plants,* **Theophrastus** (380–287 BC), from the Greek island of Lesbos, who is sometimes regarded as the father of botany, classified plants into trees, shrubs, undershrubs and herbs. An English biologist, **John Ray** (1628–1705), from Essex, was one of the first to attempt a system of modern classification of the plant and animal kingdoms. His works include *Historia Piscium* (1686), and *Historia generalis plantarum* (1686–1704) in three volumes. His *Catalogus Plantarum Angliae* (1682) contained the basic principles of plant classification into cryptograms, monocotyledons and dicotyledons. **Carolus Linnaeus** (1707–1778), a Swedish botanist who traveled widely studying plants, in his description of 11 800 species introduced the first system of classification of plants to include the term genus. His works include *Systema Natura* (1735), *Fundamenta Botanica* (1736), *Genera Plantarum* (1737) and *Classes Plantarum* (1738). **John Parkinson** (1567–1650), an English botanist from Nottinghamshire, proposed a classification of plants in his *Theatrum Botanicum* in 1640. The morphology of leaves as the basis of a classification of plants was used by **Lobelius** or **Matthias de l'Obel** (1538–1616) of The Netherlands, an eminent botanist at the botanical garden of Queen Elizabeth I (in England). A botanist from Lübeck, **Joachim Jung** (1587–1657), used flowers as a basis for classification of plants. The first English botanical work to adopt Linnean classification, *Flora Anglica* (1762) was published by a London herbalist and apothecary, **William Hudson** (1734–1793). **George Bentham** (1800–1884), a British botanist from Devon, published *Genera Plantarum* which took over 20 years to write and became a standard book on plant classification. **Stephen Ladislaus Endlicher** (1804–1849) of Austria formulated a system of plant classification in his *Genera Plantarum* (1836–1840). A system of natural classification was developed by **Adolf Engler** (1844–1930) of Germany in his *Die Natürliche Pfanzenfamilien.* A French botanist, **Phillipe Van Tieghem** (1839–1914), of Leyden, proposed a new classification of plants. A London botanist of Scottish origin, **John Scott Lennox Gilmour** (1906–1986), who founded the Classification Society in 1937, was instrumental in establishing the International Code of Nomenclature of Cultivated Plants. An American botanist, **Arthur Cronquist** (1919–1992), from San Jose, California, at the New York Botanical Garden, published *The Evolution and Classification of Flowering Plants* (1968) and *An Integrated Classification of Flowering Plants* (1981). His Cronquist system of classification came to be adopted by many workers. *See taxonomy.*

Botany [Greek: *botane*, pasture or herb] The first major monograph on botany, *Historia Plantarum*, was written by

Theophrastus (380–287 BC) around 320 BC. The first known drawings of plants were by a Greek artist, **Crateuas**, around 100 BC. The earliest printed book containing realistic plant illustrations was produced by **Otto Brunfels** (1489–1534) of Mainz, in 1530. **Carous Clusius** or **Charles De l'Ecluse** (1525–1609) of Antwerp, published several illustrative works on the plants of India and Europe. The occurrence of two sexes in plants was first observed by an Italian botanist **Prospero Alpini** (1533–1617) in 1580. **Lobelius** or **Matthias De l'Obel** (1538–1616) of The Netherlands, an eminent botanist who served as director of the botanical garden of Queen Elizabeth I (in England), used the morphology of leaves as the basis for his classification of plants. The flower Lobelia is named after him. An Italian, **Pietro Andrea Mattioli** (1501–1577), published *Commentaries on Dioscorides* in 1544. Another Italian botanist, **Andrea Cesalpini** (1519–1603), in his treatise *On Plants* (1583) took a new approach to the description of plants. **Casper Bauhin** (1560–1624) helped to clear up the confusion surrounding the names of plants with his work on botanical synonyms *Pinax Theatri botanici* (1623). One of the first English botanical works, *Anatomy of the Plants*, was published by **Nehemiah Grew** (1641–1712) in 1682. In this work he described different types of tissues in plants, and identified for the first time the male and female parts of flowering plants. **John Ray** (1628–1705), an English biologist from Essex, classified the plants into monocotyledons and dicotyledons, on the basis of the number of seed leaves, in 1667. One of the earliest monographs on botany in England, *Plantarum Umbelliferarum Distributio Nova* was published in 1672 by a Scottish botanist from Aberdeen, **Robert Morison** (1620–1683), who became professor of botany at Oxford in 1669. The first system of classification to include the genus and species was introduced by **Carolus Linnaeus** (1707–1778) in 1750 during his description of 11 800 species of plants. Another classification based on a variety of characters was suggested in 1764 by a French botanist, **Michel Adanson** (1727–1806) of Paris. He published *Les Familles naturelles des plantes* (1763), and the plant Adansonia is named after him. An early 19th century book *Opuscules Phytologigues* (1826) was published by the French botanist **Alexandre Henri Gabriel de Cassini** (1784–1832). He was the first of several generations of the Cassini family to abandon astronomy in favor of botany. A French botanist and physician, **Antoine Laurent de Jussieu** (1748–1836), of Lyons, published **Genera Plantarum** (1789) which formed the basis for the modern natural classification of plants. **Felix da Silva Avellar Brotero** (1744–1828) of Lisbon is regarded as the Portuguese Linneaus owing to his botanical terminology. His *Flora Lusitanica* (1804–1805) was in essence a sim-

plification of Linnean classification. The first work on flora covering the entire Middle East, *Flora Orientalis* (1867–1884), was published by a Swiss botanist of French origin, **Pierre Edmund Boissier** (1810–1885). Another 60 works on the flora of the Middle East – mainly Iran – was published by a German botanist, **Joseph Friedrich Nicolaus Bornmuller** (1862–1948). *See botanical classification, paleophytology, photosynthesis, plant anatomy, plant physiology.*

Bothe, Walter Wilhelm Georg (1891–1957) A German physicist who became head of the Max Planck Institute for Medical Research at Heidelberg in 1937. He shared the Nobel Prize for physics in 1954 with **Max Born** (1882–1970). *See beryllium, Geiger counter.*

Böttger, Johann Friedrich (1682–1719)   *See porcelain.*

Bouch, Sir Thomas (1822–1880)   *See bridges.*

Bouchard, Charles Jacques (1837–1915)   *See nutrition.*

Bougainville, Louis Antoine de (1729–1811) A French navigator and a mathematician at Paris who wrote an important treatise on integral calculus. He was a member of the Royal Society in London, and the plant Bougainvillaea is named after him.

Bouguer, Pierre (1698–1758)   *See heliometer, meridian, solar energy.*

Boule, Marcellin (1861–1942)   *See Neanderthal man.*

Boulliau, Ismael (*c.* 1650)   *See thermometer.*

Boulton, Matthew (1728–1809) An inventor from Birmingham and partner of **James Watt** (1736–1819) in the production of the steam engine. He was a partner in his father's metal factory in Birmingham before he took an interest in steam engines in 1764. In 1775 he went into partnership with Watt, who was a mathematical instrument maker from Greenock. Their steam engine, built in 1812, remains as the oldest preserved working steam engine.

Bourbaki Group A group of mathematicians in the 1930s, including Nicolas Bourbaki, who set out to write a treatise on pure mathematics, on strict logical development from its basic principles. The French mathematician, **André Weil** (1906–1998) and **Jean Alexandre Dieudonné** (1906–1992) were two of its founders.

Bourdon Gage   *See Bourdon, Eugene.*

Bourdon, Eugene (1808–1884) An inventor and industrialist in Paris, who devised the Bourdon gauge (Bourdon Gage) for measuring pressure in steam engines and boilers, in 1849.

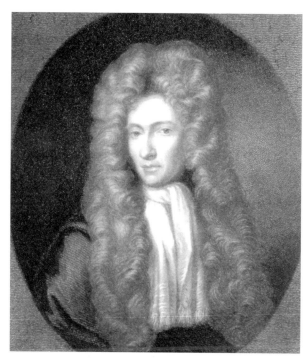

Figure 12 Robert Boyle (1627–1691). Courtesy of the National Library of Medicine

Boussingault, Jean Baptiste Joseph Dieudonné (1802–1887) *See agriculture, agronomy, biochemistry, nitrogen fixing bacteria, photosynthesis, plant physiology.*

Bouvard, Alexis (1767–1843) *See Uranus.*

Boveri, Theodor (1862–1915) *See centrosome, chromosomes.*

Bowen, Ira Sprague (1898–1973) *See cosmic rays.*

Bowen, Norman Levi (1887–1956) *See petrology.*

Bower, Frederick Orpen (1855–1948) *See ecology.*

Bowman, Isaiah (1878–1950) *See forestry.*

Boyer, Herbert Wayne (b 1936) *See genetic engineering.*

Boyle, Robert (1627–1691) The seventh son of Robert, the lord high chancellor of Ireland, who was from Lismore. He is sometimes regarded as the father of physical chemistry, and in 1659 he improved **Otto von Guericke's** (1602–1686) air pump and used it for studying the properties of air. His work led to the discovery of the fundamental law of gases relating to pressure and volume, in 1662. Some of his other contributions include: discovery of boiling point related to atmospheric pressure, preparation of acetone from acetate of lead and lime, introduction of the concept of elements, the demonstration of the necessity of air for life, discovery of the expansive power of freezing water, and

production of methyl alcohol from wood. His work *The Sceptical Chymist* was published in 1661. While in Oxford Boyle founded the Invisible College in conjunction with other notable figures such as **Christopher Wren** (1632–1723), Thomas Willis and **Seth Ward** (1617–1689), in 1655. The Invisible College promoted the science of experimentation and observation, and later became the Royal Society, through a charter from King Charles II in 1668. *See acidity, air, air pump, barometer, Boyle's law, Boyle–van't Hoff law, chemistry, electricity, Empedocles, gas laws, hydrometer, surface chemistry.*

Boyle's Law The volume of a fixed mass of gas at a constant temperature is inversely proportional to the pressure on it. It was proposed by the British chemist **Robert Boyle** (1627–1691) in 1662. A German-born French physical chemist, **Henri Victor Regnault** (1810–1878) showed that it applies only to ideal gases.

Boyle–van't Hoff Law Derived from **Robert Boyle's** (1627–1691) and **Jacobus Henricus van't Hoff's** (1852–1911) theories on the relationship between pressure and temperature of a gas.

Boys, Sir Charles Vernon (1855–1944) An English physicist and inventor from Wing in Rutland. His inventions include: an improved torsion balance which uses fused quartz fibers, an extremely sensitive radiometer capable of detecting the heat from a candle several hundred meters away, a calorimeter for measuring the calorific value of coal gas, and a camera with a moving lens. *See galvanometer, radiometer (2), torsion balance.*

Brachiosaurid [Latin: *brachium*, arm + Greek: *sauros*, lizard] One of the longest (26 meters) and tallest (6 meters) dinosaurs, believed to date from 150 million years. It was first discovered in Tanzania by a German expedition in 1909. A complete skeleton was assembled at Humboldt Museum in Berlin in 1937. *See dinosaurs.*

Bradfield, John Job Crew (1867–1943) *See bridges.*

Bradley, James (1693–1762) From Sherbourne, Gloucestershire, succeeded **Edmund Halley** (1656–1742) as Astronomer Royal in 1742. He discovered the phenomenon of aberration of light (1729) and the nutation of the earth's axis (1748). *See aberration of light, equinox, nutation.*

Bradwardine, Thomas (c. 1290–1349) *See motion.*

Bragg, Sir William Henry (1862–1942) An English physicist from Westward, Cumberland. He was educated at Trinity College, Cambridge, and became professor of mathematics in Adelaide, Australia, in 1886. He returned to England as a professor at Leeds in 1909, and started working with his Australian-born son Sir William Lawrence Bragg (1890–1971) in 1912. They constructed the first X-ray spectrometer and discovered the method of X-ray diffraction which became a key technique in the analysis of compounds such as penicillin, DNA and proteins. They were awarded the Nobel Prize for physics in 1915. William Henry Bragg's published works include *Studies on Radioactivity* (1912), *X-rays and Crystal Structure* (1915) and *Universe of Light* (1933).

Brahe, Tycho (1546–1601) A Swedish astronomer born to a noble family at Knudstrup in the south of Sweden, which was at that time a province of Denmark. He began his career in astronomy with his observation on the eclipse of the sun which occurred in August 1560. Under the sponsorship of the king of Denmark, Frederick II, he built an elaborate observatory at Hveen, which he named *Uraniborg* (the Tower of Heaven). The supernova of 1562, in Cassiopeia, is known as 'Tycho's Star' because it was carefully studied by him. He made several important discoveries and contributions to astronomy and wrote *Astronomiae Instauratae Mechanica* (1598). *See astronomy, observatories, quadrant, Rudolphine Tables, sextant, stars, supernova.*

Brahmagupta (*c.* 598–660) A Hindu mathematician from Ujjain, who lived around the 7th century. He gave the rules for dealing with negative numbers in algebra, solved quadratics, found a method for determining the volume of a prism, and wrote several formulae. *See algebra, mathematics, negative numbers, quadratic equation.*

Brakes *See air brake, car.*

Bramah, Joseph (1748–1814) An English inventor from Stainborough, near Barnsley, Yorkshire. He invented the hydraulic press capable of exerting several tons of force for shaping iron and steel, and took out 17 other patents. *See lock, toilets.*

Brande, William Thomas (1788–1866) A chemist who in 1813 succeeded **Sir Humphry Davy** (1778–1829) as professor of chemistry at the Royal Institution of Great Britain, where he delivered a series of celebrated chemistry lectures to students from 1816 to 1850. He devised the Brande's test for quinine, using chlorine water and ammonia as reagents.

Brande's Test *See Brande, William Thomas.*

Brandt, Georg (1694–1768) A Swedish chemist who studied medicine and chemistry at Leyden under Boerhaave. He investigated arsenic and its compounds and published a systematic treatise on it in 1733. He discovered cobalt in 1730, and distinguished between potash and soda. Brandt

was the first chemist to condemn alchemy and promote chemistry as a science.

Brandy [German: branntwein; burnt wine] It was first distilled from wine by the Italians in 1100. An Italian physician, **Arnold of Villanova** (1234–1311), called it the elixir of life and introduced it into the pharmacopoeia in the 13th century.

Branly, Edouard Eugène Désiré (1844–1940) A physicist who made wireless telegraphy possible. He was born in Amiens and educated at the École Normale in Paris. He qualified in medicine in 1882 but took to research in physics and published his first important paper *Variations of Electric Conductivity of Disconnected Substances under the Diverse Electric Influences* in 1890. *See broadcasting, wireless telegraphy.*

Brass An alloy of copper and zinc, first used by the Romans. During modern times, the method of making brass by adding metallic zinc to copper was patented in England by John Emerson in 1781.

Brattain, Walter Houser (1902–1987) *See semiconductors, transistor.*

Braun, Karl Ferdinand (1850–1918) A German physicist from Fulda who constructed the first cathode-ray oscilloscope (Braun tube) in 1897. He shared the Nobel Prize with **Guglielmo Marchese Marconi** (1874–1937) for his work on wireless telegraphy in 1909. *See oscilloscope, television, wireless telegraphy.*

Braun, Wernher von (1912–1977) *See rocket, space station, space travel.*

Brauner, Bohuslav (1855–1935) *See promethium.*

Breathalyzer The first device to detect the amount of alcohol in the breath was devised by **Lallamand**, **Perrin** and **Duroy** of Paris in 1860. It was introduced for testing the amount of alcohol in the blood in drivers in 1967.

Bredig Method Preparation of colloids by electrical disintegration, discovered by a German chemist, **Georg Bredig** (1868–1944).

Bredig, Georg (1868–1944) *See colloid chemistry, Bredig method.*

Breeding *See animal husbandry, hybridization.*

Breguet, Abraham-Louis (1747–1823) *See watches.*

Breit, Gregory (1899–1981) *See radar.*

Brennan, Louis (b 1852) *See torpedo.*

Brenner, Sydney (b 1927) *See codon, genetic coding.*

Breuer, Marcel Lajos (1902–1981) An Hungarian-born US architect and pioneer of modern 20th century furniture. He designed the first tubular chair in 1925 and the cantilevered chair in 1928.

Breuil, Henri Edouard Prosper (1877–1961) *See cave paintings.*

Brewery *See beer.*

Brewster, Sir David (1781–1868) *See convex lens, lighthouses, optics, stereoscope.*

Brialmont, Henri Alexis (1821–1903) *See military engineering.*

Bridges [Anglo-Saxon: *brycg*] Remnants of Mycenean bridges dating back to 1600 BC exist in Mycenae and Greece. The earliest known surviving single arch bridge, over the River Meles in Smyrna, Turkey, dates to 850 BC. The segmental arch bridge over the Chiao Shui River in China was built by **Li Ch'un** in 610 BC. Remains of Roman stone bridges built around the 2nd century were found at Corbridge, Northumberland, in England. The 700 feet long Marco Polo Bridge across the Yung-Ting River, which is still in use, was built in AD 1189. A French engineer of Swiss origin in Paris, **Jean Rodolphe Perronet** (1708–1794), was a pioneer who designed over 30 bridges including the Concorde bridges over the Seine. A Swiss engineer, Charles Labelye, built the Westminster Bridge in London between 1738 and 1750. The modern bridges in London, at Waterloo and other places, were built by a Scottish civil engineer, **John Rennie** (1761–1821), of East Linton. In 1831 his son **Sir John Rennie** (1794–1874) completed the Waterloo Bridge begun by his father in 1811. The third bridge in London, at Blackfriars, was built from 1750 to 1769 by a Scottish architect, **Robert Mylne** (1734–1811). His brother,

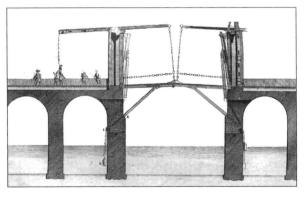

Figure 13 An early drawbridge. Owen, W. *Dictionary of Arts and Sciences*. London: Homer's Head, 1754

William Mylne, designed the North Bridge in Edinburgh. A French civil engineer, **Hubert Gautier** (1660–1737), of Nimes, in his *Traité des Ponts* (1716) recommended the reduction of bridge piers in order to minimize obstruction to water flow. The first cast iron bridge in the world was built by **Abraham Darby III** (1750–1791), over the River Severn at Coalbrookdale in England, in 1779. He was a grandson of **Abraham Darby** (1678–1717) of Dudley, Worcestershire, the first successful smelter – in 1709 – of iron with coke. Several major bridges in Britain, including the Menai Bridge joining Anglesey to the Welsh mainland, were built by a Scottish engineer from Dumfries, **Thomas Telford** (1757–1834). The wrought iron box-girder construction for bridges (used for the Menai Bridge) was introduced by a Scottish engineer, **Sir William Fairbairn** (1789–1874) from Kelso. A French civil engineer, **Claude Louis Marie Henri Navier** (1785–1836) built several bridges over the River Seine and published a treatise on bridges in three volumes from 1809 to 1816. The Tay Rail Bridge in England, which later collapsed with the loss of over 70 lives, was completed in 1877 by **Sir Thomas Bouch** (1822–1880) of Cumberland. An English engineer from Somerset, **Sir Benjamin Baker** (1840–1907), built the Forth Rail Bridge, connecting Edinburgh to Dundee, from 1883–1890. **Robert Stephenson** (1803–1859), the son of the pioneer in railways **George Stephenson** (1781–1848), built several important bridges in Britain, including the High Level Bridge over the River Tyne in Newcastle, and the Victoria bridge over the River Tweed at Berwick. The Eads Bridge (1867–1874) over the Mississippi, at St Louis, was constructed by an American pioneer in bridge building, **James Buchanan Eads** (1820–1887) of Indiana. A Scottish engineer, **William Arrol** (1839–1913), who built the Forth Rail Bridge with Benjamin Baker (1883–1890), also built London's Tower Bridge (1886–1894). The Rockville Bridge, which is the longest (1160 meters) stone arch bridge in the world, was built near Harrisberg, Pennsylvania, in 1901. The bridge over Sydney harbour in Australia was designed in 1913 by **John Job Crew Bradfield** (1867–1943) of Sandgate, Queensland, and completed in 1932. *See suspension bridges.*

Bridges, Colin Blackman (1889–1938) *See translocation.*

Bridgewater Treatises The 8th Earl of Bridgewater, **Francis Henry Egerton** (1756–1829), left a sum of 8000 GBP to be given to eight persons appointed by the president of the Royal Society to write essays on the power, wisdom, and goodness of God, as manifested in His creation. These were written in 1833–1835 by Sir Charles Bell, Thomas Chalmers, John Kidd, **William Buckland** (1784–1856),

William Prout (1785–1850), Peter M. Roget, **William Whewell** (1794–1866) and William Kirby.

Bridgman, Percy Williams (1882–1961) An American physicist from Cambridge, Massachusetts, who was awarded the Nobel Prize for physics in 1946 for his work in high pressure physics. His work enabled pressures as high as 400 000 atmospheres to be reached. *See artificial diamond, viscosity.*

Briggs, Henry (1561–1631) A mathematician from Warley Wood, Halifax, who became the first Savilian professor of mathematics at Oxford, in 1619. He proposed the base 10 for logarithms, instead of that used by **John Napier** (1550–1617), and published tables to an accuracy of 14 decimal places. His *Arithmetica logarithmica* was published in 1624.

Bright, Timothy (1551–1615) *See shorthand.*

Brindley, James (1716–1772) A son of an illiterate farmer from Thornsett, Derbyshire, who was abandoned by his father in his childhood and left to fend for himself without any education. He was apprenticed to a millwright at the age of 17 and started his career in invention by repairing a paper-making machine at the mill without any previous knowledge of engineering. His fame soon spread as an inventor and engineer, and the 3rd Duke of Bridgewater, **Francis Egerton** (1736–1803) approached him to build the first major canal in England. Brindley, at the direction of the duke, built a canal from Worsley to Manchester, and also linked Liverpool to Manchester with another canal. Following this he went on to build 365 miles of navigable canals in England. *See canals.*

Brinell Harness Test A rapid nondestructive method of estimating metal hardness, devised by a Swedish metallurgist, **Johann August Brinell** (1849–1925) in 1890.

Brinell, Johann August (1849–1925) *See Brinell Harness test.*

Brinster, Ralph Lawrence (b 1932) *See genetic engineering.*

Brisbane, Sir Thomas Markdougall (1773–1860) A Scottish astronomer and statesman from Largs, Aryshire, who established an observatory in Paramatta and contributed to a catalogue of over 7000 stars in Australia. He was governor of New South Wales in Australia and the town of Brisbane is named after him.

Brisseau-Mirbel, C.F. (1776–1854) *See protoplasm.*

British Association for the Advancement of Science Founded by **David Brewster** (1781–1868) and **Roderick Impey Murchison** (1792–1871) in 1831; **Sir George Cayley** (1771–1857) of Scarborough, sponsored the first meeting of the association, at York, in 1832. The term scientist, was coined by a British scholar, **William Whewell** (1794–1866) of Lancaster, at a meeting of the British Association for the Advancement of Science at Glasgow, in 1833. Queen Victoria presented the Kew Observatory to the Association in 1842. One of its founder members, chemist and clergyman **William Venables Vernon Harcourt** (1789–1871) of Sudbury, Derbyshire, served as its president in 1839.

British Astronomical Association An establishment for amateur astronomers founded in 1890 by a London astronomer, **Edward Walter Maunder** (1851–1928).

British Ecological Society Founded in 1917 by **Edward James Salisbury** (1886–1978) from Harpenden, Hertfordshire, who served as professor of botany at University College, London, from 1929 to 1943.

Britten, Roy John (b 1919) *See deoxyribonucleic acid.*

Britton, Nathaniel (1859–1934) An American botanist of Staten Island, New York, who was instrumental in establishing the New York Botanical Garden, and served as its director from 1896 to 1921. He published several important works on the flora of North America.

Broadcasting Dissemination of news, drama and other forms of entertainment by radio and television. Broadcasting was made possible with the invention of wireless telegraphy and the discovery of radio waves. The invention of the coherer in 1890 by professor **Edouard Eugène Désiré Branly** (1844–1940) of the Catholic University in Paris, paved the way for **Guglielmo Marchese Marconi's** (1874–1937) first regular broadcasts in England in 1922. Branly also invented the forerunner of the receiving antenna. Radio waves, discovered by a German physicist, **Heinrich Rudolf Hertz** (1857–1894), were first transmitted, over a distance of 5 kilometers, with the help of an antenna, by a Russian physicist, **Alexander Stepanovich Popov** (1859–1905), in 1897. **Reginald Aubrey Fessenden** (1866–1932), a radio-engineer from East Bolton, Quebec, devised amplitude modulation in radio-transmission, with which he was able to broadcast the first American radio program from Brant Rock, Massachusetts, on Christmas eve of 1906. First regular broadcasting in the USA started at the Westinghouse station KDKA at East Pittsburgh in 1920. The first broadcasting station in England, at Chelmsford, Essex, was installed in 1919. It was licensed to the Post Office and made its first news broadcast in February 1920. The Marconi Company in 1922 opened the London station known as LO2 which started transmitting concerts regularly. The British Broadcasting Company was established in the same year and it made the first transmission on 14 November. It became the British Broadcasting Corporation in 1925. In the same year a Scottish electrical engineer, **John Logie Baird** (1888–1946), gave a public demonstration of his television. FM or frequency modulation, with less noise interference for radio, was perfected by an electrical engineer, **Edwin Howard Armstrong** (1890–1954) of New York, in 1929. Television programs were regularly broadcast in England from Alexandra Park from 1936. The first live television pictures across the Atlantic were transmitted in 1962 by the telecommunication satellite Telstar. *See radio, television.*

Broadwood, Henry Fowler (1811–1893)　*See piano.*

Broadwood, John (1732–1812)　*See piano.*

Brocchi (1772–1826)　*See conchology.*

Broecker, Wallace (b 1931)　*See oceanography.*

Broglie, Louis Victor Pierre de (1892–1987)　*See electron, electron microscope, quantum mechanics.*

Broglie, Maurice de, 6th Duc de Broglie (1875–1960) French physicist and brother of Louis Broglie. He was pioneer in the study of X-ray spectra, and helped to establish the Einsteinian description of light in terms of photons.

Bromine [Greek: *bromos,* stench]　The element with atomic number 35, discovered in salt water by an apothecary at Montpellier, **Antoine Jerome Balard** (1802–1876), who named it muride, in 1826. He was appointed to the chair of chemistry at the Sorbonne in 1842. A German chemist, **Carl Lowig** (1803–1890), is said to have prepared a small quantity of bromine before Balard in 1825, and he published a monograph on its properties.

Brongniart, Adolphe Theodore (1801–1876)　*See paleophytology.*

Brongniart, Alexandre (1770–1847)　*See fossils, Jurassic period.*

Brønsted Theory　The Lowry–Brønsted theory of acids and bases was proposed in 1923, an acid being defined as a proton donor and a base as a proton acceptor. The theory extended the concept of acids and bases to solvents other than water – e.g. ammonia.

Brønsted, Johannes Nicolaus (1879–1947)　*See acid–base theory, acids, Lowry–Brønsted theory.*

Brontosaurus [Greek: *bronte,* thunder + *saurus,* lizard]　A plant-eating large dinosaur of about 25 meters in height. Its skeleton was reconstructed from its remains found in the Upper Jurassic strata of the western USA. Another dinosaur called apatosaurus was described before brontosaurus; it was subsequently realized that these two specimens were different examples of the same animal, hence the preferred name is aptosaurus. *See dinosaurs.*

Bronze　The term *Bronzo* for an alloy of copper and tin was first used by an Italian mining engineer **Vanocchio Biringuccio** (1460–1538) of Sienna in his *Pirotechnica* published in 1540. *See Bronze Age.*

Bronze Age　The Egyptians and Babylonians are known to have used bronze (an alloy of tin and copper) around 3000 BC and its use had spread to western Asia by 2000 BC. Bronze was in use in China at the time of Emperor Ta-Yu (2200 BC), but the Bronze Age did not reach the Neolithic or late Stone Age in Europe until around 1500 BC; bronze tools dating back to this time have been found in Mycenae, and contain 88% copper plus 12% tin. Types of bronze are still in use for making bells, ornamental purposes, and for bearings.

Brotero, Felix da Silva Avellar (1744–1828)　*See botany.*

Brouncker, Lord William (1620–1684)　An Irish mathematician in London and one of the founders of the Royal Society. He is known for his use of infinite series for quantities and for his evaluation of π.

Brouwer Theorem　A mathematical theorem on fixed points of mappings. Proposed by a Dutch mathematician, **Luitzen Egbertus Jan Brouwer** (1881–1966), who was professor of mathematics (1912–1951) at Amsterdam University.

Brouwer, Luitzen Egbertus Jan (1881–1966)　*See Brouwer theorem, intuitionism.*

Brown, Arthur Whitten (1886–1948)　*See transatlantic flight.*

Brown, Ernest William (1866–1938)　An English mathematician from Hull who became professor of mathematics (1893–1907) at Haverford College in Pennsylvania. He published accurate tables of the Moon's movements, and calculated the gravitational effects of the planet Pluto on the orbits of Uranus and Neptune.

Brown, Herbert Charles (b 1912)　*See boron.*

Brown, Robert (1773–1858)　An eminent Scottish botanist and a physician from Montrose, who served as naturalist to the ship *Investigator* on its scientific expedition (1801–1805) to Australia, captained by **Matthew Flinders** (1774–1814). He discovered the nucleus of the cell and named it. *See Brownian movement.*

Brownian Movement The constant random motion of microscopic particles (*c.* 1 micrometer diameter) when suspended in a fluid medium. It was first observed by **Robert Brown** (1773–1858) in 1827 when he was studying pollen particles suspended in water and described in his *Microscopic Observations on the Pollen of Plants* (1827). An explanation for it, on the basis of collisions between the grains and molecules of water, was given by **Christian Wiener** (1826–1896) in 1863. The complete nature of the phenomenon was explained by **M. Smoluchowski** (1872–1917) and **Albert Einstein** (1879–1955). A French physicist, **Jean Baptiste Perrin** (1870–1942) of Lille, in 1909, showed that Brownian movement obeyed the gas laws and used it to determine Avogadro's number and to demonstrate the existence of atoms. His work was translated into English by **Frederick Soddy** (1877–1965) in 1910. Perrin was awarded the Nobel Prize for physics in 1926.

Browning, John Moses (1855–1926) *See Browning pistol.*

Browning Pistol An automatic pistol invented in 1911 by **John Moses Browning** (1855–1926), a son of a gunsmith from Ogden, Utah. He also invented a breech loading single shot rifle (1879), the Browning machine gun (1917), and the Browning automatic rifle (1918).

Brownrigg, William (1711–1800) *See platinum.*

Brugsch, Heinrich Karl (1827–1894) A German Egyptologist from Berlin, who served as director of the School of Egyptology in Cairo from 1870 to 1890. He helped to decipher several papyrus writings and published a hieroglyphic dictionary.

Brunel, Isambard Kingdom (1806–1859) The only son of **Sir Marc Isambard Brunel** (1769–1849) and a pioneer of railways in England. He designed the first series of large ships, and his *Great Western*, launched in 1837, made its first transatlantic crossing in 1838. *See railway, steamships, transatlantic voyage.*

Brunel, Sir Marc Isambard (1769–1849) *See tunnel, underground railway.*

Brunelleschi, Fillipo (1377–1446) *See architecture, Italian.*

Brunfels, Otto (1489–1534) *See botany.*

Brünnich, Morton Thrane (1737–1827) *See ichthyology, zoology.*

Buache, J.N. (1741–1825) *See cartography.*

Bubble Chamber An apparatus used in nuclear physics for studying the path of short-lived subatomic particles. It was invented by a American physicist, **Donald Arthur Glaser** (b 1926), of Cleveland, Ohio, who was awarded the Nobel Prize for physics for his invention, in 1960. An American physicist, **Louis Walter Alvarez** (1911–1989), developed it for the study of particle physics, for which he was awarded the Nobel Prize for physics, in 1968. The largest bubble chamber with a diameter of 4.5 meters was installed at Weston, Illinois, in 1973.

Buch, Baron Christian Leopold von (1774–1853) *See geological map.*

Buchan, Alexander (1829–1907) A Scottish pioneer in meteorology from Kinneswood, Kinross, who served as secretary of the Scottish Meteorological Society. He published *Handy Book of Meteorology* in 1867.

Buchanan, John Young (1844–1925) *See oceanography.*

Buchner, Eduard (1860–1917) A professor of chemistry at Munich who first extracted the enzyme zymase from yeast, in 1897. He demonstrated its capability of fermenting sugar in the absence of yeast, for which he was awarded the Nobel Prize for chemistry in 1907.

Buckland, William (1784–1856) *See Bridgewater treatises, catastrophism, fossils, Ice Age.*

Buddha, Gaudama Siddartha (568–488 BC) *See philosophy.*

Buffer The German term *puffer*, to describe the ability of certain substances to resist any change in pH, was introduced by a Danish physicist, **Søren Peter Lauritz Sørenson** (1868–1939) of Copenhagen. The term became 'buffer' in English. Sørensen also introduced the concept of pH.

Buffon, George Louis Leclerc Compte de (1707–1788) A French naturalist and son of a wealthy lawyer in Montbard, Burgundy. He wrote *Histoire Naturelle* in 44 volumes while he was the director of the King's Garden (Jardin du Roi) in Paris from 1749 to 1767. His work was continued by another French naturalist, **Bernard de Laville Lacépède** (1756–1825). Buffon was one of the earliest to propose the idea of evolution with his concept that life forms in the animal kingdom were successively derived from one another. He also suggested that the earliest life forms originated from polar regions and the ocean. He translated Isaac

Newton's *Fluxions* while he was on a visit to England in 1733.

Bugatti, Ettore (1882–1947) An Italian car manufacturer and pioneer of motor racing in Europe in the 1930s. He started designing cars in 1899 and established his first factory in 1907 at Strasbourg, France.

Building Sun-dried bricks held together by mortar were used to build houses in Jericho on the west bank of the River Jordan in 9000 BC. In Catal Hüyük, an ancient city in Anatolia, Turkey, tightly packed houses were built in 6250 BC, so that there were no streets. People had to walk along the roof tops to enter their homes, and this made it difficult for enemies to invade. The earliest walled city was Uruk near the Euphrates River in Mesopotamia. Stone was used to construct buildings in the island of Guernsey in the English Channel around 4000 BC. A ziggurat in the city of Ur, the capital of Mesopotamia, shows that Sumerians were familiar with columns, domes and arches in 3500 BC. Corbeling, the building of an arch with stones or bricks, so that each layer projects out beyond the one beneath it, was practiced by the Mesopotamians around 2800 BC. The megalithic temples at Mgarr and Skorba in Malta, dating to 3250 BC, are the oldest known free-standing structures in the world. The stepped pyramid at Saqquara was built in 2780 BC. The building of the great pyramid at Giza, as the tomb of the Egyptian pharaoh, **Cheops**, started in 2700 BC. Its construction shows that the Egyptians were experts in geometry. It has a base that is perfectly square with the greatest deviation from a right angle of only 0.05 percent. The cities of Mohenjadaro and Harappa in the Indus Valley, built around 2000 BC, had a sophisticated system of roads on a gridiron plan, and advanced public health measures. Kiln-dried bricks, superior to those found in Sumeria, were used in the construction of the Indus cities. The Olmec pyramids in La Venta (Tabasco, Mexico) were built around 800 BC. The oldest continuously inhabited city in the world, Damascus, in Syria, was built around 2500 BC. The Romans developed concrete around 100 BC. Anasazi people in America started building communal villages or *Pubelos* in AD 700. The oldest surviving wooden buildings, dating to AD 715, are at the Pagoda Chumanar Gate in Japan. The tallest ancient minaret, the Qutb Minar, to the south of New Delhi, India, was built in 1194. *See architecture, cement, pyramids, structural engineering, town planning.*

Bullard, Sir Edward Crisp (1907–1980) *See oceanography.*

Bullock, William (1813–1867) *See newspapers, printing.*

Bunsen Battery A carbon–zinc electric battery invented in 1841 by the German physicist, **Robert Bunsen** (1811–1899).

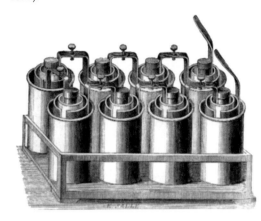

Figure 14 Bunsen battery. Lardner, Dionysius. *Handbook of Natural Philosophy, Electricity, Magnetism, and Acoustics.* London: Walton and Maberly, 1856

Bunsen Burner A laboratory gas burner in which the fuel can be mixed with varying amounts of air prior to combustion; air is admitted through a hole in the gas-tube, and the flame varies from a smoky yellow one in the absence of air to a hot, blue one when the air-hole is fully open. It was devised by the German chemist **Robert Bunsen** (1811–1899) in 1854. A similar type of burner is supposed to have been used earlier in England by **Michael Faraday** (1791–1867).

Bunsen, Robert (1811–1899) An eminent German chemist born in Göttingen where he received his doctorate of science in 1831 from the University of Göttingen. Bunsen and the German physicist **Gustav Robert Kirchhoff** in 1859 studied the lines in the sun's spectrum which had been first detected by **William Hyde Wollaston** (1766–1822) in 1802 and studied in much more detail by **Joseph von Fraunhofer** (1787–1826) in 1814, and provided an explanation for them. The sun's photosphere emits a continuous spectrum of light; the chromosphere, which lies above the photosphere, however, emits line spectra of the elements founds there. Normally these lines would be bright, but because they are silhouetted against the bright continuous spectrum they actually appear dark to an observer. Both workers while working on spectroscopy discovered the elements cesium and rubidium. Bunsen's most famous invention, the Bunsen burner, came to be used in most chemical laboratories across the world. A similar type of burner was used earlier in England by **Michael Faraday** (1791–1867). Bunsen's other inventions include: the grease-spot photometer, ice calorimeter and an actinometer. *See absorption* *spectra, actinometer, aluminum, battery, Bunsen battery, Bunsen burner, calorimeter, cesium, rubidium, spectroscopy.*

Burali-Forte, Cesare (1861–1931)   *See Burali–Forte paradox.*

Burali–Forte Paradox   To every class of ordinal numbers there corresponds an ordinal number which is greater than any element of the class. A contradiction to mathematical logic, proposed in 1897 by an Italian mathematician, **Cesare Burali-Forte** (1861–1931) of Arezzo.

Burbank, Luther (1849–1926)   *See horticulture, hybridization.*

Burbidge, Elenor Margaret (b 1923)   *See quasars.*

Burbidge, Geoffrey (b 1925)   *See quasars.*

Burdach, Karl Friedrich (1776–1847)   *See biology.*

Bürgi, Joost (1552–1632)   *See globe, logarithms.*

Burglar Alarm   The first practical device was invented in 1858 by an American, Edwin T. Holmes.

Buridan, John (*c.* 1300–1358)   *See acceleration, ballistics, dynamics, motion.*

Burks, Arthur Walter (b 1915)   *See computers.*

Burnell, Susan Jocelyn née **Bell** (b 1943)   *See pulsar.*

Burnet, Thomas (*c.* 1635–1715)   *See geogeny.*

Burning Glass   A name given to lenses used for burning. **Archimedes** (287–212 BC) is supposed to have used a lens to focus light rays and burn an enemy fleet during the Siege of Syracuse in 214 BC. The largest ever burning lens was made by a person named Parker in 1800 in England and it was exported to China. **Ehrenfried Walter von Tschirnhaus** (1651–1708), a German member of the French Académie des Sciences, constructed several powerful burning lenses, some of which are still extant. Burning mirrors were tried in physical astronomy by **George Forbes** (1849–1936) and **John Tyndall** (1820–1893) to study the heat from solar rays, but without success.

Burnside, William (1852–1927)   *See Group Theory.*

Burroughs, William Seward (1855–1898)   *See calculating machines, cash register.*

Burton, Decimus (1800–1881)   *See architecture, British.*

Bus   *See coaches, omnibus.*

Bush, Vannevar (1890–1974)   *See computers.*

Bushnell, David (1742–1824)   An American engineer from Westbrook, Maine, who is regarded as the founder of sub-

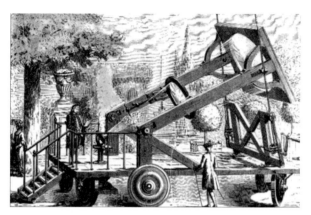

Figure 15   A 19th century French burning glass. Guillemin, Amédée. *The Applications of Physical Forces.* London: Macmillan and Co, 1877

marine engineering and submarine explosives. He developed a one-man submarine known as the *American Turtle* in 1775. Bushnell was also the first to combine a submarine and a torpedo into one unit.

Bussy, Antoine Alexandre Brutus (1794–1882)   *See beryllium.*

Butenandt, Adolf Friedrich Johann (1903–1995)   *See Ruzicka, Leopold.*

Butlerov, Alexandr Mikhailovich (1828–1886)   *See chemical structure, tautomerism.*

Bütschli, Otto (1848–1920)   *See protoplasm.*

Butter [Latin: *butryum*]   The Greek historian **Herodotus** (485–425 BC), described how the Scythians prepared butter from milk. Translators of Hebrew, about 200 years after **Hippocrates**, used the corrupted word *boutyron* for it. Hippocrates used butter as a topical medical substance under the name *pikerion*. **Aristotle** (384–322 BC) described butter as 'the fat of milk which concreted to the consistence of oil'. Methods of preparing butter or butryum have been mentioned by **Pliny the Elder** (AD 28–79) in the first century. Christians of Egypt in the 3rd century used butter as an alternative for oil to burn in their lamps.

Butterick, Ebenezer (1826–1903)   *See garment industry.*

Byerley, Perry (1897–1978)   *See earthquake.*

Byrd, Richard Evelyn (1888–1957)   *See North Pole, South Pole.*

Byte   A unit of sufficient computer memory to store a single character of data. It usually contains eight bits. A single eight-bit byte can specify 256 values, such as the decimal numbers from 0 to 255. *See bit.*

C

Cabot, Sebastian (1475–1557) *See cartography*.

Cadmium An element discovered and named in 1817 by a German professor of chemistry at Göttingen, **Friedrich Stromeyer** (1776–1835). Cadmium, a soft bluish metal with atomic number 48, is used in solder, nickel–cadmium batteries, in bearing alloys and its compounds are used as phosphorescent coatings in TV tubes.

Caecus, Appius Claudius (*c*. 300 BC) *See water supply*.

Caesalpino, Andrea (1525–1603) *See mycology*.

Cagniard, Charles de la Tour (1777–1859) *See fermentology*.

Cagnola, Luigi Marchese (1762–1833) *See architecture, Italian*.

Cahours, Auguste (1813–1891) *See amyl alcohol*.

Cailletet, Louis Paul (1832–1913) *See Eiffel Tower, liquefaction of gases*.

Caisson [French: *caisson*, coffer] A device similar to a diving bell used for underwater construction work. It was developed by **Edmund Halley** (1656–1742) in 1716.

Cajori Florian (1859–1930) A Swiss-born American historian of science who published *History of Mathematical Notations* (1929) and *A History of physics* (1899).

Calcium [Latin: *calx*, lime] A soft gray metallic element belonging to group 2 of the periodic table, with atomic number 20. It was first isolated by **Sir Humphry Davy** (1778–1829) in 1808.

Calculating Machine Around 8000 BC the Mesopotamians used clay tokens to record the numbers of animals and measures of grain. In 1597 **Galilei Galileo** (1564–1642) invented a sector compass for calculating compound interest on money, and other complex problems. In 1617 a Scottish mathematician, **John Napier** (1550–1617), invented rods made of bone for the purpose of simple multiplication. In 1623 a German engineer, **Wilhelm Schickardt** (1592–1635) built a calculating device based on the principle of Napier's bones. The first claim to a calculating mechanical device was made by Johann Ciermans, who described an apparatus with wheels, for mechanical

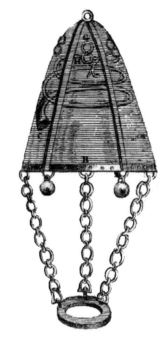

Figure 16 An early 17th century caisson. Owen, W. *Dictionary of Arts and Sciences*. London: Homer's Head, 1754

multiplication and division, in his *Disciplinae Mathematicae* published in 1640. A calculating machine that could add and subtract was devised by **Blaise Pascal** (1623–1662) in 1641. He sold his machines on a commercial basis and seven of these machines have survived. Another machine for addition and subtraction was invented by **Samuel Moreland** (1625–1696), who was a master mechanic to Charles II of England (1630–1685) in 1666. He invented another machine for multiplication, and described both machines in his work *The Description and Use of Arithmetik Instruments*

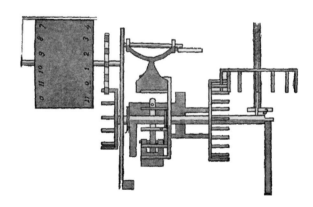

Figure 17 Pascal's calculating machine. Rolt-Wheeler, Francis. *The Science-History of the Universe, Mathematics*. London: The Waverley Book Company Limited, 1911

published in 1673. In 1694 a mathematician from Leipzig, **Gottfried Wilhelm Leibniz** (1646–1716), constructed a calculating machine that could multiply and divide. Charles Thomas of Colmar, Alsace, developed the first commercially available calculator in 1810, and 1500 of these machines were made over the next 60 years. **Charles Babbage** (1791–1871) commenced his calculating machine under the sponsorship of the British government in 1821; it was only partly completed in 1833. No further progress was made owing to the enormous additional funds that were needed despite an initial sum of 23 000 GBP already spent. This unfinished calculating machine is now exhibited at the Science Museum in London. In 1857, a Swedish engineer, **Pehr Georg Scheutz** (1785–1873) and his son Edvard Scheutz built a calculating machine for the British government. An improved machine was exhibited by Wiberg at the Paris exhibition in 1863. An adding and subtracting machine with a printer was invented by an American inventor, **William Seward Burroughs** (1855–1898) of Auburn, New York, in 1892. The first practical four-function calculator, *Millionaire,* was introduced in 1893. In 1942 an American physicist, **John Vincent Atanasoff** (1903–1995), from Hamilton, New York, built the first calculating device which used vacuum tubes. The world's first program-controlled calculator, the Harvard Mark I or Automatic Sequence-Controlled Calculator (ASCC), was built in 1943 by a New Jersey mathematician, **Howard Hathaway Aiken** (1900– 1973) and his team. A German electronic engineer, **Konrad Zuse** (1910–1995), of Berlin, built the first operational general-purpose program-controlled calculator, known as the *Z3.* The first modern pocket calculator was independently invented by Patrick Haggerty and **Jack Saint Clair Kilby** (b 1923), both of Texas Instruments, in 1971. The programmable pocket calculator was introduced by the Hewlett Packard company in 1974.

Calculation [Latin: *calculus,* small stone]   Around the 13th century, flat pieces of wood known as tally sticks first started to be used in Northern Europe for bookkeeping. These had notches corresponding to amounts of money, and they continued to be used in England until the end of the 18th century. The use of fractions is mentioned in the Ahmes papyrus (1700 BC) which is at present in the British Museum. The first use of plus and minus symbols is found in Grammateus's work in 1514. Gillis Vander Hoecke used these signs in his book published at Antwerp in 1514. The method of dividing upward, the galley method, was proposed by a Franciscan monk **Luca Paciuolo** or **Pacioli Lucas** (1445–1510) of Tuscany, in his book published in Venice in 1497. The ÷ sign was first used in its present sense

by **John Pell** (1610–1685). The = sign for equality was introduced by **Robert Recorde** (*c.* 1510–1558) in 1557. The current multiplication sign was introduced by an English mathematician and clergyman, **William Oughtred** (1575–1660) of Eton, in 1631. Logarithms were invented by the Scottish mathematician **John Napier** (1550–1617) in 1614. *See abacus, arithmetic, calculating machine, galley method, logarithms, Napier's rods, numbers.*

Calculator   *See calculating machine, computers.*

Calculus [Latin: *calculus,* small stone]   A mathematical technique in which a continuously varying quantity is treated as though it comprised an infinitely large number of infinitely small changes. Theorems relating to straight lines and distances between points were formulated by **Zeno of Elea** (463–425 BC). A scientist and philosopher, **Eudoxus** (400–360 BC), of Cnidos in Ionia, in estimating the volumes of solids, took infinitely small sections, calculated their volumes and added them together. His definition of these infinite sections contained the elements of modern calculus. Several other scientists throughout the ages, including **Archimedes** (287–212 BC), **Bonaventura Cavalieri** (1598–1647), **John Wallis** (1616–1703), **Gottfried Wilhelm Leibniz** (1646–1716) and **Sir Isaac Newton** (1642–1727) contributed to the development of calculus. The origin of the modern integral and differential calculus is obscure. Gottfried Wilhelm Leibniz first proposed the calculus in 1674 and used it for calculations in 1675. The infinitesimal calculus was first used by Sir Isaac Newton in 1666, although an account of it was printed only in 1693. The differential calculus, as an invention of Leibniz, is doubted by some historians, who believe that it may have been obtained from Newton's manuscripts. The first textbook on differential calculus, entitled *Analyse des infiniment petits,* was published by **Marquis Antoine de l'Hospital** (b 1661) of Paris in 1696. His work was borrowed from a Swiss mathematician of Dutch origin, **Jacques Bernoulli** (1654–1705), who described differential calculus in 1694. A French mathematician, **Jean de Rond d'Alembert** (1717–1783), published a paper on integral calculus in 1739 and his work over the next 9 years led to the discovery of the calculus of partial differences. Another French mathematician, **Jean Louis Lagrange** (1736–1813), founded the calculus of variations, in 1755. The functional calculus was developed by Maurice Frechet in 1906. The absolute differential calculus was developed in 1900 by two Italian mathematicians, **Tullio Levi-Civita** (1873–1941) and **Gregorio Ricci-Curbastro** (1853–1925).

Calder Hall Power Station   *See atomic power.*

Calendar [Greek: *kalendie*, proclaim] An inscribed bone dating back to 6500 BC, found in Ishango (presently Zaire), is thought to have been used for recording lunar months. Similar bone calendars from around 20 000 BC have been found in the caves of Jordan and Israel. Rounded gouges carved into a 28 000-year-old bone by Cro-Magnon man, found in the Dordogne, France, appear to represent the moon's course over a two-and-a-half month period, making this the oldest known lunar calendar. The first known annual calendar was that of the Egyptians in 4236 BC. It consisted of 365 days and 12 months based on the appearance of the brightest star in the sky, the *Sirius* or *Sothis*. Accurate calendars based on 360 days were known to the Mayans in 3114 BC. The Sumerians in 2200 BC also used 360-day calendar year. In ancient Rome, placards were used in public places to announce the important religious events every month. These placards or *Kalendie* gave origin to the present term, calendar. A Roman calendar, consisting of ten months and 304 days, was introduced by Romulus in 738 BC. One of the oldest surviving calendars, made of marble columns with the months of the year inscribed, was found in the remains of Pompeii. The Chinese calendar – in existence for over 2500 years – is based on the lunar year. The Muslim calendar begins in 622, the day after Hegira, the flight of Muhammad from Mecca to Medina. The Gregorian calendar was devised by Pope Gregory XIII on the advice of the German Astronomer, **Christoph Clavius** (1537–1612) and introduced into Catholic countries in 1582. *See date, Gregorian calendar, Julian calendar.*

Californium The element with atomic number 98, synthesized in 1950 by an American physicist, **Glenn Theodore Seaborg** (1912–1999) and his team at Berkeley, California. All its isotopes are radioactive.

Calla, Étienne (1760–1835) *See textile industry.*

Calla, François (1802–1884) Son of **Étienne Calla** (1760–1835) and one of the leading machine tool manufacturers of the 19th century in France.

Call-bells Speaking tubes for communication between various rooms in a big house and the servants' quarters were invented around 1850. This was largely replaced by a system of bells invented by a Glasgow plumber, John Black.

Callendar, Hugh Longbourne (1863–1930) *See calorimeter, thermometer.*

Callicrates (*c.* 500 BC) *See Parthenon.*

Calorescence [Latin: *calor*, heat] Absorption of light by a surface, and its conversion into heat resulting in emission of heat radiation. The phenomenon was observed and named by **John Tyndall** (1820–1893).

Calorimeter [Latin: *calor*, heat + Greek: *metron*, measure] An instrument used for measuring quantities of heat change. In 1780 **Antoine Laurent Lavoisier** (1743–1794) and **Pierre Simon Marquis de Laplace** (1749–1827) studied the heat changes in the animal body by using ice and water. In 1870 **Robert Bunsen** (1811–1899) devised an ingenious form of calorimeter in which the quantity of ice and its contraction in volume during melting were used to measure heat. Carl Voit of Munich, and a German chemist, **Max von Pettenkofer** (1818–1901) developed the differential calorimeter in 1886. A modern calorimeter capable of measuring heat production, oxygen consumption, and carbon dioxide elimination was devised by an American, Wilber Atwater, in 1892. A continuous flow type of electric calorimeter was introduced by an English physicist, **Hugh Longbourne Callendar** (1863–1930), of Gloucestershire, in 1902. A special form of calorimeter for measuring specific heat at low temperatures was designed in 1911 by a German physicist, **Walther Hermann Nernst** (1864–1941) and a German-born British physicist, **Frederick Alexander Lindemann Cherwell** (1886–1957).

Calorimetry [Latin: *calor*, heat + Greek: *metron*, measure] *See calorimeter.*

Calotype Process [Greek: *kalos,* beautiful] The art of producing a negative photograph on paper, invented by an English Victorian squire, **William Henry Fox Talbot** (1800–1877), of Wiltshire, in 1840. Talbot's process, the calotype, was patented in Britain in 1841, and in the USA in 1847. A Scottish chemist, **Robert Adamson** (1821–1848), and a photographer, **Davis Octavius Hill** (1802–1870), applied the calotype process and produced around 2500 calotypes of portraits and landscapes around 1845. *See color photography.*

Calvin, Melvin (1911–1997) *See photosynthesis.*

Cambrian period [Latin: *Cambria,* Wales] The earliest geological period of the Paleozoic era. It is estimated to have begun about 570 million years ago, and lasted for around 100 million years. Cambrian rocks are the first in the geological record to contain an abundance of fossils, and were first studied in the English Lake District by **Adam Sedgwick** (1785–1873), a geologist from Dent, Yorkshire, who coined the term Cambrian for the period in 1834. The Sedgwick Museum of Geology at Cambridge was named in his honor. *See azoic period.*

Cambridge Philosophical Society Founded in 1819 and received its royal charter in 1832.

Camera [Latin: *camera,* chamber] The history involves two aspects: the first being the development of optics, and the other the development of imprinting methods. The camera obscura was first suggested by the Arabian mathematician, **Alhazen or Ibn Al-Haitham** (AD 965–1038), of Basra, and the first description of a primitive form of camera obscura was given by the English Franciscan monk **Roger Bacon** (1214–1298) of Ilchester, in his treatise *perspectiva* in 1267. **Levi Ben Gerson** (1288–1344), a Jewish astronomer, suggested an improved version in 1310. The device is also found in the manuscripts of **Leonardo da Vinci** (1452–1519). A Venetian professor at Padua, **Daniello Barbaro**, substituted a lens for the pin hole in 1568. **Giovanni Battista della Porta** (1535–1615) described the camera obscura in more detail in 1585. In 1725 the discovery of a German anatomist, Johann Heinrich Schultz, that silver salts became black on exposure to light, made imprinting of images possible. The first printing on opaque bodies was achieved by Thomas Wedgewood in 1802. A French chemist, **Joseph Nicephore Niepce** (1765–1833), used a substance called bitumen to make the prints permanent. He also produced the first photograph on a metal (pewter) in 1826. In 1839 he went into partnership with **Louis Jacques Mande Daguerre** (1789–1851) of Cormeilles, near Lisieux, France, to perfect his process, but died 6 years before Daguerre's invention. Daguerre used sodium thiosulfate solution to remove the unchanged silver iodide and this shortened the exposure time from a few hours to a few minutes leaving a 'fixed' image. The method of producing prints from negatives by using gallic acid, known as calotype processing, was invented by an Englishman, **William Henry Fox Talbot** (1800–1877), in 1840. **George Eastman** (1854–1932) of Waterville, New York, simplified the camera (Kodak camera), and brought it within the reach of the public, in 1888. He started his experiments on photographic emulsions in 1878, and introduced the roll film in 1886. In 1914 a German microscope-designer, Oskar Barnack (1879–1936), invented the first successful miniature camera, which used 35 mm cine film. A pocket-sized camera was introduced in 1900, and 8-mm movie cameras appeared in 1932. The electronic flash was invented in 1931 by an American electrical engineer, **Harold Eugene Edgerton** (1903–1990) of Fremont, Nebraska. *See Daguerrotype, photography, Polaroid camera.*

Camera Lucida [Latin: *lucidus,* light, *camera,* a chamber] A device made of a prism, by means of which the image of an object may be projected onto a white or light surface. It was invented by **Robert Hooke** (1635–1703) in 1674. In 1807 an English physician and chemist, **William Hyde Wollaston** (1766–1822), used it to project distant landscapes onto paper, and traced their outlines.

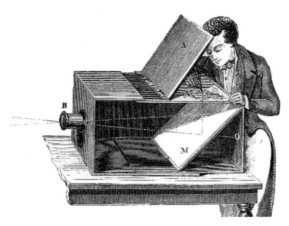

Figure 18 Camera obscura. Atkinson, E. *Elementary Treatise on Physics.* London: Longmans, Green, and Co, 1872

Camera Obscura [Latin: *camera,* chamber, *obscurus,* dark] or pinhole camera. A dark chamber with a tiny hole through which the landscape outside is projected on the opposite wall. **Giovanni Battista della Porta** (1535–1615) improved it by fixing a double convex lens to the aperture, and placing a white screen in the focus. He described the camera obscura in more detail in 1585. *See camera.*

Camerarius, Joachium or Camerer (1534–1598) A German botanist and physician who is known for his *Hortus Medicus et Philosophicus* (1588) and several other works. He provided the first proof for sexuality in plants in his *De Sexu Plantarum Epistola* published in 1594.

Camerarius, Rudolph Jacob (1665–1721) *See pollination.*

Cameron, Alastair Graham Walter (b 1925) A Canadian-born US astrophysicist who proposed that the earth's original atmosphere was blown off into space by the early solar gale, as opposed to solar breeze. He also suggested that technetium-97 might result from the decay of a nucleus of molybdenum-97 due to absorption of X-ray photons at high temperatures.

Camm, Sir Sydney (1893–1966) *See warplanes.*

Campanus, Johannes (*c.* 1205–1296) *See early printed science books.*

Campbell, Colen (1679–1726) *See architecture, British.*

Campbell, William Wallace (1862–1938) An American astronomer from Hancock County, Ohio, who is known for his study of the radial velocity of stars. In 1928 he produced a catalogue of 3000 radial velocities. *See Mars.*

Campen, Jacob van (1595–1657) *See architecture, European.*

Camphor A white crystalline cyclic ketone with a characteristic odor well known for its use in mothballs Originally derived from the wood of the Formosan camphor tree, it is now synthesized for use as a plasticizer in celluloid – a synthesis first achieved by the English chemist, **William Henry Perkin** (1860–1929) of Sudbury, Middlesex, in 1897.

Canal Rays Streams of positive ions produced in a discharge tube by making holes ('canals') in the cathode. Some of the positive ions attracted to the cathode pass through the holes and emerge on the other side as positive rays. They were first described and named by a German physicist, **Eugen Goldstein** (1850–1930), from Upper Silesia, in 1886. He was made head of the astrophysical section of the Potsdam Observatory in 1929.

Canals The oldest canals in the world, dating back to 4000 BC, were unearthed in 1968 at Mandali, Iraq. A 50-mile canal connecting Nineveh and Bavia was built by King Sennacherib of Assyria in 600 BC. **Wang Ching** (d AD 83) reconstructed the 500-mile Pien canal previously damaged by floods of the Yellow River. Another Chinese engineer, **Shen Kua** (1031–1095), reinforced the banks of Grand Canal and rebuilt it. It was originally built from Beijing to Hangzhou, in 540 BC. A Persian engineer, **Artachaies** (*c.* 500 BC), built a canal wide enough for two warships in the Athos Peninsula in northern Greece. Canal locks were known to the Chinese around AD 900, and the first one was built in Europe in 1373. The earliest canal in England, Fossdyke canal, between Lincoln and the River Trent, was built by the Romans in AD 65. The Briare Canal in France, linking the Rivers Loire and Seine, opened in 1643. The 180-mile long, Canal du Midi, connecting the Mediterranean Sea and Atlantic Ocean, was built by a French administrator and land owner, **Pierre Paul Riquet de Bonrepos** (1604–1680), in 1666. The first canal that crossed a river via an aqueduct was built over the River Irwell, in England, by an engineer, **James Brindley** (1716–1772), in 1759. He later built 365 miles of other navigable canals. In collaboration with him, the 3rd Duke of Bridgewater, **Francis Egerton** (1736–1803), who is known as the father of British inland navigation, built a 43-mile-long canal from Worsley to Runcorn and Manchester. Many important canals in England, at London Docks, Blackwall, Liverpool and Hull, were built by a Scottish civil engineer, **John Rennie** (1761–1821) of East Linton. The Forth and Clyde canals in

Scotland were built by an English engineer, **John Smeaton** (1724–1792) from Austhorpe. A major canal project, the Caledonian Canal Project, was completed by a Scottish civil engineer, **Thomas Telford** (1757–1834) who also constructed many important bridges and roads in the 18th century. **Canvass White** (1790–1834) of Whitesboro, New York, was a pioneer of canals and water supply in New York City where he was one of the project engineers to Erie Canal in 1824. The 363-mile-long Erie Canal was one of the first major engineering projects (1817–1825) in America, and it was completed under the supervision of an American civil engineer, **Benjamin Wright** (1770–1842) of Wethersfield, Connecticut. The Suez Canal in Egypt which became an important trade route between Europe and the east, was designed and built by a French civil engineer, **Ferdinand Vicompte de Lesseps** (1805–1894). Work commenced in 1860, and it opened to traffic in 1870.

Candle Clock Supposed to have been invented by Alfred the Great (849–900). It consisted of a long candle with uniform thickness, calibrated with colored bands. A wooden lantern around it protected the flame from drafts, and the time was read from the rate of burning of the candle.

Candle Power A standard lamp of ten candle power that used pentane as fuel was invented by a London chemist, **Augustus George Vernon Harcourt** (1834–1919). This was later replaced by a carbon filament electric lamp. The international unit of the candle was introduced in 1921.

Candles [Latin: *candela*] Made of a string surrounded by wax, these were used by the Romans, although a primitive form was known as early as 3500 BC. During the Middle Ages candles were a luxury in England, and as a result, the indigents had to use splinters of wood coated with fat as a substitute. Candles became available on a large scale following the researches on fatty acids by a French chemist, **Michel Eugene Chevreul** (1786–1889) in 1823.

Candolle, Alphonse Louis Pierre (1806–1893) *See taxonomy.*

Candolle, Augustin Pyrame de (1778–1841) A Swiss botanist who carried out a botanical and agricultural survey of France for the French government from 1806 to 1812. He published *Propriétés mèdicales des plantes* (1804), *Regni Vegetablis Systema Naturale* (1818–1821) and several other important botanical works. *See taxonomy.*

Canned Food An Italian biologist, **Lazzaro Spallanzani** (1729–1799), was the first to suggest, in 1765, that food could be preserved by sealing it in containers that did not allow air to penetrate. The French confectioner, **Nicolas**

François Appert (1749–1841), first used the autoclave for sterilization of food, in 1810. He used glass jars before turning to cans, and opened the first canning factory in the world in 1812. *See food industry.*

Canning, Sir Samuel (1823–1908) *See transatlantic communication.*

Cannizzaro's reaction Formation of benzoic acid and benzyl alcohol by treating benzaldehyde with potassium hydroxide, discovered by an Italian chemist, **Stanislao Cannizzaro** (1826–1910) of Rome.

Cannizzaro, Stanislao (1826–1910) An Italian organic chemist and statesman born in Palmero. He was professor of chemistry at Genoa, Palmero and Rome. He differentiated between atomic weight and molecular weight and introduced the term hydroxyl for the OH radical. He revived Avogadro's hypothesis on molecules and explained it. He was made a Senator in 1871 and died in Rome.

Cannon, Annie Jump (1863–1941) An American astronomer from Dover, Delaware, who in 1896 joined the Harvard Observatory, and classified the spectra of nearly 400 000 stars.

Cannon, Walter Bradford (1871–1945) *See fluoroscope.*

Cano, Juan Sebastian del (d 1526) *See circumnavigation.*

Canton, John (1718–1772) An English physicist born in Stroud, Gloucestershire. He did extensive research on electricity and magnets and produced the first artificial magnet. His other achievements include: the invention of an electrometer and electroscope, demonstration of the compressibility of water and the electric nature of lightning.

Cantor, Charles Robert (b 1942) *See electrophoresis.*

Cantor, Georg Ferdinand Ludwig Philip (1845–1918) A Russian-born Jewish mathematician who is regarded as the founder of modern infinite sets. His work *Beiträge zur Begründung der Transfiniten Mengenlehre* (1895–1897) was a landmark in the field.

Capillary Electrometer An instrument for magnifying minute fluctuations of electrical potential invented by a French physicist, **Gabriel Jonas Lippmann** (1845–1921) in 1875.

Car [Latin: *carrus,* wagon] Wheeled vehicles were used by Sumerians by around 3500 BC. A vehicle with four wheels covered by cloth was invented by Erichthonius of Athens in 1486 BC. The term *carrucae* referred to vehicles for travelling, used by the state officers in ancient Rome. Four-

wheeled covered carriages, *caretta,* were used by the nobility in Europe around the 12th century. **Simon Stevinus** (1548–1620) of Bruges built a two-masted sailing road wagon in 1599. Several similar sailing road vehicles were tried in the 17th and 18th centuries. In 1770 a French army engineer, **Nicholas Joseph Cugnot** (1725–1804), developed a three-wheeled steam-powered road tractor capable of six kilometers per hour, which became the first automobile. The first attempt to replace the steam engine was made in 1805 by a Swiss engineer, Isaac de Rivaz. His engine consisted of an exploding gas which pushed up a single piston in the cylinder. His invention was a failure as there was no second piston to follow up the motion. The first steam-driven road vehicle in England was built in 1829 by **Goldsworthy Gurney** (1793–1875) from Treator, Cornwall, and it operated between London and Bath at a speed of 15 miles per hour. The first horseless carriage with an internal combustion engine, instead of steam power, was built by a Belgian-born French inventor, **Jean Joseph Etienne Lenoir** (1822–1900), in 1860. Lenoir's engine used coal gas as a fuel and was found to be inefficient. **Gottlieb Daimler** (1834–1900) of Germany invented an improved internal combustion engine for a motor car in 1870 and applied it to a bicycle with success in 1886. Daimler built another engine in 1889 which doubled the power, and it was adapted by the French to the motor car. Daimler also devised the carburetor in 1876. The immediate precursor of a modern motor car was a tricycle propelled by a two-stroke monocylinder motor, built by a German engineer, **Carl Friedrich Benz** (1844–1929) from Karlsruhe, in 1883. He demonstrated the first gasoline-driven automobile, a three-wheeler, in 1886. A quadricycle was developed from this model by another German engineer, **Wilhelm Maybach** (1846–1929) of Heilbronn, in 1889. He invented the high-speed gasoline engine and the float-feed carburetor in 1893. He also designed the first Mercedes automobile in 1901, naming it after Mercedes Jellinec who was the daughter of his friend, the Austro-Hungarian consul in Nice. A steam car with pneumatic tires was invented by American brothers, Francis Edgar Stanley (1849–1918) and Freelan O. Stanley (1849–1940) in 1897. They continued to manufacture it on a commercial basis until 1917. The first car with a chassis and internal combustion engine mounted to the front was built in 1891 by two Frenchmen, **René Panhard** (1841–1908) and Emile Levassor. The first American automobile is claimed to be a model built in 1893 by an American inventor, **John Elwood Haynes** (1857–1925) of Portland, Indiana. The first experimental motor car in Britain was produced in 1895 by **Frederick William Lanchester** (1868–1948) of Lewisham, London, who founded the

Lanchester Engine Company in 1899, which produced 400 cars over the next 4 years. Louis Renault built the first fully enclosed car in 1898, and developed drum brakes in 1902. Lanchester introduced disk brakes in the same year. Spark plugs were invented in 1902. A London engineer, **Charles Stewart Rolls** (1877–1910) and **Sir Frederick Henry Royce** (1863–1933) of Cambridgeshire in England jointly built their first motor car in 1907 and by 1914 their company Rolls-Royce was producing cars that became known as the best in the world. The automatic gearbox was invented by a German engineer, Hermann Föttinger, in 1910. **André Gustav Citroën** (1878–1935) and **Walter Percy Chrysler** (1875–1940) were the first two car makers to produce aerodynamically designed cars. The first self starter for the automobile was introduced in 1911 by an American, Charles Frankelin Kettering of Ohio. The first assembly line to reduce labor costs and speed up production was established by **Henry Ford** (1863–1947) in 1913. He constructed a one-cylinder gasoline engine in 1893 and built his first motor car, the quadricycle, in 1896. He introduced the Model T Ford in 1908 and by 1924 he had produced his ten millionth automobile. The rear-view mirror for the car was introduced by an English army surgeon, John William Cockerill, in 1896. A revolutionary cheap car with an air-cooled rear engine was produced in 1934 by **Ferdinand Porsche** (1875–1951) of Germany, the Nazis naming it the Volkswagen, translated as the peoples' car. The first production Volkswagen came off the assembly lines in 1945. Porsche also invented the synchronizing gearbox and torsion-bar suspension. In England the first mass-produced affordable cars were produced by **William Richard Morris**, **Lord Nuffield** (1877–1963) at his Morris Motor Car Company in Cowley, Oxford, in 1910. The world's first gas-turbine car, Jet 1, was built by Rover in 1950. The Morris Minor, the first British motor car to pass the million mark in 1961, was developed by a British engineer, **Alec Issigonis** (1906–1988), who had emigrated from Turkey. He also designed one of the most successful British cars, the Mini, in 1959. *See automobile, automobile industry, motorcar industry, motoring.*

Car Radio   The first radio that worked on a car battery with an external aerial was invented in 1932 by the German designer, Blaupunkt, and it was fitted to an American Studebaker. Another early practical car radio was built by an American inventor, **William Powell Lear** (1902–1978) of Hannibal, Missouri.

Carathéodory, Constantin (1873–1950) A German mathematician who proposed a theory of discontinuous curves in the calculus of variations. In 1932 one of his important publications contained a simplification of a proof for the central theorems of conformal representation.

Carats [Greek: *keration*, horn-like pods]   The unit of weight for measurement of diamonds and gold, taken from the average weight of the seeds of the carob, a native tree of Africa. These seeds uniformly arranged in the pod have been used since ancient times for weighing gold. When diamonds were first discovered in India, the seeds were transported there to be used as units of weight for diamonds. The English carat was fixed at 3.1683 grains by the Board of Trade in 1888; it was replaced by the metric carat in 1914.

Carbon [Latin: *carbo*, charcoal]   Its various forms including graphite, diamond and charcoal have been known since ancient times. It was identified as a distinct element by **Antoine Laurent Lavoiser** (1743–1794) in 1788. Lavoisier demonstrated its existence in a pure form as diamond, by burning a diamond to yield carbonic acid gas. The molecular theory of structure, which explained how the carbon atoms linked together to form chains, was proposed by the German organic chemist, **Friedrich August Kekulé von Stradonitz** (1829–1896) of Darmstadt, in 1865. He also established the valency of carbon as 4. *See carbon cycle, carbon dating*.

Carbon Assimilation   *See photosynthesis*.

Carbon Cycle   A theory for generation of energy by stars, thorough a series of nuclear reactions involving carbon. Formulated in 1939 by a German-born American physicist, **Hans Albrecht Bethe** (b 1906) who was awarded the Nobel Prize for physics for his work, in 1967. *See thermonuclear fusion*.

Carbon Cyclic Ring   A German chemist, **Friedrich August Kekulé von Stradonitz** (1829–1896) deduced the cyclic six-carbon ring structure of benzene in 1865. His discovery formed the basis for the study of aromatic compounds.

Carbon Dating   A method of dating ancient objects with the use of radioactive carbon-14, introduced in 1946 by **Williard Frank Libby** (1908–1980) of Grand Valley, Colorado. In 1947 he refined the method to date objects that were 50 000 years old, and published *Radiocarbon Dating*, in 1952. He was awarded the Nobel Prize for chemistry for his work, in 1960. **Lawrence Rickard Wager** (1904–1965), a petrologist from Yorkshire, was mainly instrumental in establishing the Radiometric Age Determination Laboratory at Oxford in 1955.

Carbon Dioxide   First obtained in the 16th century, through burning charcoal, by **Jean Baptist van Helmont** (1577–1644) who named it gas. **Joseph Black** (1728–1799), a professor of chemistry at Glasgow University, rediscovered it in 1757 under the name fixed air.

Carbon Disulfide   Discovered by W.A. Lampadius of Freiberg in 1796.

Carbon Fibers   Made of polymerized long chains of carbon with strong inter-links for the purpose of industrial use, such as production of aviation engines and submarines, were first made by the British firm Courtaulds in 1964. *See polymer.*

Carbon Fixation   *See photosynthesis.*

Carbon Monoxide   Two French chemists of Dijon, **Charles Bernard Desormes** (1777–1862) and his son-in-law, **Nicolas Clement** (1779–1841), discovered the gas in 1801. A British physiologist, **John Scott Haldane** (1860–1936), demonstrated its physiological mechanism and toxic effects.

Carbon Ring Structure   *See benzene.*

Carboniferous Period   Geological period which existed 363–290 million years ago, identified by William Daniel Conybeare and Williams Phillips, in 1822. It is so named because of the delta deposit of coal on the upper-carboniferous rocks.

Carborundum or silicon carbide.   It was discovered by a French chemist **Ferdinand Frederic Henri Moissan** (1852–1907), a demonstrator at the École de Pharmacie, Paris in 1879. In 1891 an American chemist, **Edward Goodrich Acheson** (1856–1931) of Washington, Pennsylvania, developed a method of manufacturing it. He held over 69 patents, and established the Acheson Graphite Company for making artificial graphite in 1899.

Carburetor   *See car.*

Cardan, Girolomo (1501–1576)   *See algebra, early printed science books, probability theory, steam engine, water pump.*

Cards   The origin of the card game is uncertain; it appeared in Europe around AD 1200, probably brought by the Gypsies. According to the Chinese dictionary of 1678 they were invented for the amusement of concubines, during the reign of Séun-Ho, around AD 1120.

Carlson, Chester Floyd (1906–1968)   *See xerography.*

Carnegie, Andrew (1835–1919)   An industrial entrepreneur and oil magnate from Dunfermline in Scotland, who emigrated to America in 1848. He promoted literacy by establishing educational institutions and libraries across the world. He founded the Carnegie Institute of Technology in Pittsburgh in 1900, and the Carnegie Institute of Washington DC, one of the first institutes for scientific research, in 1902. He established the Carnegie Corporation of New York in 1911, and the Carnegie Endowment for International Peace in 1910.

Carnot, Nicolas Leonard Sadi (1796–1831)   A French physicist in Paris who is regarded as the founder of thermodynamics. He was the first to define work, and postulate the law of thermodynamics. His only published work *Réflexions sur la Puissance Motrice du feu et sur les Machines propres* à *Dévéloper cette Puissance* appeared in 1824. He died of cholera at the age of 36. *See thermodynamics.*

Carothers, Wallace Hume (1896–1937)   *See polymer.*

Carpenter, Nathaniel (1589–1628)   *See geography.*

Carpet Sweeper   A rotating sweeper with brushes inside a pan, invented in 1876 by Melville R. Bissell of Grand Rapids, Michigan. *See domestic appliances.*

Carrier, Willis Haviland (1876–1950)   *See air conditioner.*

Carrington, Richard Christopher (1826–1875)   *See Spörer's law, sunspots.*

Carson, Rachel (Louise) (1907–1964)   A US biologist and environmentalist who published *Silent Spring* (1962) denouncing the use of pesticides and other chemical poisons, thus raising environmental concerns. She also published a best-seller *Sea Around Us* (1951), and *The Edge of the Sea* (1955), an ecological exploration of the seashore.

Cartan, Elie Joseph (1869–1951)   *See Lie groups.*

Carter, Herbert James (1858–1940)   An English entomologist who migrated to Australia in 1881 where he described over 1000 new species. He was joint science editor of the first Australian Encyclopaedia (1925–27).

Cartesian Coordinates   Components used in coordinate geometry, to define the position of a point by its perpendicular distance from a set of two or more axes, or reference lines. It can be extended to any finite number of dimensions (axes), and is used thus in theoretical mathematics. It is named after the French mathematician, **René Descartes** (1596–1650).

Cartesian Doctrine   A theory of vortices or motions proposed in 1637 by the French philosopher **René Descartes** (1596–1650), to explain all physical phenomena.

Cartography [Latin: *charta*, a paper + Greek: *graphein,* to write] The art of map drawing. The oldest map in existence dating back to 2250 BC, a statue of Gudea of Lagash, showing the plan of the city on his lap, is at the Musée du Louvre in Paris. The earliest extant printed map is that of western China in AD 1115. The grid system, consisting of lines at right angles to each other, for specifying a point in a map, was introduced around AD 100 by Chang Heng of China. **Ptolemy** (*c.* AD 127–151) in his *Geography* described the rules for meridians and parallels used in map drawing. The earliest map of Britain was printed in 1477 in Bologna, Italy. The word atlas was used for the first time in 1585 by a Flemish geographer, **Gerardus Mercator** or **Gerard de Cremer** (1512–1594), to describe a book of maps. It is derived from the Greek god, Atlas, who is supposed to have stood on the earth and supported the heavens. The first known map, inscribed on bone, dating back to 10 000 BC, was found in Mezhirich in Russia. Sargon of Akkad, the founder of the Sumerian empire, produced the first map of Mesopotamia in 2400 BC for the purpose of land taxation. The oldest preserved map of a city, dating back to 2300 BC, is found carved on a stone from the Mesopotamian city of Lagash. **Anaximander** (611–547 BC) of Miletus was the first to draw a map of the earth giving details of its surface, and to speculate the size and distances of the heavenly bodies or stars. **Hecataeus of Miletus** developed a map of the world in around 500 BC which showed Europe and Asia as semicircles surrounded by ocean. The medieval maps called *mappa mundi* portrayed the earth as a circle with Jerusalem at its center. They were more religion orientated than accurate, but provided a stimulus for the Crusades. Mercator invented the projection used in map making that bears his name. He first used it to prepare his chart of the world in 1569. His earliest map was that of the Holy Land in 1537, followed by those of Flanders (1537–1540), the world (1538) and six sheets of Europe (1554). A Venetian navigator and cartographer, **Sebastian Cabot** (1475–1557), published an engraved map of the world in 1544, of which only one copy is extant, at the Bibliothèque Nationale in Paris. A professor of mathematics at Ingolstadt and a physician, **Peter Apian** (1495–1552) and his son Philip were pioneers of cartography in the 16th century. Peter Apian used the name America for the first time in a map in 1520. **Abraham Ortel** or **Ortelius** (1527–1598) of Antwerp in his *Theatrum Orbis Terrarum* (1570) had a collection of 70 maps. He produced a map of the world in 1564. **John Speed** (1542–1629) of Cheshire produced 54 *Maps of England and Wales* (1608–1610). One of the earliest makers of modern maps was **Jean-Baptiste Bourguignon d'Anville** (1697–1782) of Paris, whose practical maps were in use up to the 19th century. A map of the Pacific was produced by the English sea captain, **James Cook** (1728–1779) from Marton, Yorkshire, during his voyages. The first survey of all the counties of England and Wales was carried out by **Christopher Saxton** (1542–1611) from Sowood, Yorkshire, in 1579. His atlas was the first national map of any country to be published. He also published a wall map of England in 1583. A Scottish surveyor, **John Adair** (*c.* 1655–1722), prepared maps of counties in central Scotland from 1680 to 1686, and published *Description of the Sea-Coast and Islands of Scotland* (1703). Another Scottish cartographer, **Robert Gordon** (1580–1661), with his son **James Gordon** (1615–1686), edited several Scottish maps. A German cartographer, **Johann Tobias Mayer** (1723–1762) of Marbach, near Stuttgart, was one of the first to combine geographic and astronomical details to determine longitude and latitude, and produced 30 maps of Germany. A French geographer, **J.N. Buache** (1741–1825) introduced the use of contours for maps. The first map of the United States, as a new nation, was produced by Abel Buell in 1783. **Aaron Arrowsmith** (1750–1823) and his nephew **John Arrowsmith** (1790–1873), both from Winston, Durham, were eminent cartographers in London. **John Cary** (1754–1835) published the *New and Correct English Atlas* in 1787, followed by a *New Universal Atlas* in 1808. The Finnish Arctic explorer, **Nils Adolf Nordenskiöld** (1832–1901) of Helsinki, made important contributions to the history of cartography with his *Facsimile Atlas* (1889) and *Periplus* (1897). **John George Bartholomew** (1860–1920), a cartographer in Edinburgh, developed the system of color layers for contours.

Cartoons In 1917 an Austrian-born US cartoonist **Max Fleischer** (1883–1972) invented a rotoscope for transferring live action into animated cartoons by tracing. His brother **Dave Fleischer** (1894–1979), produced films which combined live action and animation. Together they produced silent cartoons synchronized with an orchestral score. Their first experimental sound-on-film cartoons appeared in the mid-1920s. Their most popular *Popeye the Sailor* was produced in 1930. The first Cinecolor cartoon, *Merrie Melodies,* was directed by **Friz Freleng** (1906–1995) of Kansas City. *See cinema.*

Cartwright, Edmund (1743–1823) An English clergyman of Nottinghamshire, educated at Oxford. He revolutionized the cotton industry with his invention of the power-loom in 1785. He took out a patent in 1790 for a wool-combing machine, which had an output equal to that of 20 hand combers. He invented an alcohol engine in 1797.

Caruso, Enrico (1873–1921)   *See musical recording.*

Carver, George Washington (1860–1943)   *See agriculture, agronomy.*

Cary, John (1754–1835)   *See cartography.*

Cascade Process   The first method used for liquefying oxygen, invented in 1877 by **Raoul Pierre Pictet** (1846–1929), a Swiss chemist from Geneva. His method involved the application of pressure, in a relatively high critical temperature, for liquefying nitrogen, hydrogen and carbon dioxide.

Cash Register   James Ritty of America designed one in 1879. The adding machine used in shop counters was invented in 1892 by an American, **William Seward Burroughs** (1855–1898) of Auburn, New York.

Caslon, William (1692–1766)   *See typography.*

Cassegrain, Guillame (*c.* 1625–1700)   A French inventor who improved the telescope designed by Sir Isaac Newton, by using an auxiliary convex mirror to reflect the image through a hole in the objective. His telescope increased the angular magnification and partly cancelled out spherical aberration.

Cassegrain, N. (1650–1675)   *See reflecting telescope.*

Cassette   *See magnetic recording.*

Cassini, Alexandre Henri Gabriel de (1784–1832)   *See botany.*

Cassini, César François Thury de (1714–1784)   *See Cassini, Giovanni Domenico.*

Cassini, Giovanni Domenico (1625–1712)   A professor of astronomy at the University of Bologna in 1650 before he became naturalized in France in 1673. He was appointed director of the Paris Observatory, and showed that the earth was flattened at its poles. He made numerous other discoveries in astronomy including the four satellites of Saturn. Cassini's calculation of the distance from the sun to the earth has been proved to be only 7 per cent in error by modern calculations. His son **Jacques Cassini** (1677–1756), also an eminent astronomer, succeeded his father as director of the Paris Observatory. The topological map of France was commenced by Jacque's son, **César François Thury de Cassini** (1714–1784) in 1744, and completed by his grandson **Jacques Dominique de Cassini** (1748–1845). *See Jupiter, parallax.*

Cassini, Jacques (1677–1756)   *See Cassini, Giovanni Domenico.*

Cassini, Jacques Dominique de (1748–1845)   *See Cassini, Giovanni Domenico.*

Castigliano, Alberto (1847–1884)   *See structural engineering.*

Castelli, Benedetto (1578–1643)   An Italian mathematician and a pupil of **Galilei Galileo** (1564–1642). He did important studies on hydrostatistics.

Castle, William Ernest (1867–1962)   *See mutation.*

Castner, Hamilton Young (1859–1899)   *See sodium.*

Cat Scanner   Computerized axial tomography used in radiology was developed independently by a British scientist, **Sir Godfrey Newbold Hounsfield** (b 1919), and a South African-born American medical physicist, **Allan Macleod Cormack** (1924–1998), in 1972. Cormack and Hounsfield shared the Nobel Prize for Physiology or Medicine in 1979.

Cataldi, Pietro Antoine (1548–1626)   *See perfect number.*

Catalysis [Greek: *kataluien,* to dissolve]   A term coined by a Swedish chemist, **Jons Jacob Berzelius** (1779–1848) in 1837. **Gottlieb Sigismond Kirchhoff** (1764–1833) in 1812 observed that starch was converted to glucose by the action of dilute acid, but the acid itself remained unchanged. During the period 1817–1823, several workers including **Johann Wolfgang Dobereiner** (1780–1849), **Eilhardt Mitscherlich** (1794–1863) and **Louis Jacques Thenard** (1777–1857) found that several metals accelerated chemical reactions without any change occurring in the metals themselves. Thenard also noted that blood fibrin accelerated the decomposition of hydrogen peroxide, an effect later explained to be due to methemoglobin. The mechanism of action of a catalyst was explained in 1854 on the basis of an intermediate compound by **Alexander William Williamson** (1824–1904), a professor of chemistry (1849–1887) at University College, London. The importance of the velocity of a catalytic reaction was emphasized by the Latvian-born physical chemist **Friedrich Wilhelm Ostwald** (1853–1932).

Catalyst   *See catalysis.*

Catapult [Greek: *kata,* against + Anglo-Saxon: *pullion,* draw]   An early form was introduced to fight the invading forces from Carthage by Dionysius the Elder, ruler of Syracuse in 406 BC. Catapults which operated on the principle of torsion were used in 395 BC by the forces of Philip of Macedon. A repeat loading catapult equipped with a spring device was designed by **Philo** of Byzantium around 240 BC. The Roman architect, **Marcus Pollio Vitruvius** (*c.* AD 100), in his treatise *On Architecture* explained the principle behind catapults or *scorpiones*. The Romans used a large catapult built of wood, known as an *onager*. Catapults were used in the First World War by the French to hurl hand grenades. *See military engineering.*

Catastrophe Theory A mathematical theory developed by René Thom in 1972. He showed that a series of gradual changes are triggered by, and also in turn trigger, large-scale or catastrophic changes or jumps. It is applicable to many fields such as biology, evolution and engineering.

Catastrophism A term coined by a British scholar, **William Whewell** (1794–1866) of Lancaster, to denote the sudden and convulsive movement in the evolution of the earth. A Swiss naturalist, **Charles Étienne Bonnet** (1720–1793) proposed a catastrophic theory of evolution. **William Buckland** (1784–1856), a professor of geology at the University of Oxford, advocated the catastrophic theory for the formation of the earth. *See geogeny.*

Cathode Refers to negative electrode. The term was coined by **Michael Faraday** (1791–1867).

Cathode Ray Tube A device for projecting a beam of electrons or cathode rays on to a fluorescent screen. Its forerunner, the Crookes tube, was invented by **Sir William Crookes** (1832–1919) in 1878. His device was an almost complete vacuum in a glass vessel through which a current was passed; it became fluorescent owing to a stream of electrons from the cathode. **Joseph John Thompson** (1856–1940) developed this in 1897. A Russian professor, **Boris Rosing** (d 1918) of St Petersburg, linked it to electric vision (television) in 1907. *See television, X-rays.*

Cathode Rays [Greek: *kathodos,* a way down] A stream of electrons produced by passing a current through a tube containing gas at very low pressure, first observed in 1859 by a German physicist and a mathematician, **Julius Plücker** (1801–1868). He shifted his interest from mathematics to physics, and became professor of physics at Bonn, in 1847. An emission from the cathode during the passage of a current was first noted by Plücker's student **Johann Wilhelm Hittorf** (1824–1914) in 1869. These rays were named cathode rays by a German physicist, **Eugen Goldstein** (1850–1930), in 1880. **Sir William Crookes** (1832–1919) in 1879 postulated that these rays were composed of small particles. Cathode rays were demonstrated to consist of a stream of negatively charged particles by a French physicist, **Jean Baptiste Perrin** (1870–1942) from Lillie, who published his work on the subject *Comptes Rendus* in 1895. The ratio of the charge on a cathode particle to its mass was determined in 1897 by **Sir John Joseph**

Thomson (1856–1940) who first called these particles corpuscles, before they were renamed electrons. A Hungarianborn Nazi German physicist, **Phillip Anton Eduard Lenard** (1862–1947) studied the electrostatic properties of cathode rays and suggested that atoms contained units of both positive and negative charge. He was awarded the Nobel Prize for physics for this work, in 1905.

Cattle Breeding *See animal husbandry.*

Cauchy, Augustin Louis (1789–1857) A French mathematician who developed the scientific treatment of mathematical series which have an infinite number of terms. In 1805 he provided the solution to the problem of Apollonius, and generalized Euler's theorem on polyhedra in 1811. He contributed to the study of wave propagation, calculus and the mathematical theory of elasticity, in his completed works of 27 volumes.

Caulx, Salomen de (1576–1626) *See steam engine, water pump.*

Cavalieri, Bonaventura (1598–1647) A Jesuit priest and professor of mathematics at Bologna who studied under **Galilei Galileo** (1564–1642). He improved the idea of indivisibles proposed by **Johannes Kepler** (1571–1630). A theorem related to mensuration of solid bodies bears his name.

Cave [Latin: *cavus,* hollow] *See cave paintings, cave exploration.*

Cave Art *See cave paintings.*

Cave Exploration An important method for the study of geology, anthropology and prehistoric culture. The world's most extensive system of caves was found at the Mammoth Cave National Park, Kentucky in 1799. In 1859 a Welsh geologist, **Sir William Boyd Dawkins** (1837–1929) commenced his exploration of caves in Somerset and found evidence of early man and animals. His exploration in Derbyshire in 1875 led to the establishment of a succession of animal and human inhabitants, and he published *Cave Hunting; or, Caves and Early Inhabitants of Europe* (1874) and *Early Man in Britain* (1880). A British cave site, the Kent's Cavern, near Torquay, Devon, has provided the evidence for a culture belonging to the Lower Paleolithic period around 300 000 years ago. In 1947 a group of Bedouin travelers from the Ta'amire tribe, while exploring one of the most intricate system of caves in the north-east shore of the Dead Sea at 'Ain Feshka, in Jordan, found 40 tall sealed clay jars. Their contents revealed archaeological findings of great historic importance, the Dead Sea Scrolls. These scrolls were bought and investigated by Athanasius Yeshue Samuel of St Mark's

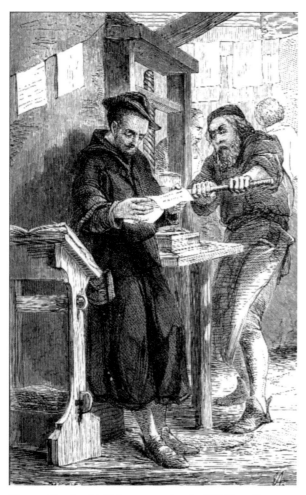

Figure 19 A mid-19th century sketch of William Caxton at his press. Fyfe, J. Hamilton. *Triumphs of Inventions and Discovery in Art and Science*. London: T. Nelson and Sons, 1878

Monastery in Old Jerusalem. They were flown to America in 1948 and were studied by William H. Brownlee and John C. Trevor. An American archaeologist and Biblical scholar, professor **William Foxell Albright** (1891–1971) of Johns Hopkins University identified them as very valuable Hebrew manuscripts dating to around 100 BC. Since then more scrolls have been recovered from other caves in the area.

Cavé, François (b 1794) *See machine tools.*

Cave Paintings The first expression of art by man, providing the earliest records of prehistoric cultures. Pictures of mammoths such as those found in the La Madeleine caves in France have revealed that early humans coexisted with species now extinct during prehistoric times. The drawing of a shaman wearing a deer mask over his face, found in a

cave at Les Trois Frères in France, is estimated to have been drawn about 39 000 years ago by Cro-Magnon man, the first humans of Europe. A bison wounded by arrows, painted about 10 000 years ago, is found at the archaeological site at Ariège in the south of France. The Altamira cave paintings by Cro-Magnon man in Spain were discovered by Maria Sautuola in 1879. A French archaeologist and pioneer of Paleolithic art, **Henri Edouard Prosper Breuil** (1877–1961), became interested in cave art in 1900, and discovered cave paintings at Combarelles and Dordogne. He published *Quatre cents siècles de l'art pariétal* (Four hundred centuries of cave art) in 1952.

Cavendish Experiment Performed by the English physicist and chemist **Henry Cavendish** (1731–1810) to calculate a mean value for the mass and density of the earth. It involved the measurement of the gravitational attraction between lead and gold spheres, using Isaac Newton's law of universal gravitation.

Cavendish Laboratory Established at Cambridge in 1874 and named after the English chemist, **Henry Cavendish** (1731–1810).

Cavendish Society Established in 1846, for the publication of research in chemistry, and named after the English chemist **Henry Cavendish** (1731–1810).

Cavendish, Charles, Lord (1703–1783) An English physicist who constructed the first maximum and minimum thermometer in 1757.

Cavendish, Henry (1731–1810) A nephew of the third Duke of Devonshire, and the eldest son of **Lord Charles Cavendish** (1703–1783). After inheriting substantial family wealth at the age of 40, he lived as a recluse devoting the rest of his life to research. He was the first to study hydrogen and gave it the name inflammable air in 1766. In 1783 he combined hydrogen and oxygen by means of an electric arc and demonstrated that water is a compound. His accuracy in measuring Newton's constant of gravitation and the density of the earth, in 1797, has not been surpassed by modern methods. *See acids, air, argon, Cavendish Laboratory, Cavendish Society, earth density, hydrogen, nitrogen, quantitative chemistry, water.*

Cavendish, Margaret The Duchess of Newcastle fought against prejudice and became the first woman member of the Royal Society in 1667. No other woman was admitted to the Royal Society until 1945.

Caventou, Joseph (1795–1878) *See chlorophyll, coffee plant.*

Caxton Society Established in the 18th century in order to publish literature of the Middle Ages. It published 16 volumes from 1844 to 1855.

Caxton, William (1412–1492) The first printer in England, from Kent, who spent some time during his youth in Europe, and learnt the new invention of printing in Flanders. In 1471 he printed his first book *Recuyell of the Historyes of Troye* which he translated from the French. He returned to England around 1472 and set up his press near Westminster Abbey. He printed the first three books in England entitled *The Game and Playe of the Chesse* (1474), *A boke of the hoole Lyf of Jason* (1475) and *The Dictes and Notable Wyse Sayenges of the Phylosophers* (1477).

Cayley, Arthur (1821–1895) An English mathematician from Richmond, Surrey, who graduated from Cambridge, where he later became the first Sadlerian professor of mathematics. He wrote nearly 300 papers on mathematics, which were collected and published in 13 volumes.

Cayley, Sir George (1771–1857) of Scarborough. A pioneer in the field of aviation who constructed the first heavier than air glider, from which he developed a man-carrying glider in 1853. He also invented a telescope, artificial limbs, caterpillar tractor and a tension wheel. The Regent Street Polytechnic in London was founded by him in 1839, and he sponsored the first meeting of the British Association for the Advancement of Science in York, in 1832. *See aerodynamics.*

Cech, Thomas (b 1947) *See ribonucleic acid.*

Celestial Mechanics A science dealing with motion and the position of objects in space. It is mainly governed by **Sir Isaac Newton's** (1642–1727) universal law of gravitation and **Johannes Kepler's** (1571–1630) laws of planetary motion.

Celestial Photography [Latin: *caelestis,* heaven] The first successful astronomical photograph, a daguerreotype of the moon, was taken by **William Cranch Bond** (1789–1859), an American watch maker from Portland, who turned his attention to astronomy. He built one of the first private observatories in America at his home and was commissioned by Harvard University to design a new observatory. He became the director of the Harvard Observatory and discovered the seventh satellite of Saturn, Hyperion, in 1848. Astronomical photography as a research tool was developed by his son **George Phillips Bond** (1825–1865) of Dorchester, Massachusetts. The first practical photographs of the Milky Way were taken in 1895 by an American astronomer, **Edward Emerson Barnard** (1857–1923) of Nashville, Tennessee. An English chemist from Derby, **Sir**

William de Wiveleslie (1844–1920), a pioneer in stellar photography, invented photographic plates that were sensitive to infrared light. The first photoheliographic telescope was invented by **Warren de la Rue** (1815–1889) of Guernsey. He took the first photograph of a solar eclipse with his device in 1860. A London astronomer, **Sir William Huggins** (1824–1910), was the first to use dry plate photography in astronomy, in 1876. An English amateur astronomer and a sanitary engineer, **Andrew Ainslie Common** (1841–1903) from Newcastle, was one of the first to apply photography to the study of nebulae, in 1881. The principle of cinematography in astronomy, a series of separate images taken in rapid succession mounted on a photographic plate, was first used in 1882 by a French astronomer, **Pierre Jules César Janssen** (1824–1907) of Paris. He published *Atlas de photographies solaires* in 1904. A German professor of astronomy in Heidelberg, **Maximilian Franz Joseph Cornelius Wolf** (1863–1932), invented a photographic method for discovering asteroids. The use of motion pictures for the study of certain aspects of astronomy was pioneered by an American astronomer, Edison Pettit (b 1890) from Nebraska. Photographic devices for studying the solar spectrum through a spectroheliograph were developed independently around 1891 by a French physicist and astronomer, **Henri Alexandres Deslandres** (1853–1948), and an American astronomer, **George Ellery Hale** (1868–1938). An astronomer, **Edward Charles Pickering** (1846–1919) of Boston, Massachusetts, did pioneer work on visual photometry and stellar photography and published the first *Photographic Map of the Entire Sky* in 1903. He also introduced the meridian photometer to measure the magnitude of stars. He worked with his brother **William Henry Pickering** (1858–1938) and produced over 300 000 photographic plates of stars for the photographic library at Harvard. A Swiss astronomer, **Wilhelm Becker** (b 1907), developed the three-color system where the brightness of stars is observed through three different color filters. This method helped to determine the distances between stars in a cluster. The modern faint object camera (FOC) and wide field planetary camera (WFPC) were developed during the 1990s.

Cell [Latin: *cella,* a small room] A term used by **Robert Hooke** (1635–1703) in his *Micrographia* (1665) to refer to the compartments that he noted in a cork under the microscope. The cell structure of plants was observed two decades later by **Marcello Malpighi** (1628–1694) and **Nehemiah Grew** (1641–1712). The nucleus was described by **Robert Brown** (1773–1858) in 1831, and the nucleolus by **Gabriel Gustav Valentine** (1810–1883) in 1836. The role of the nucleus in cell division and the formation of tissues was studied in 1838 by a German professor of botany at Jena, **Matthias Jacob Schleiden** (1804–1881). He published one of the first books on plant cytology *Grundzuge der Wissenschaftlichen Botanik* in 1842. The structure of specialized cells, such as nerve cells and smooth muscle cells, was studied by **Theodor Schwann** (1821–1902) in 1839. He coined the famous phrase *Omnis cellula e cellula* (every cell from a cell). Analysis of diseased tissue on the basis of cell formation and structure was performed by **Rudolph Virchow** (1821–1902) in his *Cellular Pathology,* published in 1858. The cell was defined as consisting of nucleated protoplasm in 1861 by **Max Johann Sigismund Schultz** (1825–1874), a professor of zoology at Bonn. The first electron-microscopic study, showing endoplasmic reticulum and mitochondria, was performed by an American cytologist of Belgian origin, **Albert Claude** (1898–1983) in 1945.

Cell Division First studied in 1838 by a German botanist, **Matthias Jacob Schleiden** (1804–1881) who proposed that new cells were budded off by the nucleus. **Rudolph Albert von Kolliker** (1871–1905) observed that the nucleus disappeared during cell division and reappeared in the daughter cells. A German botanist and professor at Bonn, **Eduard Adolf Strasburger** (1844–1912), studied the phenomenon in more detail and published *Cell Formation and Cell Division* (1875). Mitosis [Greek: *mitos*, thread], a process of nuclear division involving the longitudinal splitting of chromosomes in the cell, was described and named in 1882 by **Walther Flemming** (1843–1905). The different stages in mitosis – prophase, metaphase and anaphase – were described and named by Strasburger in 1884. In 1885, a German biologist and professor of zoology at the University of Freiburg, **August Friedrich Leopold Weismann** (1834–1914) of Frankfurt, distinguished between somatic cells and germ cells, and postulated that some form of reduction must occur during division in the germ cells (egg or sperm), in order to prevent the genetic material from doubling.

Cell Membrane Two English physiologists, **Hugh Davson** (b 1909) and **James Frederic Danielle** (1911–1984), studied the permeability of the cell membrane and published *Permeability of Natural Membranes* in 1942. Danielle did a detailed study of the structure of the cell membrane and demonstrated it to contain molecules of lipids and proteins. Researches in organic chemistry by a US chemist, **Charles Pedersen** (1904–1990), led to the understanding of metal ion transport across cell membranes in living organisms. He shared the Nobel Prize for chemistry in 1987 with **Donald James Cram** (b 1919), an American

chemist from Chester, Vermont, and a French chemist, **Jean Marie Lehn** (b 1939).

Cell Sap *See plant physiology.*

Cell Theory A term introduced by **Theodor Schwann** (1821–1902) in 1839. He also coined the phrase *Omnis cellula e cellula* (every cell from a cell). *See cell.*

Cellophane An artificial plastic material invented in 1908 by Jacques Brandenberger of Switzerland.

Celluloid First artificial plastic material prepared in 1868 by an American inventor, **John Wesley Hyatt** (1837–1920) of Starkey, New York, by adding camphor to cellulose nitrate. Hyatt's other inventions include: a knife sharpener, a water filter, a multiple-needle sewing machine and Hyatt billiard balls made of plastic. Celluloid was discovered independently by **Alexander Parkes** (1813–1890) of Birmingham in England earlier in 1862, but he failed to make it a commercial success. A Scottish electrical engineer, **Sir James Swinburne** (1858–1958), used a hard resin formed by phenol and formaldehyde to produce celluloid. He founded the Fireproof Celluloid Syndicate in 1904. An American chemist of Belgian origin, **Leo Hendrick Baekeland** (1863–1944) preceded him by one day with his discovery of the first synthetic phenolic resin.

Celluloid Photographic Film Invented by Hannibal W. Goodwin in 1887. *See camera, photography.*

Celsius, Anders (1704–1744) A Swedish astronomer, appointed to the chair of astronomy at Uppsala in 1730. He defined the boiling point of water as 100 degrees and the freezing point as 0 degrees in his paper entitled *Observationer om tvenne bestandiga grader par en Thermometer* (1742). The unit of temperature he defined was named the degree Celsius. *See thermometer.*

Cement The Egyptians used heated gypsum to build the pyramids. The Roman architect, **Marcus Pollio Vitruvius,** in AD 100 described a naturally-occurring siliceous material cement of volcanic origin, which was used in building. This material known as *pozzuolana* was rediscovered by an English engineer, **John Smeaton** (1724–1792) from Austhorpe, near Leeds, in 1756. An English bricklayer, **Joseph Aspdin** (1779–1855) of Leeds, produced a hydraulic cement (Portland cement) from clay and limestone, in 1824. **Canvass White** (1790–1834) of Whitesboro, New York, invented a new type of cement in 1820.

Cenozoic Period Geological era marking the emergence of mammals as a dominant group. It began 65 million years ago and is divided into the Tertiary and Quaternary periods.

Center of Gravity *See gravity.*

Central Heating *See heating.*

Centrifugal Force A force causing an object traveling in a curved path to move away from the center of curvature of its path. *See Clairaut Theorem, gyroscope.*

Centrifuge A machine to increase the force of gravity and speed up the rate of sedimentation, in order to separate and measure the size of small particles. It was introduced by a Swedish physical chemist, **Theodor Svedberg** (1884–1971) and J.B. Nichols in 1923. Svedberg was awarded the Nobel Prize for chemistry for his work on colloid chemistry, in 1926. Jesse W. Beams used this method first for separation of isotopes in 1935. A refrigerated centrifuge of great value in biochemistry was developed by an American immuno-chemist, **Michael Heidelberger** (1888–1991).

Centrosome [Latin: *centrum,* midpoint + Greek: *soma,* body] The term was introduced into genetics by a German biologist, **Theodor Boveri** (1862–1915). *See chromosomes.*

Cepheid Variables Stars which are used as known standard light sources for calculating distances, due to their regular fluctuation of brightness. They are named after their proto-type, *Delta Cephei,* the light variations of which were observed in 1784 by the English astronomer **John Goodricke** (1764–1786). Six were discovered in 1923 by an American astronomer, **Edwin Powell Hubble** (1889–1953) of Missouri. In 1914 **Harlow Shapley** (1885–1972) of Nashville, Missouri, used these stars to estimate distances. He served as director of the Harvard Observatory from 1921 to 1952. The relationship of its pulsation to brightness was discovered by the US astronomer **Henrietta Leavitt** (1868–1921).

Ceramics Porcelain, pottery and other products made by firing clay. *See porcelain.*

Ceres *See asteroids.*

Cerium A rare element of atomic number 58, discovered by a Swedish chemist, **Jons Jacob Berzelius** (1779–1848) in 1803. The German chemist, **Martin Heinrich Klaproth** (1743–1817) isolated cerium oxide in the same year.

CERN (*Conseil Européen pour la Recherche Nucléaire*) A nuclear research organization founded in 1954 in Switzerland by the European governments. It was subsequently renamed *Organisation Européenne pour la Recherche Nucléaire,* and houses the world's largest particle accelerator, and the Large Electron Positron Collider (LEP). *See cyclotron.*

Cesalpino, Andrea (1519–1603) An Italian physician and botanist from Arezzo, who became the professor of medicine and director of the botanical garden at Pisa in 1553. He proposed the theory of blood circulation, and classified plants for the first time on a scientific basis in his *De Plantis* (1583).

Cesaro Curves *See Cesaro, Ernesto.*

Cesaro, Ernesto (1859–1906) An Italian mathematician and professor of algebra at the University of Palermo in 1886–1891. In 1896 in his *Lezione di geometrica intrinsica* (Lessons in Intrinsic Geometry), he simplified the analytical expression and made it independent of extrinsic coordinate systems. He stressed the intrinsic qualities of the objects and described the curves that now bear his name.

Cesi, Duke Federigo (1585–1630) *See Accademia dei Lincei.*

Cesium [Latin: *caesius,* sky blue] Element with atomic number 55, discovered through spectroscopy by **Gustav Robert Kirchhoff** (1824–1887) and **Robert Bunsen** (1811–1899), in 1860.

Cesium Clock *See atomic clock.*

Ceulen, Ludolph van (1539–1610) *See pi.*

Ceva Theorem A theorem on concurrent straight lines through the vertices of a triangle. Proposed by an Italian mathematician, **Giovanni Ceva** (1647–1734) of Milan, in his *De Lineis rectis se invicem secantibus constructio statica* published in 1678. His brother, **Tommaso Ceva** (1648–1736), who was also a mathematician, published *Opuscula Mathematica,* in 1699.

Ceva, Giovanni (1647–1734) *See Ceva theorem.*

Ceva, Tommaso (1648–1736) *See Ceva theorem.*

Chabaneau, François (1754–1842) *See platinum.*

Chadwick, Roy (1893–1947) *See warplanes.*

Chadwick, Sir James (1891–1974) An English physicist, born near Macclesfield, who studied at Manchester, Berlin and Cambridge. He worked with **Lord Ernest Rutherford** (1871–1937), and in 1932 discovered a particle, similar to the proton, but with no charge on it, which was predicted in 1920 by Rutherford. Chadwick named the particle the neutron, and was awarded the Nobel Prize for physics in 1935. He published *Radiation from Radioactive Substances* (1930) with Rutherford, and built the first cyclotron in England at Liverpool, in 1935.

Chain, Sir Ernst Boris (1906–1979) German-born British biochemist. *See Fleming, Alexander, Florey, Howard Walter.*

Chain Reaction The first man-made nuclear chain reaction occurred on 2 December 1942. It resulted from an atomic pile of uranium prepared by an American nuclear scientist, **Frank Harold Spedding** (1902–1984) of Hamilton, Ontario, and his co-workers in the Manhattan Project at the University of Chicago. Their work formed the basis for Fermi's atomic pile.

Challenger One of the first ships of the British Admiralty to be assigned, in 1872, to conduct an oceanic exploration of unprecedented nature. It contained six naturalists under a Scottish marine biologist, **Sir Charles Wyville Thomson** (1830–1882), and became the first ship to cross the Antarctic Circle. It had sounding, dredging and other appliances for studying deep water, and brought back a vast collection of specimens. A preliminary account of the expedition *The Voyage of the Challenger – the Atlantic* was published in 1877 by Thomson.

Challis, James (1803–1882) *See Neptune.*

Chalmers, James (1782–1853) *See postal service.*

Chamberlain, Owen (b 1920) *See antiproton.*

Chamberlin, Thomas Chrowder (1843–1928) A professor of geology at Chicago who did fundamental work on the geology of the solar system. His publications exceeded 250 in number, and included *The Origin of the Earth* (1916), *Two Solar Families* (1928) and *Sun's Children* (1928). *See Chamberlin–Moulton hypothesis, Ice Age.*

Chamberlin–Moulton Hypothesis An alternative explanation to nebular hypothesis proposed by two American astrophysicists, **Thomas Chrowder Chamberlin** (1843–1928) and **Forest Moulton** (1872–1952).

Chambers Dictionary *See Chambers, Ephraim.*

Chambers, Ephraim (1680–1740) A British encyclopedist from Kendal who published the first edition of *A Cyclopedia, or Universal Dictionary of Arts and Sciences*, in 1728.

Chambers, Sir William (1726–1796) *See architecture, British; Kew Gardens.*

Chamisso, Adelbert von (1781–1838) A Franco-German poet and biologist who discovered and wrote about metagenesis, a peculiar lifecycle that he found in certain species of mollusks, in his work *On certain animals of the Linnean class Vermes* (1819). He is famous for his story *Peter Schlemihls wundersame Geschichte* (Peter Schlemihl's Remarkable Story).

Champollion, Jean François (1790–1832) *See hieroglyphics, Rosetta stone.*

Chance Process Modified Leblanc process where sulfur is recovered. It was invented by an industrial chemist from Birmingham, **Alexander Macomb Chance** (1844–1917).

Chance, Alexander Macomb (1844–1917) *See Chance process.*

Chance, Britton (b 1913) An American biochemist from Wilkes-Barre, Pennsylvania who demonstrated the enzyme–substrate complex in catalytic reactions, in 1946.

Chances *See probability theory.*

Chandler, Seth Carlo (1846–1913) An American astronomer from Boston who devised a telegraphic code for transmitting astronomical information. In 1884 he invented an instrument for relating the positions of the stars to a small circle at the zenith.

Chandrasekhar, Subrahmanyan (1910–1995) An eminent astrophysicist born in Lahore, India. He graduated from the Presidency College Madras and went to Cambridge, England for further studies. In 1936 he emigrated to America and worked at the University of Chicago. He proposed a theory to explain the fact that massive stars are unable to evolve into white dwarfs. The limiting stellar mass (about 1.4 solar masses) is known as the Chandrasekhar limit). He shared the Nobel Prize for physics with **William Alfred Fowler** (1911–1995), in 1983.

Chang Ssu-Hsün (c. AD 950) *See clock.*

Channel Cable The first successful submarine cross-channel cable link from Dover to Calais was established in 1851 by an English engineer, **Thomas Russell Crampton** (1816–1888).

Channel Crossing A private steam paddle ship *Rob Roy* and three British post office ships started operating in 1820 from Dover, England, to Calais in France. The London South Eastern Railway started a service between London and Folkstone in 1844, and London to Dover in 1845. In 1856 over 120 000 passengers crossed through Folkstone compared to 70 000 through Dover. The latter port became a more popular seaport for Channel crossing with the establishment of the London, Chatham and Dover Railway in 1861. The Jenkins and Churchman company started operating the *Prince Fredrick Williams* which made the Dover to Calais crossing in a record time of 83 minutes. The *Invicta* made a crossing in 72 minutes in 1882. *See Channel flight, Channel tunnel.*

Channel Flight   The first crossing of the English Channel by air was achieved in a balloon by an American physician from Boston, **John Jeffries** (1744–1819) who emigrated to England. A Frenchman, **Louis Blériot** (1872–1936) made the first cross-Channel plane flight from Baraques to Dover in his monoplane in 1909. A London pioneer of automobile engineering, **Charles Stewart Rolls** (1877–1910), made the first non-stop double crossing in 1910. He lost his life later that year in a plane crash.

Channel Tunnel   A French engineer, Albert Mathieu-Favier, submitted a plan for a Channel tunnel to Napoleon Bonaparte in 1802. In it he proposed simultaneous boring of two tunnels from England and France to meet at an artificial island in the Channel to allow for a change of horses. Although Napoleon appreciated his plan, it was not pursued. A tunnel in the form of an immersed tube was proposed by Tessier de Mottray in 1803, but he lacked the technology to execute such a task. A mining engineer, **A. Thomé de Gamond** (1807–1876) undertook geological and hydrographic studies for establishing a Channel tunnel. In 1834 he proposed a tunnel in the form of a tube but found no support for his project. Two years later he proposed an elaborate bridging system with a huge floating platform as a meeting point for bridges from both sides. In 1856 he designed a concrete tunnel of 34 kilometers, wide enough to carry two rail tracks. The French Commission for Scientific Research was assigned by Napoleon to investigate its feasibility. Several other plans by various French engineers followed, but none were practical. An English mining and railway engineer from Leeds, **John Hawkshaw** (1811–1891), studied the project and proposed a single-bore tunnel. His associate, **William Low** (1818–1886), suggested two single-track tunnels. Work on the project by the French Channel Company was sanctioned by the French government in 1875, and around the same time Hawkshaw's Channel Tunnel Company commenced work at St Margaret's Bay in England. An English statesman, **Sir Edward Watkin** (1819–1901) promoted the tunnel in England and negotiated the project with the French. He was responsible for most of the attempts to establish the tunnel until military objections stopped the project. The Channel Tunnel Defence Committee set up in 1882 by the War Office with Sir Archibald Alison reported the tunnel to be a danger to national security. Further legislative attempts for the tunnel were made in 1906 and 1913, and 22 attempts in the British Parliament took place from 1919 to 1922. Interest in the project waxed and waned for the next 50 years until the present Eurotunnel project began in 1987.

Chapman, David Leonard (1869–1958) *See Chapman–Jouguet Layer.*

Chapman, Sydney (1888–1979)   An English physical chemist from Lancashire who served as Sedeleian professor of natural philosophy (1946–1953) at Oxford. He proposed the first satisfactory theory for magnetic storms and identified a lunar atmospheric tide. He developed the theory of thermal diffusion.

Chapman–Jouguet Layer   A region behind a detonation wave in the study of explosion velocities in gases, proposed independently by an English physical chemist, **David Leonard Chapman** (1869–1958) of Norfolk and Emile Jouguet.

Chappe, Claude (1763–1805) *See semaphore.*

Chaptal, Jean Antoine Claude Chanteloup (1756–1832) *See industrial chemistry, nitrogen.*

Chardonnet, Hilaire Bernigaud Compte de (1839–1924)   A pupil of **Louis Pasteur** (1822–1895) during the time he was investigating silkworm disease. Inspired by the work of Pasteur on the subject, Chardonnet invented the process of making artificial silk in 1884. He also experimented on the effect of ultraviolet light on organisms. He invented an actinograph used for measuring solar radiation in aviation.

Chargaff, Erwin (b 1905) *See deoxyribonucleic acid.*

Charles' Law   The volume of a gas is proportional to its absolute temperature at a given constant pressure. It was proposed by **Jacques Alexandre César Charles** (1746–1823), a professor of physics at Paris in 1787. The law was discovered independently by **John Dalton** (1766–844) and **Joseph Louis Gay-Lussac** (1778–1850).

Charles, Jacques Alexandre César (1746–1823)   A professor of physics at Paris who preceded Gay-Lussac in proposing the law of expansion of gases in 1787, but failed to publish his findings. He successfully ascended the Champs de Mars in his hydrogen balloon in 1783. *See air balloon, Charles' law.*

Charney, Jule Gregory (1917–1981) *See meteorology, sand dunes.*

Charpak, Georges (b 1924)   A Polish-born French physicist who developed particle detectors, which revolutionized the study of high-energy physics. Before his invention, time-consuming bubble and spark chambers were used.

Charpentier, Johann von (1786–1855) *See Ice Age.*

Chasles, Michel (1793–1880) *See projective geometry.*

Chassepot, Antoine Alphonse (1833–1905) *See firearms.*

Chatelier, Henry Louis le (1850–1936) *See law of chemical equilibrium.*

Chatlet-Lomont, Gabrielle Emille (1706–1749) A French mathematician and physicist who, after her marriage to Compte du Chatlet-Lomont in 1725, became the mistress to the French author François Marie Arouet de Voltaire (1694–1778). She considered heat and light to be different forms of motion and published *Institutions de physique* (1740) and *Dissertation sur la nature et la propagation du feu* (1744). She produced the first French translation of Newton's *Principia*.

Chatt, Joseph (b 1914) An eminent English inorganic chemist from Durham, who classified metal atoms according to their bonding characteristics, and studied the phenomenon of nitrogen fixation in plants. His work provided a plausible mechanism for the nitrogenase reaction.

Chaucer, Geoffrey (1340–1400) An English poet and author of the *Canterbury Tales* and several other works. He wrote the earliest treatise on science in England entitled *Tractus Conclusonibus Astralabi* on the occasion of his presentation of an astrolabe to his ten-year-old son.

Chebyshev, Pafnuty Lvovich (1821–1894) A Russian mathematician and a professor at St Petersburg from 1860 to 1882. He proposed a theory of prime numbers and developed a method of approximating functions by polynomials. *See prime numbers.*

Chemical Structure A term coined in 1861 by a Russian chemist, **Alexandr Mikhailovich Butlerov** (1828–1886).

Chemical Symbols Alchemists under the influence of Chaldean astrology thought that the special properties of elements or metals were related to the planets, and used planetary signs to denote them. Silver was represented by the sign of the Moon, and lead was represented by Saturn. The modern use of chemical symbols to denote various elements in chemistry was introduced by a Swedish chemist, **Jons Jacob Berzelius** (1779–1848) in 1811. He used the first Latin letter for an element. If more than one element had the same first letter, the second letter (*cuprum* = Cu for copper, *aurum* = Au for gold, *natrium* = Na for sodium) was added.

Chemistry [Greek: *chymos*, juice] The original term *chemia* is supposed to have represented the dark soil of the Nile Valley. It was first used in AD 400 by the Alexandrian chemists to refer to activity related to the changing of matter. The first book of chemistry, apart from the beliefs of alchemy, was published by a German physician and chemist, **Andreas Libavius** or **Libau** (1540–1616) of Halle. His *Alchemia* (1597) described for the first time: stannic chloride under the name *spiritus fumans libavia*; a preparation of hydrated crystals of sugar; production of wine by fermentation and distillation. The next textbook on chemistry, dissociated from alchemy, entitled *Tyrocinium chymicum* (1610), was published by Jean Beguin of France. His work was followed by that of a Flemish physician, **Johannes Baptista Van Helmont** (1577–1644), who first described the properties of a gas and gave it the present name. The field of chemistry was further developed by a German chemist and physician, **John Rudolph Glauber** (1604–1668). He refined the method of distillation, and studied the reactions of the three main mineral acids. His work *Opera Omnia* first appeared in seven volumes in Amsterdam in 1658. The calcination of metals on exposure to air was demonstrated by Jean Rey, a physician from Paris, in the early 16th century. The principles of physics were first applied to gases by **Robert Boyle** (1627–1691), around 1662. **Joseph Priestley** (1733–1804), a clergyman and chemist from Leeds, made several discoveries in the field of chemistry and established it as a science in England. By obtaining pure oxygen through heating of a metal oxide, he helped to disprove the phlogiston theory, which had been held for over a century. The compound of chlorine and hydrogen, first known as muriatic acid, was discovered by Priestley in 1772. The first clear textbook of chemistry *Cours de Chemie* (1675) was written by a French physician and chemist, **Nicolas Lemery** (1645–1715), and it had run into 31 editions by 1756. The first systematic chemical dictionary *Dictionaire de Chyme* (1766) was published by a French chemist, **Pierre Joseph Macquer** (1718–1784) of Paris. The study of chemistry on modern lines was established in Europe by **Antoine Laurent Lavoisier** (1743–1794) of Paris. He defined an element as 'a substance that cannot be split up into a simpler form by any means' and investigated the dephlogisticated air previously described by Priestley. The use of chemical symbols in chemistry was introduced in 1811 by **Jons Jacob Berzelius** (1779–1848). **Thomas Graham** (1805–1869) established the field of colloid chemistry around 1857. **Michael Faraday** (1791–1867) was the first to liquefy carbon dioxide by using atmospheric pressure, and he condensed chlorine into a liquid, in 1823. The field of industrial chemistry was established by **Justus von Liebig** (1803–1873) of Germany. A method of determining vapor density was discovered in 1823 by **John Baptiste André Dumas** (1800–1884), a French apothecary at Geneva. The first major advance in organic chemistry was made by the German chemist, **Friedreich Wöhler** (1800–1882), who synthesized the organic compound urea from the inorganic salts, potassium cyanate and ammonium sulfate for the first time, in 1829. **Pierre-Eugène Marcellin Berthelot** (1827–1907) of Paris, produced benzene and naphthalene in 1851. The six-carbon ring structure for benzene was proposed by **Friedrich August Kekulé von Stradonitz** (1829–1896), in 1865. *See analytical chemistry, biochemistry, physical chemistry, quantitative chemistry.*

Chepman, Walter (1473–1538) *See printing.*

Cherenkov Effect Blue light emission from water caused by bombardment by gamma rays at a speed in excess of that of light. First observed in 1934 by a Soviet physicist, **Pavel Alekseyevich Cherenkov** (1904–1990). In 1937, two Soviet physicists, **Ilya Mikhailovich Frank** (1908–1990) of St Petersburg and **Igor Yevgenyevich Tamm** (1895–1971), explained it on the basis of emission of radiation related to the speed of charged particles. For their work, Cherenkov, Frank and Tamm shared the Nobel Prize for physics in 1958.

Cherenkov, Pavel Alekseyevich (1904–1990) *See Cherenkov effect.*

Chernobyl Nuclear Accident Catastrophic accidental release of radioactivity at Chernobyl, near Kiev, in the USSR on 26 April 1986. The incident, which led to 31 deaths, was initially thought to be localized and 135,000 were permanently evacuated. Subsequent studies have revealed that the radioactivity from the reactor had spread to many areas of Europe including Scotland and Northern Ireland. Another Chernobyl reactor was closed in 1991 after a fire.

Cherwell, Lord Frederick Alexander Lindemann or **Viscount** (1886–1957) *See aerodynamics, quantum theory, thermodynamics.*

Chevreul, Michel Eugene (1786–1889) A French chemist from Angers who is regarded as the father of fatty acids owing to his research on margarine, olein, stearin and other fatty acids. In 1823 he discovered that fat was composed of fatty acids and glycerol. He described one of the earliest known sterols, cholesterol, in 1815. His theory of saponification formed the basis for the use of fatty acids in many industries.

Chevrolet, Louis (1879–1941) A Swiss-born US automobile designer and pioneer of motor racing. The Chevrolet Motor Company founded by him in 1911, was later sold and incorporated into General Motors in 1916.

Chi-Square Test *See statistics.*

Child, Charles Manning (1869–1954) An American zoologist who proposed the gradient theory for regeneration, where the process occurs along the axis of the body in graded physiological stages.

Childe, Vere Gordon (1892–1957) *See prehistory.*

Childs, Borlase George (1816–1888) *See helmet.*

Chiron An unusual object orbiting between Saturn and Uranus within the solar system. It was discovered in 1977 by US astronomer Charles T Kowal (b 1940). Initially thought to be an asteroid, it is now believed to be a giant comet composed of ice with a dark crust of carbon dust.

Chittenden, Russel Henry (1856–1943) *See nutrition.*

Chladni, Ernest Florens Friedrich (1756–1827) A German physicist and musical performer, from Wittenberg, who is regarded as one of the founders of the science of acoustics. He discovered the longitudinal vibrations in a string and studied the vibration of plates in relation to their shape and weight. He published *Traité d'acoustique* in 1809.

Chlorine [Greek: *chloros*, pale green] The first of the halogens to be discovered by **Karl Wilhelm Scheele** (1742–1786) in 1774. Its bleaching action was discovered in 1785 by **Claude Louis Comte de Berthollet** (1748–1822). **Sir Humphry Davy** (1778–1829) gave it its present name in 1810. **Michael Faraday** (1791–1867) condensed the gas into liquid in 1823.

Chloroform Discovered independently, by Eugene Soubeiran of France, **Justus von Liebig** (1803–1873) of Germany, and **Samuel Guthrie** (1782–1848) from Bloomfield, Massachusetts, around in 1831. **Jean Baptiste André Dumas** (1800–1884) gave its present name in 1834. The surgeon **James Y. Simpson** (1811–1870) used it as an anaesthetic agent in 1847.

Chlorophyll [Greek: *chloros*, pale green + *phyll*, leaf] A green pigment found in leaves, first extracted using olive oil, by an English botanist and physician, **Nehemiah Grew** (1641–1712), in 1682. A clergyman and chemist from Leeds, **Joseph Priestley** (1733–1804), in 1774, and a Dutch physician, **Jan Ingenhousz** (1730–1799), in 1779, independently noted that plants which contained the pigment gave off oxygen when exposed to sunlight. Two French alkaloid chemists, **Joseph Caventou** (1795–1878) and **Pierre Pelletier** (1788–1842) named the green substance, chlorophyll, in 1817. **Julius von Sachs** (1832–1897), a professor of botany at Würzburg, proposed that the green pigment was not diffusely present in the plant tissues, but contained in special bodies. These bodies were identified and named chloroplasts by **Andreas Franz Wilhelm Schimper** (1856–1901) of Basel, in 1883. The importance of sunlight for the activity of these chloroplasts was pointed out by Sachs in 1865. The structure of chlorophyll and its components were discovered in 1905 by a German organic chemist, **Richard Willstätter** (1872–1942) from Karlsruhe. He was awarded the Nobel Prize for chemistry for his discovery in 1915. A US chemist of Russian origin, **Melvin Calvin** (1911–1997), worked out the biosynthetic pathway involved in photosynthesis, with the use of radioactive carbon tracers. He was awarded the Nobel Prize for chemistry in 1961, while he was professor of chemistry at the University of California. The first synthesis of chlorophyll was achieved in 1961 by a Boston organic chemist, **Robert Burns Woodward** (1917–1979). He was awarded the Nobel Prize for chemistry for synthesis of many biochemicals, in 1965.

Chloroplasts Structures containing chlorophyll in the leaves of plants, first described in 1865 by **Julius von Sachs** (1832–1897). They were identified, and named chloroplasts, by **Andreas Franz Wilhelm Schimper** (1856–1901) of Basel, in 1883. In 1882 a German physiologist, **T.W. Engelmann** (1843–1909), demonstrated the light reaction which occurred within the chloroplasts. A detailed study of the light reaction in isolated chloroplasts was carried out in 1937 by an English biochemist, **Robert Hill** (1899–1991).

Chordata [Greek: *chorde*, cord] Animals with a notochord [Greek: *noton*, back]. They were classified under the phylum chordata, by a lecturer on animal morphology, **Francis Maitland Balfour** (1851–1882) of Edinburgh in his *Treatise on Comparative Embryology* (1880).

Christ College, **Cambridge** Founded by Margaret, Countess of Richmond in 1506.

Christian Era A monk, the **Venerable Bede** (673–735) from Jarrow, in the north of England, was the first to establish the date of the birth of Christ as a landmark in history. It is noted by the abbreviation, AD for *Anno Domini* (the year of the Lord).

Christie, Samuel Hunter (1784–1865) *See electrical resistance.*

Christie, Sir William (b 1845) of Woolwich. The eighth Astronomer Royal to hold the post since 1675. He was educated at King's College, London before his graduation from Cambridge and was appointed to the position of Astronomer Royal at the Greenwich Observatory in 1881.

Christoffel, Elwin Bruno (1829–1900) A German mathematician who in 1869 introduced into the theory of invariants what are now known as the Christoffel symbols. His

paper on the propagation of plane waves in media with a surface discontinuity in 1877 was one of the earliest contributions to shock-wave theory.

Christofori, Bartolommeo (1655–1731) *See piano.*

Chromatography [Greek: *chroma*, color + *graphein*, to write] Its principle based on capillary action was suggested in 1850 by a German physician and industrial chemist, **Friedlib Ferdinand Runge** (1795–1867) in his third volume of Farbenchemie. The method was first studied by **Christian Friedrich Schönbein** (1799–1868), in 1861. An American chemist **David Talbot Day** (1859–1925) of East Rockport, Ohio, independently discovered the concept during his research on petroleum products. The technique was developed and named by a Russian botanist and organic chemist, **Mikhail Semenovich Tswett** (1872–1919), who used it for separating the plant pigments, carotenoids, in 1906. In 1942 two British biochemists, **Archer John Porter Martin** (b 1910) and **Richard Laurence Millington Synge** (1914–1994) of Liverpool, revived the method by using filter paper for separating amino acids. In 1950 an American biochemist, **Stanford Moore** (1913–1982) from Chicago, and a New York biochemist, **William Howard Stein** (1911–1980), invented a method of column chromatography, for identification of amino acids derived by hydrolysis from proteins. The three American biochemists, Stein, Stanford and Moore, and **Boehmer Christian Anfinsen** (1916–1995) shared the Nobel Prize for chemistry in 1972, for their work on chromatography.

Chromium [Greek: *chroma*, color] First described in 1762 by a German physician and a metallurgist, Johann Lehmann, at the Berezov mine, in Ekaterinberg. It was isolated in 1797 by a French analytical chemist, **Louis Nicholas Vauquelin** (1763–1829) of Normandy. A French chemist and physician, **Antoine François Fourcroy** (1755–1809) suggested its present name. The German chemist **Martin Heinrich Klaproth** (1743–1817) isolated it independently.

Chromolithography *See color printing.*

Chromosomes [Greek: *chroma*, color + *soma*, body] The concept of a material in the cell capable of transferring hereditary characters, the germplasm, was proposed by a German zoologist, **August Friedrich Leopold Weismann** (1834–1914). He published *Das Keimplasm* (1892) and several other works on the subject. The material was discovered (1875) and named chromatin (1879), by a German biologist, **Walther Flemming** (1843–1905) of Sachsenberg. The bodies responsible for transfer of heredity characters were recognized by a German physiologist, **Wilhelm Roux**

(1850–1924) of Halle, in 1883. A German histologist, **Wilhelm Waldeyer-Hartz** (1836–1921), named them chromosomes, in 1888. **Theodor Boveri** (1862–1915) and **Walter Stanborough Sutton** (1877–1916) independently pointed out the individuality of the chromosomes in 1890s. The modern theory of chromosomes was initiated by D.H. Wenrich who, in 1902, observed the paired occurrence of maternal and paternal chromosomes, and the linear arrangement of centromeres within the chromosome. Two American cytologists, **T.H. Montgomery** (1873–1912) and W.S. Sutton independently observed that chromosomes could be individually recognized from cell to cell by their size and shape. **Clarence Ervin McClung** (1870–1946), an American cytologist, suggested that the X or accessory chromosome was associated with sex characteristics. An American geneticist **Alfred Henry Sturtevant** (1891–1970) of Jacksonville, Illinois, produced the first chromosome map of sex-linked genes in 1911 and published a *History of Genetics* in 1965. In 1956 Joe Hin Tjio and **Albert Levan** (b 1905) showed the number of chromosomes in humans to be 46.

Chronoscope [Greek: *chronos*, time + *skopein*, look] An instrument to measure small intervals of time, invented in 1840 by **Sir Charles Wheatstone** (1801–1875). His principle was later applied to calculation of the velocity of projectiles. An improved chronoscope was constructed in 1844 by a French physicist, **Claude Servias Matthias Pouillet** (1790–1868).

Chrysler, Walter Percy (1875–1940) An American automobile manufacturer from Wamego, Kansas, who designed the first high compression engine, and introduced the Plymouth motor car. His company became the Chrysler Corporation in 1925.

Chubb, Charles (1777–1846) *See lock.*

Chubb, John (1816–1872) *See lock.*

Chuquet, Nicolas (1445–1500) *See mathematical symbols.*

Church, Alonso (b 1903) A US professor of mathematics and philosophy at Princeton who in 1936 proved that there were no algorithms for a class of quite elementary arithmetical questions. His work contained the first precise definition of a calculable function, and contributed greatly to the systematic development of the theory of algorithms.

Church, William (1778–1863) *See typography.*

Cidenas (*c.* 343 BC) *See equinox.*

Cierva, Juan de la (1895–1936) *See autogyro.*

Cinema The illusion of continuous movements was demonstrated in 1824 before the Royal Society by Peter Roget, who projected still pictures at a rate of 24 per second. The next movie-picture device was invented in 1826 by an English scientist, Henry Fitton. His *Thaumatrophical Amusement* was made up of a number of discs of pictures, which when rotated gave the impression of a moving image. A similar device but with a mirror, the *Phenakistiscope*, was designed in 1833 by a Belgian physicist, **Joseph Antoine Ferdinand Plateau** (1801–1883). A slightly more advanced *Zoetrope*, which consisted of a drum with pictures, was invented in 1860 by Pierre Desvignes of Paris. In 1877 Emile Regnaud of Paris invented the *Praxinoscope*, which showed a series of images reflected by a system of mirrors. Around the same time, an English photographer, Edward Muggeridge, while researching in America on locomotion in animals, took rapid pictures in succession with a series of cameras and viewed them through the Zoetrope. The earliest moving outlines were filmed in 1885 in New York by **Louis Aimé Augustin Le Prince** (1842–1890). The first moving projection of an actual event on a screen was achieved by an English inventor from Bristol, **William Friese-Greene** (1855–1921), in 1888. He invented a camera that could take ten photographs per second on a roll of sensitized paper. Over the next few years he developed and patented several cameras and projectors. **Thomas Alva Edison** (1847–1931) developed a motion picture machine that recorded pictures in a spiral on a cylinder. In 1889 **George Eastman** (1854–1932) of Waterville, New York, improved it with his invention of roll film. The first public viewing of movie pictures in Europe was given in Paris in 1895 by two French chemists and brothers, **Louis Jean Lumière** (1864–1948) and **Auguste Marie Louis Lumière** (1862–1954). They produced the first ever movie *La Sortie des ouvriers de l'usine Lumière* in the same year. Their first public film show in England in London was held in 1896. They developed a two-in-one machine consisting of a camera and a projector, and named it a cinematograph. The first commercial viewing of motion pictures was held at Holland Brothers Kinetoscope Parlor, in New York, in 1894. The kinetoscope used for this show was developed by **William Kennedy Laurie Dickson** (1860–1935), who was an assistant to Thomas Edison. The first building or cinema designed for the purpose of showing films was erected in Atlanta, Georgia, in 1895. Around this time two Americans, Thomas Armat and Woodville Latham invented a successful movie projector. The first attempt at talking pictures was made by a French inventor, **Leon Ernest Gaumont** (1864–1946), who synchronized pictures with a phonograph in 1901. He succeeded in demonstrating the first talking pictures at the

Académie des Sciences in Paris in 1910. He was also the first to introduce colored cinema films with the use of the three-color separation method and special lenses. **Eugene Augustin Lauste** (1857–1935) independently developed a method for sound in motion pictures and patented it in 1906. Recording of sound on film was refined by an American radio engineer, **Lee De Forest** (1873–1961) in 1922. The first public show of a talking motion picture was held at the Alhambra Cinema in Berlin in the same year. The technique of color photography in motion pictures was developed in 1914 by **Fredrick Eugene Ives** (1856–1937), an American inventor from Connecticut. The Technicolor color system was invented by another American, Herbert T. Kalmus. The largest cinema in the world, the Radio City Music Hall in New York City, opened in 1932. *CinemaScope*, which filled a wide screen, was invented by Henri Chrétien of France. A new wide-screen system was invented in 1955 by Brien O'Brien. *See cartoons, Cinerama, kinetoscope, zooprax-iscope.*

Cinemascope *See cinema.*

Cinematograph *See cinema.*

Cinerama Developed by Fred Walter in 1952. His system consisted of three cameras adjacent to each other which could film a circumferential area.

Circle The Greek philosopher, **Anaxagorus** (*c.* 500–428 BC) of Clazomenae, in Asia Minor, was the first to mention the ancient problem of squaring the circle, which involves constructing a square exactly equal in area to a given circle. **Hippocrates of Chios** (*c.* 460 BC), who was the first to write systematically on geometry, tried to square the circle. **Hippias of Elis** (*c.* 425 BC) invented a curve, quad-ratrix, to be used for squaring a circle. A celebrated mathematician from Aberdeen, **James Gregory** (1638–1675), published an original work on the hyperbola and the circle. The sign π is used for the ratio of circumference to the diameter of the circle.

Circumferentor *See surveying.*

Circumnavigation The first circumnavigation around the globe, by sea, was completed in 1522 by a Basque navigator, **Juan Sebastian del Cano** (d 1526). A German aeronautical engineer, **Hugo Eckener** (1868–1964) was the first to circumnavigate the world in an airship, the *Graf Zeppelin*, in 1929.

Cities *See towns.*

Citric Acid Cycle *See Krebs cycle.*

Citroën, André Gustav (1878–1935) A French motor manufacturer in Paris who pioneered the production of small low-priced cars.

Civil Engineering The term civil engineer was first used by a British engineer of Scottish descent, **John Smeaton** (1724–1792) from Austhorpe, near Leeds. He was a charter member of the first professional engineering society, the Society of Civil Engineers, founded in 1771. This later became the Smeatonian Society. École des Ponts et Chaussées, the first school in the world devoted to civil engineering for bridges and highways, was established in Paris in 1747. An eminent French engineer, **Bernard Forest de Belidor** (1698–1761), in his *Architecture Hydraulique* (1737–1753) dealt with many aspects of civil engineering such as transportation, water supply, fountains and pumps. The Institute of Civil Engineers of England was founded in 1818, with the Scottish engineer, **Thomas Telford** (1757–1834), as its first president.

Clairaut Theorem Relates the gravity on the surface of a rotating ellipsoid to the compression and centrifugal force at the equator. It was proposed by a French mathematician, **Alexis Claude Clairaut** (1713–1765). He predicted the return of Halley's comet in 1759.

Clairaut, Alexis Claude (1713–1765) *See Clairaut theorem.*

Claisen Condensation A group of condensation reactions in which esters are formed from acetates under the control of catalysts such as sodium ethoxide. Discovered by a German chemist, **Ludwig Claisen** (1851–1930) of Cologne.

Claisen, Ludwig (1851–1930) *See Claisen condensation.*

Clapeyron, Benoit Paul Emile (1799–1864), a French physicist born in Paris and educated at the École Polytechnique. He advanced **Sadi Carnot's** (1796–1831) work on thermodynamics in relation to the efficiency of heat engines.

Clark, William Mansfield (1884–1964) *See acidity.*

Clarke, Arthur Charles (b 1917) A science fiction writer from Minehead in Somerset. While he was a radar instructor in the Second World War he originated the idea of satellite communication. He also predicted some of the other major advancements in science and his *The Sentinel* (1951) was filmed as *2001: A Space Odyssey* (1968). He emigrated to Sri Lanka in 1956. *See space travel.*

Clarke, Frank Wigglesworth (1847–1931) An eminent American geochemist born in Boston and educated at Harvard. He was the first to present a theory for the chemical evolution of geological systems. His publications include

Data of Geochemistry (1908) and *The Composition of Earth's Crust* (1924).

Clarke, William Branwhite (1798–1878) *See gold.*

Classification of Animals Aristotle in his *Historia Animalium* used morphology or appearance, for classification of animals into groups and subgroups. In his treatise *On the Generation of Animals* he described the characteristics of viviparous and oviparous animals. His group *inanima* (bloodless animals) resembled the current group of invertebrates. He stated that all sanguinous animals (animals with blood) have a backbone, thus referring to vertebrates. *See Linnaeus, Carolus, taxonomy.*

Classification of Plants *See botanical classification, Linnaeus, Carolus, taxonomy.*

Claude, Albert (1898–1983) *See cell, electron microscope, mitochondrion.*

Claude, Georges (1870–1960) *See acetylene, neon lighting.*

Clausius, Rudolf Julius Emmanuel (1822–1888) A professor of physics at Bonn, and contemporary of **James Prescott Joule** (1818–1889). He proposed the second law of thermodynamics, which states that it is impossible to devise an engine which, working in a cycle, will convert heat from a hot body entirely into work. He also proposed a theory of electrolysis and calculated the mean speed of gas molecules in terms of pressure, in 1857.

Clavius, Christoph (1537–1612) *See calendar.*

Clayton, John (*c.* 1650) *See gas lighting.*

Clegg, Samuel (1781–1861) An engineer from Manchester who invented several systems used in the gas industry. As a chief engineer of the Charted Gas Company he illuminated the entire district of London with gas for the first time in 1814.

Clement, Joseph (1779–1844) *See machine tools.*

Clement, Nicolas (1779–1841) *See carbon monoxide, specific heat.*

Clepsydra *See waterclock.*

Clerk, Sir Dugald (1854–1932) *See internal combustion engine.*

Clerke, Agnes Mary (1842–1907) of County Cork. One of the few prominent women in the field of astronomy in the 19th century. She published several books including *Problems in Astrophysics* (1903), *The System of Stars* (1890), *Modern*

Cosmogenies (1905) and *A Popular History of Astronomy in the Nineteenth Century* (1885).

Cleve, Per Teodor (1840–1905) A Swedish chemist and geologist who developed a method for identifying the age of glacial and postglacial deposits from the diatom fossils found in them. *See holmium*

Clifford, William Kingdon (1845–1879) A mathematician from Exeter who became professor of mathematics at the University of London in 1871. His concept of the relationship between space, matter and gravity anticipated Einstein's theory of relativity. His work was cut short when he died of tuberculosis at the age of 33. His *Common Sense of the Exact Sciences* was completed after his death by his colleague, **Karl Pearson** (1857–1936) of Coldharbour, Surrey, in 1885.

Climatic Zones A Greek philosopher, **Parmenides of Elea** (*c.* 500 BC), was the first to divide the earth on the basis of its climate. **Aristotle** (384–322 BC) named the region between the tropics torrid, and the region between the tropics and Arctic circle temperate. **Posidonius** (*c.* 400 BC) divided the earth into seven climatic zones. **Polybius** of Megalopolis (204–122 BC), defined six zones, two beneath the Arctic circles, two between the Arctic circle and the tropics, and another two between the tropics and the equator. *See climatology.*

Climatology [Greek: *klino,* slope + *logy,* discourse] Study of wind, temperature, rain, humidity and other factors. Probably one of the oldest sciences; early man studied it during gathering and hunting, and later for agriculture. **Hippocrates** (460–377 BC) first studied it in relation to health. The study of climate in the past, in relation to geology, was established in the 19th century. A Scottish geologist, **James Croll** (1821–1890) published *Climate and Time* (1875) and *Discussions on Climate and Cosmology* (1886). Modern work in the field was done by a German-born US climatologist, **Helmut Eric Landberg** (1906–1985) who published *The World Survey of Climatology* in 14 volumes. *See meteorology, weather forecast.*

Clock The first device used for measuring time, a stick, struck upright on horizontal ground, was invented by **Anaximander** (611–545 BC), a pupil of **Thales** (640–546 BC). It was later developed into the sundial, a more advanced device for interpreting the movement of the shadow in relation to time. Several versions of sundials have been found in the remains of Pompeii and Tusculum. The *clepsydra* or waterclock was invented in Rome by Scipio Nascia in 158 BC. **Ctesibius** used toothed wheels to improve the device around 140 BC. The earliest clock in existence since AD 760 was owned by Pope Paul I, who later presented it to the King of France. One of the earliest mechanical clocks with an escapement mechanism was built by a Buddhist monk, **I-Hsing** (682–727) and Liang in China in 725. Their clock was the first Chinese clock to strike hours and half hours. An Archdeacon of Genoa, Pacificus, constructed a clock in AD 900. A chain drive for a mechanical clock was invented by **Chang Ssu-Hsün** of China in 976. The construction of a more elaborate and accurate armillary clock was commenced by Su Sung (1020–1101) on the order of the emperor in 1086. On completion, he wrote a detailed monograph on its construction and mechanism, in 1094. The mechanical clocks driven by weights preceded the invention of the pendulum. Elaborate mechanisms were employed in medieval cathedrals to erect clocks; one of the earliest clocks in England was installed at Canterbury Cathedral in 1292. A professor of astronomy at Padua and a physician, **Giovanni de Dondi** (1318–1389), took 18 years to construct an astronomical clock in the library of Pavia. In addition to hours and days it showed the movements of the sun, moon and planets. One of the oldest working clocks in the world, at Salisbury Cathedral in Wiltshire, England has ticked more than 500 million times since 1386. A chiming clock was erected at Westminster in 1368. Prior to the invention of portable clocks, mariners and other travelers had to depend on the astrolabe and hour glass. The pendulum was applied to the clock by **Galilei Galileo** (1564–1642) in 1639, and sundials were used until the pendulum clock was established in 1666 by a Dutch mathematician and scientist, **Christian Huygens** (1629–1695). Clocks were equipped with minute-hands for the first time in 1680. The deadbeat escapement mechanism for clocks was invented in 1710 by a London watch maker, **George Graham** (1673–1751) from Cumberland. Graham also invented the mercurial pendulum which eliminated the error due to the expansion of the metal rod. The hairspring, which replaced the function of the pendulum in controlling the stopping and starting of the escapement wheel, was invented by **Robert Hooke** (1635–1703). The great Westminster clock was completed in 1859. In 1761 **John Harrison** (1692–1776) of Foulby, Yorkshire, built the first modern English chronometer which only lost less than half a minute a month. Harrison also constructed one of the first marine chronometers, *Number One*, in 1735. Considerable refinements to the clock were made by another Englishman, **Thomas Earnshaw** (1749–1829) in 1782. *See astronomical clock, atomic clock, candle clock, escapement, pendulum, quartz clock, waterclock.*

Cloning [Greek: *klon*, twig] Asexual production of an individual from a cell with preservation of the same genetic characters. An American molecular biologist, **Gerald Meyer Rubin** (b 1950) of Boston, introduced specific cloned genes into the germ line of the fruit fly, and produced the first transgenic fruit fly. Allan Wilson of the University of California at Berkeley was the first to clone genes from an extinct species, in 1984. He used the skin of a quagga, which had been extinct for a hundred years. The first successful cloning using keratinized skin cells of adult frogs was published by an English geneticist, **John Bertrand Gurdon** (b 1933) of Hampshire, R.A. Laskey and O.R. Reeves, in 1975. In 1989, R.S. Prather and M.M. Simms published the details of the first piglet clone after nuclear transfer. The production of a sheep clone *Dolly*, from an adult somatic cell was achieved in 1996 by Edinburgh-based Ian T. Wilmut, A.K. Schnieke and colleagues. Dolly was naturally mated with a Welsh Mountain ram in 1997 and gave normal birth to a lamb on 13th April 1998. The first transgenic lamb *Polly* was cloned from a fetal cell, after introduction of a specific human gene, by the scientists at the Roslin Institute in Scotland in 1997. This opened the doors to the possibility of using cloned animals in the treatment of human disease. Following the first move by the US president Bill Clinton to ban human cloning, 19 members of the Council of Europe signed a document outlawing human cloning in 1998.

Cloth Woven in Anatolia (now part of Turkey) around 7000 BC. The oldest samples are from the city of Catal Hüyük. *See textile industry.*

Clothing Probably first used for keeping warm. Ingenious experiments were carried out in 1792, with the help of a thermometer, on how clothing preserves the body temperature, by **Benjamin Thompson** or **Count Rumford** (1753–1814).

Clothing Industry *See artificial silk, textile industry, Velcro, zip fastener.*

Cloud Chamber A chamber with strongly saturated water vapor for visualizing tracks of nuclear particles, invented in 1897 by a Scottish scientist, **Charles Thompson Rees Wilson** (1869–1959) from Glencorse, near Edinburgh. He served as the professor of natural philosophy at Cambridge from 1925 to 1934. He shared the Nobel Prize for physics, for his discovery, with **Arthur Holly Compton** (1892–1962), in 1927. The cloud chamber was further developed in 1930 by two American physicists, **Carl David Anderson** (1905–1991) of New York, and **Robert Andrews Millikan** (1868–1953) of Illinois.

Clouds The first treatise on the classification of clouds was published by a London weather diarist, Luke Howard, in 1803. The charge on raindrops from thunder clouds was first determined in 1899 by two German physicists, **Johann Phillip Julius Elster** (1854–1920) and **Hans Friedrich Geital** (1855–1923). **Sir Basil John Mason** (b 1923), the first professor of cloud physics to be appointed (1961) in England, at Imperial College, published a classic *The Physics of Cloud* (1957). A Swedish meteorologist, **Harold Percival Bergeron** (1891–1977), proposed the theory that rain is initiated by the coexistence of ice crystals and water vapor in clouds. *See artificial rain.*

Clowes, William (1779–1847) *See printing.*

Clowes, William (1807–1883) *See printing.*

Clüvier, Philip (1580–1622) *See geography.*

Coaches [Old German: *Gutsche,* couch or sofa] The oldest carriages used by ladies in England around the 15th century were called *whirlicotes,* and they were first seen in Spain in 1546. Fitz-Allen, the Earl of Arundel, introduced a light coach from Germany into England around 1580. By 1605 they were common in England, and were let for hire. They were known as hackney coaches. They became so common that by 1635, King Charles I had to issue an order limiting their numbers. They were introduced into Edinburgh in 1673. Omnibuses, a common form of transport in several cities, evolved from coaches and were first established in Paris in 1827. The first omnibus from Paddington to the Bank of England was started by **George Shillibeer** (1797–1866) in 1825. It had about 12 passengers attended by a footman or conductor and was in operation until 1829. By 1840 the total number of omnibuses in London reached 900. Omnibuses appeared in Amsterdam in 1839. A Scottish engineer from Glasgow, **John Scott Russell** (1808–1882), built steam coaches for roads and started a service between Paisley and Glasgow in 1834.

Coal This has been dug up in Europe for over 2000 years, since the Bronze Age. **Abraham Darby** (1678–1717) of Dudley, Worcestershire, was the first to find a way of obtaining coke by heating coal. In 1868 an English engineer, James Anderton, invented a steam-powered wheel-cutter for cutting coal. *See coal gas.*

Coal Gas A mixture of methane, hydrogen and carbon monoxide. The natural gas from wells was used in China as early as 900 BC. The Chinese started using coal instead of wood, for making cast iron, in AD 300. An English scientist, **John Clayton** (*c.* 1650), discovered that gas could be produced from crude coal, and stored. Coal gas was introduced for illumination by **William Murdoch** (1754–1839) of Ayrshire, who first used it in 1792 to illuminate his house at Redruth, Cornwall. Coal gas was first used on a large scale for illumination by Boulton & Watt of Soho, Birmingham, in 1798. **Samuel Clegg** (1781–1861) from Manchester, while he was a chief engineer of the Charted Gas Company, illuminated the entire district of London with gas for the first time in 1814. A London engineer, **Emerson Joseph Dowson** (b 1844) invented a method of producing coal gas for use in a gas-engine in 1879.

Coanda, Henri (1886–1972) *See jet engine.*

Cobalt Derived from *kobold,* a term for goblin, used by the miners of Saxony. The fumes of cobalt arsenite or smaltite were observed by miners in the 16th century. It was known as mundic in Cornwall, and was isolated by a Swedish chemist, **Georg Brandt** (1694–1768), in 1733.

Cochran, Jacqueline (1910–1980) *See supersonic flight.*

Cockcroft, Sir John Douglas (1897–1967) *See cyclotron.*

Cocker, Edward (1631–1677) A London mathematician and school teacher who wrote the first English work on commercial mathematics, entitled *Arithmetik, being Plain and Easy Method,* in 1678.

Cockerell, Christopher Sydney (1910–1999) *See hovercraft.*

Cockerill, William (1759–1832) *See textile industry.*

Coddington Lens A glass sphere with an equatorial groove to overcome the marginal indistinctness caused by spherical aberration. First suggested by **Sir David Brewster** (1781–1868) in 1820, and constructed by an English mathematician, **Henry Coddington** (1800–1845), in 1830.

Coddington, Henry (1800–1845) *See Coddington lens.*

Codon A term to denote a unit of three nucleotides which codes for one amino acid, proposed by a South-African born British molecular biochemist, **Sydney Brenner** (b 1927). In 1961 he discovered the codes for 20 amino acids.

Cody, Samuel Franklin (1861–1913) *See airplane.*

Coffee Plant An Italian botanist and a physician, **Prospero Alpini** (1533–1617), was the first to describe the coffee plant in Europe. A German chemist, **Friedlieb Ferdinand Runge** (1795–1867), obtained the alkaloid caffeine from its seeds in 1820. This was obtained in a pure form in 1822 by **Joseph Caventou** (1795–1878), who was professor of pharmacy at Paris.

Coherer A device that made wireless telegraphy possible by detecting radio waves from a distant transmitter. It was invented by Professor **Edouard Eugène Désiré Branly** (1844–1940) of Catholic University, in Paris. It consisted of a small glass tube of free iron filings which cohered and formed a conductor, when electromagnetic waves were passed through it. *See wireless telegraphy.*

Coke A form of charcoal obtained first by the Chinese in the 3rd century by heating coal to high temperature in the absence of air. It is used chiefly in steel making for fuelling blast furnaces. *See coal.*

Colbert, Edwin Harris (b 1905) *See tectonic theory.*

Colbert, Jean-Baptiste (1619–1683) *See Académie Royale des Sciences.*

Colding, Ludvig August (1815–1888) *See mechanical equivalent of heat.*

Colin, Jean Jacques (1784–1865) *See dyes.*

Collins, Michael (b 1930) *See astronauts.*

Collip, Bertram James (1892–1965) *See insulin.*

Colloid Chemistry [Greek: *colla,* glue + *oeidos,* form] **Thomas Graham** (1805–1869), the founder of colloid chemistry, was the first to distinguish crystalloids from colloids on the basis of diffusion, in 1857. He named the substances that passed through parchment paper, crystalloids, and those that did not pass through, as colloids. A German physical chemist, **Georg Bredig** (1868–1944), devised a method of preparing a colloidal solution or lyophobic sol, in 1898. The application of colloid chemistry to industry was pioneered by a German-born US chemist, **Herbert Max Finlay Freundlich** (1880–1941).

Colomella, Lucius Junius Moderatus (*c.* AD 100) *See agriculture.*

Color Photography Invented in 1861 by the Scottish physicist, **James Clerk Maxwell** (1831–1879). Under his instructions, Thomas Sutton, the inventor of the reflex camera, took three separate pictures with red, blue and green filters, and superimposed the transparent positives, with the aid of a magic lantern, with the same color filters. This laborious method was improved by a Frenchman, **Lois Duclos de Hauron** (1837–1920), who outlined the principles of additive and subtractive color reproduction in his *Les Couleurs en photographie* (1869). The process was refined in 1873 by a German chemist, **Hermann Wilhelm Vogel** (1834–1898) of Berlin. Vogel's orthochromatic plate contained silver bromide, which could be selectively sensitized by certain dyes when exposed to light of a specific wavelength. In 1891 **Fredrick Eugene Ives** (1856–1937), an American inventor from Litchfield, Connecticut, invented a photochromoscope that took pictures in rapid succession, using color filters. When viewed through an instrument called a *Kromscop,* these pictures merged to give full color. In 1893 **Gabriel Jonas Lippmann** (1845–1921) of Paris, developed a technique based on the interference phenomenon, for which he was awarded the Nobel Prize for physics in 1908. In 1904 two French chemists and brothers, **Louis Jean Lumière** (1864–1948) and **Auguste Marie Louis Lumière** (1862–1954), developed a single-plate system for color transparency, called autochrome. They developed a method of color printing with the use of starch, in 1907. The technique of color photography in motion pictures was pioneered by **Fredrick Eugene Ives** (1856–1937), in 1914. The first successful system, Kodachrome, was invented in 1935 by two Americans, Leopold Godowsky and Leopold Mannes.

Color Printing The Chinese used colored paper money to overcome the problem of counterfeiting in AD 1107. The use of colored ink in printing was pioneered in Europe by **Peter Schoeffer** (1425–1502) and **Johann Fust** (d 1466), around 1460. A three-color printing process was invented by Jacob Christoph Le Bon of Germany in 1710. *See color photography.*

Color Television Developed in 1940 at the laboratories of the Colombia Broadcasting System in America by a Hungarian inventor, **Peter Carl Goldmark** (1906–1977) from Budapest. His system was first used for an experimental transmission in New York. A Swedish electrical engineer, **Ernst Frederick Werner Alexanderson** (1878–1975) perfected a complete television system in 1930 and produced a successful color television receiver in 1955. A Russian-born US broadcasting pioneer, **David Sarnoff** (1891–1971), an early promoter of television broadcasting during the 1940s, was the first to manufacture color sets and transmit color programs in the 1950s. *See television.*

Colosseum Largest amphitheater in the world, capable of holding 80 000 spectators, until the construction of the Yale Bowl in 1914. It was built in Rome in AD 75 by the Emperor Titus Flavius Vespasian (d AD 79). *See theater.*

Columbus, Christopher (1442–1506) The European discoverer of America was a son of a weaver in Genoa. His nautical knowledge was attained through his marriage to a daughter of a naval commander in Lisbon. His study of cosmography caused him to believe in the existence of another continent beyond the Atlantic Ocean, and his subsequent journeys led to the discovery of the New World.

Colt Revolver Invented in 1836 by **Samuel Colt** (1814–1862), an American chemist and inventor from Hartford, Connecticut. It was first used during the Mexican war (1846–1848).

Colt, Samuel (1814–1862) An American chemist and inventor from Hartford, Connecticut, who patented the Colt revolver in 1834. He developed other firearms, and by 1855 he owned the largest private armory in the world. He also established a submarine telegraph between New York and Coney Island, in 1843.

Comet [Greek: *kometes,* star] The earliest record of a comet sighting was by the Chinese in 2296 BC. An English astronomer from Shoreditch, **Edmund Halley** (1656–1742), studied the parabolic orbit ascribed to comets by **Sir Isaac Newton** (1642–1727), and applied it to a comet which he observed in 1682. The same comet had been observed previously by a German astronomer, **Peter Apian** (1495–1552) in 1531, and by **Johannes Kepler** (1571–1630) in 1607. Halley noted that this comet had made similar appearances in 1456, 1380 and 1305, and predicted its reappearance in 1759. After its reappearance as predicted, following a 75 year interval, it was sighted again in 1835 and named Halley's comet. A method for calculating the orbits of comets was devised by a German physician and astronomer, **Heinrich Wilhelm Matthaus Olbers** (1758–1840). In 1819, another German astronomer, **Johann Franz Encke** (1791–1865), investigated a comet that first appeared in 1786. This comet, having the shortest period of return, is named after him. A French astronomer, **Jean Louis Pons** (1761–1831), discovered 37 comets between 1801 and 1827. An Italian astronomer, **Giovanni Battista Donati** (1826–1873) of Pisa, was the first to observe the spectrum of a comet, and the comet he observed in 1858 bears his name. The association between certain showers and comets was described by a British astronomer from Somerset, **William Frederick Denning** (1848–1931), who discovered five comets and some nebulae. A watch maker from Portland, **William Cranch Bond** (1789–1859), who turned to astronomy, built one of the first private observatories in America at his home and made many discoveries including 17 new comets. An Italian astronomer, **Giovanni Virginio Schiaparelli** (1835–1910) from Savigliano, Piedmont, discovered the association between comets and meteorites. The solar wind, a continuous stream of high-speed particles from the sun, which serve as a driving force behind the tails of comets, was predicted in 1951 by a

German astronomer, **Ludwig Bierman** (1907–1986), and confirmed later by the Russian space probes. In 1950, an American astronomer, **Fred Lawrence Whipple** (b 1906) of Red Oak, Iowa, explained the behavior of comets on the basis that they consisted of ice and dust.

Commercial Arithmetic *See accountancy.*

Common, Andrew Ainslie (1841–1903) *See celestial photography.*

Communication Systems *See broadcasting, facsimile machine, Internet, radar, radio telephone, telephone exchange, television, wireless telegraphy.*

Communication Technology *See electric telegraphy, facsimile machine, flag signaling, heliograph, Morse code, radar, radio, satellite, semaphore, telephone, television, wireless telegraphy.*

Compact Disc or CD. First produced in 1979 by collaboration between the Japanese company Sony and Phillips of Holland, and launched in 1982.

Comparative Anatomy A term introduced by an English botanist and physician, **Nehemiah Grew** (1641–1712) in his *Comparative Anatomy of Trunks* (1675). He published *Comparative Anatomy of the Stomach and Guts* in 1681. An early comparative study of the structure of vertebrate animals was done by a Belgian biologist, **Gerard Blaes** (1646–1682), who published *Anatome Animalium* (1681). **Pierre Belon** (1517–1574), a medical graduate from Paris, wrote one of the first books on comparative anatomy entitled the *History of Birds.*

Compass (1) The magnetic attraction of the lodestone for iron was known to the ancients. A compass needle, pivoted on a card, or floated on water, was used in the 12th century. The use of a magnetic compass for navigation was first suggested by a Chinese scientist, **Shen Kua** (1031–1095), in 1086. The earliest treatise on the compass, *Epistola de Magnete* was written in 1269 by **Peter Peregrinus** (b *c.* 1220), a friend of **Roger Bacon** (*c.* 1214–*c* 1298). The first Arabic treatise on the magnetic needle as a ship's compass was written by **Baylak al-Qibaji** (*c.* 1350) of Cairo. The variation of compass needle with time and place was described by **Henry Gellibrand** (1597–1636) in his treatise *A Discourse Mathematical on the Variation of the Magnetic Needle, together with its admirable Diminution lately discovered* (1635).

Compass (2) The term for an instrument that is used for dividing into ratios. It was known to the inhabitants of Pompeii. **Leonardo da Vinci** (1452–1519) used an adjustable compass for calculation in 1500.

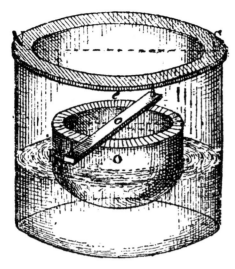

Figure 20   Floating compass of Peregrinus. Benjamin, Park. *The Intellectual Rise of Electricity*. London: Longmans, Green, & Co, 1895

Complex Number   A number written in the form a + ib, where a and b are real numbers and i is the square root of −1. A French mathematician, **Abraham de Moivre** (1667–1754) proposed a fundamental law on complex numbers which is known as de Moivre theorem. *See Argand diagram.*

Compound Microscope   Consists of several convergent lenses with one having a short focal length. The first compound microscope was probably invented by Zacharias Jansen, a spectacle maker from Middelburg, Holland, around 1590. His microscope consisted of a double convex lens for an object-piece, and a concave eye-piece. A Dutch lens maker, **Hans Lippershey** (1571–1619), independently devised a compound microscope in 1609. **Galilei Galileo** (1564–1642) was one of the first to apply the compound microscope to scientific studies. The first description of the compound microscope was given by **Robert Hooke** (1635–1703), who constructed a special microscope in 1665. Hooke's instrument had a single hemispherical lens as an object glass, and a plane convex lens for the eye-piece.

Compton Effect   A phenomenon in which electromagnetic waves such as X-rays undergo an increase in wavelength after having been scattered by electrons. It was described by an American physicist, **Arthur Holly Compton** (1892–1962) of Wooster, Ohio, who was awarded the Nobel Prize for physics for his above work, with **Charles Thomson Rees Wilson** (1869–1959), in 1927.

Compton, Arthur Holly (1892–1962)   *See cloud chamber, Compton effect, gamma rays, photoelectricity, photons.*

Computerized Axial Tomography   *See CAT scanner.*

Computer Bug   The term was first coined in 1945 by an American computer pioneer, **Grace Murray Hopper** (1906–1992), to refer to unexplained computer failures. She identified the first such failure caused by a moth that had infiltrated the circuits. She helped to invent COBOL (Computer Business Oriented Language) in 1959.

Computer Graphics   Pioneer work on the application of computer graphics to engineering was done by a German-born US scientist, **Bertram Heroz** (b 1929). He joined the Ford Motor Company in 1963, and developed the application of computer graphics to the automobile industry.

Computer Virus   A term for malignant computer program which can spread from computer to computer, usually via shared software and internet, causing damage to programs stored on the computers.

Computers   Two Frenchmen, J. Abraham and E. Bloch, were the first to apply electricity to the working of a calculating machine, in 1912. The first generation electronic calculating machines was invented in 1919 by two English scientists, W.H. Eccles and F.W. Jordan. A more accurate calculating machine or a differential analyzer was built by an American electrical engineer, **Vannevar Bush** (1890–1974) and his colleagues at the Massachusetts Institute of Technology in 1927. The IBM mark 7 machine, a large electronic machine consisting of 800 cables, was built in 1937 by an American mathematician, **Howard Hathaway Aikin** (1900–1973) of Hoboken, New Jersey. In 1938 two Americans, David Packard (1912–1996) and William R. Hewlett (b 1913) started their computer production in a garage, and expanded it to form the Hewlett–Packard computer company. The precise mathematical characterization of the intuitive concept of computability was proposed by a London mathematician, **Alan Mathison Turing** (1912–1954). He proposed the Turing Machine in his paper *On Computable Numbers* (1936), while he was at Princeton University in the USA. In theory, it was a logical machine capable of calculating any calculable number. A paper entitled *A Symbolic Analysis of Relay and Switching Circuits* (1938) by an American mathematician, **Claude Elwood Shannon** (b 1916) of Michigan, played an important role in the development of computing. He wrote *Mathematical Theory of Communications* in 1949. The first programmable electronic computer based on the concept of the Turing machine was formulated by **Max H.A. Newman** (1897–1985) and it was built by T. H. Flowers at Bletchley Park, Buckinghamshire, in 1943. It was succeeded by a more advanced computer, the Electronic Numerical Integrator and Computer (ENIAC), built by two American engineers, **John William Mauchly** (1907–1980) and **John Presper Eckert** (1919–1995) at the University of Pennsylvania. It was one of the first modern computers, weighing 30 tons and containing 18 000 vacuum tubes. ENIAC ran its first computer program on H bomb simulation for the scientists at Los Alamos, in 1945. An early paper Preliminary Discussion of the Logical Design of an Electronic Computing Instrument (1946) was jointly published by three American computer scientists, **Johann von Neumann** (1903–1957) of Hungarian origin, **Herman Heine Goldstine** (b 1913) of Chicago and **Arthur Walter Burks** (b 1915) of Minnesota. One of the earliest British electronic computers, EDSAC (Electronic Delay Storage Automatic Calculator), was built by an English mathematician, **Maurice Vincent Wilkes** (b 1913) from Dudley, and his team at Cambridge, around 1947. The EDSAC II was introduced in 1957. The first successful electrostatic random access memory (RAM) for a digital computer, using cathode-ray tubes, was built in 1946 by an electrical engineer, **Sir Frederic Calland Williams** (1911–1977) of Cheshire. A Shanghai-born US computer engineer, **An Wang** (1920–1990), invented the magnetic core memory which preceded the microchip. In 1951 he founded the Wang Laboratories in Boston, Massachusetts, and introduced a desktop computer named LOCI in 1956. The first magnetic core store or memory for an electronic digital computer was built in 1949 by an American engineer, **Jay Wright Forrester** (b 1918) of Nebraska. The first stored-program computer called the *Manchester University Mark I* was programmed by **Tom Kilburn** (b 1921) of Dewsbury, while he was at Manchester University, in 1948. He developed the storage device for the world's first electronic random access memory. The first microchip containing several transistors was invented by an American, **Jack Saint Clair Kilby** (b 1923) of Texas Instruments, in 1958. The integrated circuit, a system of interconnecting transistors on a single silicon chip, contributing to the development of microcomputers, was invented in 1959 by a US engineer, **Robert Norton Noyce** (1927–1990) of Iowa. The concept of the integrated circuit was first proposed by **Geoffry W.A. Dummer** (b 1909), in 1952. **Gilbert Hyatt** (b 1938) of Micro Computer Inc. at Van Nuys, Los Angeles, devised a single-chip microcomputer, in 1968. M.E. Hoff of Intel Corporation produced a microprocessor chip in 1969. **Kenneth Harry Olsen** (b 1926) of Bridgeport, Connecticut, established the Digital Equipment Corporation (DEC) in 1956, and launched the first successful minicomputer, PDP-8, in the early 1960s. The Virtual Address Extension (VAX) superminicomputers were designed by an American computer engineer, **Chester Gordon Bell** (b 1934). The

first voice-operated computer system that could interpret speech and answer in a synthetic voice was invented by two Americans, Thomas Martins and R.B. Cox in 1973, and it was built by the British company EMI in 1975. One of the world's fastest supercomputers, Cray I, was developed in 1976 by **Seymour R. Cray** (1925–1996) of Wisconsin. The Apple computer company was founded by **Steven Jobs** (b 1955) of San Francisco in 1976. His first successful personal computer, the Apple II in 1977 brought about a revolution in personal computers. His company introduced the first disk drive for personal computers in 1978. The first personal computer with a built-in hard drive, the PC-XT, was produced by IBM in 1983. The first 32-bit chip processor (developed from the Intel 80386) was fitted into a computer at the Compaq Company in 1986. The microcomputer language BASIC (Beginners All-purpose Symbolic Instruction Code), was developed in 1964. An American computer software scientist, **Henry William Gates** (b 1955) with another computer programmer, Paul Allen, founded the Microsoft Corporation at Redmond, Washington, in 1976. They launched the operating system, Windows, in 1981. *See calculating machines.*

Concave Diffraction Grating The use of a concave metal or glass grating eliminated the need for lenses in spectroscopy, and produced more accuracy. It was developed by an American physicist, **Henry Augustus Rowland** (1848–1901) of Homesdale, Pennsylvania. He became professor of physics at the Johns Hopkins University in Baltimore, in 1876.

Concave Lenses Came into use about two centuries after the introduction of convex lenses, in the mid-15th century. They were first used in spectacle making in AD 1500. *See spectacles.*

Conchology [Greek: *kongche*, shell + *logos*, discourse] Study of shells in relation to their origin. **James Sowerby** (1757–1822) commenced *The Mineral Conchology of Great Britain* in 1812, and it was completed in 1845, by his son, **James de Carle Sowerby** (1787–1871). An Italian geologist, **Brocchi** (1772–1826), studied the Miocene and Pliocene strata of Italy, and published *Conchiologia Fossile Subapennina* (1814).

Concrete The Romans developed concrete for building around 100 BC. Modern concrete was invented by a French civil engineer, **Louis Joseph Vicat** (1786–1861) of Nevers. Ferroconcrete or reinforced concrete was first used extensively in the building industry by a French structural engineer, **François Hennebique** (1842–1921). By 1910 over 40 000 important structures had been built using his method. Another French engineer, Eugène Freysinnet (1879–1962) pioneered the use of prestressed concrete and demonstrated the full structural potential of reinforced concrete with his innovative designs.

Condenser A device used in the steam engine for condensation of steam in order to improve the efficiency. The principle of a separate condenser which kept the engine permanently hot was invented by **Joseph Black** (1728–1799) and John Anderson in 1765. Its application to the steam engine was developed by a pioneer of the steam engine, **James Watt** (1736–1819).

Condon, Edward Uhler (1902–1974) *See alpha particles.*

Condorcet, Marie Jean Antoine Nicolas de Caritat (1743–1794) A French mathematician and scientific biographer who wrote five volumes of biographies of famous scientists and published *Essai sur le calcul integral* (1765).

Conduction Defined by **James Clerk Maxwell** (1831–1879) as a process whereby the hotter body loses heat and the colder body receives heat by means of a change occurring in the intervening medium, which does not itself become hot.

Conductivity A London physician, **Sir William Watson** (1715–1787) was one of the first to experiment on the conductivity of electricity through a rarefied gas. An Englishman, **Stephen Gray** (1666–1736), distinguished between conductors and non-conductors, in 1729. The law stating that the ratio of thermal conductivity of a pure metal to its electrical conductivity is proportional to the absolute temperature, was proposed by **G. Wiedemann** (1826–1899). **Paul Drude** (1863–1906), a professor of physics at Leipzig (1894) and Giessen (1900) assumed the conductivity of metal to be due to free electrons. A new theory of statics related to thermal and electrical conductivity of metals was developed by a German physicist from Königsberg, **Arnold Johannes Wilhelm Sommerfeld** (1868–1951). In 1911 a Dutch physicist, **Heike Kamerlingh-Onnes** (1853–1926), unexpectedly observed that the resistance of mercury disappeared when it was cooled below a certain temperature. His finding led to the discovery of superconductivity. *See superconductivity.*

Conductor The term was first used by **John Theophile Desaguliers** (1683–1749) of La Rochelle, France, in his *Dissertation on Electricity*. Desaguliers came to London with his father who was a clergyman, and became professor of philosophy at Oxford in 1710. He published several other treatises including *A Course of Experimental Philosophy* and a treatise on building chimneys that prevented smoke.

Confucianism Philosophy of social justice and harmony proposed by **K'ung Fu-Tze** (552–479 BC) whose Latinized name was **Confucius**.

Congreve, William (1772–1828) *See military engineering.*

Conical Refraction The phenomenon was correctly predicted in 1827 by an Irish mathematician, **Sir William Rowan Hamilton** (1805–1865) of Dublin, in his work on optics. It was described independently by a German mathematician, **Carl Gustav Jacob Jacobi** (1804–1851) of Potsdam, around 1829. He was also a pioneer in the study of elliptical functions and published *Fundamenta nova theoriae functionum ellipticarum* (1829).

Conics Study of curves formed by a plane intersecting a cone. A pupil of Eudoxus and a Greek mathematician, **Menaechmus** (375–325 BC), showed how to obtain an ellipse, a parabola and a hyperbola as sections of a cone. **Euclid** (*c.* 300 BC) wrote a treatise on conic sections in four books. His work was superseded by that of the Alexandrian mathematician, **Apollonius of Perga** (260–200 BC), whose work is extant. A Flemish mathematician, **Gregorius de Saint Vincent** (1584–1667), in his *Opus Geometricum* (1647) included methods for finding areas under curves, and established the relationship between the hyperbola and logarithms. His work anticipated the integral calculus developed by **Sir Isaac Newton** (1642–1727) and **Gottfried Wilhelm Leibniz** (1646–1716). **Blaise Pascal** (1623–1662) presented an essay on conics, *Essai Pour les Coniques* (1639), at the age of 16.

Conservation of Energy *See heat.*

Conservation of Mass The indestructibility of matter was known to **Democritus** more than 2000 years ago. In 520 BC, a Greek philosopher, **Parmenides**, born at a seaport, Elea, in Italy, proposed that change is illusory and nothing can be created or destroyed. **Antoine Laurent Lavoisier** (1743–1794) demonstrated this through his chemical experiments, in 1782. The theory that no change of weight or mass occurred in any chemical reaction was proposed in 1908 by a professor of physical chemistry at Berlin, **Hans Heinrich Landolt** (1831–1910). His experiments with a higher degree of accurate results helped to prove the law of conservation of mass.

Constellation A group of stars forming an identifiable area in the sky. *See stars.*

Contact Lenses The original idea of covering the cornea with a protective shell was suggested by **Leonardo da Vinci** (1452–1519). **René Descartes** (1596–1650) and an English physician, **Thomas Young** (1773–1829), made similar suggestions. In 1827 an English astronomer, **Sir John Fredrick William Herschel** (1792–1871), investigated the possibility of using a gelatinous transparent shell over the cornea, to protect it from disease of the eyelids. There was a lack of interest on the subject for the next 60 years until 1887, when Saemisch of Germany approached a glass blower and maker of artificial eyes, F.A. Muller, to make a thin glass shell suitable to be placed over the cornea for his own use. Muller made the lens as requested, and Saemisch used it for the next 20 years. In 1892 Muller made another lens for a physician, Fraenkel, who had his eyesight affected as a result of the disease called trachoma. The term contact lens (*Kontakbrille*), was introduced in 1887 by A. Eugen Fick, a physician in Zurich, who started investigating the contact lens as a refractive device. He also made several contact lenses through **Ernest Abbe** (1840–1905), an associate of Carl Zeiss.

Continental Drift *See tectonic theory.*

Convection Defined by **James Clerk Maxwell** (1831–1879), as a motion of the hot body itself carrying its heat with it.

Convex Lens Made of rock crystal dating back to 700 BC, these were found in the ruins of Nimrud near Mosul in Iraq by **Sir Austen Henry Layard** (1817–1894). **Sir David Brewster** (1781–1868) had previously reported similar findings. The oldest convex lens in existence today is from the island of Crete, dating back to the Minoan civilization around 1000 BC. The magnifying power of convex lenses and concave mirrors was described by **Lucius Annaeus Seneca** (d AD 65), around AD 50. The first scientific study of convex lenses was done by **Alhazen** or Ibn Al-Haitham (965–1038) of Basra. Convex spectacles were invented around 1270 in France, and convex lenses were produced industrially at Venice in 1300. *See spectacles.*

Cook, Frederick Albert (1865–1940) *See North Pole.*

Cook, James (1728–1779) An English sea captain from Marton, Yorkshire. He was commissioned in 1768 via the Royal Society to captain the *Endeavour* on its voyage to Tahiti to observe the transit of Venus, along with other scientists including **Joseph Banks** (1743–1820). He conducted his second expedition in 1772 and produced a map of the Pacific. He was killed by the natives of Hawaii on his third voyage. *See cartography.*

Cooke, Josiah Parsons (1827–1894) *See atomic weight.*

Cooke, Sir William Fothergill (1806–1879) *See electric telegraphy.*

Cookers An open fire with iron vessels was the first method to be used. Early man used a stick for roasting meat, and this gave way to the spit, a slender bar fixed over a fire. An automatic self-turning spit with vertical movement, assisted by pulleys, was invented by **Leonardo da Vinci** (1452–1519). Pot-cranes for moving kettles in and out of the fire were used in the 1700s. The first hot plates with concentric rings were invented by **Benjamin Thompson**, **Count Rumford** (1753–1814). In 1780 Thomas Robinson in England patented the first kitchen range consisting of a firegrate with cast-iron oven on one side, and a boiler on the other. In 1802 an English iron-founder, George Bodley, designed a closed-top cooking range, with a flue that distributed heat to all sides of the oven. A free-standing portable cooker with an iron flue came into use in America in the 1800s. Bodley joined a German businessman, Frederick Albert Winsor, and produced the first gas cooker in the 1820s. The gas range was introduced into America around 1840, and became popular in the 1860s. Electric cookers were first introduced in 1890, and took a few decades to become popular. *See pressure cooker.*

Cookworthy, William (1705–1780) *See porcelain.*

Coolridge Tube The prototype of the modern X-ray vacuum tube, invented in 1916 by an American physicist, **William David Coolridge** (1873–1975) of Hudson, Massachusetts. He replaced the cold aluminum cathode with a hot tungsten cathode.

Coolridge, Julian Lowell (1873–1954) *See probability theory.*

Coolridge, William David (1873–1975) *See Coolridge tube, tungsten.*

Cooper, Peter (1791–1883) An inventor and philanthropist of New York City, who built the first locomotive engine in Baltimore, in 1830.

Cooper, Leon Niels (b 1930) *See Bardeen–Cooper–Shrieffer theory.*

Coordinate A term introduced into mathematics by **Gottfried Wilhelm Leibniz** (1646–1716), in 1692. He also coined the terms *abscissa* and *ordinate*.

Cope, Edward Drinker (1840–1897) *See fossils.*

Copeland, William Taylor (1797–1868) *See porcelain.*

Copernicus, Nicolas (1473–1543) One of the greatest astronomers, who revolutionized the field of astronomy. He was born at Thorn, on the Vistula, in Prussia and studied astronomy at the Universities of Cracow, Bologna, Rome and Padua. He devised methods for accurately predicting the positions of the sun, moon and the planets, and improved the accuracy of astronomical calculations and tables. His great contribution was to produce a model of the solar system with the sun at its center, and the planets moving around it. It had previously been believed by European astronomers that the earth lay at the center of the universe. His legendary work *De Revolutionibus Orbium Coelestium Libri VI* was completed in 1530, and he received the first printed copy on the day of his death on May 24th. *See astronomy, heliocentric theory.*

Copier *See xerography.*

Copper [Anglo-Saxon: *coper,* Latin: *cuprum*] The first metal known to the Egyptians during the pre-dynastic times. They used the metal to make utensils 15 000 years ago, and the Sumerians around 3000 BC started using it for decorative art. Copper mines existed in Sinai around 5000 BC, and the use of the metal came into Europe around 4000 BC. Prehistoric relics made of copper dating to 2000 BC have been found in Ireland. The name *cyprium* was first used since it was initially found in Cyprus. The term was later corrupted to the Latin word *cuprum,* and is denoted by the symbol *Cu* in chemistry.

Copying In 1647 a physician from Hampshire, **William Petty** (1623–1687), made a device where two pens could simultaneously write. The pioneer of the steam engine, **James Watt** (1736–1819), invented a machine for reproducing letters and drawings. Carbon-coated paper for copying was patented in 1803 by Ralph Wedgwood. In 1880 Alexander Shapiro of Germany invented a machine which used a gelatin process. Albert Blake Dick (1856–1934) built the first mimeograph in America, around 1890. **Thomas Alva Edison** (1847–1931) patented a mimeograph. *See xerography.*

Corbeling *See building.*

Cordite A mixture of nitroglycerine and nitrocellulose, used as a propellant in artillery. *See Abel, Sir Fredrick Augustus, explosives.*

Corey, Elias James (b 1928) *See retrosynthesis.*

Coriolis Force A force caused by rotation of the earth. It governs the movement of wind in the atmosphere and currents in the ocean, and was discovered by a French physicist, **Gaspard Gustav Coriolis** (1792–1843) of Paris.

Coriolis, Gaspard Gustav (1792–1843) *See Coriolis force, kinetic energy.*

Corliss, George Henry (1817–1888) *See steam engine, textile industry.*

Cormack, Allan Macleod (1924–1998) *See CAT scanner.*

Cornell, Ezra (1804–1874) An American pioneer of the telegraph who co-founded, with Dickson White, Cornell University at Ithaca, New York, in 1868.

Cornforth, John Warcup (b 1917) *See Prelog, Vladimir, stereochemistry.*

Corona A region of luminous gas around the sun, which becomes visible during the total eclipse of the sun. *See coronagraph, solar eclipse.*

Coronagraph The first instrument for measuring the solar corona which has one-millionth of the light intensity of the solar disc. It was invented by a French astronomer, **Bernard Ferdinand Lyot** (1897–1952) of Paris, who used it to observe the solar corona during an eclipse in 1931.

Correns, Carl Franz Joseph Erich (1864–1933) *See pollination.*

Cort, Henry (1749–1800) *See iron.*

Cory, Barney Charles (1857–1921) *See ornithology.*

Cosine A mathematician, **Plato of Tivoli** (*c.* AD 1120), used the term *corda residui.* The term cosine was introduced into the language of trigonometry by an English mathematician and astronomer, **Edmund Gunter** (1581–1626) of Hertfordshire.

Cosmic Dynamics The application of classical theories of physics to the study of the origin of the earth. The principle of gravitation was used by **Sir Isaac Newton** (1642–1727) to explain the origin of the earth in 1692. An English astrophysicist, **Edward Arthur Milne** (1896–1950) of Hull, and an Irish physicist, **Sir William Hunter McCrea** (b 1904) of Dublin, were pioneers in the field.

Cosmic Radiation *See cosmic rays.*

Cosmic Rays A term coined in 1925 by an American physicist from Illinois, **Robert Andrews Millikan** (1868–1953), to denote a stream of assorted atomic particles from outside the solar system, some of which bombard the earth with great energy. They were thought to originate from bodies beyond our galaxy by a Scottish scientist, **Charles Thomson Rees Wilson** (1869–1959), in 1893. These rays were further investigated by an American astrophysicist, **Ira Sprague**

Bowen (1898–1973) of Seneca Falls, New York, in 1922. A classic paper on the theory of cosmic ray showers was published in 1937 by an Indian atomic scientist, **Homi Jehangir Bhabha** (1909–1966). In this paper he explained how cosmic rays interact with the upper atmosphere to produce the particles which are observed at ground level. In 1933, a German physicist, **Erich Rudolph Alexander Regener** (1881–1955), showed that events occurring in the stars caused cosmic rays. In 1910 an Austrian-born American physicist, **Victor Francis Hess** (1883–1964), experimented with a gold-leaf electroscope in a balloon, and proved that this mysterious radiation was not of terrestrial origin. For his work on cosmic radiation, he shared the Nobel Prize for physics in 1936, with **Carl David Anderson** (1905–1991) of New York. The cosmic microwave radiation which gave a clue to the origin of the universe was discovered in 1964 by a Munich-born US astrophysicist, **Arno Allan Penzias** (b 1933), and **Robert Woodrow Wilson** (b 1936) of Houston, Texas. An American physicist, **James Alfred Van Allen** (b 1914) of Iowa, devised a method for detecting cosmic ray intensity at various altitudes.

Cosmogeny [Greek: *cosmos,* universe + *genos,* descent] *See earth, geogeny.*

Cosmology [Greek: *cosmos,* universe + *logos,* discourse] The Greek philosopher **Anaxagorus** (*c.* 500–428 BC) of Clazomenae in Asia Minor proposed that the universe originated from a chaos of innumerable seeds, reduced to order and form, through a movement of rotation. An English philosopher and astronomer, **Thomas Wright** (1711–1786) of Durham, was one of the first to write a monograph on the theory of the universe. His work *An Original Theory or New Hypothesis of the Universe* (1750), although containing some original ideas such as that nebulae lay outside the Milky Way, retained the concept of the universe as a series of circles with a divine power at the center. A French mathematician, **Pierre Simon Marquis de Laplace** (1749–1827), proposed that the planetary bodies in the solar system were formed by the condensation of nebulous diffuse primordial matter that was previously distributed in space. A philosopher, **Immanuel Kant** (1724–1804) of Königsberg, used Isaac Newton's theory of attraction and repulsion of materials to explain the solar and other celestial systems. His *Critique Universal Natural History and Theory of Heavens* (1755) dealt with the origin and natural history of the Universe. He also proposed that the universe continued to develop. The nebular theory of Kant and Laplace was revived in 1944 by a German physicist, **Baron Carl Friedrich von Weizsäcker** (b 1912). He suggested that the multiple vortices formed by spinning gaseous mass preceded the solar system. The tidal theory of the evolution of the solar system was proposed by a London astronomer, **Sir James Hopwood Jeans** (1877–1946). He was the first to suggest that matter is continuously created throughout the universe. His theory was developed by an English geophysicist, **Sir Harold Jeffreys** (1891–1989) from Durham, who was the first to investigate the effect of radioactivity on the cooling of the earth and on mountain formation. *See Big Bang theory, earth, geogeny, Steady State theory.*

Coster, Dirk (1889–1950) *See hafnium.*

Coster, Laurens Janszoon (1370–1440) *See printing.*

Cotangent The term was introduced into the language of trigonometry by an English mathematician and astronomer, **Edmund Gunter** (1581–1626) of Hertfordshire, UK.

Cotes, Roger (1682–1716) An English mathematician and clergyman from Leicester who collaborated with **Sir Isaac Newton** (1642–1727), in the preparation of the second edition of *Principia*. His *Harmonia Mensurarum* posthumously published in 1722 contains works on logarithms.

Cotton *See mercerizing, textile chemistry, textile industry.*

Cotton, Frank Albert (b 1930) *See bonds.*

Cotton, William (1786–1866) *See textile industry.*

Cottrell Precipitator Used for precipitating particles from gases. Invented by an American chemist, **Frederick Gardner Cottrell** (1877–1948) of Oakland, California.

Cottrell, Frederick Gardner (1877–1948) *See Cottrell precipitator.*

Cotyledon *See dicotyledon, monocotyledon.*

Coulomb A unit of electric charge proposed by a French physicist, **Charles Augustus Coulomb** (1736–1806), who lived during the French revolution. The coulomb is the quantity of electricity transported by a current of 1 ampere in 1 second. Coulomb invented the torsion balance (1785), that bears his name. He was the first to postulate the law governing the attractive or repulsive forces between two charged particles in relation to their distance.

Coulomb, Charles Augustus (1736–1806) *See Coulomb, Coulomb's law, torsion balance, windmill.*

Coulomb's Law Inverse-square law for the repulsive forces of magnetism, discovered in 1750 by an English geologist, **John Michell** (1724–1793) of Nottinghamshire. It was rediscovered by a French physicist, **Charles Augustus Coulomb** (1736–1806), in around 1785.

Coulson, Charles Alfred (1910–1974) *See bonds, molecular orbital theory, valency.*

Counting *See abacus, arithmetic, numbers.*

Couper, Archibald Scott (1831–1892) *See bonds, valency.*

Courant, Richard (1888–1972) A German-born US mathematician of Jewish origin, who served as the director of the Institute of Mathematical Sciences of New York University, from 1953 to 1958. The Courant Institute of Mathematical Sciences is named after him, and his *Methoden der Mathematischen Physik* (1924–1927: *Methods of Mathematical Physics*) was an early work of reference on quantum theory.

Courtois, Bernard (1777–1838) A French chemist from Dijon who studied pharmacy at Auxerre. He isolated the first known alkaloid, morphine with another French chemist **Baron Louis Bernand Guyton de Morveau** (1737–1816) of Dijon. He took over his father's factory for manufacturing saltpeter in 1804, and accidentally discovered iodine in 1811 when he added sulfuric acid to ash of seaweed.

Cousteau, Jacques-Yves (1910–1997) *See aqualung.*

Cowan, Clyde Lorrain (1919–1974) *See neutrino.*

Cowell, Phillip Herbert (1870–1949) *See day.*

Cowling, Thomas George (1906–1990) An English physicist and mathematician from Walthamstow, Essex, who demonstrated the existence of a convective core in stars, which suggested that the sun may behave like a giant dynamo producing powerful electric currents and magnetic fields associated with sunspots.

Cox, Allan (1927–1987) *See paleomagnetism.*

Cox, William (1764–1837) *See roads.*

Coxwell, Henry Tracy (1819–1900) *See air balloon.*

Crab Nebula Cloud of gas 6000 light years from Earth, formed as a result of a supernova. It derives its name from its crablike shape. *See synchroton radiation.*

Crafts, James Mason (1839–1917) *See aromatic compounds, Friedel–Crafts reaction.*

Cram, Donald James (b 1919) An American chemist from Chester, Vermont, who is known for his work on synthetic organic chemistry. He shared the Nobel Prize for chemistry in 1987, for his work on three-dimensional highly specific molecules, with a French chemist, **Jean Marie Lehn** (b 1939) and a Korean-born US chemist, **Charles Pedersen** (1904–1990). *See cell membrane.*

Crampton, Thomas Russell (1816–1888) *See channel cable.*

Crane or hoisting machine. A Roman engineer **Marcus Pollio Vitruvius** (*c.* AD 100) in his treatise *On Architecture* described a device made of two timber pulleys and rope. The hydraulic crane was invented in 1846 by an English inventor, **William George Armstrong** (1810–1900) of Newcastle upon Tyne.

Crates of Mallus (*c.* 200 BC) *See oceanography.*

Crateuas (*c.* 100 BC) *See botany.*

Crawford, Adair (1748–1795) *See specific heat, strontium.*

Crawford, Osbert Guy Stanhope (1886–1957) *See aerial photograph.*

Cray, Seymour R. (1925–1996) *See computers, meteorology.*

Credit Card Invented by an American, Ralph Scheider in 1950, and adopted by the Diner's Club. The Bank of America created its first card in 1958.

Creed, Frederick George (1871–1957) A Canadian inventor who moved to Glasgow in 1857, where he produced the Creed teleprinter, which came to be widely used in news offices all over the world. *See telex.*

Cretaceous Period [Latin: *creta,* chalk] Last period of the Mesozoic era dating back to 146–65 million years and lasting up to 65 million years, identified by Jean Baptiste Julien Omalius d'Halloy, in 1822. Chalk was a typical finding during the second half of the period, hence its name.

Crick, Francis Harry Compton (b 1916) *See deoxyribonucleic acid.*

Critical Temperature A certain temperature above which a substance cannot be liquified by any pressure, however great. It was demonstrated by an Irish physical chemist, **Thomas Andrews** (1813–1885) of Belfast during his experiments on carbon dioxide. He worked in the laboratory of the French chemist, **John Baptiste André Dumas** (1800–1884), in Paris, before he returned in 1835 to Belfast, and became the professor of chemistry at Queen's College in 1849.

Croll, James (1821–1890) *See climatology.*

Crompton, Rookes Evelyn Bell (1845–1940) *See electric lighting.*

Crompton, Samuel (1753–1827) *See spinning mule.*

Cronin, James Watson (b 1931) *See antimatter.*

Cronquist, Arthur (1919–1992)　*See botanical classification, horticulture.*

Cronstedt, Baron Axel Fredrik (1722–1765)　*See blowpipe analysis, mineralogy, nickel, zeolite.*

Crookes Tube　*See cathode ray tube, Crookes, Sir William, X-rays.*

Crookes, Sir William (1832–1919)　A London molecular physicist and chemist who discovered thallium in 1861, and proposed the existence of the fourth stage of matter in 1873. He founded the *Chemical News* in 1859 and served as its editor. In 1878 he developed the Crookes tube, the forerunner of Roentgen's cathode or X-ray tube. *See cathode rays, cathode ray tube, fertilizers, fourth stage of matter, helium, plasma physics, radioactivity, radiometer (1), spinthariscope, thallium.*

Crop Rotation　*See agronomy.*

Cross, Frederick Charles (1855–1935)　*See artificial silk, textile chemistry.*

Crum Brown, Alexander (1838–1922)　*See benzene.*

Cryogenics　Branch of physics dealing with study of very low temperatures and its effects. Liquefaction of gases, superconductivity, cryptherapy, and refrigeration are some of its applications. *See food industry, liquefaction of gases, refrigerator, superconductivity.*

Crystallization [Greek: *krystallos*, ice]　The geometrical law of crystallization was discovered in 1781 by a French mineralogist, **René Just Haüy** (1743–1822) of St Just-en-Chaussée, Oise. He was appointed professor of mineralogy at Paris in 1802, and published a *Treatise on Crystallography* (1822). *See crystallography.*

Crystallography [Greek: *krystallos*, ice + *graphein,* to write] The study of the structure, forms and properties of crystals. The earliest account of crystals was given by **Robert Hooke** (1635–1703) in his *Micrographia* in 1665. Further work was done by **Erasmus Bartholinus** (1625–1698) of Copenhagen, who in his book, *Experimenta Crystalli Islandici Dissiaclastici* described the properties of double refraction and rhomboidal cleavage of Iceland spar or calcite. Geometrical forms of crystals were observed in 1665 by a Danish physician and geologist, **Nicolaus Steno** (1638–1687). The morphological variation of crystals in different salts was shown by a Dutch microscopist, **Anthoni van Leeuwenhoek** (1632–1723), in 1695. The earliest monograph, *Prodromus crystallographiae*, was published in 1723 by M.A. Capeller. A French pioneer, **Jean Baptiste Louis Romé de l'Isle** (1736–1790), described over 450 forms of crystals in his

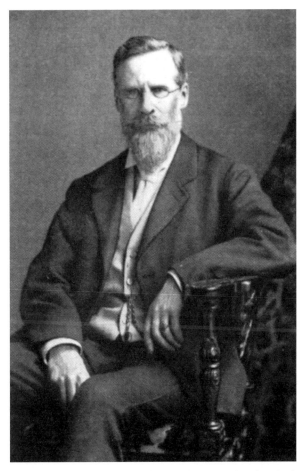

Figure 21　Sir William Crookes (1832–1919). Snyder, Carl. *New Conceptions in Science.* London: Harper and Brothers, 1903

Cristollographie (1783). **Hermann Franz Moritz Kopp** (1817–1892), one of the founders of physical chemistry, published a work on molecular volumes, crystallography and dissociation. An English mineralogist, **Mervyn Herbert Nevil Story-Maskelyne** (1823–1911) of Wiltshire, published *Morphology of Crystals* in 1895. A London chemist, **John Stuart Anderson** (1908–1990), was the first to apply electron microscopy for determining the structure of crystals. An Irish crystallographer, **John Desmond Bernal** (1901–1971), who was a professor of crystallography at Birkbeck College, London, pioneered the use of X-ray photographs for studying molecules and crystals. His work established the basis for the study of molecular biology. *See crystallography, X-ray crystalloid.*

Crystalloid [Greek: *krystallos*, ice + *eidos*, resemblance]　*See colloid chemistry, crystallography.*

Ctesibius　A scholar who studied physics at the Alexandrian school in 300 BC. He laid the foundation for the science of hydromechanics with his inventions of a hydraulic pneumatic machine, siphon and hand-operated fire engine. He invented the clepsydra or the waterclock. *See clock, fire engine, waterclock*.

Cube The Greek mathematician, **Pythagorus** (*c.* 580–500 BC), in developing his theory of arithmetic, named the product of three equal numbers, the cube.

Cugnot, Nicholas Joseph (1725–1804) *See car, steam engine*.

Culshaw, Joun (1924–1980) *See musical recording*.

Cunningham, Allan (1791–1839) A botanist and explorer of Australia, from Wimbledon, Surrey. He succeeded his brother Richard Cunningham, who was killed by the Aborigines, as colonial botanist to New South Wales. Many Australian plants are named after him, and most of his collections are preserved at Kew Gardens in London.

Curie Point The critical temperature at which a paramagnetic substance becomes ferromagnetic. It was discovered by the French physicist, **Pierre Curie** (1859–1906).

Curie, Marie (1867–1934) The daughter of Professor Sklodowska from Warsaw, Poland, who discovered radium. In 1891 she started working at the Paris faculty with **Pierre Curie** (1859–1906), whom she married in 1895. The couple, while working with **Antoine Henri Becquerel** (1852–1908), discovered polonium and radium from pitchblende in 1893. All three of them shared the Nobel Prize for physics for their discovery in 1903. Marie Curie succeeded her late husband to be the first woman professor at the Sorbonne in 1906 and was awarded the Nobel Prize for chemistry in 1911.

Curie, Pierre (1859–1906) A French physicist born in Paris. He married Marie Sklodowska (1867–1934) in 1895 and the couple worked with **Antoine Henri Becquerel** (1852–1908) to discover radioactivity in 1903. Pierre also identified α, β and γ rays and was appointed as a professor at the Sorbonne, Paris in 1904. He shared the Nobel Prize for chemistry with Becquerel and Marie Curie in 1903. He suffered radioactive injuries from his work with radioactive substances. Three years after his historic discovery he was run over by a brewer's cart and succumbed to his injuries.

Curium An element with atomic number 96, synthesized in 1944 by the American physicists, **Glenn Theodore Seaborg** (1912–1999), R.A. James, L.O. Morgan and A. Ghioso at Berkeley.

Current *See alternating current, direct current, electricity*.

Curtis, Charles Gorden (1860–1953) A Boston engineer who invented the impulse steam turbine in 1896. The modern machines, combining the use of the Curtis impulse turbine and the reaction turbine, were invented by an Irish engineer in London, **Sir Charles Algernon Parsons** (1854–1931). *See turbine*.

Curtis, Heber Doust (1872–1942) *See Mars*.

Curtis, William (1746–1799) *See scientific journals*.

Curtiss, Glen Hammond (1878–1930) *See airplane, seaplane, warplanes*.

Curtius, Theodor (1857–1928) A professor of chemistry at Heidelberg who discovered hydrazine and many other organic compounds.

Cuvier, Georges Leopold (1769–1832) A French biologist who is regarded as the founder of vertebrate paleontology. After studying at Stuttgart, became an assistant at the Natural History Museum of Paris in 1795. He published several important works on comparative anatomy and fossil bones and described over 5000 species of fish. After working initially with **Jean Baptiste Lamarck** (1744–1829), he became an opponent of Lamarck's theories. The four major divisions of the animal kingdom, the Vertebrata, Mollusca, Articulata and Radiata were proposed by Cuvier, in 1817. Cuvier held several prestigious positions including the post of Minister of the Interior, Director of Educational Reforms and Chancellor of the University of Paris. His publications include *Leçons de Anatomie Comparée* (1801–1805), *L'Anatomie des Mollusques* (1816), *Les Ossements fossiles des quadrupèdes* (1812), *Historie Naturale des Poissons* (1828–1849) and *Le Règne Animal distribue d'après son Organisation* (1817).

Cybernetics [Greek: *kubernetes*, a director] Defined in 1948 as the study of communication and control in animal and machine by an American, **Nobert Wiener** (1894–1964) of Columbia, Missouri. His concept later proved to be important in many fields including computing, physiology, mathematics and engineering. Many common terms such as feedback, input and output originate from his work. **René Descartes** (1596–1650), a French philosopher and scientist, is regarded by some as the father of cybernetics, since he was the first to compare the automaticity in animals with the automatic activity of machines such as hydraulically animated toys. An English mathematician and aircraft engineer, **John Dudley North** (1893–1968), advanced the mathematical ideas on cybernetics.

Cyberspace *See virtual reality*.

Cycloid A curve traced from a point on the rim of a wheel that rolls along a straight line. The first study was done by a French mathematician, **Pierre de Fermat** (1601–1665). An important treatise on the subject was written in 1658 by another French mathematician, **Blaise Pascal** (1623–1662) of Clermont-Ferrand.

Cyclone Produced by the movement of winds in a counterclockwise direction, around a low pressure area in the northern hemisphere. In the southern hemisphere the cyclone is produced by the movement of the wind in a clockwise direction. A Norwegian-born American meteorologist, **Jacob Aall Bonnevie Bjerknes** (1897–1975), studied the production and movement of cyclones and published *On the Structure of Moving Cyclones* in 1919. He became the first professor of meteorology at the University of California, Los Angeles. His son **Vilhelm Friman Koren Bjerknes** (1862–1951) of Stockholm, advanced the studies on the cyclone. An English meteorologist, **William Henry Dines** (1855–1927) of Oxshott, performed over 200 balloon ascents to study the relationship between pressure and temperature, and concluded that cyclonic circulation resulted from the dynamic processes in the upper layers of the troposphere or the lower stratosphere. A Finnish meteorologist, **Erik Herbert Palmen** (1898–1985), made a detailed study of tropical cyclones and determined the critical temperature for the development of cyclones.

Cyclotron An acceleration chamber which enables the bombardment of nuclei with deuterons or neutrons, for production of artificial radioactivity. A prototype particle accelerator was built by an English physicist, **Sir John Douglas Cockcroft** (1897–1967) from Yorkshire and an Irish physicist, **Ernest Thomas Sinton Walton** (1903–1995) of Dungarvan, Waterford, at the Cavendish Laboratory in 1932. They were awarded the Nobel Prize for physics in 1951. Their accelerator was superseded by a cyclotron developed in California in 1931 by **Ernest Orlando Lawrence** (1901–1958) of Canton, South Dakota. Lawrence became a professor at Berkeley, California in 1930, and was made director of the Berkeley Radiation Laboratory there in 1936. He received the Nobel Prize for physics, for his work on the cyclotron, in 1939. The first major post-war cyclotron was built in 1949 at Harwell by an English physicist, **Sir John Bertram Adams** (1920–1984) from Kingston, Surrey. Adams was a founder member of the European center for nuclear research in Geneva, the CERN (*Conseil Européen pour la Recherche Nucléaire*).

Cytogenetics [Greek: *kytos*, hollow + *genos*, offspring] The method of introducing foreign genes into bacteria in order to direct the production of a specific protein such as insulin or interferon. It was developed by an American molecular biologist and professor of biochemistry at Washington, **Paul Berg** (b 1926), around 1970. *See genetic engineering.*

Cytology [Greek: *kytos*, hollow + *logos*, discourse] The study of the cell, initiated as a science by a German professor of botany at Bonn, **Eduard Adolf Strasburger** (1844–1912). *See cell, cell division, cell theory, cytoplasm.*

Cytoplasm [Greek: *kytos*, hollow + *plasma*, mould] The term for cytoplasm, the part of the cell enclosed by the plasma membrane but excluding the nucleus, introduced by a German botanist and professor at Bonn, **Eduard Adolf Strasburger** (1844–1912) in 1882.

D

d'Abbans, Marquis Jouffroy (1751–1832) *See steamships.*

d'Anville, Jean-Baptiste Bourguignon (1697–1782) *See cartography.*

d'Arsonval, Jacques Arsène (1851–1940) *See tangent galvanometer.*

da Vinci, Leonardo (1452–1519) An artist, inventor, engineer and an anatomist from Vinci in the Valley of the Arno, between Pisa and Florence. He was an illegitimate son of a Florentine notary, Pietro da Vinci. He studied under the artist Andrea del Verrochio (1435–1488), and later became a military engineer to the Duke of Milan. He was the first to illustrate several human anatomical structures including the heart. His notebook included prototype illustrations of water gear wheels, cranks, wheels, paddle wheels, mining devices and flying machines. *See airplane, bicycle, camera, compass (1), contact lenses, cookers, differential gear, dynamics, fossils, helicopter, metallurgy, parachute, structural engineering.*

Daguerre, Louis Jacques Mande (1789–1851) *See camera, daguerrotype process, photography.*

Daguerrotype Process In 1836, a French inventor, **Louis Jacques Mande Daguerre** (1789–1851) of Cormeilles, near Lisieux, introduced a method of fixing images on copper plates coated with metallic silver, sensitized to light by iodine vapor. He used sodium thiosulfate solution to remove the unchanged silver iodide. His images had to be viewed at a right angle in relation to the source of light if the viewer wanted to see a positive picture. Around the same time an English Victorian squire, **William Henry Fox Talbot** (1800–1877) from Wiltshire, independently developed a similar type of process. In 1834 he used a weak silver chloride solution and produced outlines of leaves and lace. In the following year he discovered the negative from which unlimited positives could be made. Talbot's method was more advanced than that of Daguerre, which required a photograph to be taken each time a copy or positive was required. Both Daguerre's and Talbot's work contributed to a major advancement in the field of photography, and significantly shortened the exposure time required to make a photographic impression. Talbot's process, the calotype, was patented in Britain in 1841, and in the USA in 1847. *See photography.*

Dahl, Anders (1751–1789) A Swedish botanist and pupil of **Carolus Linnaeus** (1707–1778). The flowering plant *Dahlia*, brought into Sweden from South Africa, was named after him by another Swedish botanist, **Carl Per Thurnberg** (1743–1828).

Daimler, Gottlieb (1834–1900) A German engineer and inventor from Schorndorf near Stuttgart who developed the internal combustion engine for the motor car. In 1870 he joined **Eugen Langen** (1833–1895) and produced the first practical internal combustion engine and applied it to a bicycle with success in 1886. In 1889 he built a second two-cylinder V-engine which doubled the power, and it was adapted to the motor car. He founded the Daimler-Motoren-Gesellschaft at Cannstatt in 1890. His engines were first manufactured in England by the Daimler Motor Company, in 1896.

Dairy Farming *See animal husbandry.*

Dairy Industry Methods of preparing curd and butter were mentioned by **Pliny the Elder** (AD 28–79) in the first century. A Swedish inventor, **Carl Gustav Patrick de Latour** (1845–1913), was a pioneer in modernizing the dairy industry. In 1878 he invented the turbine-driven high-speed centrifugal cream separator for milk. Vacuum milking machines were developed around 1851, and Latour invented a new vacuum milking device in 1913. The process of pasteurization or heat treatment of milk, to destroy bacteria, was invented by **Louis Pasteur** (1822–1895). An American agricultural chemist and dairy farmer, **Stephen Moulton Babcock** (1843–1931), who taught agricultural chemistry at the Wisconsin University (1887–1913), improved the quality of dairy produce, and came to be regarded as the father of scientific dairying in America. He devised a test for measuring the fat content in milk which is named after him. An American chemist, **Mary Engle Pennington** (1872–1952) in Philadelphia, did research into the preservation of dairy products and developed standards of milk inspection that were later used by health boards across the USA.

d'Albe, Edmund Edward Fournier (1868–1933) *See facsimile machine, optophone.*

Dale, Thomas Pelham (1821–1892) *See refraction.*

d'Alembert Principle An extension of Isaac Newton's third law of motion applied to dynamics and celestial mechanics, proposed by a French mathematician, **Jean de Rond d'Alembert** (1717–1783).

d'Alembert, Jean de Rond (1717–1783) A French mathematician, who published a paper on integral calculus in

1739. His work over the next 9 years led to the discovery of the calculus of partial differences. *See d'Alembert principle.*

Dalen, Nils Gustav (1869–1937)   *See lighthouses.*

Dallam, Robert (1602–1665)   *See barrel organ.*

Dallam, Thomas (*c.* 1599–1630)   *See barrel organ.*

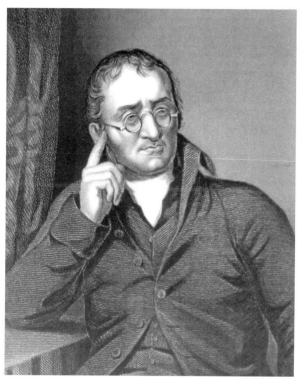

Figure 22 John Dalton (1766–1844). Courtesy of the National Library of Medicine

Dalton, John (1766–1844)   An English chemist and a son of a hand-loom weaver in Eaglesfield, Cumberland. In 1793 he obtained a post as teacher of mathematics, natural philosophy and chemistry at Manchester New College. He commenced his scientific career with the investigation of his own color blindness, and in 1787 during his study of the climate in the Lake District he became interested in gases, which led him to postulate some of the most important laws concerning them. His law of partial pressures is universally known as Dalton's Law. He developed the theory of atoms in 1801, determined the atomic weight of various elements, and published a table in 1806. Dalton's first observations on the atom, the *Inquiry into the relative weight of the ultimate particles* was submitted to the Philosophical Society, in 1803. He published his *New System of Chemical Philosophy* (1808), and came to be regarded as the father of atomic theory.

Dalton's Law   *See Dalton, John.*

Dampier, Sir William Cecil (1867–1952)   One of the descendants of **William Dampier** (1652–1715), he was born in Yeovil, Somerset and educated at Cambridge, before being appointed as secretary of the Agricultural Research Council in 1931. He published *A History of Science* (1929) and several other works.

Dampier, William (1652–1715)   An English navigator, born to a farmer's family in Yeovil. He lost his father when he was 10 years of age and took to sea at the age of sixteen and started his adventures as buccaneer before he eventually became a scientific explorer. He made observations of new plants and described them, and also wrote a classic work on meteorology entitled *Discourse on Winds*. His other important book *Voyage round the World* was published in 1697. Dampier served as the pilot in Captain Dover's ship and rescued Alexander Selkirk (1676–1721) who was marooned on the island of Juan Fernandez for a period of over 4 years. **Daniel Defoe** (1660–1731) later inspired by the experiences of Selkirk wrote *Robinson Crusoe.*

Dams   The earliest known dams dating back to 3000 BC, were discovered in 1974, in Jawa, Jordan, by the British School of Archaeology in Jerusalem. The largest concrete dam in the world, the Grand Coulee dam, on the Columbia River, in Washington State, was started in 1933 and completed in 1941.

Dana, James Dwight (1813–1895)   An American geologist from Utica, New York, who became professor of geology at Yale in 1864. Dana's publications include *System of Mineralogy* (1837), *Manual of Mineralogy* (1848), *Textbook of Geology* (1864) and *Hawaiian Volcanoes* (1890).

Dance, George (1700–1768)   A London architect who built Mansion House in 1739. His son also called George Dance (1741–1825) rebuilt the Newgate prison.

Dancer, Benjamin (1812–1887)   *See photomicrography.*

Dandy, James Edgar (1903–1976)   An English botanist from Preston who became Keeper of Botany at the Natural History Museum in London in 1927. He published several works, and the genus, *Dandya,* is named after him.

Daniell Electric Cell   A prototype of the modern battery using a zinc cathode in a double fluid cell. Invented in 1836 by **John Frederick Daniell** (1790–1845), professor of chemistry at King's College, London. Daniell also invented a hygrometer (1820) and a pyrometer (1830) and published *Introduction to Chemical Philosophy* (1839). *See battery.*

Daniell, John Frederick (1790–1845) *See Daniell electric cell.*

Danielle, James Frederic (1911–1984) An English botanist from Wembley and a pioneer in the detailed study of the structure of the cell membrane which he demonstrated to contain molecules of lipids and proteins. He published *Permeability of Natural Membranes* in 1943. *See cell membrane.*

Dantzig, George Bernard (b 1914) A US mathematician from Portland, Oregon, who in 1947 discovered that many planning problems could be formulated as linear computer programs. He also devised an algorithm, known as the simplex method, which was widely adopted for the purpose.

Darboux, Jean Gaston (1842–1917) A French mathematician from Nîmes who was professor of geometry at the Sorbonne. He proposed a new method of integration through his work on partial differential equations.

Darby, Abraham (1678–1717) *See bridges, coal.*

Darby II, Abraham (1711–1763) An iron-master and son of **Abraham Darby** (1678–1717). He was supposed to have discovered the method of producing wrought iron from coke-smelted ore.

Darby III, Abraham (1750–1791) *See bridges.*

Darlington, William (1782–1863) An American botanist from Pennsylvania. The Californian pitcher plant (*Darlingtonia*) is named after him.

Dart, Raymond Arthur (1893–1988) *See Australopithecus africanus.*

Darwin, Charles Robert (1809–1882) A British naturalist from Shrewsbury who developed the theory of the evolution of species by natural selection. He was a son of a physician, Robert Darwin, and grandson of the naturalist **Erasmus Darwin** (1731–1802). His mother was a daughter of the famous English potter, **Josiah Wedgwood** (1730–1795) of Burslam, Staffordshire. Darwin entered Edinburgh University in 1825 to study medicine, but lost interest in the subject and returned home after 2 years. He entered Cambridge University in 1828 and obtained a BA degree in 1831. At the age of 22, he was appointed as a naturalist on the *HMS Beagle* at the recommendation of J.S. Henslow, who was professor of geology at Cambridge. On his return in 1836, after 4 years on the *Beagle*, he began work on his theory of evolution and published his monumental work *On the Origin of Species by Means of Natural Selection* (1859). Darwin's other works include: *The Fertilisation of Orchids* (1862), *The Variation of Plants and Animals under Domestication* (1867), *The Descent of Man and Selection in Relation to Sex*

(1871), *Expression of the Emotions in Man and Animals* (1872), *Insectivorous Plants* (1875), *Climbing Plants* (1875), *The Effects of Cross and Self Fertilisation in the Vegetable Kingdom* (1876), *The Power of Movements in Plants* (1880) and *The formation of Vegetable Mould through action of Worms* (1881). *See evolution.*

Darwin, Erasmus (1731–1802) A physician and poet, born in Elton, near Newark in Nottinghamshire. He took his degree at St John's College, Cambridge in 1755 and later moved to Edinburgh. He proposed a theory of evolution in which he declared that all warm-blooded animals came from one living filament over a span of millions of ages. He was also a botanist and studied plant nutrition and photosynthesis. **Charles Darwin** (1809–1882), the author of the *Origin of Species by Means of Natural Selection*, was his grandson by his first marriage.

Darwin, George Howard (1845–1912) *See oceanography.*

Database Microcomputer program used for manipulating large quantities of data, the first of which appeared in 1981.

Date The first recorded date in the history of humanity refers to a solar eclipse which occurred on 28 May 585 BC. The Medes and Lydians who fought a war on this day became frightened by the eclipse and called the war off. The year 4236 BC represents the first date in the Egyptian calendar, and 3372 BC in the Mayan calendar. The Hebrew calendar treats 3760 BC as the earliest date. The Archbishop, Ussher set the date of creation of the Universe as October 23 4004 BC. The calendar based on the birth of Jesus Christ was introduced by Dionysius Exiguus in AD 525. The Archbishop, **James Ussher** (1580–1656) fixed the date of creation of the world as 23 October 4004 BC in his *Sacred Chronology* published in 1660. *See calendar.*

Daubrée, Gabriel Auguste (1814–1896) *See mineralogy.*

David, Pere Armand (1826–1900) A French naturalist who made a botanical exploration of China while he was a missionary there, and published a catalog *Plantae Davidianae* (1884–1886). The tree (*Davidia involucrata*) and a deer (*Elaphurus davidianus*) are named after him.

Davidson, Eric Harris (b 1937) *See deoxyribonucleic acid.*

Davis, Raymond (b 1914) *See neutrino.*

Davis, William Morris (1850–1935) *See rivers, soil erosion.*

Davisson, Clinton Joseph (1881–1958) *See electron diffraction.*

Davson, Hugh (b 1909) *See cell membrane.*

Davy, Edward (1806–1885) A physician from Devon who did early experiments on telegraphy and demonstrated this over a distance of one mile at Regent's Park in London. He emigrated to Australia in 1838 and practiced as a physician in Victoria. His other contributions include: Davy's blow pipe for chemical analysis, Davy's mercurial trough for gas chemistry, an electric relay and Davy's Diamond cement for repair of broken china.

Davy, Sir Humphry (1778–1829) An English chemist who made a series of epoch-making discoveries. His father was a wood carver at Penzance, and Davy apprenticed under a surgeon, J.B. Borlace in Cornwall. At the age of 17, Davy began his experiments on the inhalational effects of nitrous oxide. In 1798 he joined the Medical Pneumatic Institution founded by a physician and chemist, **Thomas Beddoes** (1760–1808), in order to study the role of inhalation of gases in the treatment of diseases. His work *Researches, Chemical and Philosophical; Chiefly Concerning Nitrous Oxide* was published in 1799. In 1801 Davy took charge of the laboratory at the Royal Institution at the invitation of **Benjamin Thompson** or **Count Rumford** (1753–1814). His *Elements of Agricultural Chemistry* (1813) was the first book to apply chemical principles to farming. In 1814, he showed that diamond was chemically identical to charcoal, and invented the safety lamp for miners in 1816. Davy was the first to decompose caustic potash by electrolysis, and discovered the earth metals sodium, potassium, magnesium, strontium and barium. *See affinity, arc light, electric lighting, electrolysis, heat.*

Davy's Lamp A safety lamp to overcome the danger of flammability in the mines, invented in 1816 by **Sir Humphry Davy** (1778–1829). It consists of a metallic gauze placed above the gas flame, in order to reduce the temperature of the gas and make it insufficient for ignition.

Dawkins, Sir William Boyd (1837–1929) *See cave exploration.*

Daws, Rutter William (1799–1868) A London astronomer who discovered many comets, and the phenomenon of double stars. He also described the *canals* in Mars for the first time. After living for a short while as a child in Sierra Leone, where his father was appointed governor in 1807, he returned to England and studied medicine before he took to astronomy.

Dawson, Charles (1864–1916) *See Piltdown Man.*

Dawson, Sir John William (1820–1899) *See paleophytology.*

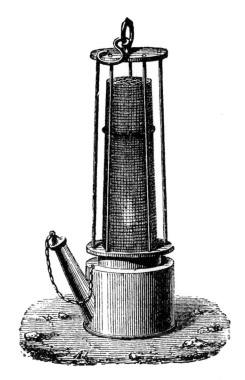

Figure 23 Davy's safety lamp. Guillemin, Amédée. *The Applications of Physical Forces.* London: Macmillan and Co, 1877

Day The Egyptians were the first to divide the day into two periods, each consisting of 12 hours. The Greek historian **Herodotus** (485–425 BC), believed that the Greeks learnt so to divide the day from the Egyptians. The Romans divided the day and night each into four parts, known as vigils and watches. These in turn were subdivided into 12 parts. Their 1st hour for the day began with sunrise and ended with the sunset at the 12th hour. The 1st hour of the night began with sunset and ended with the 12th hour at sunrise. An English astronomer, **Phillip Herbert Cowell** (1870–1949), researched the earth's rotation period and calculated that the day is lengthening by about 0.01 seconds per 1000 years. *See calendar, date.*

Day, David Talbot (1859–1925) *See petroleum.*

Day, John (1522–1584) *See music printing.*

De Broglie Waves *See quantum mechanics.*

Deacon, Sir George Edward Raven (1906–1984) *See oceanography.*

Deacon, Henry W. (1822–1877) *See Deacon's process.*

Deacon's Process Production of bleaching powder whereby hydrogen chloride mixed with air is subjected to the catalytic action of cuprous chloride, to yield chlorine, which is in turn passed over slaked lime. It was invented by a London chemist, **Henry W. Deacon** (1822–1877) in 1868, and improved by a Swiss chemist, **Ferdinand Hurter** (1844–1898), who established the first industrial research laboratory in Britain.

Dead Sea Scrolls   *See cave exploration.*

Debye, Peter Joseph Wilhelm (1884–1966)   *See X-ray crystallography.*

Decimal Notation [Latin: *decimus*, tenth] A Chinese mathematician, Liu Hsin, was the first person to use decimal notation, around AD 5. The decimal system was known in India around AD 600, and it was brought by the Arabs into Spain in 1050. It was introduced into England by **John of Halifax** or **Johannes de Sacrobosco** (*c.* 1250) in 1253. **François Viète** (1540–1603) of Pitou, France, promoted decimal representation of numbers in his *Canon mathematicus* (1579). A table of decimal notations for fractions was introduced in 1608 by a professor of mathematics at Heidelberg, **Bartholomeus Pitiscus** (1561–1613). A Flemish mathematician in Leyden, **Simon Stevinus** (1548–1620) of Bruges, introduced decimals into common usage, in his book *La Thiende* (1585).

Decoster, Pierre (1806–1861) A Belgian-born French tool manufacturer in Paris, who produced a wide variety of tools ranging from lathes to transmission gears.

Dedekind, Julius Wilhelm Richard (1831–1916)   *See Dedekind's cuts, number theory.*

Dedekind's Cuts Divides a line of infinite length representing all real numbers to define irrational numbers in terms of pairs of sequences of rational numbers. This became fundamental to the theory of numbers. It was proposed by a German mathematician, **Julius Wilhelm Richard Dedekind** (1831–1916) from Brunswick.

Dee, John (1527–1608) A London astrologer, alchemist, mathematician and spiritualist who served as an astrologer to Queen Mary I, and was imprisoned in 1555 after her death. Queen Elizabeth later made him the warden of Manchester College in 1595. Dee wrote several treatises on mathematics, astrology, logic, medicine and alchemy. He gave the preface to the first English translation of *Euclid* published by Billingsley in 1570.

Defoe, Daniel (1660–1731)   *See Dampier, William, newspapers.*

Dehmelt, Hans Georg (b 1922)   *See atomic clock, electron, Paul trap.*

Dehn, Max (1878–1952)   *See topology.*

Deijl, Harmanus van (1738–1809)   *See achromatic lens.*

Deimann (1743–1808)   *See electrolysis.*

Delambre, Jean Baptiste Joseph (1749–1822) A French mathematician and astronomer who became professor of astronomy at the Collège de France, in 1807. He wrote several works on the history of astronomy and proposed the Delambre's analogies in spherical geometry. *See meridian.*

Delisle, Joseph Nicolas (1688–1768)   *See Venus.*

Deluc, Jean André de (1727–1817) A Swiss mathematician and geologist who settled in England in 1773, and became Reader to Queen Charlotte, and a friend of George III. He was one of the first to use the term *geologie*, and published *Cosmology and Geology* (1803). *See barometer.*

Demarcay, Eugene Anatole (1852–1903) A French chemist and professor at Paris who designed a machine that achieved low temperatures by compressing gases and allowing them to expand. This later formed the basis for refrigerators. He discovered the element europium, through spectroscopy, in 1896.

Democritus (460–370 BC) A Greek philosopher from Abdera and contemporary of **Socrates** (470–399 BC). He is ranked next to **Plato** (428–348 BC) and **Aristotle** (384–322 BC). In his cosmic theory of vacuum and atoms, he was the first to state that everything in nature including the body and soul consisted of atoms, the movements of which controlled all activities. He rejected mythology and theology, and wrote scientifically on medicine and anatomy. According to **Pliny the Elder** (AD 28–79), one of his special treatises was on the anatomy of the chameleon. He is supposed to have lived to the age of 109. *See Abdera, atomic structure, conservation of mass.*

Dempster, Arthur (1886–1950)   *See mass spectrograph.*

Dendrochronology [Greek: *denron*, tree + *chronos*, time + *logos*, discourse] A method of dating ancient pieces of wood by studying its rings. Introduced and named by an American astronomer, **Andrew Ellicott Doughlass** (1867–1962) of Winsor, Vermont in 1915. He published *Climatic Cycles and Tree Growth* (1919–1936) in three volumes.

Denning, William Frederick (1848–1931)   *See comet.*

Density of the Earth   *See Cavendish, Henry.*

Denton, Sir Eric James (b 1923)   *See marine biology.*

Deoxyribonucleic Acid (DNA) In 1869, a Swiss biologist, **Friedrich Miescher** (1844–1895) of Basel, identified the substance *nuclein* in the cell, which was later found to be the nucleoprotein responsible for genetic transmission. The chemical distinction between these proteins and DNA was made in 1903 by a Russian-born American biochemist and physician, **Phoebus Aaron Theodore Levene** (1869–1940), who left Russia in 1892 and joined the Rockefeller Institute in 1905. Andrei Nikolaevitch Belozersky obtained DNA in a pure state in 1936, and demonstrated the presence of RNA and DNA in bacteria, in 1939. In the 1950s, a Czech-born biochemist, **Erwin Chargaff** (b 1905), showed that the number of adenine bases in DNA is equal to the number of thymine bases, while he was professor of biochemistry at Columbia University, New York. In 1944, a Canadian-born US bacteriologist, **Theodore Oswald Avery** (1877–1955), established DNA as the material definitely responsible for genetic transmission. In 1950 an American physicist of Russian origin, **George Gamow** (1904–1968), recognized the occurrence of four different bases in a sequence in the DNA chain as a code for directing the synthesis of proteins. The three-dimensional spiral structure (helix) was demonstrated in 1951 by B.B. Corey and **Linus Pauling** (1901–1994). The first synthesis of DNA molecules was achieved in 1957 by a New York biochemist, **Arthur Kornberg** (b 1918). He shared the Nobel Prize for Physiology or Medicine with a Spanish-born US biochemist, **Severo Ochoa** (1905–1993), in 1959. Two American molecular biologists, **Roy John Britten** (b 1919) of Washington and **Eric Harris Davidson** (b 1937) of New York, showed the existence of extra DNA with repetitive sequences, for which there was no apparent explanation. X-ray diffraction photography of DNA molecules was first performed by **Elsie Rosalind Franklin** (1920–1958) of King's College, London, around 1952. Her work led to the historic discovery of the molecular structure of DNA by **James Dewey Watson** (b 1928), a biologist from Chicago, and **Francis Harry Compton Crick** (b 1916) from Northhampton, at the Cavendish Laboratory in Cambridge, England, in 1953. The double helical structure of DNA was revealed by a New Zealand-born British biochemist, **Maurice Hugh Fredrick Wilkins** (b 1916) and his colleagues in the same year. In 1962 Crick, Watson and Wilkins shared the Nobel Prize for Physiology or Medicine. A Japanese biochemist, **Reiji Okazaki** (1930–1975), discovered the DNA–RNA fragments in 1957 that explained how DNA is synthesized simultaneously in opposite directions, but with corresponding opposite polarity. Okazaki was 14 years old when the atomic bomb was dropped on his home town, Hiroshima, and later developed leukemia. The phenomenon of DNA denaturation, which established the specificity and feasibility of nucleic acid hybridization, was discovered by an American biochemist,

Paul Mead Doty (b 1920), in 1961. The *reverse transcriptase* enzyme capable of transcribing RNA into DNA was discovered in 1970 by an American microbiologist, **David Baltimore** (b 1938) of New York, and his finding formed the basis for manipulation of the genetic code. A new method for finding the sequence of bases in nucleic acids was devised by an American molecular biologist, **Walter Gilbert** (b 1932) of Boston, Massachusetts, around 1970. The full sequence of bases in the DNA of a specific virus (ϕX174) was worked out by **Frederick Sanger** (b 1918), an English biochemist from Rendcombe, Gloucestershire, in 1977. The first genetic map was produced by an American biologist of Russian-Jewish origin, **Daniel Nathans** (b 1928) from Delaware, who used his method to locate a specific gene on the DNA. He shared the Nobel Prize for Physiology or Medicine for this work, with Sanger and Paul Berg in 1978. *See genetic engineering.*

Derham, William (1657–1735) *See velocity of sound.*

Deringer Pistol A pocket pistol, invented in 1852 by an American manufacturer of small arms, Henry Deringer from Easton, Philadelphia.

Derry, John (d 1952) *See supersonic flight.*

Desaguliers, John Theophile (1683–1749) *See conductor, insulator.*

Desargues Theorem If two triangles are placed so that the lines joining pairs of corresponding vertices pass through a single point, then the point of intersection of pairs of corresponding sides are in a single line. It was proposed by a French engineer and architect, **Gérard Desargues** (1593–1662) of Lyons, and published in 1648 by his friend Abraham Bosse.

Desargues, Gérard (1593–1662) *See Desargues theorem, projective geometry.*

Desert Dunes *See sand dunes.*

Descartes, René (1596–1650) A philosopher, mathematician and scientist, from a small French town near Tours, which is now la-Haye-Descartes. He graduated in law from Poitiers in 1616, and published *Discours de la Méthode* (1637). He reformed algebraic notation, founded coordinate geometry and made several important contributions to physiology and optics. His other publications include *Meditationes de prima Philosophia* (1641) and *Principia Philosophiae* (1644). *See Académie Royale des Sciences, analytical geometry, automation, cartesian doctrine, contact lenses, cybernetics, dioptrics, earthquake, geogeny, geometry, rainbow, solar system, tangent, velocity of light, vision.*

Desch, Cyril Henry (1874–1958) *See metallurgy, Ur.*

Descriptive Geometry Form and relative position of geometrical figures deduced by the use of transversals. Founded as a branch of geometry by a French mathematician, **Gaspard Monge** (1746–1818). His *Géométrie Descriptive* (1800) was based on the lectures he gave at the École Polytechnique in 1795.

Desfontaines, René Louiche (1750–1833) *See monocotyledons.*

Deshayes, Gerard Paul (1795–1875) *See fossils.*

Deslandres, Henri Alexandres (1853–1948) *See celestial photography.*

Desmarest, Nicolas (1725–1815) *See geology.*

Desormes, Charles Bernard (1777–1862) *See carbon monoxide, specific heat.*

Deuterium [Greek: *deuteros,* second] or ^{2}H. This isotope of hydrogen was discovered in 1932 by **Harold Clayton Urey** (1893–1981) of Walkerton, Indiana. An American chemist, **Gilbert Newton Lewis** (1875–1946) obtained deuterium oxide or heavy water in the same year. An Austrian-born US physicist, **Paul Harteck** (1902–1985), demonstrated the existence of para and ortho forms of deuterium.

Deuteron The nucleus of heavy hydrogen or deuterium atom made up of one proton and one neutron. *See cyclotron, tritium.*

Deville, Henri Étienne Sainte-Claire (1818–1881) *See aluminum, platinum, silicon.*

Devonian Period A geological period over 400 million years ago, related to the strata belonging to the paleozoic era. It was first predominantly noted in Devonshire, Great Britain. The term Devonian for the period was coined by an English geologist and clergyman, **Adam Sedgwick** (1785–1873) from northwest Yorkshire, who was professor of geology at Cambridge, from 1818 until his death.

Dewar, Michael James Stuart (b 1918) A British chemist born to Scottish parents in India. He studied molecular orbital theory in relation to organic chemistry and published *The Electronic Theory of Organic Chemistry* (1949). He became professor of chemistry at Queen Mary College, London, in 1951.

Dewar, Sir James (1843–1923) A Scottish physicist from Kincardine-on-Forth, who was educated at Edinburgh University, and studied in Europe in 1868 under **Friedrich August Kekulé** (1829–1896). He developed the theory of the pyridine ring, and invented the Dewar's flask, a device that could preserve liquefied gases for considerable periods without their undergoing evaporation. Using his flask he prepared large quantities of liquid oxygen, for the first time. He perfected the calorimeter, and in 1898 invented a method for liquefying hydrogen. *See liquefaction of gases, pyridine.*

Diadochus, Proclus (AD 410–485) *See geometry.*

Dialysis [Greek: *dia,* through + *lyein,* to loosen] The first experiments on dialysis, using different substances, were performed in 1861 by a Scottish chemist, **Thomas Graham** (1805–1869) of Glasgow. His first dialyzer was a simple device, made of parchment paper tied to the end of a large-mouthed funnel.

Diamagnetic A term first used in 1846 by **Michael Faraday** (1791–1867) to describe the effect of light on magnets. **Sir Rudolf Ernst Peierls** (1907–1995), a German-born professor of physics at Birmingham, England, developed a theory of diamagnetism related to metals. His interest in the chain reaction in nuclear physics contributed to the development of the atomic bomb.

Diamond [Greek: *adamos,* invincible] Referred to as the most valuable of stones by **Pliny the Elder** (AD 28–79). They were discovered in Golkonda, near Hyderabad in India, and **Alexander the Great** (355–323 BC) introduced them into Europe in 324 BC. Diamonds were found in Brazil by prospectors for gold in 1724, and richer deposits were found in South Africa, along the Orange River, in 1867. A geologist, **W. Guybon Atherstone** (1813–1898), was one of the first to find diamonds in the Cape colony in South Africa. **Antoine Laurent Lavoiser** (1743–1794) in 1772 demonstrated that diamond was combustible to carbon dioxide, and **Sir Humphry Davy** (1778–1829) showed that diamond was chemically identical to charcoal in 1814. Davy attributed the hardness of diamond to its symmetrical structure. An English chemist, **Smithson Tennant** (1761–1816), independently proved that diamond consisted solely of carbon. A Scotsman, James Ballantyne Hannay, claimed to have produced the first artificial diamond, in 1880. A British physicist, **Samuel Tolansky** (1907–1973) of Newcastle upon Tyne, used multiple-beam interferometry to study the properties and surface structure of diamonds and published *History and Use of Diamonds* (1962). *See artificial diamonds, carats.*

Diatoms Surface-living plants usually of a single cell, found in the sea and fresh water. First described in 1773 by a Danish biologist, **Otto Frederick Muller** (1730–1784) of

Copenhagen. He also introduced Infusoria, so called because they were found in infusions after exposure to air. This phylum of ciliated protozoa is now called Ciliophora. A Swedish botanist and a bishop, **Carl Adolf Agardh** (1785–1859), gave a general account of diatoms, and described 49 species in his *Syatema algarum* (1824).

Dicaearchus (355–285 BC)   *See geography.*

Dice   Probably the most ancient game. The Greek god Apollo is supposed to have taught their use to Hermes. They were used by the Egyptians over 3000 years ago. The term astragalus [Greek: *astragalos*, a die] was used in Homer's (*c.* 800 BC) *Iliad,* to denote the cervical vertebra, which, with the arches removed, was used for playing dice.

Dicke, Robert Henry (1916–1997)   *See Big Bang theory.*

Dicksee, Cedric Bernard (1888–1981)   *See Diesel engine.*

Dickson, Leonard Eugene (1874–1957)   *See number theory.*

Dickson, William Kennedy Laurie (1860–1935)   *See cinema.*

Dicotyledon   A botanical term for a division of flowering plants with two seed leaves, introduced in 1703, by an English biologist, **John Ray** (1628–1705) from Essex. A classification based on single-leaved seeds (monocotyledons) and two-leaved seeds (dicotyledons) was proposed by **Lobelius** or **Matthias de l'Obel** (1538–1616) of The Netherlands, in his *New Note-book of Plants.*

Dictaphone   A machine for recording dictation developed in 1885 by Charles S. Tainter.

Didumium   Discovered by a Swedish chemist, **Carl Gustav Mosander** (1797–1858) in 1842. It was later proved to be a compound of two rare elements. He also discovered lanthanum (1839), terbium (1843) and erbium (1843).

Diels, Otto (1876–1954)   *See Diels–Alder reaction.*

Diels–Alder Reaction   Used in organic chemistry to synthesize cyclic compounds. Discovered by two German chemists, **Kurt Alder** (1902–1958) and **Otto Diels** (1876–1954), who were awarded the Nobel Prize for Chemistry, in 1950. Diels was one of the first to isolate pure cholesterol from gallstones.

Diesel Engine   The forerunner of the diesel engine, a thermo-motor running on gas tar, was invented by an English chemist, **James Hargreaves** (1834–1915) of Lancashire. The modern engine based on **Sadi Carnot's** (1796–1831) principle of thermodynamics was invented in 1892 by a German engineer, **Rudolph Christian Karl**

Diesel (1858–1913). It had an injector which forced fuel oil under high pressure into the cylinder through a nozzle. Diesel's paper *The Theory and Design of Rational Heat Engine* was published in 1893. In 1933 a British engineer, **Cedric Bernard Dicksee** (1888–1981), developed it into a more suitable engine for road transport, with his invention of a compression-ignition method. *See Diesel, Rudolph Christian Karl.*

Diesel, Rudolph Christian Karl (1858–1913)   The inventor of the diesel engine, born in Paris to German parents, who migrated to England during the Franco-German war. He was first sent to Ausburgh in south Germany for education at the age of 12, where he was chosen by professor **Carl von Linde** (1842–1934), the inventor of Lind refrigerators, to do research on thermodynamics. Diesel announced his new 20-horsepower compression-ignition oil engine to the National Society of German Engineers, in 1897. His work was recognized by **William Thomson** or **Lord Kelvin** (1824–1907), on whose advice a Scottish firm acquired the right to build the diesel engine.

Dieudonné, Jean Alexandre (1906–1992)   A French mathematician from Lilie who wrote a history of algebraic geometry and algebraic topology.

Differential Gear   A system of geared wheels, for moving a given weight through a given force, was described by **Hero of Alexandria** (*c.* 100 BC). The first design for a differential gear mechanism was provided by **Leonardo da Vinci** (1452–1519). His description of a self-propelled carriage driven by a spring contained a geared mechanism, which allowed different speeds of rotation for driving the wheels. The English scientist **Robert Hooke** (1635–1703), described a stepped gear, and James White used this principle to develop a helical gear in 1808. An encyclodal form of gear teeth was first suggested by John Imison in his treatise *The School of Arts* published in 1787. **James Starley** (1831–1881) from Albourne, in Sussex, during his construction of the tricycle, invented the modern differential gear that moved the rear two wheels at different speeds.

Differential Geometry   Application of differential calculus to geometry. A French mathematican and physicist, **Gaspard Monge** (1746–1818), helped to develop it. A German mathematical physicist from Brunswick, **Carl Friedrich Gauss** (1777–1855), made further contributions. Another German mathematician, **Georg Friedrich Bernhard Riemann** (1826–1866) made significant advances and proposed a new integral for the trigonometric series. Other contributors to the field include the two Italian mathematicians, **Tullio Levi-Civita** (1873–1941) and **Gregorio Ricci-Curbastro** (1853–1925).

Diffraction *See diffraction grating, diffraction of light, electron diffraction, X-ray crystallography.*

Diffraction Grating A method which provided strong evidence for the undulatory theory of light. It is used in astronomy and atomic physics. The apparatus consists of a glass plate, with equidistant lines across it, and its action is similar to that of a prism. By analyzing the characteristic spectra of an object, the observer is able to identify the elements in the source. A diffraction grating with the use of a concave metal or glass grating was developed by an American physicist, **Henry Augustus Rowland** (1848–1901) of Homesdale, Pennsylvania.

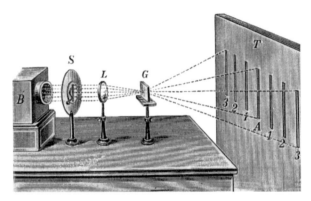

Figure 24 Apparatus for diffraction grating in the 1920s. Graetz, Leo. *Recent Developments in Atomic Theory.* London: Methuen & Co, 1923

Diffraction of Light The bending and spreading of light waves as they pass through the edge of an opaque object. Its discovery gave support to the wave theory of light. The phenomenon was first studied and explained by a Dutch mathematician and scientist, **Christian Huygens** (1629–1695). An Italian physicist, **Francesco Maria Grimaldi** (1618–1683), independently discovered the phenomenon. His theory was advanced by a French physicist, **Jean Augustine Fresnel** (1788–1827).

Diffusion The theory of diffusion of gases and liquids through minute pores was proposed in 1846, by a Scottish chemist and founder of colloid chemistry, **Thomas Graham** (1805–1869). He demonstrated the process of diffusion of fluids across a membrane as being due to osmotic pressure, at the Bakerian lecture delivered by him in 1854. *See osmosis.*

Digestion The first scientific study was carried out by a Flemish physician, **Jean Baptist van Helmont** (1577–1644). He proposed the concept of ferments in digestion that are now recognized as enzymes. Modern scientific experiments on the nature of digestion using a traumatic gastric fistula in a patient was carried out by an American physician from Connecticut, **William Beaumont** (1785–1853), in 1822. In 1889 a Russian physician from Ryazan, **Ivan Petrovich Pavlov** (1849–1936) showed that the secretions in digestion were mediated by the nervous system, through conditioned reflexes. The role of hormones was first demonstrated in 1902 by two English physicians, **Sir William Maddock Bayliss** (1860–1924) and **Ernest Henry Starling** (1866–1927).

Digges, Leonard (1520–1571) *See surveying.*

Digges, Thomas (d 1595) *See surveying.*

Dillen, Johann Jacob (1687–1747) A German botanist who emigrated to England in 1721, and became the first Sherardian Professor of Botany at Oxford in 1734. He published *Hortus Eltnamensis* (1732) and *Historia Muscorum* (1741). *See moss.*

Dines, William Henry (1855–1927) *See cyclone, meteorology.*

Dinokrates (*c.* 300 BC) *See architecture, ancient.*

Dinosaurs [Greek: *deinos,* terrible + *sauros,* lizard] An English surgeon and paleontologist, **Gideon Algernon Mantell** (1790–1852) from Sussex, started studying fossils in 1822, and discovered several types of dinosaur. In 1825 he gave the first full description of a dinosaur, which he named *Iguanodon,* due to the similarity of its teeth to those of an iguana. Some of the earliest illustrations of dinosaurs were done by an artist **John Martin** (1789–1819), for Mantell's book *The Wonders of Geology* (1838). The fossil skeleton of a *pterodactyl,* found in Bavaria in 1788, was recognized to be that of a bird, by **Friedrich Blumenbach** (1752–1840) of Göttingen, in 1807. **Georges Cuvier** (1769–1832) identified it as a flying reptile in 1812, and gave it its present name. The first evidence for it in America was found by an American paleontologist from Lockport, **Charles Othniel Marsh** (1831–1899), who published *Dinosaurs of North America* (1896). An American paleontologist, **Henry Fairfield Osborne** (1857–1935) of Fairfield, Connecticut, who served as President of the American Museum of Natural History (1908–1933), made a spectacular display of specimens of early dinosaurs. A Canadian geologist, **Joseph Burr Tyrrell** (1858–1957), discovered several fossil dinosaurs in Alberta. Fossils of dinosaur eggs and mammals were discovered in Mongolia by an American explorer from Wisconsin, **Roy Chapman Andrews** (1870–1948). The largest known dinosaur egg, belonging to *Hypselosaurus priscus*, was found in 1961 in the valley of the Durance in the south of France, and was dated at 80 million years old. The remains of a skeleton of the longest known (87 feet) dinosaur, *Diplodocus,* was found in 1899, in Wyoming, USA, and it was assembled at the Carnegie Museum, Pittsburg, Pennsylvania. Fragments of the skeleton of the earliest known dinosaur, *Herrerasaurus,* believed to be 230 million years old, were found in 1988 by a fossil hunter, Victorino Herrera, after whom the dinosaur is named. A complete skeleton of it was discovered in 1989 by Paul Sereno of the University of Chicago, on his expedition to the foothills of the Andes, in Argentina. The largest dinosaur discovered to date (167 feet), was found in Patagonia in 1999. It is yet to be named. *See brachiosaurids, Brontosaurus, Triceratops.*

Diode A two-electrode electric thermionic valve consisting of a cathode and an anode, invented by an English electrical engineer, **John Ambrose Fleming** (1849–1945) of Lancashire in 1904. *See triode.*

Diodorus Siculus (d *c.* 20 BC) *See lathe, nutrition.*

Diophantus (*c.* AD 250) An Alexandrian mathematician who was the first to use a symbol for an unknown quantity in his *Arithmetica,* which earned him the title father of algebra. His Diophantine equation brought a new understanding of the theory of numbers, and inspired Fermat's number theory. *See algebra, arithmetic, number theory.*

Diopter An instrument first used in astronomy, and later for land surveying. Archimedes, around 225 BC, used a diopter with two movable cylinders for finding the angular diameter of the sun. **Hipparchus of Bithynia** (190–120 BC) substituted a pin hole instead of a sight in one of the cylinders, and around 140 BC constructed a diopter, with which he made accurate studies of the heavenly bodies. **Hero of Alexandria** (*c.* AD 100) built an ingenious diopter. *See surveying, theodolite.*

Dioptrics [Greek: *dia,* through + *opsis,* see] A study of refracted and transmitted light in relation to the lens and the eye. A German astronomer, **Johannes Kepler** (1571–1630), published *Dioptrice* (1611). The law of refraction was discovered in 1624 by **Snellius** or **Williebrod Snell** (1591–1626), a professor of mathematics at Leyden. **René Descartes** (1596–1650) explained the mechanism of the eye in his treatise *Dioptrica* (1637), in which he compared the eye to a camera obscura. *See optics.*

Dioscorides (AD 40–90) *See arsenic, biology.*

Dip The tendency of the magnetic needle not only to turn towards the north, but also to swing down from the horizontal. The phenomenon was first studied in Europe by a London navigator and naval instrument maker, **Robert Norman** (1550–1600). His experiments formed the first step towards the idea of the magnetic field, and he published *The Newe Attractive shewing the Nature Propertie and manifold vertures of the Loadstone with the Declination of the Needle.* His work was developed by a physician **William Gilbert** (1544–1603) of Colchester, who published *De Magnete, magneticisque corporibus, et de magno magnete tellure* (1600). *See compass, magnet.*

Dipole Gradient across a molecule due to non-uniform distribution of electrons in its atoms. First suggested in 1819 by a Swedish physician and chemist, **Jons Jacob Berzelius** (1779–1848). **Peter Joseph Wilhelm Debye** (1884–1966) of Maastricht, The Netherlands, devised methods for measuring dipole moments. He first used powdered crystals in X-ray crystallography in 1916, and for his work on dipole moments and molecular structure, he was awarded the Nobel Prize for Chemistry in 1936.

Dirac, Paul Adrien Maurice (1902–1984) *See antimatter, electron, positron.*

Direct Current (DC) The first reliable source of direct electrical current, the Daniell cell, consisting of a zinc cathode and copper sulfate in a copper anode, was invented in 1836 by **John Frederick Daniell** (1790–1845), a professor of chemistry at King's College, London. In 1886, an English electrical engineer, **Rookes Evelyn Bell Crompton** (1845–1940) of Thirsk, Yorkshire, established the Kensington and Knightsbridge Electric Supply Company, which used direct current instead of alternating current, for lighting. An alternating current induction motor that enabled the alternating current (AC) to be transmitted over a much greater distance was invented by a Croatian-born US electrical engineer, **Nikola Tesla** (1856–1843). A vacuum diode for changing alternating current to direct current was invented in 1904 by an English electrical engineer **Sir John Ambrose Fleming** (1849–1945) of Lancaster.

Dirichlet, Peter Gustav Lejeune (1805–1859) *See number theory.*

Disk Brake *See car.*

Dishwasher The first hand-turned device appeared in 1865. It was improved by an American woman, W. A. Cockran of Shelbyville, Indiana, in 1879. Electric dishwashers were introduced in 1906.

Dispersion of Light   The phenomenon of dispersion of light, using a prism, was first studied by a Bohemian physician and physicist, **J.M. Marci** (1595–1667) of Kronland. **Sir Isaac Newton** (1642–1727) demonstrated the production of intense colors by making a small hole in an otherwise darkened room and letting in a ray of light thorough a prism. The mechanism was further studied in 1840 by the English physicist, **William Henry Fox Talbot** (1800–1877) from Dorset. **James Clerk Maxwell** (1831–1879) was the first to suggest a theoretical explanation for dispersion, in 1869. A similar explanation was given independently by a German physicist, Sellmeyer, in 1872. In 1860, Le Roux used iodine vapor to study the dispersion of red and violet rays. The German physicist **August Adolph Eduard Eberhard Kundt** (1839–1894), proposed a law related to dispersion of light, in 1871. Further laws related to dispersion were proposed by a Danish mathematician, **Ludwig Valentin Lorenz** (1829–1891) of Copenhagen, and **Hendrick Antoon Lorentz** (1853–1928) of Leyden. *See absorption spectra.*

Dissociation   The theory related to electrolytes in solution was proposed in 1877 by the Dutch chemist **Jacobus Henricus van't Hoff** (1852–1911), and perfected by his pupil **Svante August Arrhenius** (1859–1927), in 1883. The theory of complete dissociation was proposed by the American physical chemist, A.A. Noyes, around 1903. The other important researchers in the field in the early 20th century include **Gilbert Newton Lewis** (1875–1946) of California, and **Niels Janniksen Bjerrum** (1879–1958) of Copenhagen.

Distillation   The method for the production of spirits was introduced into Europe by the Arabs, around AD 1150. A German physician and chemist, **Andreas Libavius** or **Libau** (1540–1616) of Halle, in his *Alchemia* (1597) described the distillation of spirits of wine from grains and fruits. The German iatrochemist, **Johann Rudolph Glauber** (1604–1668), designed a distillation furnace. Distillation began to be practiced in England in the 15th century, and a Parliamentary act to prevent unlicensed persons performing it was passed in 1846. *See wine.*

Ditton, Humphrey (1675–1715)   A London mathematician from Salisbury, who made the first attempt to give a mathematical explanation for capillarity.

Diving Bell   The principle of the diving bell was mentioned by **Aristotle** (384–322 BC) in 325 BC, and its first recorded use in Europe was around AD 1509. It was used in the search for a wreck from the Spanish Armada, off the coast of Mull, in 1662. **Edmund Halley** (1656–1742) improved the

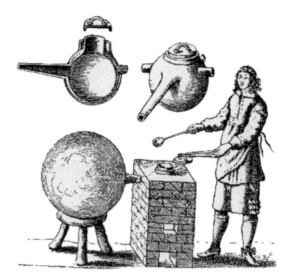

Figure 25   Glauber's furnace for distillation. Findlay, Alexander. *The Spirit of Chemistry.* London: Longmans, Green & Co, 1930

device and is supposed to have used it to become the first person to set foot on the bottom of the deep sea.

Dixon, Harold Baily (1852–1930)   A London chemist who became professor of chemistry at Owen's College, Manchester, in 1887. His main interest was gaseous explosions and flames, and he elucidated the factors affecting the velocity of explosion waves.

Dixon, H.H. (1869–1953)   *See transpiration.*

Dobell, M. Clifford (1886–1949)   *See parasitism, protozoa.*

Dobereiner Lamp   A lamp illuminated by burning hydrogen, which is obtained by the action of sulfuric acid on zinc, in the presence of a platinum sponge. It was invented in 1810 by a German professor at Jena, **Johann Wolfgang Dobereiner** (1780–1849).

Dobereiner, Johann Wolfgang (1780–1849)   A German professor of chemistry in Jena (1810–1849), who demonstrated the relationship of atomic weights between the elements calcium, barium and strontium. His work was a forerunner of the periodic table of **Dimitri Ivanovich Mendeleev**. *See atomic weight, catalysis, Dobereiner lamp, Periodic law.*

Dobzhansky, Theodosius (1900–1975)   *See genetics.*

Dodart, D. (1634–1707)   *See roots.*

Dohrn, Anton (1840–1909)   *See marine biology.*

Dolby, Raymond M. (b 1933)   *See Dolby System, magnetic recording.*

Dolby System   A method for the elimination of background sounds during magnetic recordings, invented in 1967 by **Raymond M. Dolby** (b 1933). *See musical recording.*

Dolland, John (1706–1761)   A physicist of Huguenot ancestry born in London. He lost his father at the age of 5, and taught himself optics, astronomy, physics and other subjects. Dolland built the first refracting telescope based on Newtonian principles of optics and patented it around 1752. He invented achromatic lenses in 1758. *See achromatic lens, heliometer.*

Dollfus, Audoin Charles (b 1924)   *See Saturn.*

Dollo's Law   Irreversibility of evolution, which states that once complex structures are lost they are not regained in their original form. It was proposed in 1893 by a Belgian paleontologist, **Louis Antoine Marie Joseph Dollo** (1857–1931).

Dolomieu, Déodat Guy Gratet de (1750–1801)   *See dolomite.*

Dolomite   A mineral consisting of carbonate of magnesium and calcium, named after a French geologist, **Déodat Guy Gratet de Dolomieu** (1750–1801), who was a professor at the Natural History Museum in Paris.

Domestic Appliances   *See carpet sweeper, cookers, dishwasher, electric iron, microwave oven, oven, pressure cooker, refrigerator, safety razor, sewing machine, vacuum cleaner, washing machine.*

Domestication   *See animal husbandry.*

Dometsch, Arnold (1858–1940)   *See musical instruments.*

Don, George (1764–1814)   A Scottish botanist who published *Account of Plants of Forfarshire* (1813) and *Prodromus Florae Nepalensis* (1825). His brother (1798–1856) with the same name was also a botanist who worked at the Chelsea Physic Garden in London.

Donati, Giovanni Battista (1826–1873)   *See comet.*

Donati's Comet   *See comet.*

Donders, Franciscus Cornelis (1818–1889)   *See spectacles.*

Dondi, Giovanni de (1318–1389)   *See astronomical clock.*

Donkin, Bryan (1768–1855)   *See food industry, paper, printing.*

Donnan, Fredrick George (1870–1956)   An Irish chemist born in Colombo, Ceylon (Sri Lanka). He studied science at Queen's College, Belfast, and later worked under

Friedrich Wilhelm Ostwald (1853–1932) in Leipzig, **Jacobus Henricus van't Hoff** (1852–1911) in Berlin and **William Ramsay** (1852–1916) in London. He became the first Brunner Professor of Physical Chemistry at Liverpool in 1904, and obtained international reputation as a colloid chemist. He proposed the theory of equilibrium across membranes, Donnan's equilibrium, in 1911.

Donnan's Equilibrium   A theory relating to the distribution of ions in solutions across a membrane, proposed in 1911, by **Fredrick George Donnan** (1870–1956), a Sri Lankan-born Irish chemist.

Doppler Phenomenon   The pitch of a whistle from a rapidly moving body, such as a locomotive, was observed to be higher, when the body approached the listener, by an Austrian mathematician, **Christian Doppler** (1803–1853) from Salzburg, while he was professor of mathematics at the State Technical Academy in Prague, in 1842. The Doppler phenomenon is explained by the decrease in wavelength of the sound waves as the source approaches the observer, and an increase in wavelength as it moves away. **Armand Hippolyte Louis Fizeau** (1819–1896), a French physicist, demonstrated the use of the Doppler principle in the estimation of star velocity.

Doppler, Christian (1803–1853)   *See Doppler phenomenon.*

Dorn, Friedrich Ernst (1848–1916)   *See radon.*

Dornberger, Walter Robert (1895–1980)   *See rocket.*

DOS   The first standard **D**isk **O**perating **S**ystem for personal computers, introduced by International Business Machines (IBM) in 1981. *See computers.*

Doty, Paul Mead (b 1920)   *See deoxyribonucleic acid.*

Double Star   *See binary stars.*

Doughlas, David (1798–1834)   *See horticulture.*

Doughlass, Andrew Ellicott (1867–1962)   *See dendrochronology, sunspots.*

Douglas, Donald Willis (1892–1971)   *See airplane.*

Doulton, Sir Henry (1820–1897)   The founder of the English pottery factory at Lambeth. He was born in London. His invention of impervious drainage pipes replaced the unhygienic brick gulleys, and brought about a revolution in sanitation.

Dove, Heinrich Wilhelm (1803–1879)   A German professor of philosophy at Berlin and Konigsberg. He made many optical discoveries and applied the stereoscope to the detection of forged bank notes. His work *Distribution of Heat* was published in 1853. *See paper money, storms.*

Dowson, Emerson Joseph (b 1844)   *See coal gas.*

Drake, Edwin Laurentine (1819–1880)   An American pioneer prospector of oil, from Greenville, New York. In 1859, he invented a tube to protect the drill hole down to the bed rock, at his oilwell in Tinsville, Pennsylvania. His failure to patent the invention led to its widespread use in the petroleum industry.

Draper, John William (1811–1882)   *See photography, portrait photography.*

Drebbel, Cornelis Jacobson (1570–1633)   A Dutch inventor from Alkmaar who emigrated to England in 1604. He invented a clock driven by atmospheric pressure, a thermostat to regulate the supply of air to a furnace, a new method of making sulfuric acid and a submarine, which was first tested in the River Thames, London, in 1620.

Dredges   Devices used for deepening navigable canals and clearing obstructions caused by sandbanks. The first one was patented in England in 1744, and a dredge with buckets was invented by Richard Liddell in 1753. Steam-powered dredges were introduced around 1800.

Dreyer, John Louis Emil (1852–1926)   A Danish astronomer from Copenhagen who compiled three catalogues containing more than 13 000 nebulae and star clusters. He also wrote a biography of Danish astronomer Tycho Brahe in 1890 and a history of astronomy. In 1874 he was appointed assistant at Lord Rosse's Observatory at Birr Castle in Parsonstown, Ireland. He was invited by the Royal Astronomical Society to compile a comprehensive new catalogue which he published in 1888.

Driesch, Hans Adolf Eduard (1867–1941)   *See embryology.*

Drill   *See electric drill, pneumatic drill.*

Drude, Paul (1863–1906)   *See conductivity, refraction.*

Drummond Light   *See limelight.*

Drummond, Henry (1851–1897)   A Scottish scientific explorer and teacher of spiritual philosophy, from Stirling. He published a literary and scientific work *Tropical Africa* in 1890. Drummond's Lowell lectures in Boston in 1893 were published under the title *The Ascent of Man*.

Drummond, Thomas (1794–1840)   *See limelight.*

Dry-Cleaning   A method of cleaning textiles with the use of volatile solvents devoid of water. It was first developed in France in 1849.

Du Fay, Charles François de Cisternay (1698–1739)   *See electricity.*

Dubois, Marie Eugene François Thomas (1858–1940)   *See Java Man.*

Duhamel, Henri Louis (1700–1782)   *See plant nutrition.*

Duhem, Pierre Maurice Marie (1861–1916)   A French science historian in Paris who published *L'Evolution de la Méchanique* (1903), *Origines de la statique* (1905) and several other books.

Duiller, Nicholas Faccio de (1664–1753)   *See watches.*

Dujardin, Felix (1801–1860)   *See invertebrates, protoplasm.*

Dulong and Petit Law   The product of specific heat and atomic weight is constant for all elements. It was developed from **John Dalton's** (1766–1844) idea that the heat capacity of the atoms of all gases was related to their size. A French physician, **Alexis Thérèse Petit** (1791–1820), and a French chemist, **Pierre Louis Dulong** (1785–1838), proposed the law, in 1818.

Dulong, Pierre Louis (1785–1838)   *See Dulong and Petit law.*

Dumas, Jean Baptiste André (1800–1884)   *See biochemistry, chemistry, chloroform, critical temperature, picric acid, vapor density.*

Dumbleton, John (*c.* 1340)   *See motion.*

Dummer, Geoffrey W.A. (b 1909)   *See computers.*

Dumont, Alberto Santos (1873–1932)   *See airplane.*

Dunlop, John Boyd (1840–1921)   The re-inventor of the pneumatic tire, born in Dreghorn, in Scotland. He practiced as a veterinary surgeon in Ireland, before he embarked on his studies on the means and methods of transport. The pneumatic tire, however, had been patented earlier in 1845 by a Scottish engineer, **Robert William Thomson** (1822–1873). Thomson's invention was not a success owing to the scarcity and expense of obtaining India rubber. Dunlop, unaware of Thomson's invention, produced a better version, which he patented in 1888.

Dunne, John William (1875–1945)   *See warplanes.*

Dunning, John Ray (1907–1975)   *See nuclear fission, uranium-235.*

Dunton, John (1659–1733)   *See bookshops.*

Dürer, Albrecht (1471–1528) *See early printed science books, engraving.*

Du Toit, Alexander Logie (1878–1948) *See tectonic theory.*

Dutrochet, René Joachin Henri (1776–1847) *See osmosis.*

Duve, Christian René de (b 1917) *See lysosome.*

Duwez, Pol (b 1907) A Belgian-born US scientist who in 1959 developed a method for making metallic glass from alloys at the California Institute of Technology.

Dyeing *See dyes.*

Dyes [Anglo-Saxon: *deag,* color] First made from purple murex by the Phoenicians in 1000 BC. Most of the dyes used in ancient times came from sea molluscs, plants and insects. Alizarin was used to produce Turkey red by the ancient Egyptians. The Incas were skilled in dyeing long before the Spaniards reached Peru, and they used a scarlet dye from the cochineal beetle. The Roman engineer **Marcus Pollio Vitruvius** (*c.* AD 100) described several natural materials for artificial coloring. Before the discovery of aniline dyes, an English dye chemist, **John Mercer** (1791–1866), used compounds such as manganese, antimomy and lead chromate, for dying textiles and in printing, in 1813. A French professor of chemistry at Dijon, **Jean Jacques Colin** (1784–1865), isolated the dyes alizarin and purpurin, with a French analytical chemist, **Jean-Pierre Robiquet** (1780–1840), in 1827. A German physician and chemist, **Friedlib Ferdinand Runge** (1795–1867), wrote an important work on dyes entitled *Farbenchemie* (1834, 1842, 1850) in three volumes. Coal tar remained as an unwanted waste product of the gas industry until a German chemist, **August Wilhelm von Hofmann** (1818–1892), extracted aniline from it in 1843, and established the modern dye industry. The first aniline dye, mauve, was prepared in 1856 by a London chemist, **Sir William Henry Perkin** (1838–1907), who worked with August Hofmann. The first synthesis of alizarin from anthraquinone was achieved in 1869 by two German chemists, **Karl Graebe** (1841–1927) and **Theodore Liebermann** (1842–1914). The dye from the pod of the vanilla orchid plant, used for coloring in confectionery, was discovered by a German professor of chemistry in Berlin, **Johann Karl Ferdinand Tiemann** (1848–1899). One of the first synthetic dye factories, at Blackley in England, was established in 1864 by a Berlin-born industrial chemist, **Ivan Levinstein** (1845–1916).

Dynamics [Greek: *dynamis,* power] Study of forces which by their action upon bodies bring about a change in their motion. A Greek philosopher, **Strato of Lampsacus** (Turkey), conducted experiments in 340 BC and came to the conclusion that bodies accelerate when they fall. **John Buridan** (*c.* 1300–1358) of Paris explained projectile motion and studied the cause of the acceleration of falling bodies. The study of moving bodies was established on a scientific basis by **Galilei Galileo** (1564–1642), in the early 17th century. Before his time the subject was studied by **Archimedes** (287–212 BC) and **Leonardo da Vinci** (1452–1519). Galileo conducted experiments on the movement of falling bodies, pendulums and projectiles, and introduced the concept of uniform acceleration, distinguishing it from uniform velocity.

Dynamite [Greek: *dynamis,* power] A Swedish industrial chemist and the originator of the Nobel prizes, **Alfred Bernhard Nobel** (1833–1896) of Stockholm, invented dynamite, which is a form of nitroglycerine safer to handle, and twice as powerful as gunpowder. His initial work was involved with land mines for the Russian army with the use of gunpowder. After a fatal explosion at his nitroglycerin factory where his brother was killed in 1864, he concentrated on devising a safer method for the manufacture of explosives and invented dynamite. He patented it in 1867. In 1872 he established over ten factories which manufactured dynamite across Europe. In 1873 the British government granted permission for him to build a factory to make nitroglycerin at Ardeer in Scotland. Maximum precautions were taken in this factory in order to avoid explosions, making it the only dynamite factory in the world with no record of major accidents. In 1875 he introduced a powerful explosive made of gelatinized nitroglycerine and collodion cotton. Nobel invented the first smokeless powder used for military purposes, in 1887. *See explosives.*

Dynamo [Greek: *dynamis,* power] Electricity generated by the battery was found to be too expensive for commercial purposes such as electroplating until **Michael Faraday** (1791–1867) invented an alternative, in 1831. He used a copper disk in the field of a magnet to generate electric current, and this formed the basis for the dynamo. An Italian physicist, **Leopoldo Nobili** (1784–1835), successfully used a steel magnet for producing a flow of current. Faraday's dynamo was improved by an English physicist, **Sir Charles Wheatstone** (1801–1875) and **Ernst Werner von Siemens** (1816–1892) of Berlin. Siemens' improved dynamo in 1867, contained an armature that dispensed with the need for the costly permanent magnets. The first practical dynamo based on Faraday's model was constructed by a French engineer, **Hippolyte Pixie** (1808–1835), who exhibited a generator at the French Academy of Sciences, in Paris, in 1832. The theory of the dynamo was proposed earlier in 1829 by an American physicist, **Joseph Henry** (1797–1878) of Albany, New York, but he failed to patent his invention. The first high efficiency dynamo was produced by **Thomas Alva Edison** (1847–1931), in 1876. The carbon brush for dynamos was invented by a Scottish physicist, **George Forbes** (1849–1936). In 1873, a Belgian electrical engineer, **Zenobe Theophile Gramme** (1826–1901), showed that the dynamo could function in reverse as an electric motor.

Dynamometer [Greek: *dynamis*, power + *metron*, measure] Used for measuring power in electric circuits, this was invented by a German-born British engineer, **Karl**

Wilhelm Siemens, later **Sir Charles William Siemens** (1823–1883).

Dyson, Sir Frank Watson (1868–1939) A British astronomer who established radio time-signals in broadcasting. His six-pip signal time check was adopted by the British Broadcasting Corporation in 1924. He became the Astronomer Royal in 1905.

Dysprosium A metallic element with an atomic number of 66, discovered in 1886 by a French physical chemist, **Paul Emile Lecoq de Boisbaudran** (1838–1912) of Cognac.

E

Eads, James Buchanan (1820–1887)   *See bridges.*

Eames, Charles (1907–1978) An American architect and furniture designer who is known for his innovative 'lounge chair' in the 1950s.

Early Printed Science Books The earliest books on mathematics in Europe were printed at a monastery in Subiaco, near Rome, in 1465. In 1478, a printed work on arithmetic by an anonymous writer was issued from a press in Treviso, situated on the northern trade route to Venice. The first book on commercial arithmetic was published by Borghi in Venice in 1484. The first printed translation of Euclid's *Elements,* by **Johannes Campanus** (*c.* 1205–1296), was published in 1482, and a Greek edition of it dedicated to **Cuthbert Tonstall** (1474–1559) appeared in Basel in 1533. Another edition of Euclid by Erhardt Randolt in 1482 was the first printed book to contain gold coloring. Johannes Widman's book on arithmetic, *Behède und hubsche Rechnung,* was published in Germany in 1489. Calandri's arithmetic in 1491 was the first Italian book with woodcut illustrations to explain mathematical problems. The method of downward division was described for the first time in this book. The first printed dictionary on drugs, *Synonyma medicinae,* written by Simon de Cordo (1270–1330), was published in 1473. The first printed book in pediatrics, *Libellus de aegritudinibus infantum* (Little Book of the Diseases of Children) by Paulus Begellardus or Bagellaro of Italy, based on the works of the Islamic physicians **Avicenna** (980–1037) from Bokhara, Kazakhstan and **Rhazes** (860–926) from Baghdad, was published in 1472. An Italian architect from Venice, **Leone Battista Alberti** (1404–1472), revived Roman classical architecture in his *De Re Aedificatoria* (1485). The work of the Roman physician Aulius Cornelius Celsus (*c.* AD 100), *De Medicina* (1478), became one of the earliest printed medical books. The first German mathematical text *A Treatise on Mensuration,* was published by a mathematician and engraver, **Albrecht Dürer** (1471–1528) of Nuremberg, in 1525. The *Rechenbiechlin* of the German mathematician, **Jacob Köbel** (1514), passed through 22 editions. An advanced treatise on algebra entitled *Ars Magna* (1545), published at Nurnberg by **Girolomo Cardan** (1501–1576), was the first printed book on algebra for solving equations. The first book on arithmetic in England

entitled *De Arte Svppvtandi* was published by Cuthbert Tonstall in 1522. The first important work on commercial arithmetic in Germany, entitled *Rechnung auff der Linier* (1522), was published by **Adam Riese** (1489–1559). The medical works of the Greek physician, Paul of Aegina (AD 625–690), entitled *Epitomoe medicoe libri septem,* in seven volumes, was first printed in Venice in 1528. Ptolemy's *Almagest* was translated into Latin in the 12th century and the first printed version of it appeared in Basel in 1538. An important landmark in botany, *New Krütterbuch* (New Plant Book) by a physician and botanist, Jerome Bock (1498–1554), appeared in 1539. A new edition of it with woodcut illustrations was published in 1546. The first printed monograph on ornithology, containing a description of birds mentioned by Aristotle and Pliny, was published in 1544 by an English naturalist from Cambridge, **William Turner** (1510–1568). The first treatise on algebra in English, *The Whetstone of Witte* (*c.* 1540–1542), was written by an English mathematician, **Robert Recorde** (*c.* 1510–1558). The first book on physical geology, *De Ortu et Causis Subterraneorum* (1546), was published by a German physician, **Georgius Agricola** (1494–1555). His *De Natura Fossilium* was the first book on mineralogy. The *Natural History of Plants* by Valerius Cordus (1515–1544) of Oberhessen, was published posthumously after his death, by **Conrad Gesner** (1516–1565), in 1561. Francisco Bravo's (1530–1594) *Opera Medicinalia* published in Mexico City in 1570 was the first printed medical book in the New World.

Early Science Journals   *See scientific journals.*

Early Scientific Instruments   *See abacus, air pump, astrolabe, barometer, clock, diopter, gnomon, heliostat, micrometer, microscope, odometer, quadrant, reflecting telescope, sextant, siderostat, sundial, telescope, theodolite, thermometer.*

Earnshaw, Thomas (1749–1829)   *See clock, escapement.*

Earth [Anglo-Saxon: *eorthe*] A Greek philosopher, Archelaus, who lived before the time of **Socrates** (470–399 BC), was the first to suggest that the earth was not flat. **Anaximander** (611–547 BC) of Miletus, was the first Greek to draw a map of the earth giving details of its surface, and to speculate on the size and distance of the heavenly bodies or stars. **Hipparchus**, an eminent astronomer of Bithynia in 150 BC, stated that the earth was flat at the poles. The creation of the earth was dated at 4004 BC by Archbishop James Usher in 1650. The chronology of all events including those in the bible were related to this date. A Russian scientist, **Mikhail Vasilievich Lomonosov** (1711–1765), was the first to question this date on a geological basis, pointing out that the earth was hundreds of thousands of years older. An astrophysicist, **Edward Arthur Milne** (1896–1950), came to the conclusion that the earth is about 2000 million years old. In 1779, the French naturalist, **George Louis Leclerc Compte de Buffon** (1707–1788), proposed that the earth was originally hot before cooling, and set the age of the earth at 75 000 years. Work by several geologists over the next two centuries set the age of the earth at 4.6 billion years. A Soviet chemist, **Alexander Ivanovich Oparin** (1894–1980), proposed a theory of the origin of life on earth, in 1922. His theory was based on the assumption that organisms first arose from the sea. His work *The Origin of Life on Earth* (1936) inititated the experimental search for the origin of life from either inorganic or simple organic elements. An American chemist, **Stanley Lloyd Miller** (b 1930) of Oakland, California, was one of the first experimentally to investigate the formation of organic and other matter, by simulating thunderstorms. He passed an electric discharge through mixtures of gases and noted the appearance of organic substances such as aldehydes and amino acids. His findings became accepted as a plausible explanation for the appearance of the first organic substances on earth. A landmark paper on the composition of the earth's interior, based on geochemical and seismological observations, was published in 1952 by an American geophysicist, **Albert Francis Birch** (1903–1992). *See Big Bang theory, earth density, earth mass, earth size, geogeny.*

Earth Density A London astronomer, **Nevil Maskelyne** (1732–1811), was the first to determine the density of the earth from the deflection of the plumb line at Perthshire, in 1774. Another method for determining the density of the earth was invented by **Henry Cavendish** (1731–1810) in 1798. **John Henry Poynting** (1852–1914), an English physicist from Monton, Lancashire, did experiments and published *On the Mean Density of Earth* (1893).

Earth Sciences *See agronomy, climatology, earth, earthquake, fossils, geogeny, geography, geological map, geology, glaciology, global warming, hurricane, Ice Age, meteorology, oceanography, paleomagnetism, paleontology, paleophytology, petrology, plate tectonics, rivers, sand dunes, seismology, soil erosion, soil science, storms, stratigraphy, terrestial magnetism, tides, volcanic eruptions, volcanoes, weather forecast.*

Earth Size The Greek philosopher and mathematician **Eratosthenes** (274–194 BC), was one of the first to calculate the size of the earth by a geometrical method. An astronomer of Alexandria, **Posidonius** (*c.* 400 BC), used a system of meridian circles to calculate the same.

Earthquake In 435 BC the Greek philosopher **Anaxagorus** postulated that earthquakes were produced by subterranean clouds bursting out into lightning, which shook the vault that confined them. **Aristotle**, in his *Meteorologica,* considered wind as one of the main causes of earthquakes. The Roman philosopher **Lucius Annaeus Seneca** (d AD 65) believed earthquakes to be a result of an excessive quantity of air entering the empty cavities beneath the earth. **René Descartes** (1596–1650) and **Athanasius Kircher** (1601–1680) thought that the earth contained numerous cavities underground, which were filled with water and minerals that shook the earth. **Joseph Priestley** (1733–1804), a clergyman and chemist from Leeds, believed that earthquakes occurred because of electricity. An English geologist and professor at Cambridge, **John Michell** (1724– 1793) of Nottinghamshire, was one of the first to write on the causes and phenomena of earthquakes, in 1760. An elaborate list of earthquakes that occurred from 1606 BC to AD 1842 was given by W. Mallet in 1858. **John Milne** (1859–1913) of Liverpool, a pioneer in the scientific study of earthquakes and seismology, developed an interest in earthquakes during his service as an engineer in Japan. Some of his important publications include *Earthquakes* (1883) and *Seismology* (1898). The science of seismology was established in the USA by **Perry Byerley** (1897–1978) of Clarinda, Iowa, who studied the dynamics of earthquakes. An English geophysicist, **Sir Harold Jeffreys** (1891–1989) of Durham, made an analysis of seismic travel times with the use of a mechanical calculator, and devised the Jeffreys–Bullen tables, which became a standard reference. The Richter scale, based on the amplitude of an earthquake recorded on seismograph, for measuring the strength of earthquakes, was invented by **Charles Francis Richter** (1900–1985) of Hamilton, Ohio, in 1930. *See seismograph.*

Eastman, George (1854–1932) *See camera, photography.*

Eastwood, Eric (1910–1981) *See radar.*

Echelon Grating A device with a great resolving power of light, made up of a number of quartz plates and capable of producing dispersion, invented by **Albert Abraham Michelson** (1852–1931).

Echo The term originates from the legend of Narcissus and the nymph Echo, who wasted away with unrequited love until she was reduced to only her voice. **Aristotle** (384–322 BC), in his treatise *On the Soul* stated that an echo is produced when the air is made to rebound like a ball. He also knew that an echo is always produced but not always heard. *See acoustics, velocity of sound.*

Echolocation An American zoologist, **Donald Redfield Griffin** (1864–1932) of Southampton, New York, demonstrated for the first time that bats produce ultrasound for echolocation. In 1953, he showed that they used the method for locating and capturing prey. An English zoologist, **John David Pye** (b 1932) of Nottingham, studied the use of echolocation by bats to avoid obstacles during flying.

Eckart, Carl (1902–1971) *See matrix mechanics.*

Eckener, Hugo (1868–1964) *See circumnavigation.*

Eckert, John Presper (1919–1995) *See computers.*

Eckford, Harry (1775–1832) *See sailing ships.*

Eclipse [Greek: *ekleipsis*, cessation] According to **Ptolemy of Alexandria** (*c.* AD 127–145), the first recorded eclipse occurred on 19 March 721 BC. A recent study of clay tablets, however, found in 1948 amongst the ruins of the city of Ugarit, in Syria, points to an earlier record of an eclipse, in 1223 BC. The first solar eclipse was recorded by the Babylonians in 763 BC and the Chinese recorded their first solar eclipse in 720 BC. **Thales** of Miletus (*c.* 640–546 BC) predicted and observed an eclipse on 28 May 585 BC. The Ancient Egyptians, up to 323 BC, recorded 373 eclipses of the sun, and 832 eclipses of the moon. **Anaxagoras** (*c.* 500–428 BC) correctly explained lunar and solar eclipses. A Guernsey-born British scientist and astronomer, **Warren de la Rue** (1815–1889), took the first photograph of a solar eclipse, in 1860. Two English astronomers, **Sir Richard van der Riet Woolley** (1906–1986) of Weymouth, and **Sir Frank Watson Dyson** (1868–1939), an Astronomer Royal, first for Scotland and later England, published *Eclipses of the Sun and Moon* (1937).

École des Ponts et Chaussées School of Bridges and Highways, the first school in the world for civil engineering, was established in 1747 in Paris by an administrator of highways, Daniel Trudaine and his son Philibert Trudaine.

Ecology [Greek: *oikos,* house + *logos,* discourse] The study of living animals and plants in relation to their environment and other living beings. The term *oecologie* was introduced in 1886 by **Ernst Heinrich Haeckel** (1834–1919) of Jena. In 1650, **Lobelius (Matthias de L'Obel)** (1538–1616), a Belgian botanist to King James I, noted that high mountain plants tended to be found at lower levels in cold climates. One of the first works on ecology, entitled *The Natural History and antiquities of Selborne* (1789), published by an English clergyman and naturalist, **Gilbert White** (1720–1793) of Selbourne, Hampshire, became the fourth best selling book in English and ran to 200 editions. In 1836

F.J.A.N. Unger demonstrated the dependence of plants on the chemical composition of the soil. An Austrian botanist, **Anton Joseph Kerner von Marilaun** (1831–1898), published pioneering works including *Das Pflanzenleben der Donauländer* (1863) and *Die Schutzmittel der Blüthen* (1876). The first textbook, *Plantesamfund* (1895), was published by **Johannes Eugenius Bülow Warming** (1841–1924) of Denmark. It was translated into English under the title *Ecology of the Plants,* in 1909. Another important treatise in 1898, *Pflanzengeographie* (Plant geography on a physiological basis) was written by **Andreas Franz Wilhelm Schimper** (1856–1901) of Basel. The early studies were mostly on plants, until **Charles Darwin** (1809–1882) commenced his studies on animals. Animal ecology was set on a firm footing by an English zoologist, **Charles Sutherland Elton** (1900–1991) of Liverpool, who published *Animal Ecology* (1927), *Animal Ecology and Evolution* (1930) and *The Pattern of Animal Communities* (1966). The concept of territory, where a group or individual of an animal species confined itself, was suggested by a German biologist, **Bernard Altum** (1824–1900), and advanced by a British zoologist, **H. Heliot Howard** (1873–1940). Plant ecology in Britain was pioneered by **Arthur George Tansley** (1871–1955), who was instrumental in founding the British Ecological Society, in 1913. He was editor of the *Journal of Ecology* published by the society, from 1916 to 1938. His *Practical Plant Ecology* was published in 1923, and he was knighted in 1950. Work in England on the evolution of land flora was done by **Frederick Orpen Bower** (1855–1948) of Ripon, who published *The Origin of Land Flora* (1908), *The Botany of Living Plant* (1919) and a historical work entitled *Sixty Years of Botany in Britain* (1938).

Eddington, Arthur Stanley (1882–1944) An English astronomer and professor at Cambridge, who gave the first experimental proof for Einstein's general theory of relativity, in 1919. He showed that stars whose light passed close to the sun appeared to be displaced by a minute amount which corresponded to the value calculated by Einstein. He published *Mathematical Theory of Relativity* (1923), *Space Time and Gravitation* (1920), *Stars and Atoms* (1927) and *The Expanding Universe* (1933).

Edelinck, Gerard (1649–1707) *See engraving.*

Edgerton, Harold Eugene (1903–1990) *See camera, photography.*

Edgeworth, Richard Lovell (1744–1817) *See roads, semaphore.*

Edinger, Tilly (Johanna Gabrielle Ottilie) (1897–1967) A German-born US paleontologist who demonstrated that the evolution of the brain could be studied directly from fossil cranial casts. She laid the foundations for the paleopathology with her work *Fossil Brain* (1929).

Edison, Thomas Alva (1847–1931) An ingenious American inventor born in Milan, Ohio. His family moved to Michigan in 1854 where his interest in science started with his studies on train telegraphy in 1862. His inventions include: a talking machine, a mimeograph, an electric lamp, the electrical system for New York's underground central station system and over 1000 other patents. *See cinema, dynamo, electric light bulb, electric lighting, fluoroscope, gramophone, kinetoscope, microphone, tape recorder.*

Edlefsen, Niels (1893–1971) An American physicist and a pupil of **Ernest Lawrence** (1901–1958). He built one of the first cyclotrons, in 1930.

Edlén, Bengt (b 1906) A Swedish astrophysicist and professor of physics at Lund University (1944–1973) who gave an explanation for certain lines in spectra of the solar corona that have been previously observed by astronomers since 1869 and thought to be due to a new element.

EDSAC (Electronic Delay Storage Automatic Calculator) *See computers.*

Edwards, Sir George Robert (b 1908) An English aircraft engineer from Higham Park, Essex, who designed the *Viking, Valiant* and *Viscount* planes, in the 1940s.

Egerton, Francis Henry, the 8th Earl of Bridgewater (1756–1829) *See Bridgewater Treatises.*

Egerton, Francis, the 3rd Duke of Bridgewater (1736–1803) *See canals.*

Eggen, Olin Jenck (b 1919) An American astronomer from Wisconsin who studied high-velocity stars, and classified red giants with the use of narrow and broadband photometry.

Eginhard (*c.* AD 770–840) *See sunspots.*

Ehrenberg, Christian Gottfried (1795–1876) *See mycology.*

Ehrlich, Paul (1854–1915) A German bacteriologist of Jewish origin from Strzelin who was a pioneer in chemotherapeutics. He developed the side-chain theory of receptor groups for antigen, for which he shared the Nobel Prize for Physiology or Medicine with **Elie Metchnikoff** (1845–1916) in 1908.

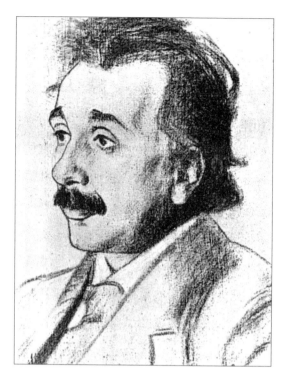

Figure 26 Albert Einstein (1879–1955), from *Relativity*. London: Methuen & Co Ltd, Translation by Robert W. Lawson, 1920

Eiffel Tower Built at a cost of 260 000 GBP for the World Exhibition of 1889 by a French engineer **Gustav Alexandre Eiffel** (1832–1923) from Dijon. At 300 m, it remained as the tallest artificial structure in the world until 1920. Over 7300 tons of iron was used for its construction, commencing in January 1887 and completed in April 1889. **Louis Paul Cailletet** (1832–1913) of Paris first tested his liquid-hydrogen apparatus for high-altitude ascents with the use of a 300 meter manometer on the Eiffel Tower. The first transatlantic call was made in 1915 between Arlington, Virginia and the Eiffel Tower, and the first television transmitter in France was installed at the tower in 1935.

Eiffel, Gustav Alexandre (1832–1923) *See Eiffel Tower.*

Eigen, Manfred (b 1927) *See flash photolysis.*

Einstein, Albert (1879–1955) A theoretical physicist and Nobel Prize winner for Physics (1921) born to Jewish parents at Ulm in Bavaria. He studied mathematics at Technical High School in Zurich from 1896 to 1900; his initial intention was to become a secondary school teacher in gymnastics. He became naturalized in Switzerland in 1901, and started working as an engineer at the Swiss Patent Office in 1902. He published his special theory of relativity while he was attached to a Swiss university, in 1905. Einstein served as professor of physics at Zurich (1909) and Prague (1911) before he was made director of the Kaiser Wilhelm Physical Institute in Berlin. He proposed theories for Brownian movement, the quantum law of emission and absorption of light. His general theory of relativity followed in 1916. One of Einstein's predictions regarding the deflection of light by cosmic masses was put to the test during the solar eclipse on May 1919, and he was proved right. He left for America in 1934, during the time of Hitler's rise to power. In 1940, he was appointed as a professor at Princeton University, New Jersey, where he continued to work on his unified field theory until his death. *See Bose–Einstein statistics, Brownian movement, ether, kinematic theory, laser, maser, photoelectricity, photons, quantum theory, relativity.*

Einsteinium An element with atomic number 99, synthesized by an American physicist, **Glenn Theodore Seaborg** (1912–1999) and his team at Berkeley. It is named after Albert Einstein.

Eisenhart, Luther Pfahler (1876–1965) An American mathematician at Princeton University who formulated a theory of the deformation of surfaces and attempted to develop his own geometry theory from that of German mathematician Georg Riemann. He wrote an account of his theory in *Transformations of Surface* (1923).

Ejection Seat A life-saving device for fighter pilots, developed by a British aeronautical engineer, **James Martin** (1893–1981), in 1944. His prototype was a powerful spring with a swinging arm, which he improved to give a demonstration of the first live ejection, in 1946. He also designed several fighter aircrafts, and founded the Martin–Baker aeronautical firm, with Valentine Henry Baker, in the 1940s.

Ekeberg, Anders Gustat (1767–1813) *See tantalum, titanium.*

Ekman, Vagn Walfrid (1874–1954) *See oceanography.*

El Malakh, Kamal (b 1918) *See boats.*

Elasticity [Greek: *elastikos,* rebounding] An English scientist, **Robert Hooke** (1635–1703) from Freshwater, in the Isle of Wight, discovered the relationship between stress and strain in elastic bodies, which is known as Hooke's law. The ratio (Poisson ratio) between the lateral and longitudinal strain in a wire, in the study of elasticity, was proposed by a French physicist and astronomer, **Siméon Denis Poisson** (1781–1840). A French civil engineer, **Claude Louis Marie Henri Navier** (1785–1836), proposed a formula for predicting the limits of elasticity in structural materials. An English geophysicist, **Augustus Edward Hough Love**

(1863–1940), published a *Treatise on the Mathematical Theory of Elasticity* (1892–1893) in two volumes.

Electric Appliances *See cookers, electric blanket, electric drill, electric food mixer, electric iron, electric light bulb, electric lighting, electric razor, electric toaster, electric typewriter, sewing machine, vacuum cleaner, washing machines.*

Electric Blanket An electric pad, the forerunner of the electric blanket, was invented in 1912 by an American physician, Sidney Russell.

Electric Chair Used for the purpose of official executions, invented in 1888 by two Americans, Harold P. Brown and E.A. Kennealley. The first person to be executed by this method was a murderer, William Kemmler, at the New York state prison, in 1890, and he took eight minutes to die. By 1915, 25 other states had accepted electrocution as a method of capital punishment.

Electric Charge The first determination of charge on a gaseous ion was determined in 1897 by an Irish physicist from Galway, **Sir John Sealy Edward Townsend** (1868–1957). He published *The Theory of Ionisation of Gases by Collision* (1910), *Electricity in Gases* (1915) and *Motions of Electrons in Gases* (1925). **Sir John Joseph Thomson** (1856–1940) of Manchester, used **Charles Thompson Rees Wilson's** (1869–1959) method to measure the charge. An American physicist from Illinois, **Robert Andrews Millikan** (1868–1953), who was professor of physics at the Californian Institute of Technology, was awarded the Nobel Prize for Physics in 1923, for improving their method.

Electric Cookers *See cookers.*

Electric Drill The first electric hand drill was invented in 1895 by Wilhelm Fein of Stuttgart, Germany. A drill with a trigger switch, the Black and Decker drill, was invented in 1917 by two Americans, S. Duncan Black and Alonso G. Decker.

Electric Food Mixer The first device came into use in 1918.

Electric Furnace Invented in 1892 by **Ferdinand Frederic Henri Moissan** (1852–1907). He became professor of chemistry at Paris in 1900 and was awarded the Nobel Prize for Chemistry in 1906 for this invention and for the isolation of fluorine.

Electric Generator *See dynamo.*

Electric Iron Until the end of the 19th century, irons filled with hot bricks or charcoal, or irons heated on a fire, were used for ironing clothes. The flat electric iron was invented by H.W. Seeley of America in 1882 and these came into use in England around 1895.

Electric Light Bulb In 1838 a Frenchman, Jobart, first observed that a carbon rod, sealed in a vacuum, lit up when an electric current was passed through it. The first incandescent lamp of this type was patented by W.E. Staite of America, in 1845. A lamp with a platinum filament was made by E.C. Shepherd of England, in 1846. The largest contribution to the development of the electric light bulb came from **Thomas Alva Edison** (1847–1931) who started his research on the subject in 1877. In 1879 he achieved the longest record of lighting – for 40 hours – and in 1880 made a 16-watt lamp which lasted for 1589 hours. An American inventor and son of an escaped slave, **Louis Howard Latimer** (1848–1928), patented an electric lamp in 1881. In 1882 he invented a cheap method of producing longer-lasting carbon filaments for an electric incandescent lamp, and published *Incandescent Electric Lighting. A Practical Description of the Edison System* (1890). An improved tungsten lamp filled with an inert gas, nitrogen, was designed in 1913 by **Irving Langmuir** (1881–1957) of Brooklyn, New York. *See electric lighting.*

Electric Lighting In 1803, the English scientist, **Sir Humphry Davy** (1778–1829), produced the first electric light, known as the arc light, by passing electricity through two carbon electrodes. Although his device produced a brilliant light, it had the disadvantage of releasing large amounts of smoke and heat. Despite its disadvantages the arc light was used to light up Paris and London in the 19th century, until it was superseded by the electric light invented by **Thomas Alva Edison** (1847–1931). In 1845 **J.W. Starr** (1822–1847) took out an American patent for a lamp in which the platinum filament was electrically heated in an evacuated glass container. He also suggested the carbon filament as an alternative. In 1876, a Russian inventor in Paris, **Pavel Nikolaivitch Jablochkoff** (1847–1894), invented a low-current arc lamp, known as the electric candle or Jablochkoff candle. By 1881, 4000 of these lamps were in service in Paris and London. In 1879, Edison made a bulb with a filament of carbonized cotton sewing thread, which did not burn out. He improved it by using a carbonized filament and gave a public demonstration in the same year. A similar incandescent electric lamp was invented independently in England by **Sir Joseph Wilson Swan** (1828–1914) of Sunderland, in 1878. Edison's first electric generation station, in London, mainly for lighting, was established in 1880, and the first electric lighting system in America was built at the Pearl Street power station, New York, in 1883. In 1886 an English electrical engineer,

Rookes Evelyn Bell Crompton (1845–1940) of Thirsk, Yorkshire, founded the Kensington and Knightsbridge Electric Supply Company, which used direct current instead of alternating current for lighting. A New York mechanic, **Peter Cooper Hewitt** (b 1861), invented a vacuum electric lamp in which the carbon filament was replaced by mercury vapor. An electric lamp with a filament of zirconium and other rare oxides, instead of carbon, was invented in 1897 by a German chemist, **Walther Hermann Nernst** (1864–1941). In 1908, an American physicist, **William David Coolridge** (1873–1975) of Hudson, Massachusetts, replaced the carbon filament with a tungsten filament. The fluorescent light tube, coated with a fluorescent material, and filled with mercury vapor, was first introduced in 1936. *See electric light bulb.*

Electric Locomotive *See locomotive.*

Electric Motor *See dynamo.*

Electric Photometry *See photoelectric cell.*

Electric Plane The first electrically propelled aircraft, equipped with a Bosch motor and nickel-cadmium batteries, was designed by an American maker of model aircraft, Fred Militky. It had a wing span of nearly 40 feet and made its first flight in 1973.

Electric Railway The first practical system based on electric traction was demonstrated by **Ernst Werner von Siemens** (1816–1892) at the Berlin Trades Exhibition, in 1879. *See tram car.*

Electric Razor The first practical device was developed in 1928 by Joseph Schick. *See safety razor.*

Electric Relay A system enabling current to be transmitted over long distances from its source was invented in 1835 by an American physicist, **Joseph Henry** (1797–1878) of Albany, New York. In 1820 he constructed powerful electromagnets, with the use of fine insulated wire wrapped around an iron core. The unit of inductance in electricity is named after him.

Electric Sewing Machine *See sewing machine.*

Electric Shaver *See safety razor.*

Electric Telegraphy A Scottish surgeon, Charles Morrison, from Renfrew, first described a method of transmitting messages through wires in the *Scots Magazine* in 1753. His biographical details are not known; he is supposed to have emigrated to Virginia and died there later. The invention of the electric battery in 1800 by **Alessandro Volta** (1745–1827) made electric telegraphy a practical possibility. In

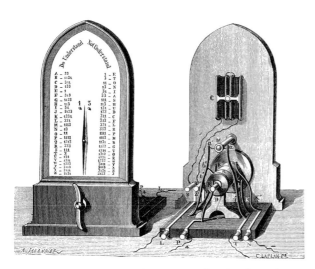

Figure 27 Cooke and Wheatstone's electric telegraph system. Guillemin, Amédée. *The Applications of Physical Forces*. London: Macmillan and Co, 1877

1819, a Danish physicist, **Hans Christian Oersted** (1777–1851), demonstrated that a magnetic needle could be deflected by an electric current, and its movements depended on the direction of the current. In 1816, an English inventor, **Sir Francis Ronalds** (1788–1873), built an electric telegraph that transmitted every requisite signal with the use of a single circuit, in his garden in Hammersmith, London. In 1837, **Sir William Fothergill Cooke** (1806–1879) of Ealing, and **Sir Charles Wheatstone** (1801–1875) built the first practical electric telegraph system and patented it in 1845. In 1837, **Samuel Morse** (1791–1872) of Charlestown, Massachusetts, developed a practical telegraph, which worked by making and breaking contact with the current, in order to produce signals that could be recorded at the end of the line, by a pen on a moving strip of paper. The transatlantic cable for telegraphy was first attempted by the Atlantic Cable Company in 1856. **Lord Kelvin** or **William Thomson** (1824–1907) successfully laid a transatlantic cable from Ireland to Newfoundland in 1866. The first message thorough this cable over a distance of 1896 miles was sent in 1858. **Thomas Alva Edison** (1847–1931) in 1872 developed duplex telegraphy for simultaneously transmitting two messages.

Electric Toaster The first device was marketed in 1909. An automatic toaster with a spring device controlled by a thermocontact was invented in 1927 by an American mechanic, Charles Strite.

Electric Transformer A device that uses induction to convert high-voltage alternating current into low-voltage, and vice versa. It was invented in 1885 by an American electrical engineer, **William Stanley** (1858–1916) of Brooklyn, New York. He also devised a long-range transmission system for delivering alternating current.

Electric Typewriter The first electric typewriter, known as the *blickensderfer,* was introduced in 1901. *See electronic typewriter, typewriter.*

Electrical Conductivity The electrical conductivity in metals was discovered in 1729 by an Englishman, **Stephen Gray** (d 1736).

Electrical Resistance The Wheatstone bridge, a device for making accurate measurements of electrical resistance, was first suggested by **Samuel Hunter Christie** (1784–1865) and popularized by an English physicist, **Sir Charles Wheatstone** (1801–1875) of Gloucester, in 1843. **Georg Simon Ohm** (1789–1854), a German professor of physics at Nuremberg (1833–1849), published the Ohm's Law relating to voltage, current, and electrical resistance, in 1827. **Gustav Robert Kirchhoff** (1824–1887) measured electrical resistance in absolute terms for the first time, in 1849. **James Prescott Joule** (1818–1889) devised a simple method of measuring the absolute value of resistance, in 1870. **Wilhelm Eduard Weber** (1804–1891) used a large coil connected in series with a tangent galvanometer. **William Thomson** or **Lord Kelvin** (1824–1907) designed a method of measuring its value, with the help of a rotating coil, around 1873.

Electricity [Greek: *elektron,* amber] The electrical property of amber, when rubbed, was observed by the Greek philosopher, **Thales** (*c.* 640–546 BC) in 600 BC. An English physician, **William Gilbert** (1544–1603) of Colchester, noticed that other substances apart from amber also produced electricity. His *De Magnete, Magneticisque Corporibus, te de Magno Magnette Tellure, Physiologia Nova* (1600) established him as the initiator of the study of modern electricity. He was also the first to introduce the term electricity. In 1629, an Italian Jesuit, Cabaeus, in his *Magnetica* made an important observation that particles that were attracted to each other often repelled after their contact. The Accademia del Cimento in Florence in 1657 arranged electrical substances in order of their attracting power when rubbed. **Otto von Guericke** (1602–1686) obtained sparks by rubbing a globe of sulfur, and produced the first frictional machine for continuous production of electricity, in 1647. **Robert Boyle** (1627–1691) made use of glass to produce a similar effect, in 1676. An Englishman, **Stephen Gray** (d 1736), discovered the electrical conductivity of metals in 1729. In 1791 **Luigi Galvani** (1737–1798) started investigating the

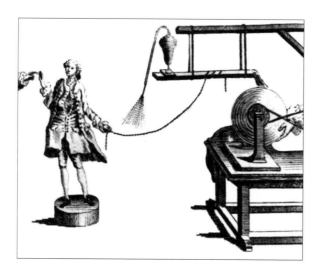

Figure 28 Early experiments on electricity. Owen, W. *Dictionary of Arts and Sciences*. London: Homer's Head, 1754

phenomenon of the twitching of frog muscle when brought into contact with two metals and discovered animal electricity. The Voltaic pile, the first primitive form of battery, consisting of zinc, silver and a moistened card, was devised in 1800 by **Alessandro Volta** (1745–1827). The positive and negative components of electricity were first demonstrated by a French chemist, **Charles François de Cisternay Du Fay** (1698–1739) of Paris. His six memoirs on electricity were published between 1733 and 1737. **André Marie Ampère** (1775–1836) deduced the formula for measuring electricity, while he was a professor at the École Polytechnique of Paris, in 1775. The magnetic effect of electric current on a needle, first observed in 1819 by a Danish physicist, **Hans Christian Oersted** (1777–1851), opened the doors to the new field of electromagnetism. **Michael Faraday** (1791–1867) discovered the phenomenon of electromagnetic rotation in 1822, and presented his first series of *Experimental Researches on Electricity* to the Royal Society in 1831. The first practical electromagnet was constructed by an English scientist, **William Sturgeon** (1783–1850) of Whittington, Lancashire, in 1825. One of the first journals on the subject, the *Annals of Electricity*, was commenced by him in 1836. The first hydroelectric machine was constructed by an English inventor, **William George Armstrong** (1810–1900) of Newcastle upon Tyne in 1840. A German-born British physicist, **Sir Arthur Schuster** (1851–1934) was the first to show that electric current is conducted by ions. Large-scale distribution of high-voltage electricity with the use of dynamos and alternators was pioneered by a Liverpool engineer of Italian origin, **Sebastian Ziani de Ferranti** (1864–1930). He patented

over 170 inventions and founded the leading electronic firm, Ferranti Ltd in 1905. *See battery, electric bulb, electric lighting, electric relay.*

Electrochemistry *See battery, electrolysis, electroplating,*

Electrolysis [Greek: *elektron*, amber + *lysis*, loosening] A term for dissociation by electricity, introduced in 1833 by **Michael Faraday** (1791–1867). A theory based on attractive and repulsive forces was proposed by a Croatian mathematical physicist and astronomer, **Ruggiero Giusseppo Boscovich** (1711–1787) from Dalmatia, and formed the basis for **Sir Humphry Davy's** (1778–1829) work on electrolysis. The decomposition of water by electric current from a powerful static machine was demonstrated by **Van Troostwijk** (1752–1837) and **Deimann** (1743–1808) in 1789. The voltaic battery was used for electrolysis of water by an English physicist, **William Nicholson** (1753–1815) of Portsmouth, and Anthony Carlisle, in 1800. The theory of electrolysis was proposed by **Theodor von Grotthus** (1785–1822) in 1805. Humphry Davy started using electricity for analysis of new elements in 1806, and reported his first experiment on electrolysis of water at the Bakerian Lecture held at the Royal Institution in the same year. **Johann Wilhelm Hittorf** (1824–1914), a professor at the academy of Munster, in Westphalia, studied the rate of movement of anions and cations during electrolysis. His method was used by **Friedreich Wilhelm Kohlrausch** (1840–1910), a professor of physics at the University of Würzburg and Berlin, to calculate ionic velocities. The understanding of the electrolytic process was advanced by **Jacobus Henricus van't Hoff** (1852–1911) and **Svante August Arrhenius** (1859–1927) in 1887. The law stating that the amount of substance decomposed by the electric current is proportional to the time of passage and the strength of the current, was proposed in 1833 by Michael Faraday. A French chemist from Châtillon-sur-Loire **Antoine-César Becquerel** (1788–1878) was the first to use electrolysis as a means of isolating metals from ores.

Electromagnet *See electricity, electric relay, electromagnetic theory.*

Electromagnetic Motor *See dynamo, induction current.*

Electromagnetic Rotation A phenomenon discovered in 1822 by **Michael Faraday** (1791–1867), who presented his initial findings in his *Experimental Researches on Electricity* to the Royal Society in 1831.

Electromagnetic Theory Related to the study of the magnetic effects caused by electric charges. The thermoelectric properties of tourmaline when heated, and its similarity to a magnet was observed by a German scientist, **Franz Ulrich**

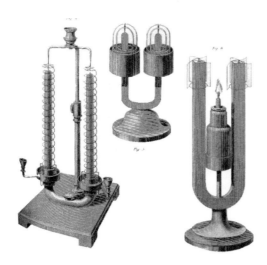

Figure 29 Early electromagnets. Partington, F. Charles. *The British Encyclopaedia of the Arts and Sciences*. London: Orr & Smith, 1835

Theodosius Aepinus (1724–1802). His *Tentamen theoriae electricitatis et magnetismi* (1759) was one of the first works linking electric and magnetic forces. In 1819 a Danish physicist, **Hans Christian Oersted** (1777–1851), observed the effect of electric current on a needle, which opened the doors to the new field of electromagnetism. Further pioneer work was done by the French physicist, **André Marie Ampère** (1775–1836), who published *Observations électro-dynamiques* in 1822. He suggested the use of the electromagnetic principle to measure electric current. An early demonstration of the magnetic field produced by the flow of electric current in a conducting coil was given by a French scientist, **Dominique François Arago** (1786–1853). The first electromagnets were constructed independently by an English physicist, **William Sturgeon** (1783–1850) of Lancashire, and **Joseph Henry** (1797–1878) of America. **Michael Faraday** (1791–1867) discovered the phenomenon of electromagnetic rotation in 1822, and presented his initial findings in his *Experimental Researches on Electricity* to the Royal Society in 1831. Faraday's work led to the development of the dynamo as a more effective alternative to the battery. Further work on the subject was published by **James Clerk Maxwell** (1831–1879) in the *Philosophical Transactions of the Royal Society* in 1865. In 1873, he predicted that by using oscillating electric currents it would be possible to generate electromagnetic waves. Maxwell's electromagnetic theory was experimentally confirmed by an English physicist, **Sir Oliver Joseph Lodge** (1851–1940), and its effects were deduced by another English physicist, **John Henry Poynting** (1852–1914) of Lancashire, who publish-

ed *On the Transfer of Energy in the Electromagnetic Field* (1884). In 1891, an Irish physicist, **George Johnston Stoney** (1826–1911) of Oakley Park, King's County, suggested that electric currents consisted of moving particles and named them electrons. *See Lenz's law.*

Electromagnetic Waves *See Compton effect, electromagnetic theory, radar, radiation pressure, radio waves.*

Electrometer [Greek: *elektron*, amber + *metron*, measure] A device for measuring electric potential, invented in 1747 by a French abbé, **Jean Antoine Nollet** (1700–1770), a professor of physics at the College de Navarre, in Paris. **Horace Benedict de Saussure** (1740–1799) of Geneva, invented a device in 1766. *See capillary electrometer, gold leaf electroscope.*

Electron An atomic particle with a negative elementary charge, and having a mass much less than that of the proton and neutron. The suggestion that electricity may be atomic is found in **Michael Faraday's** (1791–1867) work on electrolysis. The rays from the cathode were studied by **Julius Plücker** (1801–1868), **Heinrich Rudolf Hertz** (1857–1894), and **Johann Wilhelm Hittorf** (1824–1914). The term electron was first used in 1874 by an Irish physicist, **George Johnston Stoney** (1826–1911) of Oakley Park, King's County, to denote the particles of electricity that accounted for electrolysis and electric current. In 1881 **Sir John Joseph Thomson** (1856–1940) of Manchester, determined the ratio of the charge on a cathode particle to its mass. He first called these particles primordial corpuscles, before Stoney named them electrons. In 1903, **Max Abraham** (1875–1922) defined electrons as charged spherical bodies that were absolutely rigid. **Hendrik Antoon Lorentz** (1853–1928) proposed the electronic theory and used it to explain **James Clerk Maxwell's** (1831–1879) theory of electromagnetism. For this work, he shared the Nobel Prize for Physics in 1902 with his Dutch pupil **Pieter Zeeman** (1865–1943). The first measurement of the electronic charge was made in 1897 by an Irish physicist, **Sir John Sealy Edward Townsend** (1868–1957) from Galway. Two US physicists of Dutch origin, **George Eugene Uhlenbeck** (1900–1988) and **Samuel Abraham Goudsmit** (1902–1978) were the first to propose that electrons in atoms had an intrinsic spin angular momentum and orbital angular momentum. Their theory of electron spin was confirmed through **Paul Adrien Maurice Dirac's** (1902–1984) work on quantum mechanics. In 1924, a Dutch-American physicist, **Louis Victor Pierre de Broglie** (1892–1987), described the wavelike properties of the quickly orbiting electrons. A German-born US physicist, **Hans Georg Dehmelt** (b 1922), invented a device for measuring the magnetic moment of an electron, to an unprecedented accuracy of four parts in a trillion.

Electron Diffraction The diffraction of electrons by crystals was first investigated by a German-born American geophysicist, **Walter Maurice Elsasser** (1904–1991) from Baden. The American physicists, **Clinton Joseph Davisson** (1881–1958) from Bloomington, Illinois, and **Lester Halbert Germer** (1896–1971) of Chicago, developed the method in 1927. **Sir George Paget Thomson** (1892–1975) of Cambridge, a son of **Sir John Joseph Thomson** (1856–1940), independently discovered it in England. George Thompson and Davisson shared the Nobel Prize for Physics for this work, in 1937. Thompson published *Theory and Practice of Electron Diffraction* in 1939. Two other American physicists **Otto Stern** (1888–1969) and **I. Esterman** (b 1900) adapted molecular beams to study diffraction in 1929. Stern was awarded the Nobel Prize for Physics for his work on atomic physics, in 1947.

Electron Microscope In 1926, a Dutch-American physicist, **Louis Victor Pierre de Broglie** (1892–1987) from Dieppe, suggested that electrons might behave like light waves. This phenomenon was demonstrated in 1927 by an English physicist, **Sir George Paget Thomson** (1892–1975), a son of **Sir J. J. Thomson** (1856–1940). In 1873, **Ernest Abbe** (1840–1905) proposed the basic fundamental theory that led to the discovery of the electron microscope in 1934 by a German electrical engineer, **Ernst August Friedrich Ruska** (1906–1988) of Heidelberg and L. Marton. Abbe realized that, whatever improvements were made in optical microscopy, it was limited by the fact that two separate objects cannot be distinguished if the distance between them is less than half the wavelength of the light used for illumination (Abbe's law). This difficulty was overcome by the discovery of X-rays and electrons, which had a smaller wavelength than light. Ruska discovered that a magnetic coil could focus a beam of electrons, and he created the first crude electron microscope of 400 magnification, in 1932. A year later he improved its power to 12 000. Following Ruska's work, the electron microscope became commercially available in 1935 in England. Further refinements to the electron microscope were made in 1937 by a Canadian physicist, **James Hillier** (b 1915), and in 1940 he developed the high-resolution electron microscope. In 1939 a Russian-born American physicist, **Vladimir Kosma Zworykin** (1889–1982), improved it to provide 50 times more magnification than a light microscope. The first electron-microscopic study of the cell, showing structures such as the endoplasmic reticulum and mitochondria, was done by an American cytologist, **Albert Claude** (1898–1983) of

Belgian origin, in 1945. The scanning electron microscope, capable of producing three-dimensional images at a magnification of over 100 000, was developed around 1948 by an English electronic engineer, **Sir Charles Oatley** (1904–1996) of Frome in Somerset, and it came into practical use in 1969. The electron microscope was first used for detailed study of genetics in bacteria and viruses, by an American biophysicist, **Thomas Foxen Anderson** (b 1911), who was president of the Electron Microscopic Society of America. The tunneling electron microscope based on the quantum-mechanical effect or tunneling of electrons was developed in 1980 by a Swiss physicist, **Heinrich Rohrer** (b 1933) and a German physicist, **Gerd Karl Binnig** (b 1947). They shared the Nobel Prize for Physics with Ruska, for this work, in 1986. *See field-emission microscope.*

Electron Spectroscopy for Chemical Analysis (ESCA) A technique for studying the energies of electrons in atoms, developed by a Swedish physicist, **Kai Manne Börje Siegbahn** (b 1918). He was a son of **Karl Manne Georg Siegbahn** (1886–1978) who discovered X-ray spectrography. For his discovery of ESCA, Siegbahn shared the Nobel Prize for Physics in 1981, with an American physicist, **Arthur Leonard Schawlow** (1921–1999) of Mount Vernon, New York, and a Dutch-born American physicist, **Nicolaas Bloembergen** (b 1920).

Electron Spin *See electron.*

Electronic Typewriter The first typewriter capable of storing memory was developed independently in 1978, by the Italian firm Olivetti, and the Japanese company Casio. *See electric typewriter, typewriter.*

Electrophoresis A process of analysis of a substance, based on the different mobility of its components, first described in 1930 by **Arne Wilhelm Kaurin Tiselius** (1902–1971) of Stokholm. The process of gel electrophoresis, useful for examining the DNA structure of chromosomes, was developed by a New York molecular biologist, **Charles Robert Cantor** (b 1942). Another New York scientist and geneticist, **Richard Charles Lewontin** (b 1929) introduced gel electrophoresis as a means of assaying variation in protein sequences.

Electroplating The use of electrolysis to coat a metal with another metal, introduced in 1832 by an English manufacturer and inventor **George Richards Elkington** (1801–1865) of Birmingham, and his cousin, **Henry Elkington** (1810–1852). The method was refined by a London chemist **Alexander Parkes** (1813–1890) from Birmingham.

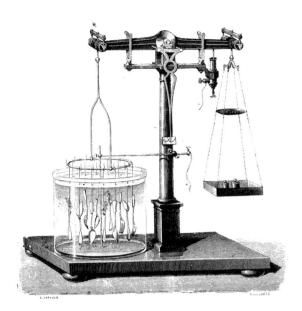

Figure 30 A 19th century balance used in gold and silver electroplating. Guillemin, Amédée. *The Applications of Physical Forces*. London: Macmillan and Co, 1877

Element [Latin: *elementum*, first principle] The concept of an element was first proposed by a Greek philosopher, **Anaxagoras** (500–428 BC) of Ionia, and the term *element* was coined by **Plato** (428–348 BC). Around 450 BC **Empedocles of Agrigento** (*c.* 490–430 BC) proposed the theory of four elements: fire, air, earth and water. The seven metallic elements, gold, silver, copper, lead, tin, iron and mercury were known to the ancients before the Christian era. The word element was first used in a modern scientific sense by **Robert Boyle** (1627–1691), in 1662. In 1789, **Antoine Lavoisier** (1743–1794) defined an element as 'a substance that cannot be split into simpler forms by any means'. As science progressed, many substances which were thought to be elements at the onset were split, to reveal their compound nature. In 1783, **Henry Cavendish** (1731–1810), demonstrated that water is a compound, and not an element as was previously thought. Of the 109 elements known at present, 94 exist naturally.

Elementary Particle *See atomic structure, atomic theory, boson, electron, meson, particle accelerator, pion, plasma physics, positron, proton, psi.*

Elevator [Latin: *elevatus*, raised] The first elevator driven by steam and equipped with a safety mechanism, was invented by an American mechanic, **Elisha Graves Otis** (1811–1861) of Halifax, Vermont. He installed his first elevator in New York's Crystal Palace Exposition in 1854.

Elkington, George Richards (1801–1865) *See electroplating.*

Elkington, Henry (1810–1852) *See electroplating.*

Ellet, Charles (1810–1862) *See suspension bridges.*

Elliptic Functions The first definitive book on the subject, *Fundamenta nova theoriae functionum ellipticarum* (1829) was published by a German mathematician, **Carl Gustav Jacob Jacobi** (1804–1851) of Potsdam. Elliptic functions were discovered independently by a Norwegian mathematician, **Niels Henrik Abel** (1802–1829).

Ellis, Alexander John (1814–1890) *See telephone.*

Ellis, C.D. (b 1895) A British physicist who was one of the first to measure the wavelength of gamma rays, with an American physicist, **Arthur Holly Compton** (1892–1962) of Ohio, around 1915.

Ellman, John (1753–1832) *See animal husbandry.*

Ellsworth, Lincoln (1880–1951) *See North Pole.*

Elsasser, Walter Maurice (1904–1991) *See electron diffraction.*

Elster, Johann Phillip Julius (1854–1920) *See clouds, photoelectric cell, solar energy.*

Elton, Charles Sutherland (1900–1991) *See ecology.*

Emanium or actinium-X. An element discovered in 1904 by a German industrial chemist, **Friedrich O. Giesel** (1852–1927).

Embedding Fixation of tissues in paraffin wax or other materials, for the protection of delicate structures, during the process of preparing sections for microscopic study. Paraffin was first used in 1860 by a German bacteriologist, **Theodor Albrecht Edwin Klebs** (1834–1913). Egg albumen was used by Paul Meyer in 1883.

Embryology [Greek: *em*, within + *bryein*, to swell + *logos*, discourse] Examination of the chick egg, in order to study the development of the embryo, is described in a Hippocratic treatise *On the Nature of the Infant.* **Aristotle** (384–322 BC) described the different stages of development of the chick in his *Historia animalium* around 350 BC. The Italian philosopher, **Aegidius Romanus** (*c.* 1245–1316) in his treatise *De Formatione Corporis Humane in Utero* discussed human fetal development, in 1276. The next important treatise *De Formato Foetu* was published by **Fabricius ab Aquapendente** (1537–1619), in 1602. The term *embryologie* was first admitted into the French language by the Académie in 1762, and came into English use in the 19th century. The embryonic development of organs from different germ layers was first proposed in 1828 by **Karl Ernst Ritter von Baer** (1792–1876), a professor of comparative anatomy and physiology at the Medico-Chirurgical Academy, in St Petersburg. In 1843, **Martin Barry** (1802–1855), an embryologist and surgeon from Edinburgh, observed the union of a spermatozoon and ovum in the rabbit and published *Researches in Embryology* (1839). Experimental embryology was pioneered by a German biologist, **Hans Adolf Eduard Driesch** (1867–1941) who divided the egg of a sea urchin into small parts, and observed the development.

Emich, F. (1860–1940) *See quantitative chemistry.*

Empedocles of Agrigento (*c.* 490–430 BC). A pupil of Pythagorus and a physician, philosopher and poet. He and his colleague **Alcmaeon** (*c.* 500 BC) enunciated the doctrine of the four elements: earth, water, fire and air. He proposed the concept that life was a gradual process, where plants evolved before animals, and imperfect forms were gradually replaced by perfect forms; he came to be regarded as the first evolutionist. He was the first to demonstrate that air has weight. *See air, evolution.*

Emulsification The principle of emulsification was used by the ancients when they employed fine earth for washing. The most common use of the principle is the application of soap for washing. The behavior of emulsions in relation to solubility and surface tension was studied independently by three American colloid chemists, Wilder D. Bancroft, **Joel Henry Hildebrand** (1881–1983) of Camden, New Jersey, and W.D. Harkins of Chicago. The soluble theory of emulsification was proposed by Bancroft in 1913, and the molecular-wedge hypothesis was put forward by Harkins and Hildebrand in 1923. A novel way of forming emulsions with the use of ultrasonic waves was invented in 1923 by a French professor of physics at the Sorbonne, **Paul Langevin** (1872–1946). *See surface chemistry.*

Encke, Johann Franz (1791–1865) *See Encke's comet.*

Encke's Comet A comet with the shortest period of return – 1206 days – first observed in 1786. A German astronomer, **Johann Franz Encke** (1791–1865), investigated it in 1819, and it was named after him.

Endlicher, Stephen Ladislaus (1804–1849) *See botanical classification.*

Energy [Greek: *energein,* to be active] The term energy was proposed in 1802 by an English Quaker physician, **Thomas Young** (1773–1829), to denote the present equivalent of kinetic energy. Pioneer work on the subject was done by a

German physicist and physiologist, **Hermann Ludwig Ferdinand von Helmholtz** (1821–1894), around 1850. In 1854, **William John Macquorn Rankine** (1820–1872) used the term energy to cover a larger area in physics. It was first used in the present scientific context by **William Thomson, Lord Kelvin** (1824–1907), later in the same year.

Engel, Johann Carl Ludwig (1778–1840) *See architecture, European.*

Engelmann, T.W. (1843–1909) *See chloroplasts.*

Engineering *See civil engineering, genetic engineering, marine engineering, mechanical engineering, military engineering, structural engineering.*

Engines *See atmospheric engine, diesel engine, gas engine, gas turbine, internal combustion engine, jet engine, rotary engine, steam engine, turbine, water turbine.*

Engler, Adolf (1844–1930) *See botanical classification.*

Engraving The art of engraving on signet rings was mentioned amongst the Israelites in 1491 BC. This method was practiced earlier by the ancient Chinese. The first attempt at printing in Europe, by taking impressions from woodcuts, was for the purpose of making playing cards for the amusement of Charles VI of France towards the end of the 14th century. One of the earliest specimens of wood engraving, a representation of St Christopher, by an unknown artist, dated 1423, was discovered in a German convent, Chartreuse of Buxheim, near Augsburg. The art of engraving on metal, in order to produce an impression on paper, was invented independently by a goldsmith in Florence, Finiguerra, and a German engraver, **Martin Schoengauer** (1450–1491). The first book with copperplate engravings was produced in 1488 by an Italian, Baccio Baldini. A mathematician, **Albrecht Dürer** (1471–1528) of Nuremberg, was one of the earliest engravers on metal. His works include *The Prodigal Son* (1500) and *Adam and Eve* (1504). He studied under another German engraver, **Michael Wolgemut** (1435–1519) in Nuremburg, and made a portrait of him. A German military officer and engraver, **Ludwig von Siegen** (1609–1675) invented the mezzotint process for engraving, in 1642. A London engraver, **William Faithorne** (1616–1691), published *The Art of Graving and Etching* in 1662. A Flemish copper engraver, **Gerard Edelinck** (1649–1707), is known for over 300 portrait engravings in Paris, around 1665. **John Faber** (1660–1721) of the Hague was a well-known engraver, and his son **John Faber** (1684–1756) worked in England and produced *The Beauties of Hampton Court.* A Frankfurt painter, Jacques

Christophe Le Blon, was the first to use mezzotint engraving for color printing, and he patented his method in England in 1719. The method of engraving on glass started in the 18th century and was perfected by Bourdier of Paris in 1799. A London engraver, **William Sharp** (1749–1824), became eminent through his engravings of historical and religious subjects. **Thomas Stothard** (1755–1834) of London engraved over 3000 of his designs around this period. The first book on typesetting and engraving, entitled *Manuel Typographique,* was published by **Pierre Simon Fournier** (1712–1768) of France, in 1764. An American inventor, **James Bogardus** (1800–1874) of Catskill, New York, invented an engraving machine and developed a method of engraving postage stamps, in 1839. A London etcher, **Sir Francis Seymour Haden** (1818–1910), founded the Royal Society of Painter-Etchers and Engravers in 1880. **Benjamin Pitman** (1822–1910) invented an electrochemical process of relief engraving in 1855. *See wood engraving.*

ENIAC (Electronic Numerical Integrator and Computer) *See computers.*

Entomology [Greek: *entomon,* insect + *logos,* discourse] Study of insects, established as a science by **Jan Swammerdam** (1637–1680), a Dutch naturalist and medical graduate of Leyden. He was one of the first microscopists to propose a system of classification of insects, and published *Historia insectorum generalis* (1669). A London naturalist, **Thomas Moufet** (1553–1604), published an important work entitled *Theatre of Insects* (1590). His work contained previous illustrations by an English clergyman and botanist, **Thomas Penny** (d 1519), who is regarded as the father of English entomology. Another founding work in entomology, *Mémoires pour servir à l'historie des insectes* (1734) was published by **René Antoine Ferchault de Reaumer** (1683–1757) of La Rochelle. A classification of insects was proposed by **Carolus Linnaeus** (1707–1778) in 1739. His contemporary, **Charles de Geer** (1720–1778) of Sweden wrote seven volumes of *Mémoirs pour servir à l'historie des Insects* (1771–1788). **Johann Christian Fabricus** (1745–1808) of Schleswig, Denmark, who is regarded as the founder of entomological taxonomy, proposed a classification based on the structure of the moth. One of the earliest English treatises on the subject, *The English Moths and Butterflies,* was written by **Benjamin Wilkes** in 1748. A French entomologist, **Pierre Andrezac Latreille** (1762–1833) was a pioneer on the classification of insects. An English naturalist and watercolor painter, **Elezar Albin** (d 1759) published *History of Insects* (1720) illustrated with his own engravings. An English naturalist from Hull, **Adrian Harvey Haworth**

(1766–1833), listed 793 species of butterflies and moths in his *Lepidopterorum Britannicorum* (1802). The Entomological Society in London was established in 1833. **Samuel Hubbard Scudder** (1837–1911) of Boston was an authority on fossil insects and he published *Butterflies of the Eastern United States and Canada* (1888–1889). Detailed accounts of the behavior of wasps and bees, and life cycles of beetles were given by a French entomologist, **Jean Henri Fabre** (1823–1915). His ten-volume *Souvenirs Entomologiques* took 30 years to complete and is regarded as a classic. Many aspects of insect physiology were first studied in detail by an English entomologist, **Vincent Brian Wigglesworth** (1899–1994) who published *The Principles of Insect Physiology* (1939). Social behavior, communication and evolution in ants was studied by an American biologist, **Edward Osborne Wilson** (b 1929), who published *The Insect Societies* (1971).

Entropy [Greek: *en,* in + *trope,* nourishment] A term first used in 1865 by a professor of physics at Bonn, **Rudolf Julius Emmanuel Clausius** (1822–1888), to denote the degradation of energy in a closed system. He used it to explain the second law of thermodynamics.

Envelope [French: *enveloppe,* covering] Used for enclosing letters, these were introduced soon after the establishment of the penny postal system, in 1840. The first patent for the production of envelopes was obtained by George Wilson in 1844. In 1845 Thomas Delarue and E. Hill of London invented a machine to fold envelopes. A Guernsey-born British scientist and astronomer, **Warren de la Rue** (1815–1889), invented an envelope-making machine in 1851.

Enzyme [Greek: *en,* in + *zume,* leaven] The term enzyme was first used in 1878 by **Willy Kuhne** (1821–1901) from Hamburg, to denote a class of organic substances that activated a chemical change. He was appointed as professor of physiology at Amsterdam (1868) and later at Heidelberg (1871). The existence of a complex between the enzyme and its substrate was demonstrated in 1943 by an American biochemist, **Britton Chance** (b 1913). An Australian chemist, **Sir John Warcup Cornforth** (b 1917), carried out a detailed study of the stereochemistry of enzymes and substrates, for which he shared the Nobel Prize for Chemistry with a Swiss chemist, **Vladimir Prelog** (b 1906), in 1975. In 1924, the British physiologist John Burdon Sanderson (1892–1964) showed that enzymes obey the laws of thermodynamics.

Eocene Period [Greek: *eos,* dawn + *cene,* recent] A geological period in the earth's history, 70 to 40 million years ago, lasting for 30 million years. It was identified and named in

1839 by a Scottish geologist, **Sir Charles Lyell** (1797–1875) from Kinnordy, Forfarshire. He published *Principles of Geology* (1830, 1832, 1833) in three volumes.

Eötvös Law *See surface tension.*

Eötvös, Baron Roland von (1848–1919) *See surface tension.*

Epalinus of Megara (*c.* 500 BC) *See water supply.*

Epicurus (342–271 BC) *See atomic theory, law of use and disuse.*

Equations *See Bernoulli's equation, Bessel equation, De Moivre's equation, Henderson–Hasselbach equation, Kolmogorov equation, London equation, Michaelis–Menten equation, polynomial equation, quadratic equation, Riccati equation, Saha's equation, Schrödinger equation, Van der Waals equation.*

Equinox One of two points in the sky that represent where the sun appears to cross the plane of the earth's equator. First observed in 160 BC by **Hipparchus of Bithynia**. The precession of the equinoxes caused by the gravitational forces of the sun and the moon (the nutation of the earth's axis) was discovered by a Babylonian astronomer, **Cidenas** (*c.* 343 BC). The Astronomer Royal **James Bradley** (1693–1762) of Sherbourne, Gloucestershire, rediscovered it in 1748.

Equivalent The proportion in which chemicals and their elements combine with each other. A concept first proposed in 1813 by an English chemist from Norfolk, **William Hyde Wollaston** (1766–1828). The English chemist, **John Dalton** (1766–1844) related it to atomic weights. *See atomic weights.*

Erard, Sebastien (1752–1831) *See piano.*

Erasistratus (310–250 BC) *See Alexandrian Museum and Library, anatomy, nutrition.*

Eratosthenes (274–194 BC) A librarian at the University of Alexandria who made significant contributions to the field of mathematics. He invented an instrument for duplicating a cube, measured the circumference of the earth and estimated the distance of the earth from the sun and the moon. He estimated the distance from the Atlantic to the eastern ocean to be 7800 miles, and the distance of Cinnamon Land or Tabrobane (Ceylon) from Thule to be 3800 miles. Eratosthenes was blinded by an eye disease and committed suicide.

Erbium An element with atomic number 68, discovered in 1843 by a Swedish chemist, **Carl Gustav Mosander** (1797–1858). It derives its name from Ytterby in Sweden.

Ercker, Lazarus (1530–1593) *See metallurgy.*

Ericsson, John (1803–1889) *See fire engine, steamships.*

Erlang Unit of telephone-traffic flow. Named after a Danish mathematician, Agner Krarup Erlang (1878–1929) who applied the theory of probabilities to study the problems connected with telephone traffic, such as congestion and waiting time.

Ernst, Richard Robert (b 1933) *See magnetic resonance imaging.*

Esaki Diode Developed in 1958 by a Japanese physicist, **Leo Esaki** (b 1925) of Osaka, who discovered tunneling in semiconductor diodes.

Esaki, Leo (b 1925) *See Esaki diode, superconductivity.*

Escalators A prototype consisting of a belt conveyer with wooden slats was invented in 1892 by Jesse W. Reno, and installed at the Old Iron Pier Company in Coney Island, in 1896. A moving staircase was patented by Charles A. Wheeler in 1892. Charles D. Seeberger bought the patent in 1898 and gave it the present name. After improving it, he had it built in 1900 by the Otis Elevator Company. It was first introduced at the Earl's Court underground station in London, in 1911.

Escapement One of the earliest mechanical clocks with an escapement mechanism was built by a Buddist monk, **I-Hsing** (682–727) and Liang in China in 725. An English clockmaker, **Thomas Tompian** (1639–1713) from Northhill, Bedfordshire, patented the cylinder escapement mechanism in 1695. A recoilless escapement was invented by **George Graham** (1673–1751) in 1715. **Thomas Mudge** (1715–1794) of London invented a detached lever escapement around 1755. In 1748 **Pierre Le Roy** (1717–1785) of Paris, invented a single-beat type of escapement. The mechanism was further refined by **Ferdinand Berthoud** (1727–1807), **John Arnold** (1736–1799) and **Thomas Earnshaw** (1749–1829). *See clock.*

Esper, Johan Friedreich (1732–1781) *See fossils.*

Espy, James Pollard (1785–1860) *See storms, weather forcast.*

Ester The term was introduced into chemistry in 1848 by a German chemist, **Leopold Gmelin** (1788–1853) of Gottingen. His *Handbuch der anorganischen Chemie* (1811) was an important early work on organic chemistry.

Esterman, I. (b 1900) *See electron diffraction.*

Etard Reaction Oxidation of toluene to benzadehyde by chromyl chloride, discovered by a French chemist, **Alexandre Léon Etard** (1852–1910).

Etard, Alexandre Léon (1852–1910) *See Etard reaction.*

Ether An invisible hypothetical substance or medium in space through which light travels in waves, proposed by an English physician, **Thomas Young** (1773–1829), in 1803. **Aristotle** (384–322 BC), in his doctrine of natural and forced motions, implied the existence of a fifth type of matter, apart from the known four elements, earth, air, fire and water. In 1888 **Albert Abraham Michelson** (1852–1931) and **Edward William Morley** (1838–1923) made an attempt to determine the velocity of the earth, by measuring the velocity of light in relation to the ether. Their work showed that the velocity of light was the same in all directions and was independent of the motion of the earth. In 1893 an English physicist, **Sir Oliver Joseph Lodge** (1851–1940) of Birmingham, proved that the ether does not exist. In 1905 **Albert Einstein** (1879–1955) discarded the ether medium in his calculations.

Ethology [Greek: *ethos*, habit + *logos*, discourse] Study of the behavior of animals in their natural environment. A science initiated by **Charles Darwin** (1809–1882) and developed by an American, **Charles Otis Whitman** (1842–1910). The behavior pattern of ants was first studied in detail by an American biologist, **Charles Henry Turner** (1867–1923) of Cincinnati. A German ornithologist, O. Heinroth (1871–1945), was one of the first to make a systemic study of natural animal behavior. An Austrian zoologist, **Konrad Zacharias Lorenz** (1903–1989), did extensive work and published *On Aggression* (1963), in which he argued that behavior in man is inherited, and that aggression can be channelled to other productive activities such as sport. A Dutch zoologist, **Nikolaas Tinbergen** (1907–1988), developed the neurophysiological aspects of animal behavior. He shared the Nobel Prize in Physiology or Medicine in 1973 with Lorenz and another Austrian zoologist, **Karl von Frisch** (1886–1982), who is best known for his study of bees. A German zoologist, **Bernhard Rensch** (b 1900), carried out research on animal behavior and sensory physiology. An American comparative psychologist and director of the Department of Animal Behavior (1936–1946) at the Museum of Natural History in New York, **Frank Ambrose Beach** (b 1911), was the first to recognize the European work on ethology and introduce it into America. The behavior of humans was described by an English ethologist, **Desmond John Morris** (b 1928) of Wiltshire, using the techniques of ethology, in his book *The Naked Ape* (1967). His *Manwatching* (1977) analyzed the behavior of the human as an animal. The chair of ethology at Cambridge was created in 1966; **William Homan Thorpe** (1902–1986) from Hastings was appointed as the first professor. He published *Learning and Instincts in Animals* in 1956. An English ethologist from Norwich, **Robert Aubrey Hinde** (b 1923), did further work especially with birds, and published *Animal Behaviour: A Synthesis of Ethology and Comparative Psycholgy* (1966). The field of cognitive ethology, the way in which non-humans think and feel, was initiated in 1981 by an American zoologist, **Donald Redfield Griffin** (1864–1932), who published *Animal Thinking* (1984).

Euclid A mathematician from Alexandria around 300 BC who wrote 13 books on mathematics, containing problems and theorems with illustrations, which remained as a standard work for over 2000 years. Euclid was held in high esteem by **Plato** (428–348 BC), and by King Ptolemy who later became his pupil. One of the earliest translations of Euclid's work into Latin was done by **Gerard of Cremona** (1147–1187) who obtained a thorough knowledge of Arabic in Toledo, Spain. Another translation of Euclid's *Elements* from an earlier Arabic version was done by **Adelard of Bath** (1090–1150) in 1142. The first printed mathematical book, a translation of Euclid's *Elements*, by a clergyman and mathematician in Paris, **Johannes Campanus** (*c.* 1205–1296) of Novara, was published in 1482. A Greek edition of Euclid appeared in Basel in 1533. An Italian version of Euclid was published by **Niccolò Fontana Tartaglia** (1499–1557) in Venice in 1543. The first English translation of Euclid, with a preface by an English alchemist, **John Dee** (1527–1608), was published in 1570 by Henry Billingsley. Another edition of Euclid's *Elements* was published in 1758 by **Robert Simpson** (1687–1768), a professor of mathematics at Glasgow University. *See Alexandrian Library, arithmetic, binomial theorem, conics, geometry, irrational numbers, law of refraction, mathematics, non-Euclidean geometry, perfect number, prime number, rational number fraction.*

Eudemus (*c.* 330 BC) *See geometry.*

Eudiometer [Greek: *eudios*, clear + *metron*, to measure] An instrument for measuring the purity or quantity of oxygen in air, devised in 1772 by a clergyman and chemist, **Joseph Priestley** (1733–1804) of Leeds.

Eudoxus (400–360 BC) A scientist and philosopher, born in Cnidos, in Ionia. He was a pupil of Plato and learnt astronomy at Heliopolis in Egypt. Eudoxus established a school and an observatory at Cnidos, and invented the theory of homoconcentric spheres, which exerted immense influence on astronomy for the next 2000 years. He compiled a map of the known areas of the world. *See calculus, musical theory, observatories.*

Eugenics [Greek: *eu*, well + *genos*, birth] Defined by **Sir Francis Galton** (1822–1911) as the study of agencies under social control that may improve or impair the racial qualities of future generations, either physically or mentally. He founded the science of eugenics and published *Hereditary Genius* (1869) and *Natural Inheritance* (1889) and endowed a chair in eugenics at London University.

Euler, Leonhard (1707–1783) A Swiss mathematician who published a large number of scientific papers, some which were still being published for the first time 50 years after his death. *See, hydrodynamics, structural engineering, trigonometry.*

Euler-Chelpin, Hans von (1873–1964) *See fermentology.*

European Atomic Energy Commission Established by the second Treaty of Rome in 1957. It promotes the cooperation of member states of the European Union in nuclear research and development of nonmilitary nuclear energy.

European Space Agency (ESA) Organization of European countries including Austria, Belgium, Denmark, France, Germany, Ireland, Italy, the Netherlands, Norway, Spain, Sweden, Switzerland, and the UK, founded in 1975 in Paris to promote space research and technology.

Europium An element with atomic number 63, discovered through spectroscopy in 1896 by a French chemist and professor at Paris, **Eugene Anatole Demarcay** (1852–1903). It was named after Europe.

Eurotunnel *See Channel Tunnel.*

Eustachio, Bartolomeo (1520–1574) *See acoustics.*

Evans, Oliver (1755–1819) *See steam engine, textile industry.*

Evans, Sir Arthur John (1851–1941) *See Minoan civilization.*

Evans, Sir John (1823–1908) *See prehistory.*

Evaporation The first set of treatises dealing with quantitative evaporation of water from lakes and seas was written in 1687 by **Edmund Halley** (1656–1742).

Evelyn, John (1620–1706) *See forestry, horticulture.*

Everest, Sir George (1790–1866) An English military engineer who served as surveyor general of India. Mount Everest is named after him.

Everett, Hugo (1930–1982) *See quantum mechanics.*

Evershed Effect Radial movements of gases in sunspots discovered in 1909 by an English astronomer, John Evershed (1864–1956).

Evolution [Latin: *evolutio*, unrolling] The term evolution was coined by a Swiss naturalist **Charles Étienne Bonnet** (1720–1793), who proposed a catastrophic theory of evolution. **Anaximander** (611–547 BC) of Miletus proposed that imperfectly organized beings developed from the action of the sun's heat on cold earth and evolved into animals. The concept that life was a gradually evolving process and plants evolved before animals, and imperfect forms were gradually replaced by perfect forms, was proposed by **Empedocles of Agrigento** around 450 BC. The Roman philosopher and poet **Lucretius** (95–55 BC), in his poem *De Rerum Natura* (On the nature of things), in 80 BC, suggested the principle of the survival of the fittest, although he erroneously thought animals directly arose from the earth. Count **George Louis Leclerc Compte de Buffon** (1707–1788) was one of the earliest in Europe to propose the idea of evolution, by stating that life forms in the animal kingdom were successively derived from one another. He also suggested that the earliest life forms originated from the polar regions and the ocean. **Benoit de Maillet** (1656–1738) in his *Telliamed* suggested the transmission of acquired characteristics. In 1763, the philosopher and physicist **Immanuel Kant** (1724–1804) of Königsberg, traced higher forms of life to simpler elementary forms. **Jean Baptiste Pierre Antoine de Monet Chevalier de Lamarck** (1744–1829) proposed that function precedes and creates structure, and that acquired characteristics are inherited. He published his theory of evolution in 1801. The pioneers of modern evolution theory were three English naturalists, **Herbert Spencer** (1820–1903), **Alfred Russell Wallace** (1823–1913) and **Charles Robert Darwin** (1809–1882). The phrase 'survival of the fittest' was coined by Spencer. Both Wallace and Darwin drew their inspiration from the work of an English clergyman, **Thomas Robert Malthus** (1766–1834), who published *An Essay on the Principle of Population or A View of its Past and Present Effects* (1798). In his treatise, Malthus argued that the only limits to the expansion of a population are space and food, implying the idea of survival of the fittest. Although Darwin commenced his work in 1838, Wallace independently came to the same conclusion, one year before Darwin published his work. Herbert Spencer was one of the earliest to propose the concept of evolution in his article *The Development Hypothesis* in the *Leader* in 1852. In his article Spencer also suggested the possibility of the transmutation of the species. The epoch making treatise *On the Origin of Species by Natural Selection* was published by Darwin after 20 years of work, in 1859. One of the pioneer works, linking Mendelian genetics and evolution, was carried out by an English geneticist,

Edmund Brisco Ford (1901–1988) from Cumberland, who published *Mendelism and Evolution* in 1931.

Ewart, James Cossar (1851–1933)　*See animal husbandry.*

Ewing, Sir James Alfred (1855–1935)　*See hysteresis.*

Ewing, William Maurice (1906–1974)　*See tectonic theory.*

Exhaustion A mathematical method of doubling and redoubling the number of sides of a regular inscribed polygon, on the assumption that, if this process continued, the difference in area between the circle and polygon would be exhausted. It was proposed by a Greek mathematician **Antiphon** (*c.* 430 BC).

Expanding Universe An American astronomer, **Edwin Powell Hubble** (1889–1953) of Missouri, showed that the amount of red shift was directly proportional to the speed of the galaxy concerned, and in 1929 discovered that galaxies recede from the earth with increasing speeds. A Dutch cosmologist and physicist, **Willem de Sitter** (1872–1934), proposed an expanding universe of constantly decreasing curvature, in relation to Einstein's equations on general relativity. A Belgian priest and astrophysicist, **Henri George Lemaître** (1894–1966), proposed expanding models based on the field equations of general relativity. In 1932 an English physicist, **Edward Arthur Milne** (1896–1950) from Hull, Yorkshire, who was professor of mathematics at Oxford, demonstrated a world model based on special relativity.

Explorer I　*See satellite.*

Explosives [Latin: *explodere,* drive away by clapping]　Explosives were a main cause of fatal accidents in mining during the early 19th century. A safer method of mining, by combining gunpowder with flax yarn, giving it a slow-burning fuse, was invented in 1831 by **William Bickford** (1774–1834) of Cornwall. The first modern explosive, nitroglycerin or *piroglicerina,* was invented in 1846 by an Italian chemist, **Ascanio Sobrero** (1812–1888), a professor of applied chemistry at Turin Technical Institute. In 1867 **Alfred Bernhard Nobel** (1833–1896) used it for making dynamite in civil engineering. The production of the highly explosive gun-cotton, by treating cotton with a mixture of nitric acid and sulfuric acid, was discovered in 1846 by **Christian Friedrich Schönbein** (1799–1868) of Basel. Another explosive, trinitrotoluene (TNT), was invented in 1863 by a Swedish chemist, J. Wilbrand. In 1884, a French chemist, Paul Vieille, invented smokeless gunpowder. A new product, ballistite, consisting of nitrocellulose and nitroglycerin, was produced in 1887 by Nobel. An English

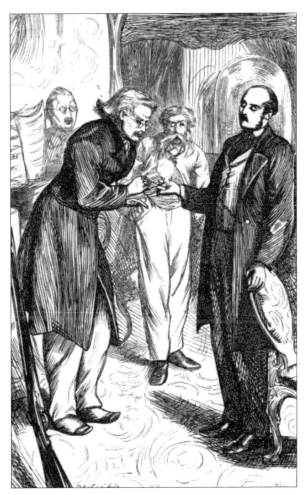

Figure 31　Schönbein demonstrating the properties of gun-cotton in England to Prince Albert in 1846. Temple, Ralph and Chandos. *Invention and Discovery.* London: Hodder and Stoughton, 1893

chemist from Woolwich, **Sir Fredrick Augustus Abel** (1827–1902), invented cordite, a paste of gun-cotton and nitroglycerin, and it was adopted as a standard explosive by the British Army in 1891. He published *Gun-cotton* (1866) and *Electricity Applied to Explosive Purposes* (1884). Picric acid was first obtained in 1771 by an English chemist, **Peter Woulfe** (1727–1803), and adapted as an explosive in France in 1885. Explosives for British military use were developed by a British chemist, **Robert Robertson** (1869–1949), who produced a new explosive, *Amatol,* from trinitrotoluene and ammonium nitrate. In 1887, a professor of chemistry at Owen's College, Manchester, **Harold Baily Dixon** (1852–1930), studied gaseous explosions and flames, and elucidated the factors affecting the velocity of explosion waves. *See dynamite.*

Extraterrestrial Life   A German theologian and philosopher, **Nicholas Krebs** (b 1401), also known as **Nicholas of Cusa**, suggested that the earth was not the only place in the universe that supported life. The founder of the Royal Society, **John Wilkins** (1614–1672), in his *Discovery of a World in the Moon* (1638), gave an imaginary account of a journey to the moon and a description of its inhabitants. A French astronomer, **Nicolas Camille Flammarion** (1842–1925) was the first to consider the possibility of life forms in the universe in his book *La Pluralité des Mondes Habités* (1862). With the start of many alleged UFO (unidentified flying object) sightings around 1947, several books on encounters with extraterrestrial beings started to be published. Some of the early books in the 20th century include *The Riddle of the Flying Saucers* (1950) by Gerald Heard, *Flying Saucers are Real* (1950) by Donald E. Keyhoe

and *Inside the Spaceships* (1955) by George Adamski. Frank Scully's *Behind the Flying Saucers* in 1950 became a best-seller. An astronomer Frank Drake in 1960 used the facilities at the National Radio Astronomy Observatory, Green Bank, West Virginia, to try and detect radio signals from intellegence beyond our solar system. This project was known as *Ozma*. The Search for Extraterrestrial Intelligence (SETI) is a NASA research program, first proposed in 1959. Large radio telescopes are used to detect artificially generated radio signals that might be coming from interstellar space. In 1973, the Ancient Astronomer Society was organized in Chicago, on the theory that many of the projects during early civilization were achieved with help from extraterrestrial beings. *See science fiction, space travel.*

Eyde, Samuel (1866–1940)   *See nitric acid.*

F

Faber, Johannes (1574–1629) *See microscope.*

Faber, John (1660–1721) *See engraving.*

Faber, John (1684–1756) *See engraving.*

Fabre, Jean Henri (1823–1915) *See bees, entomology.*

Fabricius, ab Aquapendente (1537–1619) *See embryology.*

Fabricius, David (1564–1617) *See variable star.*

Fabricius, Johannes (1587–1615) *See sunspots.*

Fabricus, Johann Christian (1745–1808) *See entomology.*

Fabry, Charles Marie Paul (1867–1945) *See interferometer, ozone, ozone layer.*

Facsimile Machine or fax. [Latin: *facere*, make + *similis*, like] The idea of transmitting optical signals, via electricity, was first conceived by **Sir Humphry Davy** (1778–1829) in 1826. He managed to decipher electrical signals by using potassium iodide. In 1842, a Scottish clockmaker, Alexander Bain, managed to transmit graphic signs over short distances. Another system, using potassium cyanate to decipher pictures by decomposition, was devised by an Italian monk, Giovanni Casselli, in 1855. His device, the pantelograph, was installed between Paris and Amiens in 1856. An English physicist and barrister, Shelford Bidwell, devised a picture-transmission system, in 1881. In 1884, a German, **Paul Nipkow** (1860–1940) of Lauenberg, devised a mechanical scanning disk, and used it in conjunction with a photoelectric selenium cell, but the resulting images were poor. The first transmission of a photograph via electric wires was effected from Munich to Berlin, by a German, Arthur Korn, in 1907. A quicker automatic method of transmission was invented by Edouard Belin in 1925. Another system was developed during the 1920s by the Siemen's firm in Germany. A London inventor, **Edmund Edward Fournier d'Albe** (1868–1933), was the first to transmit a portrait by telephotography, in 1923. The modern system of the fax linked to the telephone was developed by several companies, including RCA, Western Union and the American Telephone and Telegraph Company (AT&T).

Fahlberg, Constantin (1850–1910) *See saccharin.*

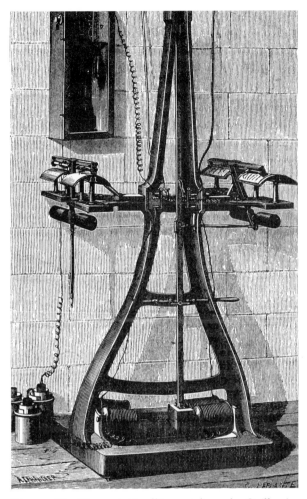

Figure 32 Giovanni Caselli's pantelograph. Guillemin, Amédée. *The Applications of Physical Forces*. London: Macmillan and Co, 1877

Fahrenheit Scale A scale of thermometry proposed by **Gabriel Daniel Fahrenheit** (1686–1736), and named after him. In order to avoid negative measurements he used 32 degrees for the temperature of a mixture of water and ice, and 212 degrees for the boiling point of water.

Fahrenheit, Gabriel Daniel (1686–1736) An experimental philosopher and son of a wealthy merchant from Danzig, in Prussia. He settled in Amsterdam in 1717 where he learned the trade of scientific instrument making. In 1720, he improved the thermometer by making use of mercury instead of spirits of wine. He introduced a scale for measurement of temperature that avoided negative values. *See Fahrenheit scale.*

Fairbairn, Sir William (1789–1874) *See bridges.*

Fairey, Sir Richard (1887–1956) A London aircraft designer and founder of the Fairey Aviation Company in 1915.

Some of the aircraft he produced include the *Fantome*, *Delta*, *Swordfish*, *Firefly*, *Albacore* and *Barracuda*.

Fairfax, John (1804–1877) *See newspapers.*

Faithorne, William (1616–1691) *See engraving.*

Fajans, Kasimir (1887–1975) *See bonds, isotopes.*

Falconer, Hugh (1808–1865) *See tea.*

Falling Bodies *See acceleration, dynamics.*

Faraday, Michael (1791–1867) An eminent English physicist, born in Newington, Surrey. At the age of 12, he started his working life as an errand boy to a bookseller who promoted him to the position of bookbinder's apprentice in 1804. While at this job at the age of 21 he started attending **Sir Humphry Davy's** (1778–1829) lectures, became interested in chemistry and joined the Royal Institution as a laboratory assistant in 1813. He published his observations on ether in *The Quarterly Journal of Science and Arts* in 1818. At the Royal Institution Faraday made many important discoveries in the fields of both chemistry and physics. He pioneered the work on electrolysis and introduced the terms electrode, cathode and anode. He liquefied carbon dioxide by using atmospheric pressure in 1823, and condensed chlorine into liquid in the same year. Faraday also discovered the phenomenon of electromagnetic rotation in 1822, and presented his first series of *Experimental Researches on Electricity* to the Royal Society in 1831. He succeeded Davy at the Royal Institute in 1825. *See anode, benzene, Bunsen burner, chlorine, diamagnetic, electricity, electrolysis, induction current, liquefaction of gases, refrigerator, Royal Institution of London, Zeeman effect.*

Farina, Battista (1893–1966) An Italian car designer from Turin who started his career at the Fiat factory. He studied production designs at the Ford factory in the USA and established his own bodywork company in 1930.

Farina, Johann Maria (1685–1766) An Italian perfumer from Novara who settled in Cologne, where he invented eau-de-Cologne.

Farman, Henri (1874–1958) *See airlines.*

Farman, Maurice (1878–1964) *See airlines.*

Farming *See agricultural instruments, agriculture, agronomy, animal husbandry, fertilizers.*

Farr, William (1807–1883) *See vital statistics.*

Faulds, Henry (1844–1930) *See fingerprints.*

Fax *See facsimile machine.*

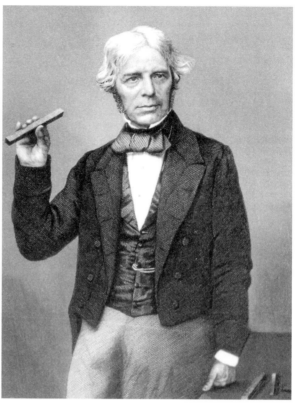

Figure 33 Michael Faraday (1791–1867). Courtesy of the National Library of Medicine

Faye, Hervé Auguste Étienne (1814–1902) *See Faye's comet.*

Faye's Comet First observed by a French astronomer, **Hervé Auguste Étienne Faye** (1814–1902) on 22 November 1843. It is calculated to have made its first appearance in 1747.

Fedden, Sir Roy (1885–1973) An English aviation engineer from Bristol who designed several aero-engines including the *Pegasus* and the *Taurus*. He was responsible for the development of the sleeve-valve engine.

Federal Aviation Administration (FAA) A US agency established in 1958 under the name Federal Aviation Agency for control of air traffic and supervision of air safety. It was given its present name when it became part of US Department of Transportation in 1967.

Feller, William (1906–1970) *See probability theory.*

Fellows, Sir Charles (1799–1860) *See Xanthus.*

Femtochemistry A study of chemical reactions that take place on a time scale of a small fraction of a second, pioneered by an American physical chemist, **Richard Barry Bernstein** (1923–1990) of Long Island, New York, in 1955.

Fenning, William Frederick (1919–1988) *See atomic power.*

Ferdinand, Harry (1901–1982) *See musical synthesizer.*

Ferguson, Harry George (1710–1776) A Scottish astronomer from Rothiamy, Banffshire. He published *Astronomy Explained on Newton's Principles* (1756) and *Lectures on Mechanics, Hydrostatics, Pneumatics, and Optics* (1760).

Ferguson, Henry George (1884–1960) *See agricultural instruments.*

Fermat, Pierre de (1601–1665) *See Académie Royale des Sciences, analytical geometry, cycloid, Fermat's last theorem, Fermat's theory, number theory.*

Fermat's Last Theorem The most famous unsolved problem in mathematics until recently on integers, proposed in 1637 by a French mathematician, **Pierre de Fermat** (1601–1665): the equation $x^n + y^n = z^n$ has no integer solutions for any n greater than 2. Several mathematicians of repute including the French mathematician, **Sophie Germain** (1776–1831), an Italian-born French mathematician, **Joseph Louis Lagrange** (1736–1813), and a German mathematician, **Ernst Eduard Kummer** (1810–1893) attempted its proof. An English mathematician and a professor at Princeton University, **Andrew Wiles** (b 1953), after seven years of trying, solved it in 1993. His revised work was published in the journal *Annals of Mathematics* in 1995.

Fermat's Theory of numbers. Every natural number is the sum of at most three triangular numbers. First proposed in 1636 by a French mathematician, **Pierre de Fermat** (1601–1665) of Mountauban, in his letter to a Franciscan friar and mathematician, **Marin Merssene** (1588–1648) of Paris. Although Fermat made significant contributions he did not publish any of his work. His theory was publicly stated in 1665 by a French mathematician, **Blaise Pascal** (1623–1662) of Clermont-Ferrand, and proved by **Carl Friedrich Gauss** (1777–1855) of Brunswick, in 1801.

Fermentology [Latin: *fermentum,* leaven + *logos,* discourse] The study of organisms and the process which produces fermentation. It started with the invention of the microscope, and the first description with drawings of yeast cells was submitted to the Royal Society of London in 1680 by a Dutch microscopist, **Anthoni van Leeuwenhoek** (1632–1723). The Swedish botanist, **Carolus Linnaeus** (1707–1778), despite his suspicions that fermentation was caused by microscopic living organisms, failed to prove it. The process was first explained on a chemical basis by **Antoine**

Laurent Lavoisier (1743–1794). The equation for fermentation, involving the decomposition of the hexose molecule, was proposed by **Joseph Louis Gay-Lussac** (1778–1850), in 1810. In 1837, a French Chemist, **Charles de la Tour Cagniard** (1777–1859), showed that the spherical bodies in the yeast beer belonged to the vegetable kingdom, and were capable of reproducing. His theory was proved by **Theodor Schwann** (1810–1882). The final proof for fermentation by living organisms was provided by **Louis Pasteur** (1822–1895) in 1857. The mechanism of fermentation of sugars, and the role of enzymes in the process, was studied by an English biochemist, **Arthur Harden** (1865–1940) of Manchester. He shared the Nobel Prize for Chemistry, for his work with **Hans von Euler-Chelpin** (1873–1964), in 1929.

Fermi, Enrico (1901–1954) *See atomic bomb, Fermi National Accelerator Laboratory, nuclear reactor, neutrino, Wigner theorem.*

Fermi National Accelerator Laboratory (Fermilab) US center for study of particle physics established in 1972 at Batavia, Illinois, near Chicago, and named after Italian-born US physicist Enrico Fermi (1901–1954). It houses the world's most powerful particle accelerator capable of boosting protons and antiprotons to speeds near that of light.

Fermion A subatomic particle whose spin can only take values that are half-integers. All elementary particles are either fermions or bosons. The Austrian-US physicist Wolfgang Pauli in 1925 formulated that no two fermions in the same system (such as an atom) can possess the same position, energy state, spin, or other quantized property.

Fermium An element with an atomic number of 100, synthesized by an American physicist, **Glenn Theodore Seaborg** (b 1912) and his team at Berkeley, California.

Ferranti, Sebastian Ziani de (1864–1930) *See electricity.*

Ferrari, Enzo (1898–1988) An Italian racing car driver and automobile designer from Modena. In 1929, he founded a company and designed his own cars, which were successful in many motor racing events.

Ferrel, William (1720–1760) *See tides.*

Fertilization [Latin: *fertilis,* fertile] In 1779, an Italian biologist, **Lazzaro Spallanzani** (1729–1799), observed that a sperm must make physical contact with an egg for fertilization to take place. In 1875, a German biologist, **Oscar Hertwig** (1849–1922), while working on the eggs and spermatozoa of the sea urchin in his small laboratory in the Mediterranean, proved that the process involved the union of two nuclei. The penetration of an ovum by a spermatozoon was first observed in 1877 by Hermann Fol of Geneva. Fertilization in mammals was described in 1883 by a Belgian cytologist, and pupil of Hertwig, **Edouard Joseph Louis-Marie van Beneden** (1846–1910). The process in seed plants was described in 1884 by a German botanist and professor at Bonn, **Eduard Adolf Strasburger** (1844–1912).

Fertilizers [Latin: *fertilis*, fertile]   A German chemist, **Justus von Liebig** (1803–1873) was the first to point out that plants needed elements other than water and carbon dioxide to thrive, and published *Chemistry in its Application to Agriculture and Physiology* (1840). A French statesman and chemist, **Jean Antoine Claude Chaptal** (1756–1832) of Nogaret, published *Chimie appliquée à l'agriculture* (The Application of Chemistry to Agriculture) in 1803. In 1898, **Sir William Crookes** (1832–1919) warned of the possibility of famine unless the soil was cultivated and enriched to replace the depleted nitrogen. Pioneering work in England on nitrogen fertilizers was done by **Sir Joseph Henry Gilbert** (1817–1901) from Hull. **Sir John Edward Russell** (1872–1965) published *Soil Conditions and Plant Growth* in 1912. A German agriculturalist in Scotland, **Augustus Voelcker** (1822–1884), made significant advances in soil research and artificial fertilizers. In 1857, he served as consultant chemist to the Royal Agricultural Society of England. Haber's process for making cheap fertilizers, by extracting nitrogen from the air, in order to generate ammonia, was invented by a Polish professor of physical chemistry (1906–1911) at Karlsruhe, **Fritz Haber** (1868–1934), in 1908. A German chemist, **Carl Bosch** (1874–1940), devised a method for the industrial synthesis of ammonia in 1914, which enabled the cheap production of agricultural fertilizers.

Fessenden, Reginald Aubrey (1866–1932) A radio-engineer from East Bolton, Quebec. He patented over 500 inventions, including a method of the amplitude modulation for radio transmission. He broadcast the first American radio program with his transmitter, from Brant Rock, Massachusetts on Christmas eve of 1906.

Feynman Diagrams A method of representing particle interactions in electrodynamics. Devised by a New York physicist, **Richard Phillips Feynman** (1918–1988). He shared the Nobel Prize in 1965, for developing the theory of quantum electrodynamics, with **Julian Schwinger** (1918–1994) of New York, and **Sin-Itero Tomanaga** (1906–1979), a professor of physics at Tokyo University.

Feynman, Richard Phillips (1918–1988) A New York physicist who studied at the Massachusetts Institute of Technology and at Princeton. During World War II, he worked at Los Alamos, New Mexico, on the behavior of neutrons in atomic explosions. Feynman was professor of theoretical physics at the California Institute of Technology from 1950, where Feynman Lectures on Physics became a standard work in 1963. *See Feynman diagrams, nanotechnology, proton.*

Fibonacci, Leonardo (*c.* 1172–1250) of Pisa. A distinguished Italian mathematician of the Middle Ages who introduced the Indian system of decimals into Europe. He discovered the Fibonacci sequence of integrals and wrote *Liber Quadratorum* in 1225. *See abacus, accountancy, algebra, negative numbers, quadrant, zero.*

Field-Emission Microscope Used for the study of atomic structure, and invented by a Berlin-born US physicist, **Erwin Wilhelm Mueller** (1911–1977) in 1936. It consists of a fine needle point in a vacuum which emits electrons. When the electrons strike a fluorescent screen, a magnification up to one million times is produced.

Field-Ion Microscope The first device that enabled photographs to be taken from a direct view of atoms and heat-stable molecules. It was invented in 1951 by a Berlin-born US physicist, **Erwin Wilhelm Mueller** (1911–1977).

Fighter Planes *See warplanes.*

Finck, Thomas (1561–1646) *See tangent.*

Fingerprints A Czech physiologist, **Johannes Evangelista Purkinje** (1787–1869), was the first to classify fingerprints, in 1832. **Henry Faulds** (1844–1930) published a fingerprint method of identification, in *Nature,* on 28th October 1880. **Francis Galton** (1822–1911) published a work on the use of fingerprints for identification, in 1892. In 1900 Sir Edward Richard Henry introduced a complete system of identification of humans by fingerprints.

Finley, James (1762–1828) *See suspension bridges.*

Finsch, Friedrich Hermann Otto (1839–1917) *See ornithology.*

Fiorelli, Gieuseppe (1823–1896) *See Pompeii.*

Fire The origin of its discovery by man is not known, and early humans were capable of creating fire which helped them to live through the Ice Age over 400 000 years ago. It was one of man's earliest discoveries to keep him warm and cook his food. The remains of a man-made fire found in China is estimated to be 500 000 years old.

Fire Alarm The modern fire alarm system for a city, by applying the principle of electric telegraphy, was first introduced in 1851 by William F. Channing and Moses Farmer.

Fire Engine   A hand-operated fire engine was invented in 300 BC by an Alexandrian scholar, **Ctesibius**. He used the principle of hydromechanics to construct a hydraulic pneumatic machine and a siphon for his fire engine. In 1672, two Dutchmen with the same name, Jan Van der Heide, made a significant advance through their invention of a leather hose with a jet at the end, for projecting water. Their method was introduced into Denmark and other places in 1697 by Gottfried Fuchs, a director of fire apparatus in Copenhagen. The first steam driven fire engine was built in 1830 by a Swedish-born inventor, **John Ericsson** (1802–1889), who migrated to England in 1826.

Fire Escape   Based on a ladder, this was invented by a person named Davis who received a prize of 50 guineas from the Royal Society of Arts for his invention, in 1810. His device consisted of three ladders, fitted in a telescopic manner, on a low carriage with four wheels.

Fire Extinguisher   The first device that did not contain water was invented in 1866 by a Frenchman, François Carlier. It consisted of a mixture of bicarbonate of soda and sulfuric acid.

Firearms   Cannons were the first firearms to be invented. In 1120 the Arabs constructed a cannon, known as *Madfaa,* which consisted of a wooden bowl containing gunpowder, with the cannon ball placed at its rim. The first known gun, a small cannon, was made in China in 1277. A German monk, **Berthholdus or Bertholet, Michael Schwartz** (*c.* 1320) used gunpowder for firearms. The first attempt to control guns was made by Henry V, who tried to prohibit the manufacture of gunpowder in 1414. The wheel-lock, which coordinated trigger action and ignition, was invented around 1520 in Nuremberg. Small firearms in the form of pistols were used by the British cavalry in 1544. The cartridge containing both the powder and the ball was invented in 1585 by Gustavus Adolphi of Sweden. The revolving loader was invented in 1718 by an Englishman, James Puckle. The percussion-cap was invented in 1807 by a Scottish clergyman, **Alexander John Forsyth** (1769–1843) from Belhelvie, Aberdeenshire. A detonating mercury percussion cap was invented by J. Shaw of Philadelphia, in 1814. **Sir William George Armstrong** (1810–1900) of Newcastle upon Tyne, in Great Britain, developed the rifled cannon. The Colt revolver, first used during the Mexican war, was invented in 1836 by **Samuel Colt** (1814–1862), an American chemist and inventor from Hartford, Connecticut. The first cast steel cannon was developed by a German metallurgist, **Alfred Krupp** (1812–1887) of Essen, in 1847. He produced an all-steel gun, in 1863. The Gatling

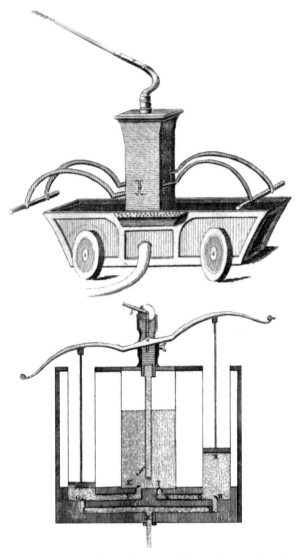

Figure 34   An early hand-operated fire engine and its principle. Owen, W. *Dictionary of Arts and Sciences*. London: Homer's Head, 1754

machine gun with ten revolving barrels was invented by **Jordan Richard Gatling** (1818–1903), a medical practitioner from North Carolina, during the American civil war, in 1862. **Benjamin Berkeley Hotchkiss** (1826–1885) of Watertown, Connecticut, invented a revolving-barrel machine gun (1872) and a magazine rifle (1875). In 1863 **Antoine Alphonse Chassepot** (1833–1905) of Paris, invented a rifle that was adopted by the French army, and named after him. Pistols were manufactured on a large scale in America during the mid-19th century and they were first imported to England in 1853. **John Moses Browning** (1855–1926), a son of a gunsmith from Ogden, Utah, invented the breech-loading single-shot rifle (1879), the

Browning automatic pistol (1911), the Browning machine gun (1917) and the Browning automatic rifle (1918). An English engineer, **William Ellis Metford** (1824–1899) from Taunton, designed a breech-loading rifle in 1871, and it was modified by a Scottish-born US inventor, **James Paris Lee** (1831–1904), and came to be known as the Lee–Metford rifle. Two Americans, **Daniel Baird Wesson** (1825–1906) and **Horace Smith** (1808–1893) devised a new type of repeating mechanism for small arms in 1854, and founded the Smith and Wesson firm for firearms at Springfield in 1857. The Maxim machine gun was made by **Sir Hiram Stevens Maxim** (1840–1916), an American inventor from Sangersville, Maine, in 1883. His son, **Hiral Percy Maxim** (1869–1936), developed the silencer for rifles. **John Anderson** (1726–1796), a professor of oriental languages at Glasgow University and the founder of the Andersonian College in Glasgow, invented a gun with an air chamber to absorb the recoil, in 1791. The Deringer pocket pistol was invented in 1852 by an American, Henry Deringer of Philadelphia. The Remington breech-loading rifle was developed by an American inventor, **Philo Remington** (1816–1889) of Litchfield, New York. The submachine gun, known as the 'tommy gun', was patented in 1920 by a retired army officer, **John Taliaferro Thompson** (1860–1940), and it was first used for military purposes by the US Marines in Nicaragua, in 1925.

Fischer, Edmund Henry (b 1920) An American biochemist born in Shanghai, China and educated in Geneva and Basel, before he emigrated to America in 1953. In 1955, while working with **Hans Adolf Krebs** (1900–1982), he showed that the phosphorylation and dephosphorylation processes were the key factors in the activation of glycogen phosphorylase by adenylic acid. Fischer and Krebs shared the Nobel Prize for Physiology or Medicine for their work, in 1992.

Fischer, Emil Hermann (1852–1919) A German chemist, born in Euskirchen, in Prussia, and educated at Bonn and Strasburg. He became a chemist to Bayer at Munich and discovered a new compound of hydrogen and nitrogen, which he named hydraxane (phenylhydrazine), in 1875. In 1889, he succeeded in breaking down some of the albumin substances into compounds of ammonia or amino acids. He successfully linked together 18 amino acids in 1902, and was awarded the Nobel Prize for Chemistry, for his work on the synthesis of sugars and purine compounds, in the same year.

Fischer, Ernst Otto (b 1918) An organic chemist from Munich who shared the Nobel Prize for Chemistry in 1973

with **Geoffrey Wilkinson** (1921–1996), for their work on organometallic compounds of transition metals.

Fischer, Hermann Otto Lawrence (1888–1960) A German organic chemist and eldest of the three sons of **Emil Hermann Fischer** (1852–1919). His main contribution was in the synthesis and structure of carbohydrates.

Fischer, Johann Bernard von Erlach (1656–1723) *See architecture, European.*

Fisher, Hans (1881–1945) A German organic chemist who determined the molecular weights of three important biological pigments, chlorophyll, bilirubin and hemoglobin. He was awarded the Nobel Prize for Chemistry in 1930, for his work on hemoglobin.

Fisher, Sir Ronald Aylmer (1890–1962) A professor of genetics and a statistician from East Finchley, London, who did pioneering work on blood groups as possible genetic markers. His work *Statistical Methods for Research Workers* (1925) was the first standard work on the application of statistics in research. In 1933, he was appointed professor of eugenics at University College London, and was made professor of genetics at Cambridge, in 1943. He published *The Theory of Inbreeding* in 1949.

Fisheries *See marine biology, icthyology.*

Fisk, Ernest Thomas (1886–1965) *See wireless telegraphy.*

Fission *See nuclear fission.*

Fitch, John (1743–1798) *See steamships.*

Fitch, Val Lodgson (b 1923) *See antimatter.*

Fittig, Rudolf (1835–1910) A German organic chemist, and professor of chemistry at Tubingen (1869) and Strasbourg (1876). He synthesized toluene, anthrene and several other organic compounds.

Fitzgerald, George Francis (1851–1901) *See Fitzgerald–Lorentz contraction.*

Fitzgerald–Lorentz Contraction In 1887, the American physicist, **Edward William Morley** (1838–1923) of Newark, New Jersey, and **Albert Abraham Michelson** (1852–1931), during their famous Michelson–Morley experiment for studying motion through the ether, failed to detect certain expected changes. This negative result was explained independently, on the basis of contraction of the apparatus in the direction of motion, by an Irish physicist, **George Francis Fitzgerald** (1851–1901) and a Dutch physicist, **Hendrik Antoon Lorentz** (1853–1928) of

Arnhem, in 1904. Lorentz was awarded the Nobel Prize for Physics in 1902.

Fitzroy, Robert (1805–1865) The commander of the *Beagle,* which carried **Charles Robert Darwin** (1809–1882) on his voyage. He was born in Ampton Hill, Suffolk, and became the first director of the London Meteorological Office in 1855. In 1863, he invented the Fitzroy barometer, and published *The Weather Book,* which contained sophisticated pictures of storms, similar to the present satellite pictures.

Fixatives [Latin: *fixus,* fixed] Various chemicals used for preserving animal and plant tissues in order to study them with minimal damage. Chromic acid was used by A. Hannover for fixing tissues in 1840. Acetic acid was used to fix nuclei by a A. Corti in 1851 and by **Robert Remak** (1815–1865) in 1854. Potassium dichromate was introduced as a cytological fixative by **Heinrich Muller** (1820–1864) in 1859. F. Blum introduced formalin in 1893.

Fizeau, Armand Hippolyte Louis (1819–1896) A French physicist born into a wealthy family in Paris. In 1849 he made one of the first measurements of the velocity of light in the laboratory without using astronomical distances or phenomena. He also demonstrated the use of the Doppler principle in the estimation of star velocity. He took the first daguerreotype photograph of the sun in 1845. *See photo-engraving.*

Flag Signalling First came into use in Europe around 1600. An Irish naval commander, **Sir Home Riggs Popham** (1762–1820), invented a code that was used at Trafalgar for Nelson's message. In 1817, an English novelist and naval officer, **Frederick Marryat** (1792–1848), simplified the code, and it was adapted officially for signalling. In 1858, an American army signal officer, Albert Myer, used a system of flags by day and lamps by night, to transmit Morse code. A similar system was independently invented in England in the same year.

Flammarion, Nicolas Camille (1842–1925) A French astronomer who founded the French Astronomical Society in 1887, and made many important planetary and lunar observations. *See extraterrestrial life.*

Flamsteed, John (1646–1719) An English astronomer from Denby, near Derby, who was the first Astronomer Royal to the Greenwich observatory, designed by **Sir Christopher Wren** (1632–1723). He published a famous catalog of stars and made several original observations in astronomy. *See observatories, stars, Uranus.*

Flash Photolysis Use of a brief flash of intense light to bring about a photochemical reaction. It was developed by two English chemists, **Ronald George Reyford Norrish** (1897–1978) and **Sir George Porter** (b 1920). They shared the Nobel Prize for Chemistry (1967) for their work, with **Manfred Eigen** (b 1927) of Germany, in 1967.

Fleischer, Dave (1894–1979) *See cartoon.*

Fleischer, Max (1883–1972) *See cartoon.*

Fleischmann, Martin (b 1927) *See nuclear fusion.*

Fleming, Alexander (1881–1955) A Scottish bacteriologist from Loudoun in Ayrshire who discovered penicillin. He received his education at Kilmarnock and worked as a shipping clerk for five years until 1902. He later qualified as a surgeon from St Mary's Hospital in Paddington in London and spent the rest of his career there. In 1928 he noticed by chance that *Penicillium* mold inhibited the growth of staphylococci grown on his culture plate. The clinical efficacy of penicillin was demonstrated by **Howard Walter Florey** (1895–1968), **Ernst Boris Chain** (1906–1979) and **Edward Penley Abraham** (b 1913).

Fleming, Sir John Ambrose (1849–1945) *See alternator, thermionic valve.*

Fleming, Williamina Paton Stevens (1857–1911) A Scottish astronomer from Dundee who emigrated to the US in 1878 where she worked with **Edward Pickering** (1846–1919) to produce the first catalogue classifying stellar spectra. She discovered 59 nebulae, and more than 300 variable stars.

Fleming, Sir Sanford (1827–1915) *See railway.*

Flemming, Walther (1843–1905) *See cell division, chromosomes, mitosis.*

Flett, Sir John Smith (1869–1947) A Scottish petrologist and physician from Orkney who published several works on petrology including *The Old Red Sand Stone of the Orkneys* (1898).

Flettner, Anton (b 1885) *See remote control.*

Flinders, Matthew (1774–1814) *See Brown, Robert.*

Flint Tools First observed by Horace, **Pliny the Elder** (AD 28–79) and Diodorus, who believed that they were produced by lightning, and named them *ceraunia* [Greek: *ceruvos*; thunder]. **Georgius Agricola** (1558) and **Conrad Gesner** (1516–1565) described some stone axes and stone arrowheads, but failed to give an adequate explanation for their origin. The first correct explanation for thunder-bolts or *ceraunia* was given by Michel Mercati in 1593. In 1797 an English archaeologist, John Frere, discovered stone flints and bones of large animals at Hoxne, Suffolk, and recognized that these were from the remote past. His findings were ignored for nearly half a century until **Jacques Boucher de Perthes** (1788–1868) announced similar findings at Abbeville in 1838. *See arrow.*

Floating Bodies   *See hydrodynamics, hydrometer, hydrostatistics.*

Float-Feed Carburetter   *See car.*

Floating Compass   *See compass.*

Floppy Disks   Introduced in 1970 for storing data for computers. *See computers.*

Florey, Howard Walter (1898–1968)   An Australian-born pathologist from Adelaide who was appointed as professor of pathology at Oxford in 1935. While working with **Sir Ernst Boris Chain** (1906–1979) he produced a pure extract of penicillin from the mold *Penicillium notatum* in 1940. Their work led to the practical commercial production of penicillin. Florey shared the Nobel Prize for Physiology or Medicine with **Alexander Fleming** (1881–1955) and Chain in 1945.

Flory, Paul John (1910–1985)   *See polymer.*

Flower [Latin: *flora*, goddess of flowers]   **Theophrastus** (380–287 BC) from the Greek island of Lesbos, in his treatise *History of Plants,* gave an account of flowers, including their position, growth, morphology and structure. A botanist from Lübeck, **Joachim Jung** (1587–1657), first used them as a basis for classification of plants. They were first suggested to be the sexual organs in plants by a London physician and botanist **Nehemiah Grew** (1641–1712), in 1682. **Carolus Linnaeus** (1707–1778) based his system of classification of plants on the free male parts of flowers. A similar system was previously proposed by a French botanist, **Joseph Pitton de Tournefort** (1656–1708). The largest flower known, *Rafflesia arnoldi,* was named after a botanist, Joseph Arnold (1782–1818) and the British colonial administrator **Sir Thomas Stamford Raffles** (1781–1826), by **Robert Brown** (1773–1858). An important work related to sex in plants and entitled *On the Embryology of Flowering Plants* (1849) was published by **Wilhelm Friedrich Benedikt Hofmeister** (1824–1877) of Saxony. **Charles Robert Darwin** (1809–1882) published *The Different Forms of Flowers* in 1859. *See pollination.*

Flower, Sir William Henry (1831–1899)   An English zoologist and anatomist from Stratford-upon-Avon, who served as Hunterian professor of comparative anatomy and physi-

ology, in 1869. He became the first director of natural history at the British Museum, and held the post from 1884 to 1898.

Fludd, Robert (1574–1637)   *See thermometer.*

Fluorescence   A term coined by an Irish physicist, **Sir George Gabriel Stokes** (1819–1903), who gave the first explanation for the phenomenon, in 1852. He used the method to study ultraviolet spectra.

Fluorescent Paint   Invented in 1933, under the name, *Dayglo,* by two American brothers, Joe Switzer and Bob Switzer.

Fluorine [Latin: *fluo*, flow]   Named by **Sir Humphry Davy** (1778–1829) in 1813. The presence of fluorine in fluorspar, giving it a fluorescent effect, was first noted by a German physician, **Georgius Agricola** (1494–1555) in 1529. The corrosive effect of hydrofluoric acid was observed in 1670 by an artist in Nuremburg, Herr Swanhardt. A French chemist, **Edmond Frémy** (1814–1894) of Versailles, who was an assistant to **Joseph Louis Gay-Lussac** (1778–1850), although prepared it, but was unable to collect it. It was isolated through electrolysis in 1886 by **Ferdinand Frederic Henri Moissan** (1852–1907), a demonstrator at the École de Pharmacie, Paris.

Fluoroscope [Latin: *fluo,* flow + Greek: *skopein,* view]   The first X-ray fluoroscope was constructed by **Thomas Alva Edison** (1847–1931) and it was exhibited at the New York city electrical exhibition in 1896. **Walter Bradford Cannon** (1871–1945) of Harvard University first used fluoroscopy for studying the act of deglutition in animals in 1898.

Flute   The modern flute was developed in 1847 by **Theobold Boehm** (1794–1881), who became a member of the Bavarian Court Orchestra, in 1818. He established a factory for making flutes in Munich in 1828, and began improving the flute in 1831.

Fluxions   An earlier term for differential calculus. *See calculus.*

Flying Saucers   *See extraterrestrial life, science fiction.*

Foam Rubber   First produced by the Dunlop Rubber Company in 1929.

Fock, Vladimir Alexandrovich (1898–1974)   *See Schrödinger equation.*

Fokker, Anton Herman Gerard (1890–1939)   *See warplanes.*

Fontana, Carlo (1638–1714) A Swiss-born Italian architect who designed many major works in Rome, including the Piazza di San Pietro.

Fontana, Franciscus An Italian astronomer in the 17th century and one of the first to use a telescope to observe the markings on the surface of Mars, in 1636.

Fontenelle, Bernard le Bovier de (1657–1757) *See Académie Royale des Sciences.*

Food Industry Water-powered machines for sifting flour were used by the Chinese around AD 530. The modern food industry became established with the discovery of refrigeration. A mixture of snow and saltpeter as a refrigerating compound was first used by an Italian, Zimara, in 1660. The first artificial ice was made in 1810 by freezing water under an air pump by a Scottish physicist and professor of natural philosophy at Edinburgh (1819), **Sir John Leslie** (1766–1832) from Largo, Fifeshire. Leslie's invention led to the use of steam machines and electricity for mass production of ice. Following this, cold storage rooms for preserving food were established around 1830. A method of preserving meat and vegetables by excluding air from their containers was discovered by a French confectioner, **Nicolas François Appert** (1749–1841). A British engineer, **Bryan Donkin** (1768–1855) of Northumberland, modified Appert's bottling process and used metal cans instead of glass bottles. **Joseph Louis Gay-Lussac** (1778–1850) examined Appert's bottles and found that they were devoid of oxygen, and came to the conclusion that oxygen caused putrefaction. Appert was one of the first to use the autoclave for the sterilization of food, in 1810, and he opened the first canning factory in the world in 1812. Modern refrigeration began with the invention of the compression method using ammonia, by a French engineer, Ferdinand Carre in 1857. An English-born Australian food industrialist, **Thomas Sutcliffe Mort** (1816–1878), built one of the largest refrigeration plants for the preservation of food at Darling Harbour, Sydney, in 1875. **Phillip Danworth Armour** (1832–1901) of Stockbridge, New York pioneered the large-scale packing and transport of meat in America and across the world. Freon, a non-toxic and non-flammable agent for domestic refrigerators, was introduced in 1930 by an American scientist, **Thomas Midgley** (1889– 1844) of Beaver Falls, Pennsylvania. The plastic bottle for storage, in place of the glass bottle, in order to avoid breakage, was invented in 1888 by a Swiss chemist, G.W.A. Kahlbaum. A US food manufacturer of German origin, Henry John Heinz (1844–1919), was a pioneer of packaged food in America, and he established the F. & J.

Heinz food packaging company in 1876. The first breakfast cereal was made from shredded wheat by Henry Perky of Denver, Colorado in 1893. **William Kellogg** (1852–1943), a physician from Tyrone in Michigan, introduced the method of flaking maize into crisp flakes, in 1894. These corn flakes were first marketed through the mail by Kellogg's food company in 1898. Kellogg established an industrial plant at Gloucester, Massachusetts, in 1923. The production of uncooked frozen food on a commercial scale was introduced by an American leather merchant, **Clarence Birdseye** (1886–1956) of Brooklyn, New York in 1917. Sliced bread was introduced into the market in 1930. Pre-cooked frozen food on a large scale was first introduced by Birdseye's rival, Findus, in 1939.

Forbes, Edward (1815–1854) *See marine biology, oceanography.*

Forbes, George (1849–1936) *See dynamo, Pluto, velocity of light.*

Forbes, James David (1809–1868) *See radiation of heat.*

Ford, Edmund Brisco (1901–1988) *See evolution.*

Ford, Henry (1863–1947) A pioneer of the motor car industry who founded the Ford Motor Company in 1903. He introduced his model-T chassis in 1909. He published *Today and Tomorrow* (1926) and *Moving Forward* (1931). *See car.*

Forest, Lee de (1873–1961) A physicist and pioneer in radio and wireless telegraphy from Iowa, who patented over 300 related inventions, which earned him the title of the father of radio in America. *See cinema, radio, thermionic valve.*

Forestry An English horticulturist, **John Evelyn** (1620–1706) of Wotton, Surrey, was one of the first to write a treatise on the subject in England entitled *Sylva or a Discourse of Forrest Trees* (1664). Owing to concern over the destruction of forests and extravagant use of timber, this book received a lot of attention, and was approved by Charles II (1630–1685). Another early treatise *The Manner of Raising, Make and Keep Woods; and improving Forest and Fruit Trees* was published by Moses Cook, around 1679. A French botanist, **Jean Baptiste Christophe Aublet** (1723–1788), who spent two years in French Guyana, published *Histoire des plantes de la Guiane française* (1775) which established the field of tropical forest botany on the American continent. An American botanist, **François Michaux** (1770–1852), wrote the first book on American forest trees in 1810–1813. A Canadian-born US geographer, **Isaiah Bowman** (1878– 1950), published *Forest Physiography* in 1911.

Fork The table fork for eating has been in use for less than four centuries. The ancient Greeks used the term *creagra* for a fork used by cooks to take the meat from the boiling pot. Table forks or *forchetta* were first known in Italy by the end of 15th century. Galeotus Martinus, an Italian at the court of Matthias Corvinus, the King of Hungary from 1458 to 1490, mentioned the use of table forks during this period. They were introduced into France at the end of the 16th century.

Forrest, George (1873–1932) A Scottish botanist from Falkirk who explored Tibet, Burma and China. He discovered several plants which now bear his name.

Forrester, Jay Wright (b 1918) *See computers.*

Forschammer, Johan Georg (1794–1865) *See oceanography.*

Forsyth, Alexander John (1769–1843) *See firearms.*

Forsyth, Andrew Russell (1858–1942) A Scottish mathematician from Glasgow who published *Theory of Functions* (1893) which incorporated various thinking on the subject across Europe. He formulated a theorem that generalized a large number of identities between double theta functions.

Fortification *See military engineering.*

Fortin Barometer A portable barometer constructed by a French scientific instrument maker, **Nicolas Jean Fortin** (1750–1831) in 1797.

Fortin, Nicolas Jean (1750–1831) French instrument maker. *See Fortin barometer.*

Fortran (**For**mula **Tran**slation) The first software computer language, suggested by an American computer programmer, **John Backus** (b 1924), and developed by International Business Machines (IBM) in 1957.

Fortune, Robert (1813–1880) *See tea.*

Fossils [Latin: *fossilis,* dug up] A term introduced in 1546, by a German physician and naturalist, **Georgius Agricola** (1494–1555), to refer to the remains of plants or animals dug out of the earth, which had changed into a stony consistency. A Greek philosopher, **Anaximander** (611–547 BC) of Miletus, first observed fossil seashells in the mountains, and inferred that the earth's surface must have fallen and risen from the sea, in the past. **Xenophanes of Colophon** (*c.* 560–478 BC), Ionia, held a similar view. For a long time fossils and shells were attributed to Noah's flood. During the Middle Ages, the Islamic physician **Avicenna** (980–1037) and **Albertus Magnus** (1192–1280) believed that fossils were substances of a non-organic nature. This view was opposed by **Leonardo da Vinci** (1452–1519) and an

Italian physician **Girolamo Fracastoro** (1483–1553), who attributed fossils to extinct organisms. The first work on fossils in relation to geology was carried out by **Conrad Gesner** (1516–1565), a Zurich physician, in 1565. His work *Hortorum Germaniae Descripto Historia Animalium* (1551–1621) published in five volumes earned him the name of the Modern Pliny. In 1691, **John Ray** (1628–1705), an English biologist from Essex, suggested that fossils were remains of animals from the past. **Johan Friedreich Esper** (1732–1781) gave an illustrative account of human and animal bone fossils, which were found in 1770, at the Gailenreuth Cave. An English physician and naturalist, and one of the original members of the Royal Society, **Christopher Merrett** (1614–1695), published a work on British flora and fossils entitled *Pinax rerum Naturalium Britannicarum, continens Vegetalia, Animalia, et Fossilia* in 1667. The study of fossils in paleontology was established as a branch of science by **Georges Cuvier** (1769–1832) of Paris, around 1800. Certain layers of the earth were shown to have characteristic series of fossils by a civil engineer, **William Smith** (1769–1839) in his *Stratigraphical Organised System of Fossils* (1817). The first English book devoted to fossils was published by **Martin Lister** (1638–1712) in 1678. **William Buckland** (1784–1856), a professor of geology at the University of Oxford, discovered several fossil remains of animals such as the hippopotamus, rhinoceros and elephant, in a cave near Kirkdale in Yorkshire, and published *Reliquiae Diluvianiae* (Relics of the flood) in 1823. A significant study of fossils in the Paris basin was done by a French geologist, **Gerard Paul Deshayes** (1795–1875), who collected over 40 000 specimens. A French naturalist, **Alexandre Brongniart** (1770–1847), was one of the first to relate the age rocks or strata to fossils. An American Quaker paleontologist, **Edward Drinker Cope** (1840–1897), was a prolific collector of fossils in North America, and published over 1400 papers and books. He sold his lifelong collection of fossils to the American Museum of Natural History. Several fossils of dinosaur eggs and mammals in Mongolia were discovered by an American explorer from Wisconsin, **Roy Chapman Andrews** (1870–1948). A method using radioisotopes to identify amino acids in fossils was devised by an American physical chemist, **Philip Hauge Abelson** (b 1913) from Tacoma, Washington, around 1960. The origin of early humans in Africa was brought to light through the discovery of several hominid fossils by a British anthropologist in Kenya, **Louis Seymour Bazett Leakey** (1903–1972).

Foucault, Jean Bernard Léon (1819–1868) *See gyroscope, heliostat, siderostat, sunspots, velocity of light.*

Fountain Pen *See pen.*

Fourcroy, Antoine François (1755–1809) *See chromium, nutrition.*

Fourdrinier, Henry (1766–1854) *See paper.*

Fourdrinier, Sealy (d 1847) *See paper.*

Fourier, Jean Baptiste Joseph (1768–1830) A French applied mathematician who in 1807 proposed that, with certain constraints, any mathematical function can be represented by trigonometrical series. This principle formed the basis of Fourier analysis, used in many different fields of physics today. He laid the groundwork for the later development of dimensional analysis and linear programming. He also investigated probability theory and the theory of errors. He accompanied Napoleon on his Egyptian campaign in 1798–1801. *See Fourier Series.*

Fourier Series Any function of a variable, whether it be continuous or discontinuous, can be expanded in a series of sines of multiples of the variable. Proposed by a French physicist, **Jean Baptiste Joseph Fourier** (1768–1830) from Auxerre, Bourgogne, in his *Théorie analytique de la chaleur* (1822). Light, sound and other wavelike forms of energy can be studied using this method, and a developed version of it is now called harmonic analysis.

Fourier Theorem Application of Fourier series to the investigation of energy from heat, sound or light, propagated in the form of waves. It was developed by a French physicist, **Jean Baptiste Joseph Fourier** (1768–1830) from Auxerre.

Fourneyron, Benoit (1802–1867) *See hydroelectric schemes.*

Fournier d'Albe, Edmund Edward (1868–1933) *See facsimile machine, optophone.*

Fournier, Pierre Simon (1712–1768) *See engraving, printing.*

Fourth Stage of Matter In physics an ionized gas having an equal number of positively charged ions and free electrons, known as a plasma. In thermonuclear reactions the plasma produced is confined through the use of magnetic fields. Referred to as the fourth stage of matter, its existence was demonstrated in 1873 by a London molecular physicist and chemist, **Sir William Crookes** (1832–1919). The Aurora Borealis or the Nothern Lights is considered to be a natural plasma.

Four-Stroke Engine *See internal combustion engine.*

Fowler, Sir John (1817–1898) *See underground railways.*

Fowler, Sir Ralph Howard (1889–1944) An English physicist from Essex, who became professor of theoretical physics at Cambridge, in 1932. He made several important contributions to statistical mechanics and quantum theory.

Fowler, William Alfred (1911–1995) *See helium.*

Fox, Sir Charles (1810–1874) A civil engineer from Derby who built the Crystal Palace in London. His two sons **Sir Douglas Charles Fox** (1840–1921) and **Sir Francis Fox** (1844–1927) were also engineers who contributed, with their father, to the construction of the English railways.

Fox, Sir Douglas Charles (1840–1921) *See Fox, Sir Charles.*

Fox, Sir Francis (1844–1927) *See Fox, Sir Charles.*

Fracastoro, Girolamo (1483–1553) *See fossils.*

Fractal [Latin: *fractus*, broken] A term coined by a Lithuanian mathematician, **Benoit Mandelbrot** (b 1924), to describe irregular geometrical shapes in nature, such as trees, coastlines and the vascular system, that repeat themselves endlessly on a decreasing scale. In computing, fractals are used in creating models for geographical and biological processes, and in computer art. Sets of curves with such properties were first developed in Germany by **Georg Cantor** (1845–1918) and **Karl Weierstrass** (1815–1897). Fractal compression is a modern method of storing digitally processed picture images and it uses less than a quarter of the data produced by breaking down images into pixels. The technique was first used commercially in 1993.

Fraction [Latin: *fractus*, broken] In Greece, an arithmetic fraction was considered as the ratio of two numbers. The Egyptians considered it to be a part of a number. *See calculation.*

Fraenkel, Abraham (1891–1965) An Israeli mathematician who, with the German mathematician **Ernst Friedrich Ferdinand Zermelo** (1871–1953), proposed the Zermelo–Fraenkel set theory, related to modern mathematical logic. *See Zermelo–Fraenkel theory.*

Fraenkel-Conrat, Heinz (b 1910) *See bacteriophage.*

Francis, James Bicheno (1815–1892) *See hydroelectric schemes.*

Francium An element originally known as actinium K, discovered in 1939 by a French physicist, **Marguerite Catherine Perey** (1909–1975). She became the first woman member of the French Academy of Sciences, in 1962.

Franck, James (1882–1964) *See Hertz, Gustav Ludwig, quantum theory.*

Frank, Albert Bernhard (1839–1900) *See mycorrhiza.*

Frank, Ilya Mikhailovich (1908–1990) *See Cherenkov effect.*

Frankland, Sir Edward (1825–1899) An eminent organic chemist from Churchtown, Lancashire, who developed the theory of valency in 1852. He discovered the presence of helium in the sun's atmosphere, through spectroscopy, with **Sir Norman Joseph Lockyer** (1836–1920), in 1868. *See valency.*

Franklin, Benjamin (1706–1790) An American scientist and statesman from Boston, Massachusetts, who invented the bifocal lens in 1785, and investigated the electrical phenomenon of lightning. He made many important contributions to diverse fields such as medicine, navigation, optics and electricity. He founded the American Philosophical Society in 1743 and helped to draft the Declaration of Independence in 1776. *See kite, lightning, storms.*

Franklin, Elsie Rosalind (1920–1958) *See deoxyribonucleic acid.*

Frasch, Herman (1851–1914) *See sulfur.*

Fraser–Darling Effect The enhancing effect of other species of birds on the breeding of colonial birds, observed by an English ecologist, **Sir Frank Fraser Darling** (1903–1979) of Chesterfield.

Fraser-Darling, Sir Frank (1903–1979) *See Fraser–Darling effect.*

Fraunhofer Lines *See absorption spectra.*

Fraunhofer, Joseph von (1787–1826) *See absorption spectra, astrophysics.*

Frederick II (1197–1250) *See ornithology.*

Fredholm Theory Related to integral equations, derived in 1900 by a Swedish mathematician, **Erik Invar Fredholm** (1866–1927) of Stockholm. He became professor of theoretical physics at Stockholm in 1906.

Fredholm, Erik Invar (1866–1927) *See Fredholm theory.*

Free Electron Laser A device for producing photon emission beams by passing electrons through a magnetic field, invented by an American physicist, John Madey, around 1972. His invention provided the laser system for precise surgery, and was also used in the *star wars* program of the Strategic Defence Initiative of the USA. *See laser.*

Freeman, Sir Ralph (1880–1950) *See suspension bridges.*

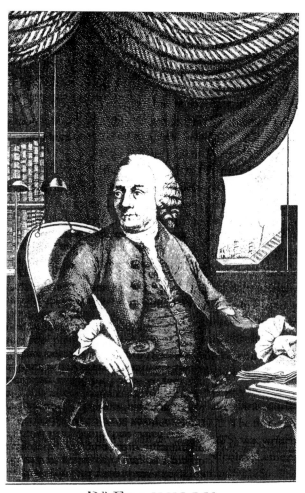

DR FRANKLIN.

Figure 35 Benjamin Franklin (1706–1790). Benjamin, Park. *The Intellectual Rise of Electricity.* London: Longmans, Green, & Co, 1895

Freesia A genus of plants native to South Africa named after a Swedish botanist, **Elias Magnus Fries** (1794–1878). He was a professor of botany at Lund and Uppsala, and proposed a system of classification of plants based on morphology.

Freeze Drying A method of fixing tissues by dehydration at low temperatures, invented in 1894 by **Richard Altman** (1852–1900).

Freezing Point The depression of freezing point was shown to be proportional to the concentration of particles in solution, by a professor of chemistry at the University of Grenoble, **François Marie Raoult** (1830–1901), in 1883. The freezing point was demonstrated in 1778 by an English chemist, **Sir Charles Blagden** (1748–1820) of Gloucestershire.

Frege, Ludwig Friedrich Gottlob (1848–1925) *See mathematical logic.*

Freleng, Friz (1906–1995) *See cartoons.*

Frémy, Edmond (1814–1894) *See fluorine.*

Frequency Modulation (FM) A method by which radio waves are altered for the transmission of broadcasting signals. It is constant in amplitude and varies the frequency of the carrier wave in accordance with the transmitted signal. It has an advantage over AM or amplitude modulation in having a better signal-to-noise ratio. Its use for radio was perfected by an electrical engineer, **Edwin Howard Armstrong** (1890–1954) of New York, in 1929. His method virtually eleminated the problem of interference from static.

Fresenius, Karl Remigius (1818–1897) A German pioneer of analytical chemistry, born in Frankfurt, and educated at Bonn. He studied under **Justus von Liebig** (1803–1873) at Giessen, and designed a systematic way of identifying compounds, by precipitating various radicals through precipitating reactions. His work was published in English under the title *Elementary Instruction in Qualitative Analysis* in 1841.

Fresnel, Jean Augustine (1788–1827) A French physicist who developed the transverse-wave theory of light. He also invented the compound lighthouse-lens, and published a monumental work on optics, *Oeuvres Complètes* (1860) in three volumes. *See light, lighthouses, polarization.*

Freundlich, Herbert Max Finlay (1880–1941) *See colloid chemistry.*

Freysinnet, Eugène (1879–1962) *See concrete.*

Friedel, Charles (1832–1899) *See aromatic compounds, Friedel–Crafts reaction.*

Friedel–Crafts Reaction Use of aluminum chloride as a catalyst for halogenating an aromatic compound. Discovered by a French professor of organic chemistry at the Sorbonne, **Charles Friedel** (1832–1899), and an American chemist, **James Mason Crafts** (1839–1917) of Boston, Massachusetts.

Friedman, Herbert (b 1916) *See X-ray astronomy.*

Friedman, Jerome Isaac (b 1928) *See quarks.*

Friedmann, Alexsandr Alexandrovich (1888–1925) A Russian mathematician from St Petersburg. In 1922, he derived several solutions to Einstein's field equation in the general theroy of relativity. All of his solutions suggested that space and time were uniform at all points and in every direction, although the mean density and radius of the universe varied with time. This provided support for theories of an expanding or contracting universe.

Friends of the Earth (FOE) An international group established in the UK in 1971 to protect the environment. They address issues such as pollution, destruction of rainforests, and promote recycling of waste and energy conservation.

Fries, Elias Magnus (1794–1878) *See Freesia, mycology.*

Friese-Greene, William (1855–1921) *See cinema.*

Frisch, Karl von (1886–1982) *See ethology, imprinting.*

Frisch, Otto Robert (1904–1979) *See atomic bomb.*

Frisius, Reiner Gemma (1508–1555) *See surveying.*

Frobenius, Georg Ferdinand (1849–1917) A German mathematician in Berlin who formulated the concept of the abstract group and the theory of group representations. His methods were used by a London mathematician, **William Burnside** (1852–1927) to develop quantum mechanics.

Frobenius, Joannes (1460–1527) A German printer who established a printing press at Basel in 1491, from where he published over 300 works.

Froebel, Friedrich Wilhelm August (1782–1852) A German educationist who established the kindergarten system of child education. The first such school was opened by him in 1837 at Blankenburg.

Fröhlich, Herbert (1905–1991) A German-born British physicist who applied solid-state theory to the methods of quantum field theory, in the application of quantum theory to particle interactions. He also made important contributions to the understanding of superconductivity. After being dismissed by the Nazis from his teaching post in Munich in 1933, he emigrated to England and became professor of theoretical physics at Liverpool University in 1948.

Frontier Orbitals Interaction of two of the electronic orbitals of the reacting molecules in a chemical reaction. Its theory is widely used in rationalizing organic reactivity. It was described by a Japanese chemist, **Kenichi Fukui** (b 1918), who shared the Nobel Prize for Chemistry in 1981, with a Polish-born US chemist **Roald Hoffmann** (b 1937).

Frontius, Sextus Julius (*c.* AD 35–103) *See water supply.*

Froude, William (1810–1879) *See law of comparison, marine engineering.*

Frozen Sections   A technique of freezing tissues in order to produce fine microscopic sections, first used in 1818 by **Pieter de Riemer** (1760–1831). A French chemist and physician, **François Vincent Raspail** (1794–1878), revived the method in 1825. *See embedding.*

Fry, Peter W. (d 1860)   *See portrait photography.*

Fuchs, Johan Nepomuk von (1774–1856)   *See waterglass.*

Fuchs, Klaus Emil Julius (1911–1988)   A German-born British physicist and spy who revealed nuclear secrets to the Russians, while he was head of theoretical physics at the atomic project at Harwell, after 1946. After receiving a 14-year sentence in 1950 he was released in 1959 and became an East German citizen.

Fuchs, Leonhard (1501–1566)   *See Fuchsia.*

Fuchsia   A genus of plants named after the German botanist, **Leonhard Fuchs** (1501–1566). He became professor of medicine at Tubingen in 1535 and published an illustrated book on botany, *Historia stirpium* (1542).

Fuel Cell or Grove cell.   A device with a platinum plate, capable of producing electricity by combining hydrogen and oxygen. It was invented in 1839 by a physicist and lawyer, **Sir William Robert Grove** (1811–1896) of Swansea, Wales. Grove's invention, although ideal in theory, was not found practical. The Bunsen cell, an improved form of it, contained a plate of carbon instead of platinum. Bunsen was the first to demonstrate the dissociation of water. A British scientist, F.T. Bacon, invented a successful fuel cell in 1959, and first demonstrated it in Cambridge, to drive a fork-lift truck.

Fukui, Kenichi (b 1918)   *See frontier orbitals.*

Fulton, Robert (1765–1815)   *See submarines, torpedo.*

Fungus   *See mycology.*

Funk, Casimir (1884–1967)   *See vitamins.*

Furlong   A unit of measurement of length (220 yards), originating in Anglo-Saxon England.

Fusion   *See nuclear fusion.*

Fust, Johann (d 1466)   *See printing.*

Fysh, Wilbot Hudson (1895–1974)   *See airlines.*

G

Gabelsberger, Franz Xavior (1789–1848) *See shorthand.*

Gabor, Denis (1900–1979) *See hologram.*

Gabriel Synthesis A method used for synthesis of primary amines from potassium phthalimide and alkaline halides, followed by hydrolysis. It was invented in 1887 by a German chemist **Siegmund Gabriel** (1851–1924).

Gabriel, Jacques Ange (1698–1782) *See architecture, European.*

Gabriel, Siegmund (1851–1924) *See Gabriel synthesis.*

Gadolin, Johan (1760–1852) A Finnish chemist, born in Turku. He investigated the rare metals of the earth and isolated yttrium from a black mineral from Ytterby, Sweden, in 1794. The rare metal gadolinium is named after him. He was appointed professor of chemistry at Uppsala in 1797.

Gadolinium A rare earth element of atomic number 64, isolated in a pure state in 1886 by a chemist **Charles Gallisard de Marignac** (1817–1894) of Stockholm. He named it after the Finnish chemist, **Johan Gadolin** (1760–1852). A Swedish chemist, **Carl Gustav Mosander** (1797–1858), first fractionated gadolinium from a natural ore.

Gagarin, Yuri Alekseyevich (1934–1968) *See astronauts, satellite.*

Gahn, Johan Gottlieb (1745–1818) A Swedish chemist who discovered selenium, and isolated metallic manganese. He demonstrated the phosphoric acid content of bone, with **Karl Wilhelm Scheele** (1742–1786).

Gaia Hypothesis The earth considered as a constantly self-regulating system of interacting physical, chemical and biological processes to maintain the conditions necessary for preserving life. Proposed in 1972 by an English chemist, **James Ephraim Lovelock** (b 1919) from Letchworth, Hertfordshire. He published *Gaia* (1979) and *The Ages of Gaia* (1988).

Galaxy [Greek: *galaxias*, Milky Way] A term for a cluster of stars, gas and dust. Out of millions of galaxies only four galaxies (Milky Way, Large and Small Magellanic Clouds, and Andromeda Nebula) are visible to the naked eye from the earth. The Greek philosopher **Democritus** (460–370 BC) recognized that a galaxy consisted of stars. **Galilei Galileo** (1564–1642) constructed a telescope in 1609, and managed to visualize the stars in the galaxy. The theory that stars are contained in spherical giant clusters in the Milky Way was proposed in 1761 by a Swiss mathematician, **Johann Heinrich Lambert** (1728–1777). The first ever observation of a spiral galaxy was made in 1845 by an Irish astronomer, **William Parsons, Lord Rosse** (1800–1867), with his giant metal-mirror telescope. The first correct description of the shape of the Milky Way was given by **Sir William Herschel** (1738–1822) in 1785. The first practical photographs of the Milky Way were taken in 1895 by **Edward Emerson Barnard** (1857–1923). A Dutch astronomer, **Jacobus Cornelius Kapteyn** (1851–1922) of Groningen, with his assistant **Pieter Johannes van Rhijn** (b 1886), demonstrated in 1904 that there are two streams of stars in our galaxy moving in different directions. In 1920, an American astronomer, **Vesto Melvin Slipher** (1875–1969) of Indiana, while working at Flagstaff in Arizona, discovered that light from certain distant galaxies exhibited a Doppler shift to the red end of the spectrum. **Edwin Hubble** (1889–1953) showed that the amount of the red-shift was directly proportional to the speed of the galaxy concerned, and in 1929 discovered that galaxies recede from the earth with increasing speeds. In 1924, he provided proof that the galaxies were star systems separate from our own galaxy. An important study of the dynamics of spiral galaxies was done by a Swedish astronomer, **Bertil Lindblad** (1895–1965). In 1957, an American astronomer, **Nicholas Ulrich Mayall** (b 1906), developed a system of classification for galaxies, based on their composite spectra. *See Andromeda nebula, Magellanic Clouds, Milky Way.*

Galen (AD 130–200) A Roman physician from Pergamum in Asia Minor. His works on physiology and anatomy dominated the field of medicine for nearly 1500 years.

Galileo (Galilei Galileo) (1564–1642) An Italian mathematician and scientist, born to a noble family in Pisa. He first studied medicine and later turned to mathematics and physics. At the age of 25 he became professor of mathematics at Pisa, and he moved to Padua in 1592. He constructed one of the first telescopes, based on a Dutch pattern, and used it to discover the black spots on the sun, the hills and valleys of the moon, and the Milky Way. The satellites of Jupiter were discovered by him in 1610. His scientific ideas that were not in conformity with the church earned him a short period of imprisonment and his books were publicly burnt. His principal works include: *The Operations of the compass, Nuncus Siderius, On the trepidation of the Moon, Discourse on*

Solar Spots, Mathematical discourses and demonstrations, and *Treatise of the Mundane System.* Galileo came to be regarded as the father of the science of moving bodies or dynamics, owing to his experiments on the movement of falling bodies, pendulums and projectiles. He introduced the concept of uniform acceleration and distinguished it from uniform velocity. His invention of the pendulum was applied to clocks by his son Vincenzo Galilei. *See acceleration, astronomy, barometer, clock, compound microscope, galaxy, gravity, hydrostatics, ice, Jupiter, Moon, motion, pendulum, pitch, Saturn, stars, sunspots, telescope, thermometer.*

Galilei, Vincenzo (1520–1591) An Italian mathematician and music theorist, and father of **Galilei Galileo** (1564–1642).

Galle, Johann Gottfried (1812–1910) *See Neptune.*

Galley Method A method of dividing upward, and scratching out the number as soon as it is used. It is called the galley method because its final form resembles a boat under full sail. A Franciscan monk, **Luca Paciuolo** or **Lucas Pacioli** (1445–1510) of Tuscany, first proposed the method in his book on arithmetic, published in Venice in 1497.

Gallium [*gallia,* Gaul in France] An element of atomic number 31. First observed spectroscopically by a French

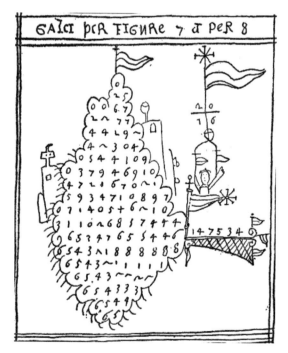

Figure 36 Galley method. Fyfe, J. Hamilton. *Triumphs of Inventions and Discovery in Art and Science.* London: T. Nelson and Sons, 1878

physical chemist, **Paul Emile Lecoq de Boisbaudran** (1838–1912) of Cognac, Charante, in 1875. He isolated the substance later in the same year and named it gallium in honor of his native country. He also published a spectroscopic study of 35 other elements, entitled *Spectres lumineux* (1874). Gallium was the first element to be discovered, based on the prediction from periodic table proposed by **Dmitri Ivanovich Mendeleev** (1834–1907).

Galois, Evariste (1811–1832) *See algebra, group theory.*

Galton, Francis (1822–1911) *See eugenics, fingerprints.*

Galvani, Luigi (1737–1798) An Italian physician from Bologna who established animal electricity on a scientific basis. In 1786, he started his studies on bioelectric effects using frogs' legs, and in 1791 came to the conclusion that the muscle or the nerve generated electricity. His work led to the construction of the voltaic pile in 1800 by **Alessandro Volta** (1745–1827), a professor of physics at Pavia. Galvani published his work *Aloysis Galvani de Viribus Electricitatis in Motu Musculari Commentarius* in 1791. He became depressed after the death of his wife in 1790 and died nine years later.

Galvanism Alternative term for electricity, named after **Luigi Galvani** (1737–1798), an Italian physician, who first demonstrated the presence of electricity in animal tissue, in 1791. *See electricity.*

Galvanometer An instrument for detecting small changes in electric current. In 1820, a Danish physicist, **Hans Christian Oersted** (1777–1851), discovered that an electric current flowing through a wire was associated with a magnetic field. The use of this principle for the measurement of electric current was first suggested by a French physicist, **André Marie Ampère** (1775–1836). In this instrument, a magnetic needle is pivoted at the center of a coil, and the current flowing through it is measured by its deflection. A string galvanometer was invented in 1820 by a German physicist, **Johann Salomo Schweigger** (1779–1857) of Erlangen. An English physicist and physician, **William Sturgeon** (1783–1850) of Lancashire, constructed the first moving-coil galvanometer, in 1836. A micro-radiometer combining a thermocouple and a galvanometer was invented in 1888 by an English physicist, **Sir Charles Vernon Boys** (1855–1944).

Gambey, Henri Prudence (1787–1847) *See machine tools.*

Games Theory A theory applicable to both games of chance, and games of skill such as chess, was put forward by a Hungarian-born American mathematician and physicist, **Johann von Neumann** (1903–1957) and **Oskar**

Morgenstern (1902–1977), in *The Theory of Games and Economic Behavior* (1944). An earlier work (1921–1927) on the theory of games, including the game of bridge, was written by a French mathematician, **Emile Felix Edouard Justin Borel** (1871–1956). A British psychologist **John Maynard Smith** (b 1920) applied game theory to animal behavior and developed a mathematical technique for studying the evolution of behavior. He published *The Theory of Evolution* (1958) and *Evolution and the Theory of Games* (1982).

Gamete [Greek: *gamete*, wife + *gametes*, husband] The term refers to the ovum of the female or the sperm of the male. Around 300 BC the fertilization of the ovum was thought to take place by a mystic process called 'aura seminalis'. It was believed that the ovum was complete in itself and was capable of producing an embryo, after a suitable stimulus was received. This view, preformation, was held until the 16th century. In 1779 an Italian biologist, **Lazzaro Spallanzani** (1729–1799), observed that a sperm must make physical contact with the egg for fertilization to take place. In 1875, a German biologist, **Oscar Hertwig** (1849–1922), while working on the eggs and spermatozoa of the sea urchin, in his small laboratory in the Mediterranean, proved that the process involved the union of the nuclei of the two gametes. The process of reproduction by the fusion of two gametes during fertilization was described by **August Friedrich Leopold Weismann** (1834–1914) of Jena in 1891.

Gamma or γ The third letter of the Greek alphabet which is sometimes used to denote the third member of a group or series.

Gamma Rays or γ rays. Following the discovery of the radiation properties of uranium by **Lord Ernest Rutherford** (1871–1937) in 1899, a new type of ray, known as the γ ray, and more penetrant than α, β or X-rays, was discovered in 1900 by a French physicist, **Paul Ulrich Villard** (1860–1934) of Lyons. The wavelength of gamma rays was first measured by an American physicist, **Arthur Holly Compton** (1892–1962) of Ohio, and a British physicist, **C.D. Ellis** (b 1895), around 1915.

Gamond, A. Thomé de (1807–1876) *See Channel tunnel.*

Gamow, George (1904–1968) *See alpha particles, Big Bang theory, deoxyribonucleic acid.*

Garbett, Samuel (1717–1805) *See lead chamber process.*

Gardening *See horticulture.*

Garment Industry The standard paper patterns used for designing garments were invented in 1859 by an American taylor, **Ebenezer Butterick** (1826–1903). *See textile industry.*

Garnerin, André Jacques (1769–1823) *See parachute.*

Garnerin, Jean Baptiste Olivier (1766–1849) *See parachute.*

Garrod, Dorothy Annie Elizabeth (1892–1968) An English archaeologist and the first woman to hold a professorial chair at Cambridge, in 1939. She was an expert on the Old Stone Age.

Garstang, Walter (1868–1949) *See pedomorphosis.*

Garstin, Sir William Edmund (1849–1925) *See water supply.*

Gas [Dutch: *geest*, ghost or spirit] The term gas was coined by **Jean Baptist van Helmont** (1577–1644) to refer to carbon dioxide. A Swiss alchemist and physician, **Paracelsus** or **Theophrastus Bombastus van Hohenheim** (1493–1541), used the Greek term *chaos* for air. The fundamental law of gases related to pressure and volume was proposed by **Robert Boyle** (1627–1691) in 1662. Hydrogen, nitrogen, oxygen, nitric oxide and carbon monoxide were initially known as permanent gases, owing to the initial difficulty in liquefying them. This was later overcome with the discovery of the critical temperature of gases. A systematic study of the diffusion of gases was performed by a Scottish chemist, **Thomas Graham** (1805–1869) of Glasgow. *See ammonia, argon, bromine, chlorine, fluorine, gas laws, halogens, helium, hydrogen, hydrogen sulphide, krypton, nitrogen, nitrous oxide, oxygen, ozone, xenon.*

Gas Chamber Used for the purpose of capital punishment, invented by an American major, D. A. Turner from the US Army Corps. The first person to be executed by this method was a murderer Gee Jon, from the Nevada State prison, who took 10 minutes to die, in 1924.

Gas Engine An engine powered by a mixture of air and oxygen, ignited through sparks from a Ruhmkorff coil with a current supply from a Bunsen battery. A Belgian-born French inventor, **Jean Joseph Etienne Lenoir** (1822–1900) first used it in 1860, instead of steam power, for the first horseless carriage. It was a forerunner of the internal combustion engine. A German engineer, **Nikolaus August Otto** (1832–1891), and **Eugen Langen** (1833–1895), developed it for use in the motor car.

Gas Laws Four fundamental universal gas laws: **Robert Boyle** (1627–1691) stated that the volume and pressure varied inversely if the temperature remained constant

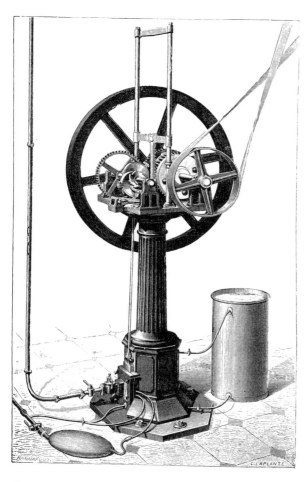

Figure 37 Otto and Langen's gas engine. Guillemin, Amédée. *The Applications of Physical Forces*. London: Macmillan and Co, 1877

(1662); **Joseph Louis Gay-Lussac** (1778–1850) proposed that the volume varied directly with the temperature if the pressure remained constant (1808); **Jacobus Henricus van't Hoff** (1852–1911) pointed out that solutions and gases behaved similarly (1877); and **Amedeo Avogadro** (1776–1856) proposed that equal volumes of all gases under the same conditions of temperature and pressure contained the same number of molecules (1811). Boyle's experiments were repeated at different temperatures by an Irish physicist, **Thomas Andrews** (1813–1885). A deviation of Boyle's law was investigated by a French physicist, **Emile Hilaire Amagat** (1841–1915), who published *The Laws of gases* in 1899. *See Charles' Law.*

Gas Lighting A Yorkshire clergyman, scientist and contemporary of Robert Boyle, **John Clayton** (*c.* 1650) was the first to realize, in 1739, that gas could be distilled from crude oil and stored. Gas lighting with the use of gas from coal was invented by **William Murdoch** (1754–1839) of Ayshire, who installed it in his house in Redruth, Cornwall, in 1792. The artificial gas obtained from sawdust was first used on a large scale in 1799 for illumination by a French engineer, **Phillipe Lebon** (1767–1804), in Paris. Coal gas was first used industrially as an illuminant by the Boulton and Watt company in Soho, Birmingham. William Murdoch illuminated the streets of London for the first time in 1807. In 1812, the city of London, as a whole, was first lit up with gas by the London Gas Light and Coke Company, founded in 1810 by a German pioneer of gas lighting, **Frederick Albert Winzer** (1763–1830).

Gas Turbine A gas turbine is any engine that uses gas to turn a turbine. In principle, air is drawn into the engine by a fan (the compressor) and is mixed with fuel and ignited (in the combustion chamber). The resultant combustion forces the hot gases out of the engine past a turbine. This turbine can power generators, pumps or propellors or, in the case of jet engines, develop thrust by accelerating the turbine exhaust through a nozzle. The concept of modern gas turbines was developed by an American aeronautical engineer, **Edward Story Taylor** (1903–1991). He founded the Gas Turbine Laboratory at the Massachusetts Institute of Technology, in 1946. A turbojet engine that passes all the air drawn in through the combustion chambers and expels it in a high-velocity jet was developed by an English engineer from Kent, **Stanley Hooker** (1907–1984). His engine was more efficient at high speeds and was adapted for high-speed military aircrafts. The world's first gas turbine car, Jet 1, was built by the Rover Company, in 1950.

Gascoigne, William (1621–1644) *See micrometer.*

Gasoline In 1886, **Carl Friedrich Benz** (1844–1929) of Karlsruhe demonstrated the first gasoline-driven car, a three-wheeler. **Thomas Midgley** (1889–1944), an American inventor from Beaver Falls, Pennsylvania, devised the octane rating method for gasoline. The first unleaded gasoline in the United Kingdom went on sale in 1986. *See octane rating, petroleum.*

Gassendi, Pierre (1592–1655) *See Académie Royale des Sciences, atomic theory, Mercury (planet).*

Gates, Henry William (b 1955) *See computers.*

Gatling Gun Made of ten revolving barrels, this was invented in 1862, during the American civil war, by a medical practitioner from North Carolina, **Jordan Richard Gatling** (1818–1903).

Gatling, Jordan Richard (1818–1903) A medical practitioner from Hertford County, North Carolina, who invented a gun (Gatling gun) which was used in the American civil war. He also devised a steam plough (1857) and a machine for sowing seeds (1850).

Gatterman Reaction Synthesis of aldehydes by formylation with a mixture of hydrogen chloride and hydrogen cyanide, invented by an industrial organic chemist, **Ludwig Gatterman** (1860–1920).

Gatterman, Ludwig (1860–1920) *See Gatterman reaction.*

Gaudin, M.A.A. (1804–1880) *See Avogadro's law.*

Gauging A method of measuring any vessel in relation to its capacity for wine or other liquids, established by law in 1352 by King Edward III.

Gaumont, Leon Ernest (1864–1946) *See cinema.*

Gauss, Carl Friedrich (1777–1855) A German mathematical physicist from Brunswick who invented a scientific system for units of magnetism and electricity. In 1839, he proposed the general theory of attraction of forces, in relation to the inverse square of distances. He published *Disquisitiones arithmeticae* (1801) containing new advances in number theory, and made several landmark contributions to mathematics and astronomy. *See bifilar magnetometer, hyperbolic geometry, law of quadratic reciprocity, non-Euclidean geometry.*

Gautier, Hubert (1660–1737) *See bridges, structural engineering.*

Gay-Lussac, Joseph Louis (1778–1850) An eminent French chemist, born in Saint Leonard, Haute Vienne. He became an assistant to **Claude Berthollet** (1748–1822) in 1800. In 1808, he proposed the law of gases, which states that volume varies directly with temperature, if pressure remains constant. This is known as Charles' Law in England. Gay-Lussac prepared hydroiodic acid, iodic acid and cyanogen. *See air, boron, fermentology, fluorine, gas laws, Gay-Lussac's law, law of combination of gases, silicon.*

Gay-Lussac's Law In AD 100, **Hero of Alexandria** noted that air expanded on heating, and he used this to effect the automatic closing and opening of a temple door. A French physicist, **Jacques Alexandre Charles** (1746–1823), found that oxygen, hydrogen, carbon dioxide and air expanded equally between 0 and 80 degrees Celsius. In 1802, the French chemist **Joseph Louis Gay-Lussac** (1778–1850) observed that a volume of a gas varies not only with pressure, but also, and to a very marked extent, with the temperature. He determined the amount of expansion

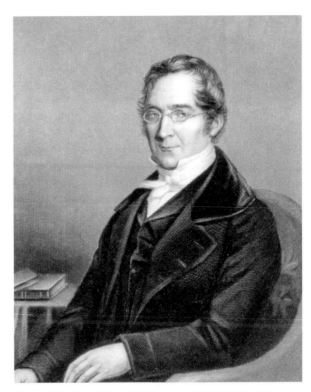

Figure 38 Joseph Louis Gay-Lussac (1778–1850). Courtesy of the National Library of Medicine

that took place and proposed the law that, at constant pressure, the volume of a given mass of gas is proportional to the absolute temperature. This law was later named after him.

Gear *See differential gear.*

Geber or Abu Musa Jabir ibn Hayyan A Persian chemist and founder of alchemy. He was born at Tus near Meshed in AD 721 and served at the Court of Harun Al-Rashid. Geber is credited with the discovery of nitric acid and aqua regia. The word gibberish was derived from his name, to denote the unintelligible jargon used by the alchemists.

Geddes, Sir Patrick (1854–1932) *See town planning.*

Geer, Baron Gerhard Jacob de (1858–1943) *See geochronology, Ice Age.*

Geer, Charles de (1720–1778) *See entomology.*

Geiger Counter An ionization chamber for measuring radiation or alpha and beta particles, developed in 1928 by two German professors, **Hans Wilhem Geiger** (1882–1945) and Erwin Walther Müller of Tübingen University. Another German physicist, **Walter Wilhelm Georg Bothe** (1891–1957), developed an electric circuit for scintillation counting, which replaced the laborious process of visual counting used by Geiger. For this work, Bothe shared the Nobel Prize with **Max Born** (1882–1970), in 1954.

Geiger, Hans Wilhem (1882–1945) *See Geiger counter.*

Geikie, James (1839–1915) Scottish geologist and brother of **Sir Archibald Geikie** (1835–1924). He succeeded his brother as professor of geology at Edinburgh (1882–1914) and was the first to suggest multiple glaciation. He published *Prehistoric Europe* (1881), *Earth Sculpture or the Origin of Land Forms* (1898) and *The Great Ice Age* (1874).

Geikie, Sir Archibald (1835–1924) A Scottish geologist from Edinburgh. In 1871, he was appointed to the first chair of geology at Edinburgh University, a post which he held for over ten years. He published *Outlines of Geology* (1879) and *Text-book of Geology* (1882), both of which passed through several editions.

Geissler Tube First effective vacuum device in which rarefied gases could be visualized when electricity was passed through. First demonstrated by a German physicist, **Julius Plücker** (1801–1868), and developed in 1855 by a German physicist, **Heinreich Geissler** (1814–1879) of Saxony. **Sir William Crookes** (1832–1919) modified the Geissler tube in 1861, and used it to demonstrate cathode rays.

Geital, Hans Friedrich (1855–1923) *See clouds, photoelectric cell, solar energy.*

Gelfand, Izrail Moiseyevich (b 1913) *See Lie groups.*

Gellibrand, Henry (1597–1636) *See compass (1), magnetic needle.*

Gell-Mann, Murray (b 1929) *See quarks.*

Geminus (*c.* 300 BC) An astronomer and pupil of **Posidonius of Alexandria**, who wrote *Elements of Astronomy*, which described and defined the day and the month. *See month.*

Gemmology One of the first works on the physical structure of gem stones, in relation to their identification and cutting, *Traité des Caractères Physiques des Pierres Précieuses* (1817) was published by a French crystallographer and mineralogist, **René Just Haüy** (1743–1822).

Gene [Greek: *genesis*, descent] A term for genetic material, coined in 1909 by a Danish botanist, **Wilhelm Ludwig Johannsen** (1857–1927) of Copenhagen. *See chromosomes, genetic coding, genetic engineering, genetics.*

Genentech The first company to use genetic engineering through recombinant DNA techniques, started in 1977 by Herbert Boyer and Robert Swanson.

General Electric An American electrical company founded in 1878 in New Jersey to back the experiments of the inventor **Thomas Edison**. Initially known as the Edison Electric Light, it merged with another company in 1892 to form General Electric.

Genetic Coding Study on the subject was advanced by the isolation of transfer RNA by a Boston biochemist, **Mahlon Bush Hoagland** (b 1921) in the late 1950s. The Nobel Prize in 1968 for Physiology or Medicine, for deciphering the chemistry of the genetic code, was shared by **Robert William Holley** (b 1922) of Illinois, **Marshall Warren Nirenberg** (b 1927) of New York City, and an Indian-born US chemist, **Har Gobind Khorana** (b 1922) from Raipur, Punjab. In 1967 Mary Weiss and Howard Green attempted sequencing of human genes through a method known as somatic cell hybridisation. In 1960, a South African scientist **Sydney Brenner** (b 1927) discovered the messenger RNA that provided the link between the DNA and the ribosomes on which proteins are synthesised. In the late 1970s an American geneticist, **Phillip Leder** (b 1934) of Washington DC, discovered the mechanism of coding in genes. **Walter Gilbert** (b 1932) and Allan Maxam in 1977 devised a method for sequencing DNA with the use of chemicals rather than enzymes. *See Human Genome Project.*

Genetic Engineering The process of transduction involving the transfer of genetic material from one bacterial strain of salmonella to another was demonstrated in 1952 by an American geneticist, **Norton David Zinder** (b 1928) and **Joshua Lederberg** (b 1925). Two French molecular biologists, **François Jacob** (b 1920) and **Elie Léo Wollman** (b 1917), independently demonstrated the direct transfer of genetic material in *Escherichia coli*, in 1956. The Nobel Prize for Physiology or Medicine, for the study of gene control of enzyme production in bacteria, was shared by **André Michel Lwoff** (1902–1994), **Jacques Lucien Monod** (1910–1976) and François Jacob, in 1965. The synthesis of DNA in growing populations of *E. coli* was first studied in detail in 1958 by **Matthew Stanley Meselson** (b 1930) of Denver, Colorado, and **Franklin William Stahl** (b 1929), a molecular biologist and professor at the University of Missouri. The method of inserting new genetic information into viral DNA was developed in 1972 by David Archer Jackson and Robert Symons. The fusion of a segment of human DNA, synthesized in the laboratory, into the bacterium *E. coli* was first performed in 1973 by **Herbert Wayne**

Boyer (b 1936) of Pittsburgh, Pennsylvania, and Stanley H. Cohen, and their experiments opened the doors to the immense possibilities in biogenetic engineering. The method of obtaining enzymes from bacteria, capable of splitting genes to generate genetically active fragments, was discovered by an American molecular biologist, **Hamilton Othanel Smith** (b 1931) in the 1970s. The first successful introduction of a human gene into the germline of a mouse (transgenic mice) was achieved by an American molecular biologist from New Jersey, **Ralph Lawrence Brinster** (b 1932), and a New York geneticist, **Richard de Forest Palmiter** (b 1942), in the late 1970s. In 1975, an American molecular biologist, **Richard Axel** (b 1946), showed that DNA, when combined with chromatin, could be cleaved at specific regions by staphylococcal nucleases. This contributed to the understanding of gene regulation. In 1979, Axel developed the technique of introducing a cloned viral gene into a mammalian tissue culture. The first transfer of genes between cells of different mammalian species was achieved in 1978 by an American molecular biologist, **Paul Berg** (b 1926) from Brooklyn, New York. The first field trials on genetically engineered organisms were conducted in 1985 by the biotechnological company Agracetus, in Wisconsin. In 1980, the US Supreme Court made a ruling that genetically engineered life forms could be patented. The world's first license to market living organisms produced by genetic engineering was issued in 1986 by the US Department of Agriculture.

Genetic Fingerprinting Involves the identification of certain core sequences in DNA, and is unique to each person. Discovered in 1984 by an English molecular biochemist, **Alec John Jeffreys** (b 1950) of Oxford. The technique involves digesting a DNA sample from an individual with the use of specific endonuclease enzymes, and subjecting it to electrophoresis on agarose gel. The first conviction of a criminal in England, based on genetic fingerprinting, was achieved in 1987.

Genetics [Greek: *genesis*, descent] A term coined in 1906 by **William Bateson** (1861–1926), a British geneticist from Whitby, Yorkshire. The science of genetics was founded by an Augustinian monk, **Gregor Mendel** (1822–1884), who worked on hybridization of pea plants in 1856, and published his epoch-making work in 1865. His work went unheeded until Bateson published *Mendel's Principles of Heredity* in 1902. The constant number of chromosomes for each cell in a given body, also characteristic of each species, was pointed out in 1887 by a Belgian cytologist, **Edouard Joseph Louis-Marie van Beneden** (1846–1910). Sex-linked inheritance was demonstrated by a geneticist

Thomas Hunt Morgan (1866–1945) of Lexington, Kentucky, during his work on the *Drosophila* fruitfly, in 1910. He published *The Mechanism of Mendelian Heredity* (1915), *The Theory of Gene* (1926) and *Embryology and Genetics* (1933), and was awarded the Nobel Prize in Medicine or Physiology in 1933, for his work on the hereditary functions of chromosomes. Evolutionary genetics was established as a special branch of genetics by a Russian-born US geneticist, **Theodosius Dobzhansky** (1900–1975), who published *Genetics and Origin of Species* (1937). The first chair of genetics was created at Cambridge in 1912, by an anonymous donor, in memory of the British Prime Minister (1902 to 1905), Arthur James Balfour (1848–1930), and his brother the biologist **Francis Maitland Balfour** (1851–1882). A contemporary of Bateson, **Reginald Crundall Punnett** (1875–1967) of Tonbridge, was appointed as its first professor. He published *Mendelism* in 1905.

Gennes, Pierre-Gilles de (b 1932) *See polymer.*

Genth, Frederick August (1820–1893) A German-born American mineralogist and professor of chemistry and mineralogy at Pennsylvania in 1872, who discovered cobalt-ammonium compounds and several new minerals.

Genus *See binomial nomenclature, botany, Linnaeus, Carolus.*

Geocentric Theory Proposes earth as the center of the universe with motion of heavenly bodies around it. A belief held by many ancient astronomers including **Heraklides of Pontus** (388–315 BC). Although an alternative heliocentric theory was proposed by **Aristarchos** (*c.* 320–250 BC) of Samos, the geocentric theory prevailed for 1800 years. **Ptolemy's** (*c.* AD 127–151) *Mathematical Syntaxis,* known as *Almagest* [Greek: *megiste,* the greatest] to the Arabs, was based on the geocentric concept. *See heliocentric theory.*

Geochronology [Greek: *ge,* earth + *chronos,* time + *logos,* discourse] A chronological study of the geological strata of the the earth. Pioneered by **Baron Gerhard Jacob de Geer** (1858–1943), who founded the Geochronological Institute of Stockholm and became its first director, in 1912. He published *Geochronologica Suecia* in 1940. An English geologist, **Arthur Holmes** (1890–1965), pioneered the measurement of radioactive constituents in the strata, for estimating age.

Geodesic Dome A hemispherical lightweight triangulated structure formed of short rods arranged in triangles. It allows large spaces to be enclosed using the minimum of materials, and was patented in 1954 by an American engineer Buckminster Fuller.

Geoffroy, Etienne François (1672–1731) *See acids.*

Geogeny [Greek: *ge*, earth + *genos*, descent] or geogony. The study of the origin of the earth. In 568 BC **Anaximander** (611–547 BC) of Miletus made the first attempt at a model of the earth according to scientific principles. He believed that the earth was a cylinder with north-south curvature. Around 450 BC a Pythagorian philosopher, **Philolaus**, believed that the earth rotated around a central fire, the sun. A modern study of the origin of earth, as part of the solar system, was commenced by **René Descartes** (1596–1650), around 1640. According to his *Principles of Philosophy* (1644), the origin of the earth was a glowing mass like the sun. Descartes also described the formation of various layers of the earth. **Athanasius Kircher** (1601–1680) of Geysen, in his *Subterranean World* (1665), postulated that numerous volcanoes and thermal springs, fed by the sea, existed under the earth's surface. According to an English clergyman, **Thomas Burnet** (*c.* 1635–1715) of Yorkshire, in his *Telluris Theorica Sacra* (Sacred Theory of the Earth, 1680–1689), the origin of the earth was a chaotic mixture of oil, water and sand. **Gottfried Wilhelm Leibniz** (1646–1716) proposed the theory that the earth was originally an incandescent mass that cooled and contracted with an outer crust formation, in his *Acta Eruditorum* (1697). The philosopher and physicist, **Immanuel Kant** (1724–1804) of Königsberg, in his nebular hypothesis, suggested the possible development of stars, suns and planets by slow contraction of diffuse and incandescent clouds. The origin of the earth as water, and the theory of the great flood of Noah, was proposed by **John Woodward** (1665–1728), a professor of medicine at Gresham College, in his *An Essay towards the Natural History of Earth* (1695). The principle of gravitation was used in 1692 by **Sir Isaac Newton** (1642–1727) to explain the origin of the earth. An American chemist, **Stanley Lloyd Miller** (b 1930) of Oakland, California was one of the first to investigate the formation of organic matter experimentally, by simulating thunderstorms. He passed an electric discharge through mixtures of gases, and noted the appearance of new organic substances such as aldehydes and amino acids. His findings became accepted as a plausible explanation for the appearance of the first organic substances on the earth.

Geography [Greek: *ge*, earth + *graphein*, to write] **Ptolemy** (*c.* AD 127–151) defined geography as a representation, by a map, of the portion of the earth known to us, together with its general features. The geographical map was invented by **Anaximander** (611–547 BC) of Miletus, in 568 BC. **Hecataeus of Miletus** (now Turkey), around 500 BC, developed a map of the world, which showed Europe and

Asia as semicircles surrounded by the ocean. **Dicaearchus** (355–285 BC), a pupil of **Aristotle** (384–322 BC), gave a physical description of the world accompanied by a world map. He was also the first to draw a parallel of latitude across a map. **Hipparchus** of Bithynia (190–120 BC) tried to deduce geography on a mathematical basis in 138 BC. Great attention and technical details were applied to the construction of maps by **Polybius** (204–122 BC) of Alexandria, who lived around the time of the destruction of Carthage, in 146 BC. **Eratosthenes** (274–194 BC) in his *Third Book of Geography* established a map of the inhabited world and divided it into two parts by drawing a line from west to east. A Greek geographer and native of Pontius, **Strabo** (*c.* 63 BC–AD 21) wrote *Geographica,* consisting of 17 books of which the first two dealt with geographical science. The rest were on the physical, political and economic geography of Europe, Asia and Africa. One of the first maps from the Middle Ages is found in the 7th century Cordex of **St Isidore of Seville** (AD 560–636). Modern maps were introduced into Europe in AD 1201 by the Moors from Spain, and they were brought to England in 1489 by Bartholomew Columbus in his attempt to illustrate his brother's theory of the Western continent. The first survey of all the counties of England and Wales was done by **Christopher Saxton** (1542–1611) from Sowood, Yorkshire, in 1579. His atlas was the first national map of any country to be published, and he published a wall map of England in 1583. A German Franciscan monk, **Sebastian Münster** (1489–1552), produced *Cosmographia: Beschreibung aller Lender* (1544), the first popular account of the world for laymen. His other books on geography include *Germaniae descriptio* (1530), *Mappa Europae* (1536) and *Rhaetia* (1538). An English geographer, **Nathaniel Carpenter** (1589–1628) of Oxford, published an important work, in 1625. *Geographia Generalis* by a German physician, **Bernhard Varen** or **Varenius** (1622–1650), remained in use for over a century. Another German geographer, **Philip Clüvier** (1580–1622) from Danzig, made a study of ancient geography in Italy, and published *Inriductio in universum, tam veterem quam novam* (1624). The Royal Geographical Society of London was established in 1830. *See cartography.*

Geological Map The first practical geological map was suggested before the Royal Society in 1684, by an English physician, **Martin Lister** (1638–1712). In 1751 **Jean Etiene Guettard** (1715–1786) of France wrote a treatise on minerals and rocks, combined with a geological map of France. A French naturalist, **Nicolas Desmarest** (1725–1815), published a geological map of the Auvergne, in 1774. The first geological map of England, based on fossil strata, was published in 1825 by an engineer, **William Smith** (1769–1839) of Churchill, Oxfordshire. Smith produced 21 other colored geological maps of English counties (1819–1824), and came to be regarded as the father of English geology. In 1824 **Baron Christian Leopold von Buch** (1774–1853) produced the first geological map of Germany consisting of 42 sheets. The first complete geological map of Ireland was produced in 1838 by a soldier and engineer, **Richard John Griffith** (1784–1878). He revised his map in 1855, and received his knighthood in 1858. A geological map of the Mississippi region of America was prepared by **William Maclure** (1763–1840) from Ayr, in Scotland, who settled in Virginia, and it was published by the American Philosophical Society in 1809. Maclure became known as the father of American geology, and published *Observations on the Geology of the United States of America* (1817). An American geophysicist, **Alexander Dallas Bache** (1806–1867), who was a great grandson of **Benjamin Franklin** (1706–1790), had the entire US coast mapped out, while he was superintendent of the US Coast Survey. The first geological map of South Africa was produced in 1856 by a Scottish geologist **Andrew G. Bain** (1797–1864). *See geology.*

Geology [Greek: *ge,* earth + *logos,* discourse] A science that seeks to explain the structure and origin of the earth and the successive changes in its scene and life. Around 500 BC, **Pythagorus** observed the physical changes in the land, and its eruptions, and described it as a fiery state of earth. **Leonardo da Vinci** (1452–1519) observed the changes in the land in relation to time and events. The first book on physical geology *De Ortu et Causis Subterraneorum* (1546) was published by a German physician, **Georgius Agricola** (1494–1555). The first work on fossils, in relation to geology, was carried out by **Conrad Gesner** (1516–1565), in 1565. A systematic observation of the strata of the earth was made by George Owen in his work on the *History of Pembrokeshire* (1570). **Robert Hooke** (1635–1703) in 1688 contributed to the study of earthquakes. A systematic study was done by a professor of medicine at Gresham College, **John Woodward** (1665–1728), who published *An Essay toward Nature and History of Earth* (1695). His geological collection formed the basis of Sedgwick Museum, Cambridge. **John Whitehurst** (1713–1788) of London proposed the theory of orderly deposition of strata in his *An Inquiry into the Original State and Formation of Earth* (1788). A Scottish natural philosopher, **James Hutton** (1726–1797) of Edinburgh, after an exhaustive study, published *The Theory of the Earth* (1785), in which he stated that the strata of earth had once been lakes and seas. A similar study in the

Alps was done in 1779 by a Swiss geologist **Horace Benedict de Saussure** (1740–1799) of Geneva, who was the first to introduce the term *geology* into scientific nomenclature. Volcanic geology was pioneered by a French naturalist, **Nicolas Desmarest** (1725–1815), who published a geological map of the Auvergne, in 1774. The Geological Society of London was established in 1807, initially with 13 members. The first important book in England *An Introduction to Geology* (1813) was published by an agriculturist, **Robert Bakewell** (1725–1795) from Leicestershire. **William Smith** (1769–1839) of Churchill, Oxfordshire, published the first geological map of England in 1815, and 21 other geologically colored maps of English counties, from 1819 to 1824. Through these contributions, he came to be regarded as the father of English geology. Experimental geology was initiated by **Sir James Hall** (1761–1832) of Berwickshire, England. He studied the effect of heat on limestone and other materials of the geological strata. The International Union of Geological Sciences was founded in 1878, and held its first meeting at Paris in 1878. A Scottish-born geologist, **William Maclure** (1763–1840) from Ayr, is regarded as the father of geology in America. His *Observations on the Geology of United States* (1817) was one of the first books on the subject to be published in America. The first state-funded geological survey of Massachusetts (1830), directed by **Edward Hitchcock** (1793–1864) of Deerfield, Massachusetts, resulted in the publication *The Geology of Massachusetts* (1833). Another pioneer of geology in America, **James Hall** (1811–1898), served as the first president of the Geological Society of America, founded in 1888. He published 13 volumes (1847–1894) on the paleontology of New York State. An American geologist from Rochester, **Grove Karl Gilbert** (1843–1918), studied the mountains of Utah, and stated the law of unequal slopes related to the denudation of a ridge between two valleys. **John Wesley Powell** (1834–1902) of Mount Morris, New York, made an important geological study of the Grand Canyon. He directed the US Geological and Geographical Survey of Territories, and helped to map out various regions from 1874 to 1880. *See geological map.*

Geometry [Greek: *ge,* earth + *metron,* measure] According to the Greek historian **Herodotus** (485–425 BC), geometry originated from the need of people to establish the boundaries of their properties obliterated by the Nile, and for the purpose of taxation. **Thales** (640–546 BC) of Miletus, the first of the Greek philosophers, initiated the science of geometry around 600 BC. **Pythagoras** (*c.* 580–500 BC) made geometry a part of a liberal education. **Hippocrates of Chios** (*c.* 460 BC) was the first to write systematically on geometry; he tried to square the circle. **Euclid**, a Greek scholar at the Alexandrian School, wrote his legendary treatise *Elements of Geometry* around 300 BC and the system of Euclidean geometry came to dominate the field for the next 2000 years. **Archimedes** (287–212 BC) helped to revive geometry. **Eudemus** (*c.* 330 BC), a pupil of **Aristotle** (384–322 BC) wrote a history. **Apollonius of Perga** (260–200 BC) wrote eight books, which included an important work on conic sections. Out of these, four survive in the original Greek, and three others in Arabic translation. The first book of **Ptolemy of Alexandria** (*c.* AD 127–145) dealt with trigonometry, degrees, minutes and seconds, in relation to astronomy. **Proclus Diadochus** (AD 410–485), amongst his other works, wrote an important commentary on Euclid's *Elements*, which has served as a valuable work on the history of geometry. **Pappus**, an Alexandrian mathematician in the 3rd century, who made several contributions to geometry, was one of the first to propose the analytical method, which was developed by **René Descartes** (1596–1650). Geometry started to be taught in Europe in the 13th century. The books on geometry and astronomy were thought to be infected with magic, and were destroyed by a Royal decree, in England, in 1552. René Descartes published his work on analytical geometry in 1627, and Simpson's first edition of Euclid appeared in 1756. Non-Euclidean geometry was invented in 1773 by Girolamo Saccheri, and independently developed in 1820 by a Russian professor of mathematics at Kazan, **Nikolai Lobachevski** (1792–1856), and in 1840 by a Hungarian mathematician, **Janos Bolyai** (1802–1860). A Swiss mathematician, **Jakob Steiner** (1796–1863), is regarded as the founder of projective geometry, which was independently developed by a French mathematician, **Michel Chasles** (1793–1880), who published a classic paper *Aperçu historique sur l'origine et la développement des méthodes en geometrie* (1837). *See analytical geometry, descriptive geometry, mathematics.*

Geothermal Energy [Greek: *ge*, earth + *therme*, heat] The use of earth's heat to produce power. Hot springs have been used as a source of heat energy since ancient times. **Charles Babbage** (1792–1871) in 1832 suggested the volcanoes and glaciers of Iceland as alternative sources of energy. The first trial use of geothermal energy was demonstrated in 1818 by a Frenchman, François de Larderel, at his village, near Tuscany. This village, later named Laderelle, was chosen as a pilot station for production geothermal energy, by Prince Giovanni Conti, in 1903. Geothermal energy was converted to electrical energy for the first time at this site, and used to light four lamps.

Gerard of Cremona (1147–1187) The most prolific translator of Arabic works into Latin in the 12th century. He obtained a thorough knowledge of Arabic at Toledo in central Spain.

Gerbert (d 1003) A French teacher and mathematician from Aurillac who taught at Rheims from 972 until he was elected Pope (Pope Sylvester II) in 999. He dealt with Hindu numerals, the astrolabe and abacus, and devised an instrument to measure the zenith distance. *See abacus, astrolabe, barrel organ.*

Gergonne, Joseph Diez (1771–1859) *See projective geometry.*

Gerhardt, Charles Frederic (1816–1856) of Strasbourg. An eminent chemist who studied at Leipzig, before he was appointed professor of chemistry at Montpellier, in 1841. He was later professor at Paris, in 1848, and gave the name phenol to carbolic acid. He proposed the concept of the chemical radical, and was the first to prepare acetanilide, in 1852. He was also one of the first to classify organic compounds. *See amines.*

Gerlach, Joseph von (1820–1896) *See staining.*

Gerlach, Walther (1889–1979) *See molecular beams.*

Germain, Sophie (1776–1831) *See Fermat's last theorem.*

Germanium An element of atomic number 32, with properties between those of metals and non-metals. It was discovered in 1886 by a German chemist from Freiberg, **Clemens Alexander Winkler** (1838–1904), and named after his country.

Germer, Lester Halbert (1896–1971) *See electron diffraction.*

Germination The founder of botany, **Theophrastus** (380–287 BC) in his *Historia Plantarum* (History of plants) described the process of germination of plants from their seeds. His description includes the morphology of different species of seedlings and their duration of germination.

Germplasm *See chromosomes.*

Gesner, Conrad (1516–1565) A Swiss naturalist and physician in Zurich whose work *Hortorum Germaniae Descripto Historia Animalium* (1551–1621), published in five volumes, earned him the name of the modern Pliny. He is regarded as the founder of bibliography, owing to his *Bibliotheca Universalis* (1545–1549), containing a bibliography of almost all the Latin, Greek and Hebrew writers. *See early printed science books, flint tools, fossils.*

Giaconni, Ricardo (b 1931) *See X-ray astronomy.*

Giaever, Ivar (b 1929) *See superconductivity.*

Giauque, William François (1895–1982) A chemist from Niagara Falls, Ontario, who discovered the oxygen isotopes. He was awarded the Nobel Prize for Chemistry for his work on chemical thermodynamics, in 1949. *See oxygen.*

Gibb, Alexander (1804–1867) *See Gibb, Alexander (1872–1958).*

Gibb, Easton (1841–1916) *See Gibb, Alexander (1872–1958).*

Gibb, Sir Alexander (1872–1958) Fifth generation of a line of Scottish master masons who developed one of the largest civil engineering works, which built bridges, hydroelectric schemes and harbors across the world. His father **Easton Gibb** (1841–1916) built the Kew Bridge over the River Thames. His grandfather **Alexander Gibb** (1804–1867) worked with **George Stephenson** (1781–1848) and built several railways in Scotland and England.

Gibbs, Josiah Willard (1839–1903) *See Gibbs-Donnan equilibrium, physical chemistry, thermodynamics.*

Gibbs, William Francis (1886–1967) *See warships.*

Gibbs–Donnan Equilibrium A phenomenon related to the movement of ions across a membrane, proposed by an American physicist, **Josiah Willard Gibbs** (1839–1903) of New Haven, Connecticut. It was studied experimentally by a Srilankan-born Irish chemist, **Fredrick George Donnan** (1870–1956). Gibbs also proposed the phase rule related to heterogeneous equilibria, and published *On the Equilibrium of Heterogeneous Substances* (1876–1878). A Dutch physical chemist, **Hendrik Willem Bakhuis Roozeboom** (1856–1907), developed Gibb's phase rule for practical applications.

Gibbs-Smith Charles Harvard (1909–1981) *See airplane.*

Gibson, James (1904–1979) *See perception.*

Giesel, Friedrich O. (1852–1927) *See emanium.*

Giffard, Henri (1825–1882) *See airships, air balloon.*

Gilbert, Cass (1859–1934) *See architecture, American.*

Gilbert, Grove Karl (1843–1918) An American geologist from Rochester, New York who worked for the US Geological Survey in Utah, and studied the ancient lakes of the Great Basin. He published a *Monograph on Lake Bonneville* in 1890.

Gilbert, Sir Joseph Henry (1817–1901) *See agriculture, nitrogen-fixing bacteria, roots.*

Gilbert, Walter (b 1932) *See deoxyribonucleic acid, genetic coding.*

Gilbert, William (1544–1603) An English physician from Colchester and a pioneer in the study of electricity. He developed the idea of the magnetic field, first observed through the dip of a compass needle by **Robert Norman** (1550–1600) of London. Gilbert demonstrated that other substances apart from amber also produced electricity. He conducted some of the earliest scientific experiments on electricity lasting for 17 years and published *De Magnete, Magneticisque Corporibus, te de Magno Magnette Tellure, Physiologia Nova* (1600), the first major scientific work to be published in England. He introduced the term *electrics,* from which **Sir Thomas Browne** (1605–1682) derived the term *electricity,* in 1646.

Gilbreth, Frank Bunker (1868–1924) *See management.*

Gilbreth, Lilian Evelyn née **Molder** (1879–1972) *See management.*

Gilchrist, Percy Carlyle (1851–1935) *See steel.*

Gill, Sir David (1843–1914) A Scottish astronomer from Aberdeen who became Astronomer Royal at the Cape of Good Hope, in 1879. He used a heliometer to measure solar and stellar parallaxes, and was a pioneer in the use of photography in astronomy. He followed the suggestion of a German astronomer, **Johann Gottfried Galle** (1812–1910), to use minor planets for solar determination, and obtained the distance to the sun.

Gillespie, Ronald James (b 1924) *See valency.*

Gillette Blade The first safety razor, invented in 1901 by a travelling salesman, **King Camp Gillette** (1855–1932) from Fond Du Lac, Wisconsin. His first batch of 51 razors were sold in 1903, and by 1908 his company had produced over 300 000 razors and 14 million blades. Gillette was a sociologist, and published *Gillette's Industrial Solution* (1900) and *The People's Corporation* (1934). *See safety razor.*

Gillette, King Camp (1855–1932) *See Gillette blade.*

Gillott, Joseph (1799–1873) *See pen.*

Gilmour, John Scott Lennox (1906–1986) *See botanical classification.*

Gimson, Ernest William (1864–1919) An English architect from Leicester whose name is more associated with his furniture designs.

Gin A machine in the textile industry, which gathered cotton while simultaneously separating it from the seed. Invented in 1793 by an American from Westboro, Massachusetts, **Eli Whitney** (1765–1825).

Ginzberg, Vitalii Lazarevich (b 1916) *See astrophysics.*

Giotto (*c.* 1266–1337) *See architecture, Italian.*

Girard, Albert (1595–1632) *See mathematical symbols.*

Glaciology [Latin: *glacialis,* icy + *logos,* discourse] Study of ice in relation to geology, the earth's regions, and its climate. The first detailed study of the Ice Age was done by **Jean Louis Rodolphi Agassiz** (1807–1873) of Switzerland, around 1836. A study into the sequence of past Ice Ages by a German glaciologist, **Albrecht Penck** (1858–1945), served as a basis for later work on the European Pleistocene. The modern field of radioglaciology, with the use of electromagnetic waves, was established by an American geophysicist, **Charles Raymond Bentley** (b 1929) of Rochester, New York. He used the method to study the physical characteristics of ice in Antarctica and the ocean floors. A French earth scientist and glaciologist, **Louis Antonin François Lliboutry** (b 1922), made glaciological studies in France and the Chilean Andes, and was mainly instrumental in establishing the Laboratory of Glaciology and Environmental Geophysics. **Sigurdur Thorarinsson** (1912–1983) of Iceland, made the first determination of glacier mass balance, in relation to climatic changes. An Australian glaciologist, **Gordon de Quetteville** (b 1921) of Melbourne, pioneered the use of the radio-echo sounding technique in glaciology. **John Frederick Nye** (b 1923) of Hove, Sussex, in England, suggested a theory of glacier motion, around 1950. The first observations on the basal sliding of glaciers, in relation to existing theories, were made in 1964 by a Californian glaciologist, **Walter Barclay Kamb** (b 1931) from San Jose. **Hans Rothlisberger** (b 1923) of Switzerland, studied the rate of melting caused by the frictional heat of running water, and the rate of conduit closure caused by ice (Rothlisberger canal). He was president of the International Glaciology Society (1984–1987) and published *Seismic Explorations in Cold Regions* (1972). *See Ice Age.*

Gladstone, John Hall (1827–1902) *See refraction.*

Glaisher, James (1809–1903) *See air balloon, aurora borealis.*

Glaser, Donald Arthur (b 1926) *See bubble chamber.*

Glashow, Sheldon Lee (b 1932) *See quantum chromodynamics.*

Glass A term originating from the Celtic word, *glas,* meaning gray or green. According to **Pliny the Elder** (AD 28–79),

glass making was accidentally discovered by the Phoenicians, who found that saltpeter that washed ashore from shipwrecks became converted to transparent stone (crude glass), when exposed to fire. A process of toughening glass, known to the Romans, was described by Petronius, in AD 100. The Romans introduced the technique of glass making into Britain, and glass remained a precious product there up to the 15th century. Home owners during this time removed their glass window panes and locked them up for safety whenever they stayed away from home. The first book devoted to the manufacture of glass, *De Arte Ventraria,* was published in Venice by a Florentine priest, Antonio Neri, in 1612. His book was translated into English (*The Art of Glass*) by Christopher Hemet, in 1662. The art of making colored glass, with the use of cobalt blue, was discovered in 1540 by Christoph Schrurer of Neudeck, in Germany. The production of red or ruby glass, with the use of iron and gold, was discovered by the German alchemist, **John Rudolph Glauber** (1604–1668), around 1665. A Russian scientist and professor of chemistry at St Petersburg, **Mikhail Vasilievich Lomonosov** (1711–1765), studied glass making and established a glasswork for making colored glass. A method of producing fine-quality optical glass, free of optical distortion and air bubbles, was invented by a Swiss glass maker, **Pierre Louis Guinand** (1744–1824). The one-process method, by blowing, for production of glass

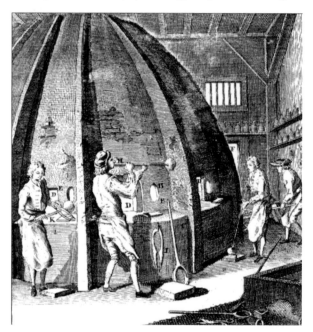

Figure 39 Glass makers in the 16th century. Owen, W. *Dictionary of Arts and Sciences.* London: Homer's Head, London, 1754

cylinders, was invented in 1896 by J.H. Lubbers. An English inventor, **Sir Lionel Alexander Bethune Pilkington** (1920–1995), developed a method of producing high-quality glass with a uniform thickness and absence of defects. His technique involved pouring glass straight from the furnace onto a bath of molten tin.

Glauber, John Rudolph (1604–1668) A German alchemist and physician, born in Carlstadt. He discovered a neutral purgative salt, sodium sulfate, which is known as Glauber's salt. He produced sulfuric acid and nitric acid, and published a work on chemistry. *See acids, chemistry, distillation, glass, nitric acid, sulfuric acid*.

Glauber, Roy Jay (b 1925) *See quantum optics*.

Glenn, John Herschel (b 1921) An American astronaut from Cambridge, Ohio, who was the first to orbit the earth. He made a three-orbit flight in the *Friendship 7* space capsule in 1962. With his other astronauts he published *Into Orbit* in 1962.

Gliders *See aerodynamics, airplane*.

Global Warming An American oceanographer, **Roger Randall Dougan Revelle** (1909–1991) of Seattle, Washington, was one of the first to warn of the effects of global warming. At the Scripps Institution of Oceanography, at La Jolla, he studied the effects of the release of carbon dioxide and heat on the atmosphere. He constructed a device that could measure the upward flow of heat from the ocean floor, and developed the theory of sea-floor spreading. *See greenhouse effect*.

Globe [Latin: *globus*, ball] A term used for spherical maps of the earth (terrestrial globe) or the universe (celestial globe). The first global map of the earth, excluding the New World and Pacific Ocean was constructed by a geographer and navigator, **Martin Behaim** (1440–1506) of Nürnberg, in 1492. A Swiss clock-maker and mathematician, **Joost Bürgi** (1552–1632), is supposed to have invented the celestial globe. The first globe of the earth, including the Americas, was made in 1515 by a German geographer and mathematician, **Johanes Schoner** (1477–1547) of Carlstadt, and he published a treatise on the use of globes. Some of the early terrestrial (1541) and celestial (1551) globes were constructed by the Flemish cartographer, **Gerardus Mercator** (1512–1594). An English geographer, **Richard Hakluyt** (1552–1616) from Hertfordshire, introduced the use of globes into English schools.

Globe Map *See globe*.

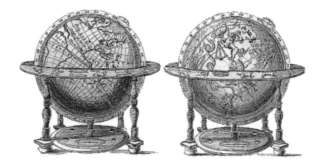

Figure 40 Terrestrial and celestial globes. Owen, W. *Dictionary of Arts and Sciences*. London: Homer's Head, London, 1754

Glycol An organic compound discovered in 1856 by a French chemist, **Charles Adolphe Wurtz** (1817–1884).

Gmelin, Johann Fredrick (1748–1805) *See metabolism*.

Gmelin, Johann Georg (1709–1755) A botanist, physician and chemist from Tübingen who became professor of chemistry and natural history at St Petersburg, in 1731. He published several botanical works including *Flora Siberica* (1748–1749) and *Reisen durch Sibirien* (1751–1752).

Gmelin, Leopold (1788–1853) Son of a physician from Tübingen, **Johann Fredrick Gmelin** (1748–1805). *See ester, ketone, lithium*.

Gmelin, Samuel Gottlieb (1745–1774) A botanist and nephew of **Johann Georg Gmelin** (1709–1755) whose *Flora Siberica* (1748–1749) he edited. He published *Historia Fucorum* (1768) and several other works.

Gnomon An L-shaped sundial with a vertical needle, used by the Egyptians, around 1500 BC. It was first applied to astronomy by a Greek philosopher, **Anaximander** (611–547 BC), to determine equinoxes.

Goddard, Robert Hutchings (1882–1945) *See rocket*.

Gödel's Theorem Demonstrates the existence of formally unprovable elements, within any formal system of arithmetic. Proposed in 1931 by a US mathematician of Czechoslovakian origin, **Kurt Gödel** (1906–1978).

Godwin, Sir Harry (1901–1985) *See pollen analysis*.

Goeppert-Mayer, Maria (1906–1972) *See atomic nucleus*.

Goethe, Johann Wolfgang von (1749–1832) *See morphology*.

Gold [Sanskrit: *jval*, to shine] Called *aurum* in Latin, and designated by the symbol *Au*. One of the earliest metals to be identified, owing to its glittering nature in river beds and soil. Gold was popular in Egypt as early as 3500 BC before the time of the first dynasty. Dusratta, the king of Mitani in 1400 BC, wrote to Amenophis III, the king of Egypt, 'the gods have done well in making gold as plentiful as dust in the land of Egypt'. **Pliny the Elder** (AD 28–79) wrote a chapter on gold around AD 50 in which he described the properties and uses of the metal. The Incas of Peru used gold lavishly in their temples and royal palaces before the time of the Spanish conquest in the 16th century. Gold was found in County Wicklow in Ireland in the 16th century, and a manuscript in the British Museum dating back to 1603 gives a prospector's reasons for believing that gold was present in Crawford Moor, in Lanarkshire. Gold was discovered by accident in California, by Captain Suter, while he was erecting a sawmill in 1847. It was first discovered in Australia in 1841 by an English geologist and clergyman, **William Branwhite Clarke** (1798–1878) in the alluvium of Macquarie. An American geologist, **Josiah Dwight Whitney** (1819–1896), investigated the source of gold in California and Nevada, and published *Auriferous Gravels of the Sierra Nevada* (1879–1880). Mount Whitney in California is named after him.

Gold Gilding The Roman encyclopedist, **Pliny the Elder** (AD 28–79), mentioned the practice of beating gold into thin leaves, for gilding. The use of gold varnish for leather tapestry was described in 1680 by an Italian artist, Antonio Cento of Palermo. The invention is attributed to the ancient Sicilians in *The Inventions of Sicilians* published in 1704. This book also describes the preparation of gold varnish. Homer's *Odyssey* refers to gold gilding of the horns of the cow, brought by Nestor, as an offering to Minerva. The method was extensively employed for gilding wooden frames and other articles in the 17th and 18th centuries. The method is supposed to have been introduced into England in 1633 by George Evelyn of Salop.

Gold Leaf Electroscope A sensitive electrometer based on the degree of repulsion between two pieces of gold leaf, when charged. Invented in 1787 by an English physicist and clergyman, **Abraham Bennett** (1750–1799). It was based on the principle of the portable electrometer constructed earlier by an Italian engineer in London, **Tiberius Cavallo** (1749–1809).

Gold, Thomas (b 1920) *See pulsar, steady-state theory.*

Goldberg, Leo (1913–1981) A New York astrophysicist who with his colleagues designed an instrument to photograph the sun using monochromatic light. This device which could function either as a spectrograph or a spectro-

heliograph formed part of the equipment of Orbital Solar Observatory IV, launched 1967.

Goldmark, Peter Carl (1906–1977) *See color television, gramophone.*

Goldschmidt Process Reduction of metallic oxides, using fine aluminum powder, fired by magnesium ribbon. Named after a German chemist in Berlin, **Johann Hans Goldschmidt** (1861–1923), who invented the process in 1894.

Goldschmidt, Johann Hans (1861–1923) *See Goldschmidt process.*

Goldschmidt, Richard Benedikt (1878–1958) A geneticist who gave up his professorship at Berlin in 1921, to become the director of the Kaiser Wilhelm Institute. He emigrated to America in 1934, and became professor of zoology at the University of California, where he conducted experiments on the geographical and environmental influence on genes and mutation. He published *Die Lehre von der Vererbung* (1927), *Die Sexuellen Zwischenstufen* (1931), *Physiological Genetics* (1938), *The Material Basis of Evolution* (1940) and several other works.

Goldschmidt, Victor Moritz (1888–1947) A Swiss geochemist who made an X-ray study of binary elements in the field of crystallography and petrology. His work *Geochemistry* was published posthumously in 1951.

Goldstein, Eugen (1850–1930) *See canal rays, cathode rays.*

Goldstine, Herman Heine (b 1913) *See computers.*

Gomberg, Moses (1886–1947) A Russian-born US chemist who discovered trivalent carbon. He was professor of chemistry at Michigan, and became the president of the American Chemical Society, in 1931.

Gondwanaland The southern landmass formed 200 million years ago by the splitting of the single world continent Pangaea. It fragmented into the present continents of South America, Africa, Australia, and Antarctica, which drifted slowly to their present positions.

Goniometer [Greek: *gonia*, angle + *metron*, to measure] Invented in the 18th century to measure the angles in rocks and crystals. **Jacques Babinet** (1794–1872) designed one, and F.J. Wollaston invented another, in 1817.

Goniometry [Greek: *gonia*, angle + *metron*, measure] The application of algebra to trigonometry, pioneered by a French mathematician, **François Viète** (1540–1603), who published *In Artem Analyticam Isagoge* (1591).

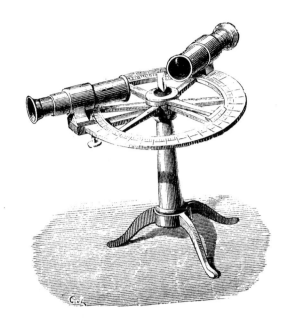

Figure 41 Babinet's goniometer. Guillemin, Amédée. *The Applications of Physical Forces*. London: Macmillan and Co, 1877

Goodricke, John (1764–1786) A British astronomer who emigrated from Groningen. He was awarded the Copley Medal in 1783 for his work on variable stars.

Goodyear, Charles (1800–1860) A hardware merchant from New Haven, Connecticut. In 1939, he discovered the method of making a moldable form of melted rubber, which he called 'vulcanizing' after the Greek god of fire, Vulcan. *See vulcanization.*

Goppert-Mayer, Maria (1906–1972) *See atomic nucleus.*

Göransson, Göran Frederik (1819–1900) *See Bessemer process.*

Gordan, Paul Albert (1837–1912) A Polish professor of mathematics at the University of Erlangen who proposed the theorem of finiteness, in 1868. In this he proved the existence of a finite fundamental system of variants and covariants for all binary quantics.

Gordon, Andrew (1712–1751) A professor of philosophy from Aberdeen who published *Phenomena Electricitasis Exposita, Physica Experimentalis Elementa,* and several other works on philosophy and science. He was the first to use a cylinder instead of a globe for electrical apparatus.

Gordon, James (1615–1686) *See cartography.*

Gordon, Robert (1580–1661) *See cartography.*

Gossage, William (1799–1877) *See Leblanc process.*

Gosse, Phillip Henry (1810–1888) *See aquarium, marine biology.*

Gosset, William Sealy (1876–1937) *See statistics.*

Goudsmit, Samuel Abraham (1902–1978) *See electron.*

Gould, Benjamin Apthorp (1824–1896) *See American scientific journals.*

Gould, John (1804–1881) *See ornithology.*

Graaf, Robert Jemison van de (1901–1967) *See Van de Graaf generator.*

Graebe, Karl (1841–1927) *See aromatic compounds, dyes.*

Graham, George (1673–1751) *See escapement, pendulum.*

Graham, Thomas (1805–1869) An eminent Scottish chemist, born in Glasgow, who studied chemistry there and at Edinburgh. He became a professor at Anderson's College in 1830, and proposed the law of diffusion of gases in 1831. In 1837, he moved to London as professor of chemistry at University College, and was appointed as the first president of the Chemical Society in 1841. He founded the field of colloid chemistry with his work on solutions in 1849, and conducted the first experiments on dialysis. He published *Liquid Diffusion applied to Analysis* (1861) and other treatises. *See colloid chemistry, dialysis, diffusion, gas, osmosis.*

Graham-White, Claude (1879–1959) The first English pilot to receive a British certificate of proficiency in aviation in 1910. He was instrumental in establishing the aerodrome at Hendon in London in 1911.

Gramme, Zenobe Theophile (1826–1901) *See alternating current, dynamo.*

Gramophone Prior to the invention of the gramophone by **Thomas Alva Edison** (1847–1931), the term phonograph was used for a machine that printed the notes played on a piano and other key instruments, onto paper. The principle of the gramophone was first suggested to the French Academy of Sciences in 1877 by a French poet and scientist, Charles Cros (1842–1888). It was independently invented by an Englishman, Fenby, in 1862. Leon Scott de Martinville, an American of French origin, was the first to make graphic recordings of speech, by using a vibrating membrane and a stylus, in 1857. The first patent for an apparatus that transmitted recorded sound on tin foil was obtained by **Thomas Alva Edison** (1847–1931), in 1877. In 1885, two Americans, Chichester A. Bell and Charles S. Tainter, used waxed paper tape, instead of tin foil. A rival claim to the invention was made by Charles Cros in the same year, and the origin of the invention still remains obscure. **Emile Berliner** (1851–1929), an inventor from Hanover, who emigrated in 1870 to America, invented the flat disk gramophone record in 1888, which was found to be superior to Edison's cylinder. In 1895, with his associate **Eldridge R. Johnson** (1866–1945), Berliner developed a method of making several copies of records in hard rubber, from a single master disk. A few years later he replaced hard rubber with shellac-based pressing, which was developed into 78 rpm records. Johnson established the Victor Talking Machine Company in 1901. In 1906, he made the first phonograph, which had its horn hidden in the cabinet. The modern long-playing microgroove record was invented in 1948 by a Hungarian-born American inventor, **Peter Carl Goldmark** (1906–1977). *See automatic musical instruments, magnetic recording.*

Granit, Ragnar (1900–1991) *See vision.*

Grant, Verne Edwin (b 1917) *See pollination.*

Graphical User Interface (GUI) An interface where programs and files appear as icons and user options are selected from pull-down menus. The data are displayed in windows which the operator can manipulate in various ways. The concept was developed by the Xerox Corporation in the 1970s, and popularized through the Apple Macintosh computers in the 1980s.

Graphite [Greek: *graphein*, to write] It was initially mistaken for lead, which is used for writing, hence its name. The main source of graphite was Ceylon or Sri Lanka and Madagascar in the early 1900s. A method of making artificial graphite on a commercial basis was developed in 1896 by an American chemist, **Edward Goodrich Acheson** (1856–1931).

Graphotype A method of obtaining blocks for surface printing, invented in 1860 by Witt Clinton Hitchcock. Fitz-Cook demonstrated the method to the Society of Arts, in 1865.

Grassmann, Hermann Gunther (1809–1877) A German mathematician who proposed a new theory of *n*-dimensional geometry, which had the elements of quaternions and matrices. He was also a philologist who studied Sanskrit and other Indo-European languages.

Graunt, John (1620–1674) *See vital statistics.*

Gravity [Latin; *gravis*, heavy] Considered to be an innate power by the Greeks. **Lucius Annaeus Seneca** (d AD 65) spoke of the moon attracting the waters by this power. In 1586, **Simon Stevinus** (1548–1620) of Leyden, performed some key experiments which led to the understanding of gravity. He dropped two objects of different weights from

the same height and noted that they took the same time to strike the ground. The astronomer **Johannes Kepler** (1571–1630) investigated this phenomenon in 1615, and **Robert Hooke** (1635–1703) studied the system of gravitation, in 1674. The principles of gravitation were demonstrated by **Galilei Galileo** (1564–1642) in Florence, in 1633. **Paul Guldin** or **Guldinus** (1577–1643) in his *Centrobaryca* (1635–1642) determined the center of gravity of curves, surfaces and solids. The Law of Gravitation was formulated by **Sir Isaac Newton** (1642–1727) in 1670, who published his findings in 1687.

Gray, Asa (1810–1888) An American botanist from Sauquot, New York, and a leading authority on taxonomy. He was an advocate of Darwin's theory of evolution, and is regarded as the founder of systematic botany in America. He wrote one of the first textbooks on botany, *Elements of Botany* (1836). He became professor of natural history at Harvard University in 1842 and published a *Manual of the Botany of the Northern United States* (1848).

Gray, Elisha (1835–1901) The inventor of the telephone, born at Barnesville, in Ohio. He was unaware of Alexander Graham Bell's invention, and independently built the telephone. When he visited the patent office in Washington, on 14 February 1876, he found that Alexander Bell had already patented the device, at the same office, a few hours earlier. Although Gray was bitter with disappointment, he went on to make several other contributions to telegraphy and communication.

Gray, George Robert (1808–1872) A London ornithologist and entomologist, who published *Entomology of Australia* (1833) and three volumes of the *Genera of Birds* (1844–1849).

Gray, John Edward (1800–1875) An English zoologist from Staffordshire who served as the Keeper of Zoology (1840–1874) at the British Museum. He was a prolific writer, with over 1000 publications including *The Natural Arrangement of British Plants* (1821) and the *Handbook of British Waterweeds* (1864).

Gray, Robert (1825–1887) Founder of Glasgow Natural History Society in 1851. He published *Birds of the West of Scotland* in 1871.

Gray, Stephen (1666–1736) One of the earliest experimenters on electricity, from London. In 1728, he started following up the discoveries on electricity made by an English physician, **William Gilbert** (1544–1603) of Colchester, and demonstrated the flow of electricity from one object to another. In 1696 he described the water droplet method for use in microscopy. *See conductivity.*

Greathead Shield *See underground railways.*

Greathead, Henry (1787–1816) *See shipping.*

Greathead, James Henry (1844–1896) *See underground railways.*

Green, George (1793–1841) *See potential.*

Green, Michael Boris (b 1946) *See superstring theory.*

Green's Functions *See potential.*

Greenhouse Effect The rise of earth's temperature due to reemitted solar radiation from the earth being trapped by pollutant gases such as carbon dioxide, methane and chlorofluorocarbons. It was first predicted in 1827 by French mathematician **Joseph Fourier** (1768–1830), and the term was introduced by Swedish scientist **Svante Arrhenius** (1859–1927). Petroleum-fuel consumption, agricultural byproducts and forest fires are the main causes of the phenomenon. According to the United Nations Environment Programme, by 2025, average world temperatures will have risen by 1.5°C with a consequent rise of 20 cm in sea level. To halt global warming or the greenhouse effect, emissions would probably need to be cut by 60%. *See ozone layer.*

Greenway, Francis Howard (1777–1837) *See architecture, Australian.*

Greenwich Mean Time (GMT) Local time on the zero line of longitude which passes through the Old Royal Observatory at Greenwich, London. First determined at the Greenwich observatory, with the help of **Sir George Biddle Airy's** (1801–1892) telescope, positioned on the line of zero longitude. He set about installing an electric clock at Greenwich, which sent an electric pulse to Lewisham Station from where it was relayed to post offices all over Britain. In 1862 hourly signals were sent from Greenwich to the newly installed Big Ben in London. It became Britain's legal time in 1880, and was introduced at the International Meridian Conference in Washington DC, in 1884. An engineer for the Atlantic Telegraph Company, Cromwell Fleetwood Varley, invented an instrument, the chronopher, which enabled the first transmission of Greenwich Mean Time by telegraph, twice daily to all parts of Britain around 1852. GMT was replaced in 1986 by coordinated universal time (UTC), but continues to be used to measure longitudes and the world's standard time zones.

Greenwich Observatory Founded in 1675 on the summit of Flamsteed Hill, by King Charles II, at the instigation of **Sir Christopher Wren** (1632–1723) and Sir Jonas Moore. **John Flamsteed** (1646–1719) was appointed as its first Astronomer Royal in 1675. In 1767, the Astronomer Royal, **Nevil Maskelyne** (1732–1811), instituted the publication of annual nautical almanac, as a result of which Greenwich came into steady use as the zero longitude on many maps and charts. The observatory was considerably modernized in 1811 by the then Astronomer Royal, **John Pond** (1767–1836), who improved the accuracy of many instruments there. The tenth Astronomer Royal, **Sir Harold Spencer Jones** (1890–1960), improved the accuracy of time measurement at Greenwich, with the introduction of quartz-crystal clocks.

Gregg, John Robert (1867–1948) *See shorthand.*

Gregor, William (1761–1817) *See titanium.*

Gregorian Calendar Received its name from Pope Gregory I, who improved the calendar in AD 590. In 1582, on the advice of an astronomer, **Christoph Clavius** (b 1537), Pope **Gregory XIII** designed a new Gregorian calendar. It excluded the leap year found in the Julian calendar, and was adopted in Great Britain in 1752.

Gregory, David (1659–1708) A Scottish mathematician in the tradition of his uncle **James Gregory** (1638–1675) of Edinburgh. His *Astronomiae Physicae & Geometricae Elementa* (1701), was the first textbook on gravitational principles. *See achromatic lens.*

Gregory, James (1638–1675) A celebrated mathematician from Aberdeen. He announced his invention of a reflecting telescope in his *Optica Promota, feu abdita Radiorum Reflexorum and Refractorum Mysteria, Geometrice Enucleata* in 1668. While he was in Padua, he published an original work on the hyperbola and the circle. He became professor of mathematics at St Andrew's in 1668, and one year before his death moved to Edinburgh as professor of mathematics. He made important contributions to the discovery of differential and integral calculus.

Gregory, John Walter (1864–1932) A London geologist who served as the first professor of geology at the University of Melbourne from 1900 to 1904, before he became a professor at Glasgow University. He published over 300 papers and books on geology including *The Dead Heart of Australia* (1906) and *Elements of Economic Geology* (1927).

Gresham College Founded in 1575 by **Sir Thomas Gresham** (1519–1579), who was financial adviser to Queen Elizabeth I (1533–1603) and founder of the Royal Exchange. On his death, he left a certain proportion of his property to establish lectures in divinity, astronomy, geometry, civil law and physic. These lectures commenced at Gresham's house in 1597. The founders of the Royal Society used the college as a meeting place in 1645. The buildings were demolished, and an excise office was erected at the site in 1768, and the lectures were moved to a room over the Royal Exchange. A new building for Gresham College, at Basinghall Street, opened for lectures in 1843.

Gresham, Sir Thomas (1519–1579) *See Gresham College.*

Gresley, Sir Herbert Nigel (1876–1941) *See locomotive.*

Grew, Nehemiah (1641–1712) A London physician and botanist who was educated at Leyden and Cambridge. He was the first to suggest that flowers were the sexual organs of plants, and he published *Anatomy of the Plants* (1682). *See botany, cell, chlorophyll, comparative anatomy, flower, gymnosperms.*

Grid An electrode in the path of the electrons in a valve. *See thermionic valve.*

Grid System *See cartography.*

Griess, Peter Johann (1829–1888) *See azo dye, textile chemistry.*

Griffin, Donald Redfield (1864–1932) *See echolocation, ethology.*

Griffin, Walter Burley (1876–1937) *See town planning.*

Griffith, Richard John (1784–1878) *See geological map.*

Grignard, François Auguste Victor (1871–1935) *See hydrogenation.*

Grimaldi, Francesco Maria (1618–1663) *See light, optics.*

Groma *See surveying.*

Grosse, Aristid V. (b 1905) *See fission, uranium-235.*

Grosseteste, Robert (1175–1253) *See optics, rainbow.*

Grotthus, Theodor von (1785–1822) *See electrolysis.*

Group Theory Investigation and classification of the properties of the mathematical structures known as groups. The first theory was suggested by a French mathematician, **Evariste Galois** (1811–1832). **Marie Ennemond Camille Jordan** (1838–1922), in his *Traité des substitutions et des équations algébraiques* (1870), related equations and groups of substitutions. The first book on Group Theory in English was published in 1897 by a London mathematician, **William Burnside** (1852–1927).

Grove Cell *See fuel cell.*

Grove, Sir William Robert (1811–1896) An English judge and scientist who devised a new form of voltaic cell, which

is named after him. He also gave one of the earliest accounts of the principle of conservation of energy in his treatise *The correlation of Physical Forces* (1846). He served as professor of physics at the London Institution from 1841 to 1864, after which he took to study of the law.

Grubb, Sir Howard (1844–1931) *See periscope, submarines.*

Grumann, Leroy Randle (1895–1982) *See warplanes.*

Gryphius, Sebastian (1493–1556) An early German printer from Swabia who established his press in Lyons in 1528, and published more than 300 works.

Guarini, Guarino (1624–1683) An Italian mathematician and architect from Modena who published several books on astromomy and mathematics. His *Architectura Civile*, published posthumously in 1737, relates geometry to architecture.

Guericke, Otto von (1602–1686) A burgomaster of Magdeburgh in Germany, and an eminent scientist. His inventions include an air pump, an apparatus for generating electrical charge, a weather glass and several other ingenious devices. He published several treatises on experimental philosophy. *See air pump, atmospheric pressure, barometer, electricity, thermometer, vacuum, velocity of sound.*

Guettard, Jean Etienne (1715–1786) *See geological map, transpiration.*

Guicciardini, Francesco (1482–1540) *See insurance.*

Guillaume, Charles Edouard (1861–1938) A Swiss physicist and winner of the Nobel Prize for Physics in 1920, for his work on nickel and steel alloys. He discovered a new alloy of nickel and steel, called Invar, not affected by temperature changes, which therefore was very useful in making precision instruments. *See Invar, steel.*

Guillotine A machine for quick and painless execution by decapitation, devised in 1789 by a physician in Paris, **Joseph Ignace Guillotine** (1738–1814).

Guillotine, Joseph Ignace (1738–1814) *See guillotine.*

Guinand, Pierre Louis (1744–1824) *See glass.*

Guldberg, Cato Maximillian (1836–1902) A Norwegian chemist from Oslo who, in 1865, proposed the law of mass action, which related the speed of a reaction to the concentrations of the reactants.

Guldin, Paul or **Guldinus** (1577–1643) *See gravity.*

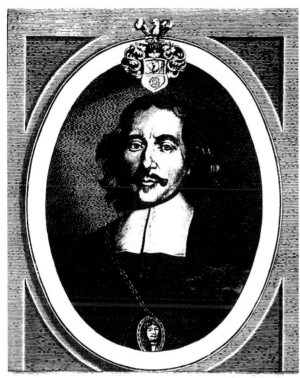

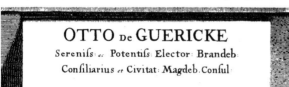

OTTO De GUERICKE
Serenifs *a* Potentifs Elector Brandeb.
Confiliarius *et* Civitat Magdeb Conful

Figure 42 Otto von Guericke (1602–1686). Benjamin, Park. *The Intellectual Rise of Electricity*. London: Longmans, Green, & Co, 1895

Gulf Stream A current of warm water that flows through the north Atlantic to the west coast of Europe. *See oceanography.*

Gun-Cotton A highly explosive product obtained by treating cotton or cellulose with a mixture of nitric acid and sulfuric acid, invented in 1846, by **Christian Friedrich Schönbein** (1799–1868) of Basel. **Sir Fredrick Augustus Abel** (1827–1902), an English chemist from Woolwich, used a paste of gun-cotton and nitroglycerin to develop, the cordite, which was adapted as a standard explosive by British Army, in 1891. He published *Gun-cotton* in 1866.

Gunpowder The English Franciscan monk, **Roger Bacon** (*c*. 1214–*c*. 1298) of Ilchester, has been credited with the discovery of gunpowder, probably because he had mentioned its composition in his treatise *De Nulliate magiae* (1242). It is also believed to have been invented by a German Franciscan monk, **Bertholet Michael Schwartz** or

Berthholdus (*c*. 1320) of Brunswick. Casper Weinde of Schemnitz first used it for ground blasting in mines, in 1627, and it was introduced for mining in Cornwall, in 1689. An American-born physicist in England, **Count Benjamin Thompson Rumford** (1753–1814) studied various gunpowders in relation to their force and effectiveness in propelling a cannon-ball.

Guns *See firearms.*

Gunsalus, Irwin Clyde (b 1912) *See radioisotope studies.*

Gunter, Edmund (1581–1626) *See cosine, cotangent, logarithms, slide rule.*

Gurdon, John Bertrand (b 1933) *See cloning.*

Gurevich Mikhail Iosifovich (1893–1976) *See warplanes.*

Gurney, Goldsworthy (1793–1875) *See car, limelight.*

Gutenberg, Beno (1889–1960) *See Richter Scale.*

Gutenberg Bible The first book to be printed by movable type, in two volumes, from 1452 to 1455. It involved the setting of three million type characters by hand, and was printed by **Johannes Gutenberg (Gensfleisch)** (1400–1468) of Mainz. It had 1284 pages, set in two columns, each with 42 lines. *See printing, movable type printing.*

Gutenberg, Johannes (Gensfleisch) (1400–1468) of Mainz. A pioneer of movable type printing. He had to leave his native place at the age of 10 with his mother, owing to political riots, and settled in Strasburg. He worked there as a mechanic around 1434 and formed a partnership for a press with a moneylender and printer, **Johann Fust** (d 1466) in 1450. Together they printed the famous Latin Bible in 1456, but after a legal battle they split up and Gutenberg acquired the press. He then worked with a skilled metal worker, **Peter Schoeffer** (1425–1502) until 1462, and established another press in 1463. Following the establishment of Gutenberg's press, the knowledge and art of printing spread rapidly to Italy, Germany and other parts of Europe. Gutenberg however, despite his pioneering works, did not include his name or the mark of his press in his books. He died a poor man in 1468. *See Gutenberg Bible, movable type printing, printing.*

Guthnick, Paul (1879–1947) *See photoelectric cell.*

Guthrie, Peter (1831–1901) *See knot theory.*

Guthrie, Samuel (1782–1848) *See chloroform.*

Gutta Percha Solidified juice of a tree (*Isonandra percha*) similar in composition and properties to India rubber. It was

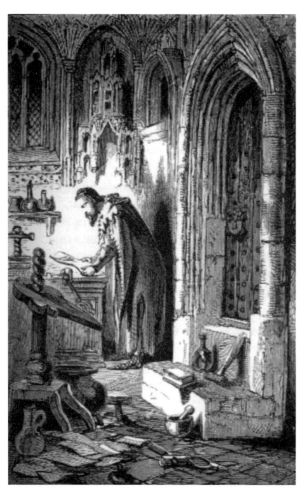

Figure 43 Gutenberg secretly experimenting at the abandoned monastry of St Arbogaste. Fyfe, J. Hamilton. *Triumphs of Inventions and Discovery in Art and Science*. London: T. Nelson and Sons, 1878

introduced into Europe from Borneo and Malacca in 1822. It is a non-conductor of electricity and is largely used as an insulating agent.

Guzmon, Laurenço de or **Bartolomeu de Gusmao** (1685–1724) *See air balloon.*

Gymnosperms [Greek: *gymnos*, naked + *sperma*, seed] A term for a group of plants, including pines and cypresses, proposed by an English botanist and physician, **Nehemiah Grew** (1641–1712).

Gyroscope [Latin: *gyrus*, circle + *skopein*, to view] An instrument used for measuring centrifugal and centripetal forces, in the study of the laws of gravitation. It was invented in 1852 by Fessel of Cologne, and improved by **Sir Charles Wheatstone** (1801–1875) and **Jean Bernard Léon Foucault** (1819–1868). The theory of the gyroscope was developed in 1906 by a German physicist, **Arnold Johannes Wilhelm Sommerfeld** (1868–1951) of Konigsberg, who was director of the Institute of Technical Physics, in Munich. The gyroscopic compass was invented independently by H. Anschutz-Kaempfe in 1908, and by an American electrical engineer, **Elmer Ambrose Sperry** (1860–1930) of Cortland county, New York, in 1911. Its principle is used in the guidance and control of space vehicles.

Gyrostabilizer A device to counteract a ship's roll and stabilize it, developed by an American electrical engineer, **Elmer Ambrose Sperry** (1860–1930) of Cortland county, New York. **Hermann Anschutz Kaempfe** (1872–1931), of Germany, independently developed one, which he fitted to a German ship, *Deutschland,* in 1908.

H

H Bomb or hydrogen bomb. The first bomb that worked on the principle of thermonuclear fusion was developed in 1952 by an American physicist, **Edward Teller** (b 1908) of Hungarian origin. A Polish mathematician, **Stanislaw Ulam** (1909–1985), is thought to have contributed originally to the design of the bomb. A Russian physicist, **Andrey Dmitriyevich Sakharov** (1921–1989) of Moscow, contributed to the development of the Soviet hydrogen bomb which was first exploded in 1949. He later campaigned for a nuclear test-ban treaty and was awarded the Nobel Prize for Peace in 1975. Sakharov also proposed controlled thermonuclear fusion for the generation of thermonuclear power for peaceful use. Further work on the hydrogen bomb was carried out in Russia by **Igor Vasilevich Kurchatov** (1903–1963) in 1953. A London physicist, **Baron William George Penney** (1909–1991) was instrumental in the British developing their hydrogen bomb in 1957. *See thermonuclear fusion.*

Haak, Theodore (d 1690) A German-born writer from Neuhausen who studied at Oxford, where he was one of the founders of the Royal Society.

Haas, William (d 1800) *See printing.*

Haber Process A method of making cheap fertilizers, by extracting nitrogen from the air and combining it with hydrogen under pressure at high temperature, in order to generate ammonia. Invented in 1908 by a Polish professor of physical chemistry at Karlsruhe, **Fritz Haber** (1868–1934). He was awarded the Nobel Prize for chemistry for this achievement, in 1918.

Haber, Fritz (1868–1934) *See agriculture, Haber process.*

Hackworth, Timothy (1786–1850) *See locomotive.*

Hadamard, Jacques (1865–1963) *See prime number.*

Haden, Sir Francis Seymour (1818–1910) *See engraving.*

Hadfield, Robert Abbot (1858–1940) *See stainless steel.*

Hadley, George (1685–1768) A London meteorologist, and one of the first members of the Royal Society. *See wind.*

Hadley, John (1682–1744) A London mathematician and astronomer who perfected the reflecting telescope, and in 1731 invented a reflecting quadrant, which bears his name.

Hadron-Electron Ring Accelerator (HERA) World's most powerful collider of protons and electron (accelerator) built underground at Hamburg, Germany. It began operating in 1992.

Haeckel, Ernst Heinrich (1834–1919) A German zoologist who is regarded as the founder of modern morphology. He was born in Potsdam, and studied medicine at Würzburg, Berlin and Vienna, before he relinquished medicine in 1862 to became a professor of zoology at Jena. He published *Generelle Morphologie* (1866), *Natural History of Creation* (1868) and *Anthropogenie* (1874). He coined the terms 'ontogeny', 'phylogeny' and 'ecology'. The Phyletic Museum he left behind in Jena contains a most illustrative collection on evolution. Haeckel introduced Darwinism into Germany. *See ecology, Pithecanthropus, recapitulation theory.*

Hafnium [Latin: *Hafnia*, Copenhagen] An element of atomic number 72, discovered in 1923 at the Bohr Institute of Theoretical Physics in Copenhagen, by a Dutch physicist, **Dirk Coster** (1889–1950), who was later professor of physics and meteorology at Groningen, and a Hungarian chemist, **Georg Charles von Hevesy** (1885–1966). A French professor of chemistry at the Sorbonne, **Georges Urbain** (1872–1938), independently discovered it around the same time.

Hagenbeck, Carl (1844–1913) *See zoo.*

Hahn, Otto (1879–1968) *See atomic bomb, fission, hahnium, protactinium.*

Hahn, Phillip Matthew (1739–1790) A mechanical genius from the University of Tübingen who invented a clock showing the course of the earth and the planets, and a calculating machine.

Hahnium An element with an atomic number 105, named after the German nuclear physicist **Otto Hahn** (1879–1968).

Hakluyt, Richard (1552–1616) *See globe.*

Haldane, John Burdon Sanderson (1892–1964) Son of the Scottish physiologist, **John Scott Haldane** (1860–1936). He carried out research on underwater respiratory physiology and submarine safety during World War ll. He published *Everything has a History* in 1951. He was a committed Marxist but left the Communist Party in 1956 and emigrated to India in 1957. A biography, *Portrait of Haldane,* was written by Eric Ashby (1904–1992), a London-born Australian botanist, in 1974.

Haldane, John Scott (1860–1936) *See carbon monoxide.*

Hale, George Ellery (1868–1938) An American astronomer from Chicago, who developed the spectroheliograph. He did important studies on sunspots, and was appointed as professor of astrophysics at Chicago, in 1892. He founded the *Astrophysical Journal. See celestial photography, Mount Wilson Observatory.*

Hales, Stephen (1696–1761) *See plant growth, plant physiology, roots.*

Hall, Asaph (1829–1907) *See Mars, Saturn.*

Hall, Charles Martin (1863–1914) *See aluminum.*

Hall, Chester More (1703–1771) *See achromatic lens, telescope.*

Hall Effect Production of a voltage across a conductor carrying a current at a right angle to a surrounding magnetic field. It was discovered in 1897 by the US physicist Edwin Hall (1855–1938) and is employed in the Hall-probe used for measuring the strengths of magnetic fields and in magnetic switches.

Hall, James (1811–1898) *See geology.*

Hall, Philip (1904–1982) A London mathematician and professor of mathematics at Cambridge (1953–1967) whose main interest was group theory. In 1933 he developed his theory of regular groups, and postulated a general structure theory for finite soluble groups in 1937.

Hall, Sir James (1761–1832) A British geologist from Dunglass, Haddingtonshire, and one of the first to study volcanoes. He was the author of *An Essay on the Origin, Principles,* and *History of Gothic Architecture. See geology, volcanoes.*

Halley, Edmund (1656–1742) An astronomer from Shoreditch who succeeded **John Flamsteed** (1646–1719) as Astronomer Royal in 1721. He was the first to detect the acceleration of the moon's mean motion. In 1676, he compiled the first catalog of stars in the southern hemisphere. He studied the parabolic orbits ascribed to the comets by **Sir Isaac Newton** (1642–1727), and applied these studies to a comet that he observed in 1682. The same comet had been observed by a German astronomer, **Regiomontanus** (1436–1476) in 1482, **Peter Apian** (1495–1552) in 1531 and **Johannes Kepler** (1571–1630) in 1607. Halley noted that this comet had made similar appearances in 1305 and

1380, and predicted its reappearance in 1759. After its reappearance as predicted following a 75-year interval, it was sighted again in 1835 and named Halley's comet. The Chinese are thought to have first observed Halley's comet in 240 BC. *See astronomy, aurora borealis, comet, diving bell, evaporation, meteorology, Moon, Newton, Isaac, nutation, Royal Society of London, Sirius, statistics, wind.*

Halley's Comet *See Halley, Edmund.*

Halliburton, William Dobinson (1860–1931) *See biochemistry.*

Hallstrom, Sir Edward John Lees (1886–1970) *See refrigerator.*

Halogens [Greek: *hals*, salt + *genos*, descent] A term coined by **Jons Jacob Berzelius** (1779–1848) since these (chlorine, bromine, iodine and fluorine), in their compound forms, were found in seawater or sea salt. A German physical chemist, **Ernst August Max Bodenstein** (1871–1942), who is regarded as the father of gas kinetics, carried out an important study of the reactions between halogens and hydrogen. *See chlorine, bromine, iodine, fluorine.*

Hamberger, George Albert (1622–1765) A mathematician from Beyerberg, Franconia who became professor of natural philosophy and mathematics at Jena. He wrote several works on hydraulics, optics and other subjects.

Hamilton, Robert (1753–1829) *See accountancy.*

Hamilton, Sir William (1730–1803) A Scottish naturalist who served as ambassador to the court of Naples, where he published his observations on Mount Vesuvius, Mount Etna and other volcanoes. He presented many of his geological collections to the British Museum.

Hamilton, Sir William Rowan (1805–1865) A professor of astronomy at Dublin and a pioneer in the application of mathematics to astronomy. He was made Astronomer Royal in 1827, and published a work on optics entitled *Theory of Systems of Rays* (1823) and *Lectures on Quarternions* (1853). *See conical refraction, quantum mechanics, quaternions.*

Hammet, Louis Plack (1894–1987) *See physical chemistry.*

Hammick Reaction Decarboxylation of quinaldinic acid by aldehydes and ketones. Studied by and named after a London organic chemist Dalziel Llewellyn Hammick (1887–1966).

Hanbury-Brown, Robert (b 1916) *See andromeda nebula.*

Hancock, Thomas (1786–1865) *See Macintosh cloth, vulcanization.*

Handley-Page, Sir Fredrick (1885–1962) *See warplanes.*

Hankel Functions A solution to the Bessel differential equation, orginally proposed in relation to planetary motions. Devised by a German mathematician and historian, **Hermann Hankel** (1839–1873).

Hankel, Hermann (1839–1873) *See Hankel functions.*

Hansard Usually refers to the printed proceedings of the House of Commons in London, UK. Named after an English printer, **Luke Hansard** (1752–1828) from Norwich, who was initially a compositor at the House of Commons printing office, owned by Hughes. He acquired the business in 1798, and printed the official reports of the proceedings of the Parliament from 1774 to 1889.

Hansard, Luke (1752–1828) *See Hansard.*

Hansteen, Kristoph (1784–1883) *See magnetic theory.*

Hantzsch, Arthur Rudolf (1857–1935) *See physical chemistry.*

Harcourt, Augustus George Vernon (1834–1919) *See candle power.*

Harcourt, William Venables Vernon (1789–1871) *See British Association for the Advancement of Science.*

Hard Water The soap test for hard water, was devised by a Scottish scientist, **Clark Thomas** (1801–1867), professor of chemistry at Marischal College, Aberdeen. He developed a process for softening hard water, in 1833.

Harden, Arthur (1865–1940) *See zymase.*

Hardy, Alister Clavering (1896–1985) *See plankton.*

Hardy, Godfrey Harold (1877–1947) An English Savilian professor of mathematics at Oxford (1920–1931), and Sadleirian professor of mathematics at Cambridge (1931–1942), who published *A Mathematician's Apology* (1940). *See Ramanujan, Srinivasan.*

Hare, Robert (1781–1858) *See oxyhydrogen blowpipe.*

Hargrave, Lawrence (1850–1915) *See airplane.*

Hargreaves, James (1720–1778) Inventor of the spinning jenny in 1764. *See spinning mule.*

Hargreaves, James (1834–1915) *See Diesel engine.*

Harington, Sir John (1561–1612) *See toilets.*

Harker, Alfred (1859–1939) *See petrology.*

Harland, Sir Edwards James (1831–1896) *See warships.*

Harmonics *See musical theory.*

Harriot, Thomas (1560–1621) *See algebra, mathematical symbols, snowflakes.*

Harris, Henry (b 1925) *See heterokaryon.*

Harris, John (1667–1719) An English clergyman from Shropshire, who wrote one of the first dictionaries of science (*Dictionary of Arts and Sciences*), which explained over 8000 scientific terms.

Harrison, John (1692–1776) An English clockmaker from Foulby, Yorkshire. He built a clock at the age of 20, which is now exhibited at the Kensington Museum, London. Harrison designed the first marine chronometer, in 1728. The English explorer **Captain James Cook** (1728–1779) made his longitude determination with Harrison's No. 4 chronometer. *See clock, marine chronometer, shipping.*

Harrison, Ross Granville (1870–1959) *See tissue culture.*

Harteck, Paul (1902–1985) *See deuterium.*

Hartline, Halden Keffer (1903–1983) *See vision.*

Hartree, Douglas Rayner (1897–1958) An English mathematician, born in Cambridge. He became professor of mathematical physics there in 1946. He devised an early analog computer.

Harvard College, now University. In Cambridge, Massachusetts it was founded in 1636. It was named after a London clergyman from Southwark, **John Harvard** (1607–1638) who went to Charlestown, Massachusetts to preach, in 1637. He bequeathed his library of 300 volumes and a sum of 779 GBP to the college.

Harvard College Observatory The first official observatory in America, founded in 1839. **William Cranch Bond** (1789–1859) of Portland, Maine, served as its first director.

Harvard, John (1607–1638) *See Harvard College.*

Harvey, Sir William (1678–1757) The discoverer of the circulation of the blood. From Folkstone, Kent, he was a physician at St Bartholomew's Hospital, London.

Harvey, William Henry (1811–1866) *See algae.*

Hassel, Odd (1897–1981) *See stereochemistry.*

Hasselbach, K.A. (1874–1962) *See Henderson–Hasselbach equation.*

Hassium Element of atomic number 108, discovered in 1984 at Darmstadt, Germany and named after the German state of Hessen.

Hauptman, Herbert Aaron (b 1917) *See X-ray crystallography*.

Hauron, Lois Duclos de (1837–1920) *See color photography*.

Hausdorf, Felix (1868–1942) *See topology*.

Hausmann, George Eugene (1809–1891) *See town planning*.

Haüy, René Just (1743–1822) *See crystallization, gemmology*.

Havilland, Geoffrey de (1882–1965) *See jet engine, transatlantic flight*.

Hawking, Stephen William (b 1942) An English theoretical physicist from Oxford and the author of *A Brief History of Time*. He became the Lucasian professor of mathematics at Cambridge University, a post once held by Sir Isaac Newton. He proposed the idea that the universe began as a singularity. *See black hole*.

Hawksbee's Electrical Machine An early machine for generating electricity, invented by an English physicist, **Francis Hawksbee** (d 1713).

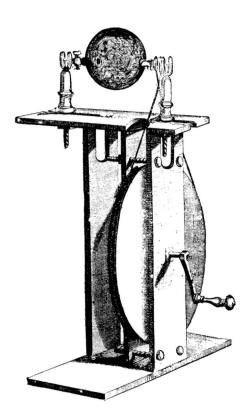

Figure 44 Hawksbee's electric machine. Benjamin, Park. *The Intellectual Rise of Electricity*. London: Longmans, Green, & Co, 1895

Hawksbee, Francis (d 1713) An English physicist and curator of experiments at the Royal Society, London. He conducted early experiments on electricity in 1705, and invented a glass electrical machine. He invented an air pump that bears his name. His son **Francis Hawksbee** (1687–1763) was also an experimenter on electricity.

Hawkshaw, John (1811–1891) *See Channel tunnel, underground railways*.

Haworth, Adrian Harvey (1766–1833) *See entomology*.

Haworth, Sir Walter Norman (1883–1950) An English chemist from Lancashire, who shared the Nobel Prize for Chemistry, for his synthesis of vitamin C and research on carbohydrates, with Paul Karrer, in 1937.

Hayashi, Chusiro (b 1920) *See Hertzsprung–Russell diagram*.

Hayashi Forbidden Zone *See Hertzsprung–Russell diagram*.

Hayden, Ferdinand Vandeveer (1829–1887) An American geologist and army surgeon from Westfield, Massachusetts, who served as professor of geology (1865–1872) at Pennsylvania University. He was one of the early geological explorers of western North America, and was instrumental in establishing Yellowstone National Park.

Hayes, Charles (1678–1760) An English mathematican who published a treatise on fluxions and other mathematical works.

Haynes, John Elwood (1857–1925) *See car*.

Hayward, Nathaniel (1808–1868) *See vulcanization*.

Hearing Aid The first electrical hearing aid was invented in 1902 by Millar Hutchinson of New York.

Hearst, William Randolph (1863–1951) *See newspapers*.

Heat [Anglo-Saxon: *haetu*] The English philosopher and scientist **Francis Bacon** (1561–1626) in his *Novum Organum* (1620) stated the essence of heat to be motion and nothing else. The first systematic experiments on heat were performed by **Benjamin Thompson, Count Rumford** (1753–1814), who in 1796 observed the production of heat by mechanical means, during the boring of a cannon. He came to the important conclusion that heat was a form of energy. **Sir Humphry Davy** (1778–1829) held the view that heat was a result of vibration of corpuscles. A Quaker physician and scientist, **Thomas Young** (1773–1829), concluded from his experiments that heat was a form of motion. Karl Friedrich Mohr, in his short memoir *On the Nature of Heat* (1837), was the first to suggest diverse forms of energy that included heat. The conversion of kinetic energy into heat and its reconversion into mechanical energy (later interpreted as conservation of energy) was demonstrated by a German physician and physicist, **Julius Robert von Mayer** (1814–1878), in 1842. In 1840 **James Prescott Joule** (1818–1889), a British natural philosopher from Salford, proposed (the Joule effect) that heat produced in a wire by an electric current is proportional to the resistance and square of the electric current. He also demonstrated the conversion of work into heat in 1845. **Rudolf Julius Emmanuel Clausius** (1822–1888) a professor of physics at Bonn, and contemporary of Joule, proposed the law of thermodynamics that established that energy has a constant tendency to move in the direction of dissipation rather than concentration. *See thermodynamics.*

Heat Pump   A device for tranferring heat from one object to another which is already at a higher temperature. First suggested by **William Thomson** or **Lord Kelvin** (1824–1907). Its principle is currently used in refrigerators.

Heath, Thomas Little (1861–1940) An English mathematical historian from Lincolnshire. He published *History of Greek Mathematics* (1921), *Diophantus of Alexandria: A Study in the History of Greek Algebra* (1885) and *Aristarchus of Samos, the Ancient Copernicus* (1913).

Heathcoat, John (1783–1861)   *See textile industry.*

Heating   Lighting a fire to keep warm has been practiced since prehistoric times. Simple oil lamps were used by the early Egyptians. The Romans around 100 BC used a system of under-floor channels to distribute warm air from a furnace. A similar system with a heater in the basement was in operation in America in the 1800s. The first alternative to fire, steam heat, was used by the pioneer of the steam engine, **James Watt** (1736–1819) to heat his office in 1784. The first steam central heating system was installed in 1817 at a Watford silk factory in England. An elaborate method for warming and ventilating public theaters was invented by the Marquess of Chabanne in 1819. An essay on steam heating was published by an English engineer, **Thomas Tredgold** (1788–1829) in 1824. The system of hot water circulation for central heating was patented in 1829 by Henry Cruges and Charles Fox in England. A French industrialist, Léon Duvoir, independently patented it in France in 1834. **Neil Arnott** (1788–1874), an English inventor and physician, wrote a treatise on the subject, in 1838. The first commission on ventilation and warming was appointed in England, in 1859.

Heaviside Layer   *See ionosphere.*

Heaviside, Oliver (1850–1925)   *See Heaviside layer, ionosphere.*

Heavy Hydrogen   *See deuterium.*

Heavy Water   First produced in 1933, by the combination of deuterium and oxygen; became valuable as a moderator in nuclear fusion. *See heavy water reactor.*

Heavy Water Reactor   The first heavy water reactor for large-scale production came into operation at the Argonne National Laboratory, near Chicago, in 1944.

Hecataeus of Miletus (*c.* 500 BC)   *See cartography, geography.*

Hedley, William (1779–1843)   *See railway.*

Hedwig, Johannes (1730–1799)   *See algae, moss.*

Heezen, Bruce Charles (1924–1977)   *See oceanography.*

Hegel, Georg Wilhelm Friedrich (1770–1831) An eminent German philosopher of Stuttgart who published *Encyclopädie der philosophischen Wissenschaften in Grundrisse* (Encyclopedia of Philosophical Sciences, comprising logic and the nature of the mind), in 1817.

Heidelberg University   One of the oldest continuously surviving universities, founded in Germany in 1386.

Heidelberger, Michael (1888–1991)   *See centrifuge.*

Heine Theorem   A classic theorem on uniform continuity of continuous functions, proof of which was provided by a German mathematician Heinrich Eduard Heine (1812–1881).

Heinkel, Ernst Heinrich (1888–1958)   *See warplanes.*

Heisenberg Uncertainty Principle   Formulated in 1927 by **Werner Karl Heisenberg**, the principle that the uncertainty of the position of a particle times the uncertainty of its momentum approximately equals Plauck's constant. The more certain we are of the position of a particle, the less certain we are of its momentum.

Heisenberg, Werner Karl (1901–1976)   *See matrix mechanics, quantum mechanics.*

Helicopter [Greek: *helico,* spiral]   An aircraft propelled by a vertical axle. The first design was given by **Leonardo da Vinci** (1452–1519) in 1500. In 1907, a French bicycle dealer, Paul Cornu, demonstrated the first helicopter that could take off vertically, carrying a human. However, his machine broke up a few seconds after the attempted take-off. Louis Bréguet and Jacques Bréguet performed the first piloted flight in their helicopter in the same year. A practical helicopter was developed by a German engineer, Heinrich Focke-Achgelis, in 1936. The first practical helicopter for mass production was designed by a Russian-born US engineer, **Igor Ivan Sikorsky** (1889–1972), in 1939. He began building helicopters in 1909 and founded the Sikorsky Aero Engineering Corporation, which became United Aircraft Corporation, in 1923. His first production helicopter was flown in 1943. The first solo round-the-world helicopter flight was made by Dick Smith of Australia in a Bell helicopter in 1983. *See autogyro.*

Heliocentric Theory [Greek: *helios,* sun] **Aristarchos** (*c.* 320–250 BC) of Samos, proposed the sun as the center of the universe, with the six known planets at that time revolving around it. The geocentric theory (Earth as the center of the universe, with the planets and sun revolving around it), proposed by **Heraklides of Pontius** (388–315 BC), prevailed for nearly 2000 years, until **Nicholas Copernicus** (1473–1543) revived the heliocentric theory in his *Nicolai Copernici Torinensis de Revolutionibus Orbium Coelestium Libri VI* (1543). A Dominican monk, Giordano Bruno (1548–1600), advocated the Copernican theory and developed it. He recognized that the earth rotates on its axis and is flattened at the poles. **Johannes Kepler** (1571–1630), a German astronomer, confirmed the theory.

Heliograph [Greek: *helios,* sun + *graphein,* to write] The intermittent reflection of sunlight by mirrors and other devices has been used as a method for transmitting messages since ancient times. It was first adapted for signalling Morse code around the 1830s. A heliograph with adjustable mirrors and a shutter to interrupt the sun's rays, so as to represent the dots and dashes of Morse code, was invented around 1860.

Heliometer [Greek: *helios,* sun + *metron,* to measure] A telescopic instrument for measuring the diameter of the sun, moon, planet and stars and the angular distances between them. Invented in 1754, by a London instrument maker, **John Dolland** (1706–1761). A French astronomer and mathematician, **Pierre Bouguer** (1698–1758) in 1748 invented a heliometer for measuring the light from the sun. In 1849, a heliometer made by **Johann Georg Repsold** (1770–1830) of Hamburg was installed at the Radcliff Observatory, in Oxford, England. He also designed a special pendulum that is named after him.

Heliostat An optical instrument or a solar microscope, used for keeping the inclination of solar rays constant. It was invented and named by William James Gravesande in the 17th century. A French physicist, **Jean Bernard Léon Foucault** (1819–1868) designed a heliostat.

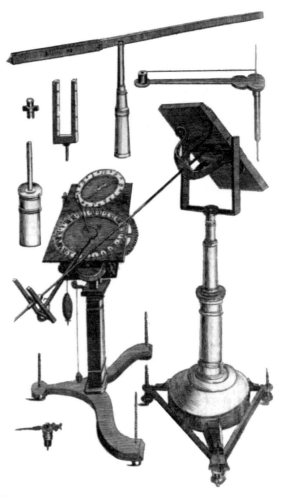

Figure 45 Heliostat. Owen, W. *Dictionary of Arts and Sciences.* London: Homer's Head, 1754

Helium [Greek: *helios,* sun] A yellow line in the spectrum of the sun was first noted in 1868 by a French astronomer, **Pierre Jules César Janssen** (1824–1907). This was thought to be due to a new element, and it was named helium by two English physicists, **Sir Norman Joseph Lockyer** (1836–1920) of Rugby, and **Edward Frankland** (1825–1899) of Churchtown, Lancashire. An English physicist, **William Crookes** (1832–1919), identified the gas in 1895. It was found to be a disintegration product of radium by **Sir William Ramsay** (1852–1916) and **Frederick Soddy** (1877–1965) in 1903. Helium was first liquefied by a Dutch physicist, **Heike Kamerlingh Onnes** (1853–1926) in 1908, and solidified by a Dutch professor of physics at Leyden, **Wilhelmus Henrikus Keesome** (b 1876), in 1926. A Canadian physicist, **John Cunningham McLennan** (1867–1935) of Ontario, used a method to liquefy it in 1932. The properties of liquid helium at extremely low temperature were studied by a Russian physicist, **Pyotr Leonidovich Kapitza** (1894–1984) in 1941. He was awarded the Faraday Medal (1942), the Stalin Prize for Physics (1941, 1943) and the Order of Lenin (1943). The Nobel Prize for Physics in 1978 was shared by him, **Robert Woodrow Wilson** (b 1936) and **Arno Allan Penzias** (b 1933). An English astrophysicist, **Fred Hoyle** (b 1915) of Yorkshire, proposed that for helium to be converted to heavier elements in the stellar core, an excited state of helium must exist. This was proved by an American physicist, **William Alfred Fowler** (1911–1995), and it formed a crucial link in stellar evolution. Fowler shared the Nobel Prize for Physics in 1983, for this work and for nucleosynthesis, with **Subrahmanyan Chandrasekha**r (1910– 1993). A Soviet physicist, **Lev Davidovich Landau** (1908– 1968) from Baku, developed a theory to explain the properties of liquid helium.

Hell, Maximillian (1720–1792) A Hungarian astronomer born in Chemnitz. He served as Director of the observatory there and published several works.

Helmet [Old French: *helmet*, head covering] The police helmet was invented in 1861 by **Borlase George Childs** (1816–1888) from Cornwall, who served as a surgeon to city of London police for 40 years.

Helmholtz, Hermann Ludwig Ferdinand von (1821– 1894) *See acoustics, energy, tangent gavanometer.*

Helmont, Jean Baptist van (1577–1644) or Johannes Baptista Van Helmont. Born in Brussels and studied at the University of Louvain. After serving as a surgeon for a short period, he gave up his practice and travelled widely in Europe in a futile search for the philosopher's stone. During his travels he met several alchemists from whom he learnt the art of alchemy. In 1609, he settled in Vilvorden, near Brussels, where his work on chemistry formed the basis for iatrochemistry. Helmont was the first to recognize carbon dioxide obtained by burning charcoal, and he coined the term *gas. See carbon dioxide, chemistry.*

Helriegel, Hermann (1831–1895) *See nitrogen-fixing bacteria.*

Henckel, John Frederic (1679–1744) *See porcelain.*

Henderson, Lawrence Joseph (1879–1942) *See Henderson–Hasselbach equation.*

Henderson, Thomas (1798–1844) A Scottish astronomer from Dundee, who became the Director of Royal Observatory at Cape of Good Hope in 1831. He became first Astronomer Royal of Scotland, in 1834.

Henderson–Hasselbach Equation Used for calculation of pH value of blood and other fluids. It was proposed by an American biochemist at Harvard, **Lawrence Joseph Henderson** (1879–1942) and a Danish biochemist, **K.A. Hasselbach** (1874–1962).

Hendrik, Christian (1761–1836) *See mycology.*

Hennebique, François (1842–1921) *See concrete.*

Henry of Hesse or **Heinreich von Langenstein** (1325– 1397) A German philosopher and one of the founders of the University of Vienna. He wrote several treatises on a variety of subjects including astronomy, astrology and theology.

Henry, Joseph (1797–1878) An American physicist from Albany, New York, who became the first director and secretary of the Smithsonian Institution, in 1846. He demonstrated the first electromagnetic telegraph to the National Academy of Sciences, in 1831, and was elected to the American Philosophical Society in 1835. *See academy, dynamo, induction current.*

Henry, William (1775–1836) *See Henry's law.*

Henry's Law The amount of gas dissolved by a given amount of water at a given temperature is proportional to the pressure. Proposed in 1803 by an English chemist and physician, **William Henry** (1775–1836) of Manchester.

Hensen, Victor (1835–1924) *See marine biology.*

Henslowe, Philip (d 1616) *See theater.*

Hephaistos God of fire in Greek mythology and patron of craftsmen. Homer (*c.* 800 BC) mentioned his skills in metallurgy.

Heraclitus (540–475 BC) A philosopher from Ephesus, who proposed fire as fundamental to creation of the world. He is said to have left Ephesus and lived on herbs and roots in the mountains, up to the age of 60. He was known as the weeping philosopher, owing to his habit of weeping at the follies of his fellow men.

Heraklides of Pontius (388–315 BC) A Greek astronomer who proposed that the earth turns on its axis once every 24 hours. *See geocentric theory, heliocentric theory.*

Herapath, John (1790–1868) *See railway, scientific journals.*

Herbig, George Howard (b 1920) *See Herbig–Haro objects.*

Herbig–Haro Objects Small convoluted luminous nebulae, connected with newly formed stars. Discovered and described by an American astronomer, **George Howard Herbig** (b 1920) from West Virginia.

Herbrand, Jacques (1908–1931) A French mathematical prodigy who at the age of 20 published his first paper on mathematical logic for the Paris Academy of Sciences. His doctorate thesis containing the Herbrand theorem in 1929 has found applications in many fields.

Herman, the Cripple (1013–1054) *See astrolabe.*

Hermann, James (1678–1733) A mathematician from Basel who became professor of mathematics at Padua. He published a work on the forces of fluids and solids, and several other treatises.

Hermite, Charles (1822–1901) *See quadratic equation.*

Hero of Alexandria A scientist around AD 100 who is regarded as the father of mechanical engineering. He invented the diopter, the steam turbine and several other scientific devices. He also proposed the concept of the air thermometer. His works include *Metrica* (on mensuration), *On the Diopter* (on engineering), *Mechanics, Catoptrics* (on light) and *Pneumatics*. *See automatic musical instruments, differential gear, diopter, Gay-Lussac's law, lamp, mechanical engineering, odometer, physics, steam engine, surveying, theodolite, thermometer, turbine, water siphon.*

Herodotus (485–425 BC) A Greek historian who is regarded as the father of history. His history, based on evidence, includes that of Greek, Egyptian and Persian culture. *See butter, day, geometry, hour, numbers.*

Herophilos of Chalcedon A Greek anatomist of the Alexandrian School, who was the first to perform public dissections to learn human anatomy, around 250 BC. He recognized the brain as the center of the nervous system. *See Alexandrian Museum and Library.*

Héroult Process An electrolytic method used for extracting aluminum from cryolite. Devised by a French metallurgist, **Paul Louis Toussaint Héroult** (1863–1914) of Normandy. He also designed a furnace (Héroult furnace) for production of steel. A similar method was described in America by **Charles Martin Hall** (1863–1914).

Héroult, Paul Louis Toussaint (1863–1914) *See aluminum, Héroult process.*

Heroz, Bertram (b 1929) *See computer graphics.*

Herschbach, Dudley Robert (b 1932) *See Polanyi, John Charles.*

Herschel, Caroline Lucretia (1750–1848) *See Andromeda nebula.*

Herschel, Clemens (1842–1930) *See hydraulics.*

Herschel, Sir John Fredrick William (1792–1871) A son of **Sir William Herschel** (1738–1822), born in Slough, Berkshire. He revised and completed the catalogs of stars commenced by his father, and published *General catalogue of Nebulae* (1864). *See absorption spectra, actinometer, contact lenses.*

Herschel, Sir William (1738–1822) An astronomer, born in Hanover, who came to England to train as a musician. He started his study of astronomy with a hired telescope, and discovered the planet Uranus in 1781. Six years later he detected two satellites, and by the end of his career he had discovered over 2500 nebulae and 806 stars. He proposed the dynamic theory of stars, extending the law of gravitation to stars, and their relation to each other in elliptical orbits. He was the first to recognize the advantages of larger apertures for telescopes. *See galaxy, infrared radiation, Milky Way, nebulae, Uranus.*

Hertwig, Oscar (1849–1922) *See fertilization.*

Hertz A unit of frequency equal to one complete vibration or cycle per second. Named after the discoverer of radio waves, **Heinrich Rudolf Hertz** (1857–1894).

Hertz, Gustav Ludwig (1887–1975) A German physicist and nephew of **Heinrich Rudolf Hertz** (1857–1894). He worked with a German-born US scientist, **James Franck** (1882–1964), on the energy levels of the atom, and shared the Nobel Prize for Physics with him in 1925.

Hertz, Heinrich Rudolf (1857–1894) A professor of physics from Homberg at the Carlsruhe Polytechnic during the period 1885 to 1889. He discovered the waves from electric discharge in 1886 which led to the discovery of the electron. *See electron, Hertz, radar, radio, radio waves.*

Hertzsprung, Ejnar (1873–1967) *See Hertzsprung–Russell diagram.*

Hertzsprung–Russell Diagram Plotting of luminosities of stars against their spectral types. Devised independently by a Danish astronomer, **Ejnar Hertzsprung** (1873–1967) and **Henry Russsel** (1877–1957) of Oyster Bay, New York. The diagram helped to establish the evolution and distance of stars. Hertzsprung was also a pioneer in celestial photography. Early analysis of the Hertzsprung–Russell diagram through stellar magnitudes was carried out by an English astronomer from Gloucestershire, **Roderick Oliver Redman** (1905–1975), who became professor of astrophysics at

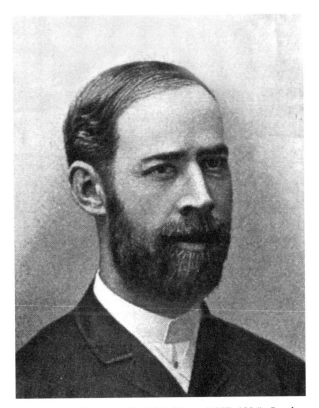

Figure 46   Heinreich Rudolph Hertz (1857–1894). Snyder, Carl. *New Conceptions in Science*. London: Harper and Brothers, 1903

Cambridge, in England, in 1947. A zone in the Hertzsprung–Russell diagram, showing logarithmic variation of stellar luminosity as a function of surface temperature, through which stars cannot pass (Hayashi forbidden zone), was demonstrated in 1961, by a Japanese astrophysicist, **Chusiro Hayashi** (b 1920).

Herzberg, Gerhard (b 1904)   *See spectroscopy.*

Hess, Germain Henry (1802–1850)   *See Hess's law.*

Hess, Harry Hammond (1906–1969)   *See tectonic theory.*

Hess, Victor Francis (1883–1964)   *See antimatter, cosmic rays.*

Hesse, William (d 1597)   An astronomer who built an observatory at Cassel. His *Observations* were printed in Leyden in 1618.

Hess's Law   Heat change in a given chemical reaction depends on the initial and final stages of the system, and is independent of the path followed, provided heat is the only form of energy to enter or leave the system. Proposed in 1840 by a Swiss-born Russian chemist, **Germain Henry Hess** (1802–1850).

Heterokaryon [Greek: *heteros,* other + *karyon,* nut]   Cells in which the cytoplasm, but not the nucleus, is fused. First produced experimentally in 1965 by an Australian-born British geneticist, **Henry Harris** (b 1925).

Hevelius, Johannes (1611–1687)   *See azimuth, moon, stars.*

Hevesy, Georg Charles von (1885–1966)   *See hafnium, isotopes, radioisotope studies.*

Hewish, Antony (b 1924)   *See pulsar.*

Hewitt, Peter Cooper (b 1861)   *See electric lighting.*

Hey, James Stanley (b 1909)   *See meteors, radioastronomy.*

Heyrovsky, Jaroslav (1890–1967)   *See polarography.*

Heytesbury, William (1310–1380)   *See motion.*

Hieroglyphics [Greek: *hieros,* sacred + *glyphein,* engrave]   The expression of ideas or thoughts through the drawing of objects was done by Athotes in 2112 BC. An earlier form of it by the Egyptians dating back to 3000 BC was found in King Narmar's Palette. **Pythagorus** (*c.* 580–500 BC) was the last of the ancient Greek philosophers to use hieroglyphics. Hieroglyphic art was used mainly by the Egyptians, and the first attempt to decipher them was made by **Jean François Champollion** (1790–1832), the French founder of Egyptology. Much of the Egyptian history and culture was made known through his work, and he published *Précis du Système Hiéroglyphique* (1824).

Higgs Boson   A theoretical elementary particle postulated in 1964 by **Peter Ware Higgs** (b 1929) of the University of Edinburgh and Thomas Kibble (b 1932) of Imperial College, London. Its presence has not yet been proved.

Higgs, Peter Ware (b 1929)   *See Higgs Boson, quantum electrodynamics.*

Higgins, William (1763–1825)   An Irish physicist who proposed the elements of chemical atomic theory in his *Comparative View of the Phlogistic and Antiphlogistic Theories* (1789).

Hilbert Space   A concept of infinite dimensional space proposed by a German mathematician and theoretical physicist, **David Hilbert** (1862–1943) of Konigsberg. In 1901 he listed 23 major unsolved mathematical problems, some of which still remain unsolved.

Hilbert, David (1862–1943)   *See Hilbert space.*

Hildebrand, Joel Henry (1881–1983)   *See aqualung, emulsification.*

Hill, Davis Octavius (1802–1870)   *See calotype process.*

Hill, John (1716–1775) *See microtome, staining.*

Hill, Robert (1899–1991) *See chloroplasts.*

Hill, Sir Rowland (1795–1879) *See postal service.*

Hillebrand, William Francis (1853–1925) *See petrology.*

Hillier, James (b 1915) *See electron microscope.*

Hinde, Robert Aubrey (b 1923) *See ethology.*

Hinshelwood, Sir Cyril Norman (1897–1967) A London chemist who shared the Nobel Prize for Chemistry in 1956, for his work on chain reaction mechanisms, with **Nikolai Semenov** (1896–1986). He developed the equation for the hydrogen–oxygen reaction, and wrote *The Chemical Kinetics of the Bacterial Cell* (1946) and *Growth Function and Regulation in Bacterial Cells* (1966). He was elected a Fellow of the Royal Society in 1929, and knighted in 1948.

Hinton, Christopher (1901–1983) *See atomic power.*

Hipparchus of Bithynia (190–120 BC) An eminent astronomer in Asia Minor who discovered several stars, predicted eclipses, and laid the foundation for trigonometry and geography. He was the first to recognize that the earth was flattened at the poles, and he completed a star catalog. *See astrolabe, astronomy, diopter, equinox, moon.*

Hippasus of Metapontium (*c.* 450 BC) *See musical theory.*

Hippias of Elis (*c.* 425 BC) *See circle.*

Hippocrates of Chios (*c.* 460 BC) Founder of the mathematical school at Athens, from the Ionian island of Chios, and a contemporary of **Socrates** (470–399 BC). He was one of the first specialists in mathematics, and solved many of the complex mathematical problems faced by the mathematicians of his time. He compiled a work on *Elements of Geometry.*

Hippocrates of Cos (*c.* 460–377 BC) Founder of modern medicine based on observations. He was born on the island of Cos, where a medical school had existed since 600 BC. He compiled an ethical code for young physicians, the Hippocratic Oath.

Hire, Phillipe de la (1640–1718) *See structural engineering.*

Hirn, Gustav Adolphe (1815–1890) *See thermodynamics.*

His, Wilhelm (1831–1904) *See microtome.*

Histochemistry A method of identifying cell constituents with the use of chemicals. In 1807, D.H.F. Link of Göttingen devised the first histochemical test for tannins, with the use of iron sulfate. Microscopy was added to the technique by a French chemist and physician, **François Vincent Raspail** (1794–1878), in 1825.

Hitchcock, Edward (1793–1864) *See geology.*

Hittorf, Johann Wilhelm (1824–1914) *See cathode rays, electrolysis, electron, X-rays.*

Hjelm, Peter Jacob (1746–1813) *See molybdenum.*

Hoagland, Mahlon Bush (b 1921) *See genetic coding, ribonucleic acid.*

Hobbes, Thomas (1588–1679) An English philosopher from Malmsbury, educated at Magdalen College, Oxford. He published several treatises on philosophy, mathematics and other subjects.

Hodgkinson, Eaton (1789–1861) An English engineer from Cheshire who is known for his work on the strength of materials. He was appointed professor of mechanical physics at the University of London in 1847. *See mechanical engineering.*

Hodometer *See odometer.*

Hoe, Richard March (1812–1886) *See newspapers.*

Hoe, Robert (1839–1909) *See newspapers.*

Hofmann, August Wilhelm von (1818–1892) *See amines, aniline, benzene, dyes, industrial chemistry.*

Hoffman, Samuel Kurtz (b 1902) *See rocket.*

Hoffmann, Roald (b 1937) *See frontier orbitals.*

Hofmeister, Wilhelm Friedrich Benedikt (1824–1877) *See flower, pollination.*

Hofstadter, Robert (1915–1990) *See quarks.*

Hogben, Lancelot Thomas (1895–1975) *See statistics.*

Hohenheim, Theophrastus Bombastus von (1493–1541) *See Paracelsus.*

Hohlfeld (1711–1771) See odometer.

Holden, Sir Edward Wheewall (1896–1978) An Australian pioneer of motor chassis manufacturing, born in Adelaide. He introduced automatic production into Australia, and by 1929 his company had become one of the world's largest builders of car bodies. His first Holden car appeared in 1946.

Holden, Sir Isaac (1807–1897) *See matches.*

Holland, John Phillip (1840–1914) *See submarines.*

Hollerith, Hermann (1860–1929) *See International Business Machines.*

Holley, Robert William (b 1922) *See genetic coding.*

Holmes, Arthur (1890–1965) *See geochronology, petrology, tectonic theory.*

Holmes, William Henry (1846–1933) *See prehistory.*

Holmium A metallic element of atomic number 67. Discovered in 1879 by a Swedish chemist and geologist **Per Teodor Cleve** (1840–1905).

Holocene Period [Greek: *holos*, whole] A geological period starting from 8000 BC to the present. During this period glaciers retreated as the climate became warmer.

Hologram [Greek: *holos*, whole + *graphein*, to write] A three-dimensional image produced by a special method of photographic recording. It was invented in 1947 by a Hungarian physicist, **Denis Gabor** (1900–1979) of Budapest, while he was in England. He made his discovery while he was researching to improve the resolution of the electron microscope, and named it holography. He was awarded the Nobel Prize for Physics for his invention, in 1971. His method involved the production of two images in line, which could not be separated, and it was improved by an American electrical scientist, **Emmett Norman Leith** (b 1927) of Detroit, who produced the first laser hologram. A Russian scientist, **Yuri Ostrovski** (1926–1992), developed the use of holographic techniques for measuring mechanical vibrations, and published several papers on this. A holographic computer capable of producing three-dimensional images was invented in 1988 by an American, Dana Anderson, of Colorado University.

Holography *See hologram.*

Homberg, Wilhelm (1652–1715) *See borax, phosphorus, zinc.*

Home Appliances *See carpet sweeper, cookers, dishwasher, electric iron, microwave oven, oven, pressure cooker, refrigerator, safety razor, sewing machine, vacuum cleaner, washing machines.*

Hominids [Latin: *homo*, man + *oidos*, shape] The earliest human-like creature was named *Australopithecus*. A hominid jaw bone, estimated to be 4 million years old, was found in 1984, near Lake Baringo, Kenya, by Kitalam Chepboi. A 40% complete hominid skeleton, 3 millions years old, was found in 1974 in the Afar region of Ethiopia by **Donald Carl Johanson** (b 1943). It belonged to a female who died at the age of 40, and was nick-named, *Lucy*. A fossil skull, nearly 1.75 million years old, was found in Tanzania by an English archaeologist, **Mary Douglas Leakey** (1913–

1997), in 1959. It was initially named *Zinjanthropus*, but was later reclassified as *Australopithecus*. Mary's husband, **Louis Seymour Bazett Leakey** (1903–1972), found several important hominid fossils in East Africa. Their son **Richard Erskin Leakey** (b 1944) continues their work and has found several other important hominid remains in Africa. *See human race.*

Homo erectus [Latin: *homo*, man + *erectus*, upright] The earliest complete skeleton of this species, 1.6 million years old, belonging to a 12-year-old boy, was found in Kenya in 1985 by Kamoya Kimeu.

Homo habilis [Latin: *homo*, man + *habilis*, handy] A term for the earliest species of true humans or *Homo*, dating back 1.7 million years, coined in 1960 by a South African anatomist and physical anthropologist from Durban, **Phillip Valentine Tobias** (b 1925), and **Louis Seymour Bazett Leakey** (1903–1972) of Kenya. The earliest known fossils of this human, 1.9 million years old, were discovered by Bernard Ngeneo in Kenya in 1972.

Homo sapiens [Latin: *homo*, man + *sapiens*, wisdom] A term for the first modern man, who appeared shortly after the first Neanderthal man or *Homo neanderthalensis*, about 100 000 years ago. A part of a skull belonging to this species was found in 1936 in Britain, in Kent, by Alvan T. Marston. Findings of fossils in 1988 by French and Israeli scientists in a cave in Israel suggest that modern *Homo sapiens* is at least 92 000 years old. Carbon dating of a jaw bone found in 1980, in Britain, in a cave in Torquay, Devon, has revealed it to be 31 000 years old.

Homology [Greek; *homoios*, alike + *logos*, discourse] A concept that organs fulfilling different pupuses (e.g. the wing of a bird and the arm of a human) could be equivalent structures, being derived from the same part of the embryo. Proposed by **Geoffry Etienne Saint-Hilaire** (1772–1844), a French zoologist, and rival of **Georges Cuvier** (1769–1832) at the Jardin des Plantes, in Paris. The term homology was introduced by **Thomas Henry Huxley** (1825–1895).

Honda, Soichiro (1906–1992) *See motorcycle.*

Hood, Raymond Mathewson (1881–1934) *See architecture, American.*

Hooke, Robert (1635–1703) A scientist and pioneer microscopist, born in Freshwater, on the Isle of Wight. He became the first curator of experiments at the Royal Society of London, and performed the first experiment demonstrating artificial respiration in animals, in 1667. In his experiments he kept the animals alive by blowing air through their lungs, with bellows. He invented the camera lucida (1674) and gave the first description of a compound microscope, in 1667. He was the first to adopt the term cell, in biology, to denote the compartments of cork observed under a microscope, in 1665. He contributed to the subject of geology with his work on earthquakes in 1688. *See absorption of heat, air, air pump, artificial silk, camera lucida, clock, compound microscope, crystallography, differential gear, elasticity, geology, Hooke's law, hygrometer, light, meteorology, mycology, oceanography, radiation of heat, Royal Society of London, siderostat, surface chemistry, textile chemistry, velocity of light, watches.*

Hooker, Sir Joseph Dalton (1817–1911)   An English botanist from Suffolk who succeeded his father as director of Kew Gardens, in 1865. He published *Flora of British India* (1872–1897) and *A Handbook to the Flora of Ceylon* (1898). *See plant anatomy, plant physiology.*

Hooker, Sir William Jackson (1785–1865)   *See Kew Gardens, scientific journals.*

Hooker, Stanley (1907–1984)   *See gas turbine, jet engine.*

Hooke's Law   Stress placed on an elastic body is proportional to the strain produced. Discovered by the English scientist, **Robert Hooke** (1635–1703). *See elasticity.*

Hoover, William Henry (1849–1932)   *See vacuum cleaner.*

Hope, Thomas Charles (1766–1844)   *See strontium, water.*

Hopf, Heinz (1894–1971)   *See topology.*

Hopkins, Sir Fredrick Gowland (1851–1947)   *See nutrition.*

Hopkins, Smith B. (b 1873)   *See illinium.*

Hopper, Grace Murray (1906–1992)   *See computer bug.*

Hopton, Arthur (1588–1614)   An English mathematician from Somerset who published *A Treatise on Geodetical Staff, The Topographical Glass* and *A Concordance of Years.*

Hormones [Greek: *hormon,* to rouse]   The term was coined in 1902 by two English physiologists, **Sir William Maddock Bayliss** (1860–1924) and **Ernest Henry Starling** (1866–1927), during their study of intestinal mucous secretions. The concept of internal secretions or hormones directly secreted into the body fluids or blood, without being conveyed through a duct, and having an effect on the organism remote from its original site, was first suggested in 1746 by a French physician, **Théophile de Bordeu** (1722– 1776). The first experimental demonstration of such a substance was given by **Arnold Berthhold** (1801–1863), in 1849.

Horology [Greek: *hora,* time + *logos,* discourse]   A science of measuring and marking the times of the day. The earliest instruments used for this purpose were clepsydra, gnomon and the sundial. One of the first devices, consisting of wheels and pinions to measure time, was constructed in 1364 for Charles V of France by a German, Henry de Wyck. **Galilei Galileo** (1564–1642) of Pisa, first observed the principle of pendulum, from the oscillations of a suspended lamp in the cathedral at Pisa in 1583. His observation that the oscillations were equal in time whatever their range, led to its use for measuring time. **Christian Huyghens** (1629–1693), a Dutch physicist from Hague, while at Accademia del Cimento, continued Galileo's work and invented a bifilar pendulum in 1656, and patented a pendulum clock in 1657. Huygen's description of the mechanism of the pendulum clock is found in his book *Horologium Oscillatorium* published in 1673. In 1725, a Parisian clock and instrument maker, **Antoine Thiout** (1692–1767), proposed an equation-clock showing solar time rather than mean time, and published *Traité de l'Horlogerie* (1741). The British Horological Institute at Clerkenwell, London, was established in 1858. *See clocks, date, day, gnomon, hour, sundial.*

Horrocks, Jeremiah (1618–1641)   *See parallax, Venus.*

Horsepower   A unit of power first proposed in 1784 by a Scottish pioneer of the steam engine, **James Watt** (1736–1819) of Greenock, and his partner **Matthew Boulton** (1728–1809) from Birmingham.

Horsley, Samuel (b 1733)   A London mathematician and clergyman who published an edition of Newton's works in 1775. He was secretary to the Royal Society of London, and published several works on mathematics and other branches of science.

Horticulture [Latin: *hortus,* garden + *cultus,* cultivated]   One of the ancient sciences. **André Lenotre** (1613–1700) of Paris is regarded as the father of modern French landscape gardening; he designed several important gardens in Paris and London. An English natural philosopher **John Evelyn** (1620–1706) of Wotton, Surrey, was one of the first to improve horticulture in England by introducing several exotic plants. *The Manner of Raising, Make and Keep Woods; and improving Forrest and Fruit Trees* (1679) by Moses Cook contained advice on maintaining avenues, walks, hedges and lawns. A gardener and naturalist, **John Tradescant** (1567–1637), and his son (1608–1662) with the same name, introduced many plants into English gardens. A Scottish horticulturilist, **John Claudius Loudon** (1783–1843) of Cambuslang, founded the *Gardener's Magazine* in 1826, and remained its editor until his death. He compiled an

Encyclopaedia of Gardening in 1822. Many new species of North American flowering plants were discovered by a Scottish plant collector for the London Horticultural Society, **David Doughlas** (1798–1834) from Perthshire. He commenced his botanical explorations of North America around 1825. An Irish gardener, **William Robinson** (1838–1935) from County Down published 18 books on the subject including *The English Flower Garden* (1883). He founded and edited three journals, *The Garden* (1872), *Gardening Illustrated* (1879) and *Flora and Sylva* (1903). **Luther Burbank** (1849–1926) from Lancaster, Massachusetts, was a pioneer of modern horticulture in America, and he improved several horticultural crops such as roses and lilies through his experiments on hybridization. An American botanist, **Albert Francis Blakeslee** (1847–1954) from Genesco, New York, studied the effects of various chemicals on plants during his investigation of polyploidy, in 1937. His work made it possible commercially to produce giant-cell varieties of some well-known flowering plants. He was professor of agricultural botany at the Connecticut Agricultural College from 1904 to 1914. A London horticulturist, **Gertrude Jekyll** (1843–1932), designed over 300 gardens and published *Wood and Garden* (1899), *Home and Garden* (1900), and several other works. A massive index of all the flowering plants, *Index Kewensis* was begun by a London botanist, **Benjamin Daydon Jackson** (1846–1927), and its first volume was published in 1892. An American horticulturist, **Liberty Hyde Bailey** (1858–1954) of South Haven, Michigan, made important contributions and published *Standard Cyclopedia of Horticulture* (1914–1917) and *Manual of Cultivated Plants* (1923). The Royal Dutch Society for the Advancement of Horticulture was established in 1842 by two German botanists and physicians, **Karel Lodewijk Blume** (1796–1862) and **Philipp Franz von Siebold** (1796–1866). Modern work on flowering plants was done by an American botanist, **Arthur Cronquist** (1919–1992) from San Jose, California, at the New York Botanical Garden. He published *The Evolution and Classification of Flowering Plants* (1968) and *An Integrated Classification of Flowering Plants* (1981) and his Cronquist system of classification was adopted by many workers.

Hosiery Knitted or woven underwear, and stockings or socks. *See knitting.*

Hot-Air Engine *See Stirling engine.*

Hotchkiss, Benjamin Berkeley (1826–1885) *See firearms.*

Houghton, Sir John Theodore (b 1931) *See meteorology.*

Hounsfield, Sir Godfrey Newbold (b 1919) The inventor of the CAT scanner was born in Newark, UK and educated at City and Guilds College, London. After serving as a radar engineer during the Second World War, he joined Thorn-EMI in 1952, and became a director in the medical research department there in 1972. He developed the CAT scanner, for which he shared the Nobel Prize in Medicine or Physiology with **Allan Macleod Cormack** (1924–1998) of Johannesburg, in 1979.

Hour [Latin: *hora*] According to **Herodotus** (485–425 BC), the Greeks learnt to divide the day into 12 parts from the Egyptians. The Romans divided the day and night each into four parts known as vigils and watches. These in turn were subdivided into 12 parts separately for day and night. The first hour of the day began with sunrise and ended at sunset at the 12th hour. The first hour of the night began with sunset and ended with the 12th at sunrise.

Houston, Edwin James (1847–1914) *See arc light.*

Hovercraft The idea of a sea vehicle that could travel on a cushion of air (air cushion vehicle) was proposed in 1877 by an English engineer, **John Thornycroft** (1843–1928). The first hovercraft was invented by an English radio-engineer, **Christopher Sydney Cockerell** (1910–1999) from Cambridge, in 1955. His hovercraft, made of balsa-wood and powered by a small engine, reached a speed of 12 miles per hour over land and water. A practical model was built and flown by the aircraft firm Saunders-Roe Ltd in 1959. The first public transport by hovercraft was established across the Dee estuary, Scotland, in 1962.

Howard, H. Heliot (1873–1940) *See ecology.*

Howe, Elias (1819–1867) *See sewing machine.*

Hoyle, Fred (b 1915) *See helium, steady-state theory.*

Hubble Space Telescope One of the largest space telescopes, weighing 11 tonnes, placed in orbit in a US space shuttle, in 1990, at Cape Canaveral, Florida. It is named after the American astronomer, **Edwin Powell Hubble** (1889–1953) of Missouri.

Hubble, Edwin Powell (1889–1953) *See Andromeda nebula, Big Bang theory, expanding universe, Hubble Space Telescope.*

Hubel, David Hunter (b 1926) *See vision.*

Huber, François (1750–1831) *See bees.*

Hückel, Erich (1896–1980) *See aromatic compounds.*

Hudalrichus Regius (*c.* 1500) *See perfect number.*

Hudde, Johann (1633–1704) *See negative numbers.*

Hudson, Henry (*c.* 1550–1611) *See volcanic eruptions.*

Hudson, Sir William (1896–1978) *See hydroelectric schemes.*

Hudson, William (1734–1793) *See botanical classification.*

Huggins, Sir William (1824–1910) *See astrophysics, celestial photography, nebulae, spectroscopy,*

Hughes, David Edward (1830–1900) The inventor of the microphone, born to a Welsh family in London. At the age of seven he accompanied his family to Virginia, and he received his education at St Joseph's College, Kentucky. At the age of 26, Hughes invented a type printing telegraph, which was bought by the French government. On his return to England he established a laboratory in London and invented the microphone in 1857. Upon his death he left the major proportion of his wealth to London hospitals. *See musical recording.*

Hughes, E.D. (1906–1963) An English chemist and one of the first to use isotopes in the study of chemical reactions.

Hull, Gordon (1870–1956) An American physicist who contributed to the development of the light quantum hypothesis, which interprets light as a momentum-bearing stream of particles, similar to concentrations of energy.

Hulst, Hendrik Christofel, van de (b 1918) *See radioastronomy.*

Human Genome Organization (HUGO) An international group set up in 1989 for coordinating activities on the human genome project.

Human Genome Project A project launched in 1985 to determine the exact sequence of all 3×10^9 base pairs in the human genome. This has set the platform for diseases to be treated on a genetic basis. The first complete decoding or sequencing of a genome (chromosome 22) was achieved in November 1999. The Human Genome Diversity (HGD) program has set out to ensure that a wide variety of humanity are sampled under informed conditions, with a view to unraveling human past history.

Human Race Human line branched off from the ape about 6 million years ago. The evidence for the earliest forms or hominids is mostly found in Africa suggesting the origin of human race there. The earliest species to be identified so far is *Ardipithecus ramidus*. The tooth of this hominid found in Aramis, Ethiopia indicates its existence about 4.4 million years ago. Stone implements found in Ethiopia and neighboring regions reveal early man's capability to devise things

2.5 million years ago. The first early skull outside Africa was found in 1891 in Trinil, Indonesia. This *Homo erectus* species about 1.7 million years ago was the first to use fire and migrate out of Africa. One million year old skeletal remains of a *Homo antecessor* found in Gran Dollina, Spain may be the last common ancestor of Neanderthal man and the modern human of Europe. *See evolution, Hominids, Homo sapiens, Java man, Neanderthal man, prehistory, Stone Age.*

Humason, Milton (1891–1972) An American astronomer who worked with **Edwin Hubble** (1889–1953) to show that the amount of the red-shift is directly proportional to the speed of the galaxy concerned. Their work in 1929 led to the discovery that galaxies recede from the earth with increasing speeds.

Humboldt, Friedrich Heinrich Alexander von (1769–1859) A German botanist from Berlin who is regarded as the founder of plant geography. He defined isothermal lines, and completed his work *Kosmos* (1845–1847) at the age of 78.

Hunter, I.M. (1915–1975) *See nuclear fusion.*

Huntington, Collis Porter (1821–1900) *See railway.*

Huntsman, Benjamin (1704–1776) *See steel.*

Hurricane Any wind with a speed of over 75 miles per hour or a force of 12 on the Beaufort scale. *See Beaufort scale, meteorology, storm.*

Hurter, Ferdinand (1844–1898) *See Deacon's process.*

Hussey, Obed (1792–1860) *See agricultural instruments.*

Hutton, Charles (1737–1823) A mathematician from Newcastle upon Tyne who published *Mathematical and Philosophical Dictionary* (1796) and *Course of Mathematics* (1798).

Hutton, James (1726–1797) *See geology.*

Huxley, Thomas Henry (1825–1895) A London biologist and physician born in Ealing, Middlesex. He served as surgeon to *HMS Rattlesnake* on its expedition to the South Seas. He advocated Darwin's theory of evolution and refuted **Richard Owen's** (1804–1892) and **Lorenz Oken's** (1779–1851) theory regarding the vertebrate skull. He published *Zoological Evidence as to Man's Place in Nature* (1863), *Evolution and Ethics* (1893) and several other books. *See homology, Isis.*

Huygens, Christian (1629–1695) An astronomer and physicist from the Hague. At the age of 16 he studied law at Leyden and graduated in mathematics from the University of Breda. He constructed a 12-foot telescope in 1656 with the help of which he discovered the sixth satellite of Saturn, Titan. He published *The System of Saturn* or *Systema Saturnium* (1659), and made several other important contributions to astronomy. While at the Accademia del Cimento, he invented a bifilar pendulum (1656) and he patented a pendulum clock in 1657. Huygens' description of the pendulum clock is found in his work *Horologium Oscillatorium* (1673). The undulatory theory of light was proposed by Huygens in his *Treatise in Light*, in 1690.

Hyatt, Gilbert (b 1938) *See computers.*

Hyatt, John Wesley (1837–1920) *See celluloid, sewing machine.*

Hybridization [Latin: *hybrida,* cross] The Dominican priest and scientist, **Albertus Magnus** (1192–1280), believed that some existing types of plants, by grafting, could be changed into new species. Early scientific work was done in 1760 by **Joseph Gottlieb Kolreuter** (1733–1806), the director of botanical gardens at Carlsruhe. He made a large number of crosses between different species and varieties of plants. In 1822, an English naturalist, **Thomas Andrew Knight** (1759–1838), in his attempt to produce improved varieties of fruit trees, raised a large number of hybrids. In the 1850s a French botanist, **Charles Naudin** (1815–1899), experimented with plant hybridization and proposed the theory of disjunction. The founder of genetics, **Gregor Johann Mendel** (1822–1884), worked on hybridization of pea plants, while he was a monk at an Augustinian monastery in Brünn, growing about 30 000 plants which he artificially fertilized, to examine the inheritance of specific characteristics. A hybrid corn program in 1909 by G.H. Shull, with use of self-fertilized lines, led to an abundance of food in the USA. Various advantageous strains of wheat were produced by an English agricultural botanist, **Sir Rowland Harry Biffen** (1874–1949) of Cheltenham, who became the first professor of agricultural botany at Cambridge, in 1908. He was knighted in 1925. **Luther Burbank** (1849–1926) from Lancaster, Massachusetts, was a pioneer in America who improved several agricultural and horticultural crops such as blackberries, tomatoes, plums, corn, roses and lilies. **George Ledyard Stebbins** (b 1906) of Lawrence, New York, artificially induced polypoidy for creating fertile hybrids. He applied evolution theory to botany and published *Variation and Evolution in Plants* (1950). Other landmarks in the field include *Plant Breeding* (1907) by **Hugo Marie de Vries** (1848–1935), and *Practical Plant Breeding* (1937) by W.J.C. Lawrence.

Hydraulic Cement *See cement.*

Hydraulic Devices A mechanical device that uses an incompressible fluid, such as oil, to transmit a force applied to a piston of small area, to a piston of larger area. The first hydraulic press was patented in 1785 by **Joseph Bramah** (1748–1814), and the hydraulic crane was invented in 1846 by **Sir William George Armstrong** (1810–1900) of Newcastle upon Tyne.

Hydraulics Generally refers to the study of the effect of pressure on a liquid system for engineering purposes. In 1797, an Italian physicist, **Giovanni Battista Venturi** (1746–1822), described the decrease in pressure of a fluid in a pipe with tapering diameter, known as the Venturi effect. A Venturi flow-meter based on the principle was invented by an American engineer, **Clemens Herschel** (1842–1930). *See hydraulic devices, hydrodynamics.*

Hydrodynamics [Greek: *hydros,* water + *dynos,* power] Study of the effect of forces and movement in liquids. It was initiated by **Archimedes** (287–212 BC), who discovered the principles of flotation while he was contemplating on an experiment to determine the content of gold in king Hiero's crown. A French priest, **Edmé Mariotte** (1620–1684), studied the effect of pressure on the flow of a liquid through an orifice and published *Traité du mouvement des eaux et des autres corps fluides* (1686). **Daniel Bernoulli** (1700–1782), in his *Hydrodynamica* (1738), explored the relationship between pressure, velocity and density in flowing fluids. In the above work he formulated the laws for the flow of liquids through pipes of various diameters. Motion in a perfectly compressible fluid was analyzed by the Swiss mathematician **Leonhard Euler** (1707–1883) in his study of tidal fluctuations. An English applied mathematician, **Horace Lamb** (1849–1934) of Stockport, Cheshire, published an important work, *A Treatise on the Motion of Fluids* (1879), which was issued as a new edition under the title *Hydrodynamics* in 1895. The motion of water in parallel channels at different velocities was studied around 1880 by an Irish engineer, **Osborne Reynolds** (1842–1912) of Belfast, who extended his findings to river channels and water turbines.

Hydroelectric Schemes Water wheels were an important source for power in industry during the early 19th century, but their design was low in efficiency. **Benoit Fourneyron** (1802–1867), a French engineer from the Loire, invented the radial turbines in 1827 that improved the efficiency of the machine to 65%, and in 1833 he achieved an efficiency of 75% with a 50 horse-power turbine. Fourneyron's turbines were used in the hydroelectric scheme for the Niagara Falls in 1895. An English engineer from South Leigh, Oxfordshire, **James Bicheno Francis** (1815–1892), who emigrated to America in 1833, designed the inward-flow turbine that bears his name. He was chief engineer to the locks and canals on the Merrimack River. Another English inventor, **William George Armstrong** (1810–1900) of Newcastle upon Tyne, built a hydroelectric machine in 1840. The Pelton wheel, having 90% efficiency and used all over the world for high hydropower generation, was invented in 1880 by an American engineer, **Lester Allen Pelton** (1829–1918) from Vermillion, Ohio. One of the first hydroelectric plants in America was established at Appleton, Wisconsin, in 1882. The Kaplan propeller turbine, which could operate with the lowest possible rate of flow of water, was invented in 1913 by an Austrian engineer, **Viktor Kaplan** (1876–1934). The first few major hydroelectric schemes in Scotland were completed by a Scottish industrialist and electrical engineer, **George Balfour** (1872–1841). One of the world's largest schemes, involving 16 dams and seven power stations over 150 kilometers of water, in New South Wales, Australia, was started in 1949 under the direction of a New Zealand hydroelectric engineer, **Sir William Hudson** (1896–1978), and completed ahead of time in 1973.

Hydrogen [Greek: *hydros,* water + *gen,* to produce] First obtained under the name of combustible air by a Swiss alchemist and physician, **Paracelsus** or **Theophrastus Bombastus von Hohenheim** (1493–1541) in the 16th century. Its properties were described by **Henry Cavendish** (1731–1810), who named it inflammable air, in 1766. **Antoine Laurent Lavoisier** (1743–1794) named it hydrogen, and described the properties of hydrogen, nitrogen and oxygen in the air, in his *Elementary Treatise on Chemistry* (1789). **Jaques Alexandre César Charles** (1746–1823) was the first to use hydrogen in balloons, in 1783. The production of water by the combination of hydrogen with oxygen was demonstrated by **James Watt** (1736–1819), in 1781. The structure of the hydrogen atom, consisting of a positively charged central nucleus or proton, surrounded by a single travelling electron, was first demonstrated in 1926 by a Danish physicist, **Niels Hendrik David Bohr** (1885–1962). Heavy hydrogen or deuterium was discovered in 1932 by **Harold Clayton Urey** (1893–1981) of Walkerton, Indiana, and his coworkers. He was appointed professor of chemistry at Columbia University, New York, in 1934 and was awarded the Nobel Prize for Chemistry for his discovery, in the same year.

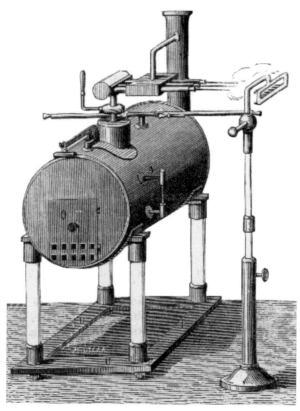

Figure 47 Armstrong's hydroelectric machine. Lardner, Dionysius. *Handbook of Natural Philosophy, Electricity, Magnetism, and Acoustics.* London: Walton and Maberly, 1856

Hydrogen Bomb *See H bomb.*

Hydrogen Convection Zone Discovered in 1931 by a German astrophysicist, **Albrecht Otto Johannes Unsöld** (b 1905). The existence of this atmospheric zone explains the transport of heat energy upwards to the sun's photosphere.

Hydrogen Sulfide According to the historian and alchemist Zosimos (*c.* AD 400), an ancient Egyptian craftsman noticed the unpleasant smell of the gas while boiling slaked lime with sulfur. **Karl Wilhelm Scheele** (1742–1786) prepared the gas by treating hydrochloric acid with ferrous sulfide. A French chemist, **Paul Sabatier** (1854–1941), was the first to prepare a pure form. He was made professor of chemistry at Toulouse in 1884 and published *La Catalyse en Chimie Organique* (1912). He shared the Nobel Prize for Chemistry with **François Auguste Victor Grignard** (1871–1935) for their work on heterogeneous catalysis, in 1912.

Hydrogenation [Greek: *hydor*, water + *genos*, descent] A process of converting liquid oils into fats for manufacturing magarine, soap and other products, invented by a French chemist, **Paul Sabatier** (1854–1941) and his assistant **Jean Baptiste Senderens** (1856–1936). Sabatier shared the Nobel Prize for Chemistry in 1912, for this work, with **François Auguste Victor Grignard** (1871–1935).

Hydrometer [Greek: *hydor*, water + *metron*, to measure] The method of measuring the density of liquids with a floating device was discovered by **Archimedes** (287–212 BC). His discovery is mentioned in the letters of Bishop Synesius of Cyrene (*c.* AD 370–415), written to his friend and teacher **Hypatia** in the 5th century. **Robert Boyle** (1627–1691) described a hydrometer in 1675.

Hydrostatics [Greek: *hydor*, water + *statokos*, causing to stand] Study of the behavior of liquids under the action of forces and pressures when the liquid is at rest. In 250 BC **Archimedes** (287–212 BC) discovered the pressure exerted by fluids on an immersed body and the laws related to flotation. The subject was revived and established on a modern basis by **Simon Stevinus** (1548–1620) of The Netherlands, in 1586. His *Principles of Hydrostatics* was the first systematic treatise on the subject since the time of Archimedes. A French priest and one of the founder members of the Académie des Sciences, **Edmé Mariotte** (1620–1684), advanced the theories on hydromechanics in his *Traité du mouvement des eaux* (1686) and it became an important landmark. **Galilei Galileo** (1564–1642) made significant contributions to the subject, and the theory of oscillation of fluids was explained in 1714 by **Sir Isaac Newton** (1642–1727).

Hydrostatic Balance A balance based on Archimedes' law of flotation. It was used in the early 18th century for determining the specific gravity of fluids and solids.

Hygrometer [Greek: *hygros*, wet + *metron*, to measure] An instrument for measuring the moisture in the atmosphere. It was first constructed at the Accademia del Cimento in the 17th century. **Robert Hooke** (1635–1703) constructed a hygrometer, using the beard of a wild oat, in 1655. Another one was invented by a French mathematician, **Guillaume Amontons** (1663–1705) in 1698. **Horace Benedict de Saussure** (1740–1799) of Geneva constructed a hygroscope for studying the weather.

Hyman, Libbie Henrietta (1888–1969) *See invertebrates.*

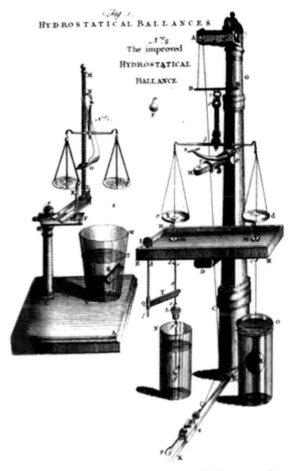

Figure 48 Hydrostatic balance. Owen, W. *Dictionary of Arts and Sciences.* London: Homer's Head, 1754

Hypatia (*c.* AD 370–415) A Greek philosopher and mathematician who was a daughter of another celebrated mathematician, Theon of Alexandria. She was murdered by a Christian mob at the instigation of Cyril, the bishop of Alexandria, who was jealous of her influence. *See hydrometer.*

Hyperbolic Geometry A system of non-Euclidean geometry, proposed independently by **Carl Friedrich Gauss** (1777–1855) of Brunswick, **Nikolai Ivanovich Lobaschevsky** (1793–1856) of Russia and **Janos Bolyai** (1802–1860) of Hungary. It was developed by a German mathematician, **Georg Friedrich Bernhard Riemann** (1826–1866).

Hyperion The seventh satellite of Saturn, discovered in 1848 by an American astronomer, **William Cranch Bond** (1789–1859) who was Director of the Harvard Observatory, and an English astronomer from Bolton, **William Lassell**

(1799–1880). **George Phillips Bond** (1825–1865) of Dorchester, Massachussetts, a pioneer in celestial photography, was the son of Cranch Bond.

Hypsicles (*c*. AD 200) A mathematican of Alexandria during the reign of Marcus Aurelius. He is known for his treatise *Anaphoricus,* which is extant.

Hypsometer [Greek: *hupsos*, top + *metron*, to measure] A thermometrical barometer for measuring altitudes.

Invented in 1817 by **William Hyde Wollaston**, and improved in 1847 by a German-born French physicist, **Henri Victor Regnault** (1810–1878).

Hysteresis [Greek: *husteros*, coming after] A term first used in 1890 by a Scottish physicist, **Sir James Alfred Ewing** (1855–1935), to refer to the ability of certain metals, similar to iron, to retain their magnetization after the magnetizing field was removed.

I

Iapetus Ocean The ocean that existed during early Paleozoic times between the two land masses that were to become Europe and North America later. Both continents moved together obliterating the ocean during late Paleozoic times and separated out again giving way to the Atlantic Ocean.

Icarus An asteroid discovered in 1949. It was the first asteroid observed to approach closer to the sun than the planet Mercury. In 1968 it passed 4 million miles close to the earth.

Ice Age The term 'Ice Age' was first used by botanist Karl Schimper in 1837. Of a series of nearly twenty Ice Ages which occurred over a period of 2300 million years, the most recent was around 16 000 BC. The first person to propose the theory of Ice Ages preceding historic times was a Swiss civil engineer, Ignace Venetz, in 1821. A teacher, A. Bernardi, from a small forestry school in The Netherlands, was the first to publish his findings on the theory of the Ice Age in 1832. Four years later, **Jean Louis Rodolphe Agassiz** (1807–1873) of Switzerland, travelled to the Alps with another geologist, **Johann von Charpentier** (1786–1855), with the intention of disproving the glacial theory. But Agassiz during his studies became convinced of the glacial period, and presented his findings to the Geological Society of London, in 1840. His work entitled *Etudes sur les Glaciers* was published in the same year. **William Buckland** (1784–1856), who at that time was president of the Geological Society, supported Agassiz' views. Agassiz later settled in Massachusetts in 1846 and contributed further papers on the subject. In 1865, he unearthed evidence of an Ice Age in one of the hottest places in the world, equatorial Brazil. A study in America on the glacial period was done by professor **Thomas Chrowder Chamberlin** (1843–1928) from Illinois, who occupied the Chair of geology at Beloit College from 1873 to 1882, and published *Our Glacial Drift* around 1880 and *The Origin of Earth* (1916). He also founded and edited the *Journal of Geology*. **Sir Joseph Prestwich** (1812–1896), a professor of geology at Oxford from 1874 to 1888, was an authority on the quaternary or recent Ice Age and he published several papers on the subject. A Swedish geologist, **Baron Gerhard Jacob de Geer** (1858–1943), studied the annual deposits of sediments under the glacial meltwater, and established a chronology dating back 15 000

years. He founded the Geochronological Institute of Stockholm and became its first director in 1912. *See glaciology.*

Ice Demonstrated to be lighter than water by **Galilei Galileo** (1564–1642) in 1597. The trade in ice making was first begun in 1803 by a person named Tudor, from Boston. By 1841, 16 ice-making companies were operating in Boston. *See refrigeration.*

Ice Calorimeter A device used for measuring the specific heat of substances. A Scottish chemist, **Joseph Black** (1728–1799), devised the first one, made of a block of ice with a cavity at its center. A French chemist, **Antoine Laurent Lavoisier** (1743–1794), and a French mathematician **Pierre Simon Marquis de Laplace** (1749–1827), independently replaced the block of ice with more complicated apparatus.

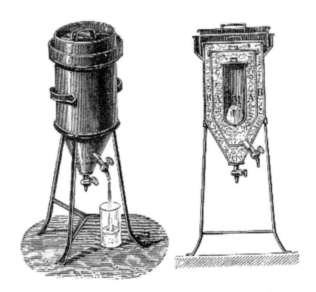

Figure 49 An early 19th century ice calorimeter. Atkinson, E. *Elementary Treatise on Physics.* London: Longmans, Green, and Co, 1872

Ichthyology [Greek: *ichthus*, fish + *logos*, discourse] A branch of biology dealing with the study of fishes. One of the first books on the subject, an illustrated monograph on Mediterranean fish, was published by a French naturalist **Guillaume Rondelet** (1507–1566). A Swedish naturalist, **Peter Artedi** (1705–1735) made a systematic study and published *Icthyologia* which earned him the title 'the father of ichthyology'. A Danish naturalist, **Morton Thrane Brünnich** (1737–1827), published a book on Mediterranean fish entitled *Icthyologia Massiliensis* (1768). Modern writers include **Baron Georges Cuvier** (1769–1832), **Sir Richard Owen** (1804–1892) and **Jean Louis Rodolphe**

Agassiz (1807–1873). A London naturalist, **William Yarrell** (1784–1856), published a classic work *British Fishes* (1836–1859). Agassiz proposed a new classification of fishes based on the characteristics of their skin. George Brown Goode (1851–1896) of New Albany, Indiana, wrote *The Oceanic Ichthyology* (1895) and *American Fishes* (1888). A Scottish zoologist, **Sir D'Arcy Wentworth Thompson** (1860–1948) of Edinburgh, published a *Glossary of Greek Fishes* (1945). *See marine biology.*

Ichthyosaurus [Greek: *ichthus,* fish + *saurus,* lizard] The fossil skeleton of the dinosaur which is now in the British Museum of Natural History was discovered in 1811 by an English paleontologist, **Mary Anning** (1799–1847) of Lyme Regis.

Iconoscope [Greek: *eikon,* image + *skopein,* to look] The first all-electronic television camera tube with no moving parts was invented by a Russian-born American electronic engineer, **Vladimir Kosma Zworykin** (1889–1982) in 1928. It used a beam of electrons to scan and electrically store an optical image, before converting it to electrical signals for transmission.

Ictinus (*c.* 500 BC) *See Parthenon.*

I-Hsing (682–727) *See clock.*

Illinium Predicted element no 61 in the periodic table, discovered and named in 1926 by an American chemist, **Smith B. Hopkins** (b 1873) who became professor of chemistry at the University of Illinois in 1912.

Ilyushin, Sergei Vladimirovich (1894–1977) *See warplanes.*

Image Photon Counting System (IPCS) Used in astronomy to study distant quasars, invented in the 1960s by a London astronomer, **Alexander Boksenberg** (b 1936).

Impact In 1668, the London architect and scientist, **Sir Christopher Wren** (1632–1723), discovered the laws of impact of elastic bodies, and published his findings in the *Philosophical Transactions of the Royal Society.* The Society received an account of the laws of central elastic impact from **Christian Huygens** (1629–1695) in 1669. More systematic experiments on impact were described by a French priest, **Edmé Mariotte** (1620–1684) in his *Traité de la percussion ou choc des corps* (1677).

Imprinting A process of learning that takes place soon after birth. During this highly impressionable period a pattern is set for the recognition of and reaction to particular objects. The study of imprinting was initiated by a physician and

zoologist, **Konrad Zacharias Lorenz** (1903–1989) of Vienna. He shared the Nobel Prize with a Dutch-born British ethologist, **Nikolaas Tinbergen** (1907–1988), and **Karl von Frisch** (1886–1982), in 1974. *See ethology.*

Incandescence Emission of light by a substance, owing to its heat. See *electric light bulb, lamp, neon lighting.*

Inch [Latin: *uncia,* thumb] First defined by an act of parliament in England in 1824. The act specified 39.13929 inches as the length of a seconds pendulum in the latitude of London, vibrating *in vacuo* at sea level at a temperature of 62 degrees Fahrenheit. *See units and measures.*

Indium [Latin: *indicum,* indigo] An element with an atomic number of 49, discovered in 1863 by a German physicist, **Ferdinand Reich** (1799–1882) and a German metallurgist, **Hieronymus Theodor Richter** (1824–1898). It was so named because of the specific color of its spectrum.

Induction Current Discovered by **Michael Faraday** (1791–1867) who published his findings in *Experimental Researches* in 1831. An American physicist, **Joseph Henry** (1797–1878) from Albany, New York independently discovered the phenomenon, and constructed the first electromagnetic motor in 1829. The unit of inductance is named in his honor. An alternating current induction motor that enabled alternating current to be transmitted over a much greater distance than direct current was invented by a Croatian-born US electrical engineer, **Nikola Tesla** (1856–1943).

Inductometer An instrument to compare specific inductive capacities of various substances, first devised by **Michael Faraday** (1791–1867).

Indus Valley Civilization Excavations carried out at Mohanjadaro and Harappa in the Indus Valley region (now Pakistan), in the 1920s, by an English archaeologist, **Sir John Hubert Marshall** (1876–1958), produced evidence for an advanced civilization that had existed around 2600 BC. The brick-built cities uncovered in this region showed an advanced system of town planning. Following the invasion by the Aryans in 2150 BC, the civilization came to an end in 1500 BC.

Industrial Chemistry One of the first chemical treatises to include industrial chemistry was written in 1540 by an Italian mining engineer **Vanocchio Biringuccio** (1460–1538) of Sienna. In his work *Pirotechnica,* Biringuccio clearly set out the economic advantages of chemical production on a large scale. The first modern scientific book on industrial chemistry, *Chemistry applied to the Arts* (1807), was published by a French statesman and chemist, **Jean Antoine Claude**

Chaptal (1756–1832) of Nogaret. Industrial chemistry became established with the discovery of aniline in coal tar by **August Wilhelm von Hofmann** (1818–1892) of Giessen, in 1843. He was the first professor of chemistry in London, and in 1865 became the professor of chemistry at Berlin, and founded the German Chemical Society. The coal tar industry was established by Hofmann, and it led to the development of the dye industry, and the production of benzene and other hydrocarbons on a commercial scale.

Inert Gases [Latin: *iners*, inactive] *See argon, helium, krypton, xenon.*

Inertia [Latin: *iners*, inactive] The measure of reluctance of a body to become affected by a dynamic force. Defined by **Sir Isaac Newton's** (1642–1727) in his enunciation of the second law of motion. The term moment of inertia was introduced by a Swiss mathematician, **Leonhard Euler** (1707–1883).

Inferometer [Latin: *inferus*, beneath + *meter*, measure] A device for measuring distances by observing the interference patterns of a light beam, invented in 1881 by an American physicist of Polish origin, **Albert Abraham Michelson** (1852–1931).

Infinite Series A term in mathematics introduced by the Scottish mathematician, **James Gregory** (1638–1675).

Infinitesimal Calculus Original name for calculus. So named because it is thought to rely on infinitely small quantities. *See calculus.*

Information Superhighway A term was first used 1993 by US vice president Al Gore in a speech outlining plans to build a high-speed national data communications network.

Information Technology *See broadcasting, fax, internet, radio, radar, telephone, telephone exchange, television, wireless telegraphy.*

Infrared Radiation [Latin: *infra*, below] The invisible electromagnetic part of the visible light spectrum, beyond the red. It corresponds to wavelengths between those of microwaves and invisible light. Discovered in 1800 by **Sir William Herschel** (1738–1822), who showed that infrared rays were more effective for heating than sunlight. Infrared and ultraviolet rays were incorporated into the theory of electromagnetc fields by **James Clerk Maxwell** (1831–1879), in 1873. The reflection of radiation from the infrared part of the spectrum was investigated in 1897 by a German physicist, **Heinrich Rubens** (1865–1922) from Wiesbaden. *See ultraviolet rays.*

Infusoria *See diatoms.*

Ingenhousz, Jan (1730–1799) *See chlorophyll, photosynthesis, plant physiology.*

Ingold, Sir Christopher Kelk (1893–1970) *See aromatic compounds.*

Ingram, Herbert (1811–1860) *See newspapers.*

Ink *See writing devices.*

Inman, William (1825–1881) *See transatlantic voyage.*

Insects *See entomology.*

Institute of Civil Engineers of England. Founded in 1818 with a Scottish engineer, **Thomas Telford** (1757–1834) from Westkirk, Dumfries, as its first president.

Insulator [Latin: *insula,* island] A term introduced by **John Theophile Desaguliers** (1683–1749) of La Rochelle, France, in his *Dissertation on Electricity*. Desaguliers came to London with his father, who was a clergyman, and in 1710 became professor of philosophy at Oxford. *See gutta percha.*

Insulin [Latin: *insula*, island] A hormone from the pancreas that regulates blood sugar levels. It was named by an English physiologist **Sir Edward Albert Sharpey-Schafer** (1850–1935) in 1916. It was first isolated by two Canadians, **Frederick Banting** (1891–1941) and **Charles Herbert Best** (1899–1978), under the direction of a Scottish professor, **John James Rickard Macleod** (1876–1935), in 1922. **Bertram James Collip** (1892–1965), a chemist from Alberta, obtained a purified extract of insulin in 1923. The sequence of amino acids in the protein chain of insulin was deduced by an English biochemist **Frederick Sanger** (b 1918), who was awarded the Nobel Prize for Chemistry, in 1958.

Insurance The first mention of the practice was by an Italian historian, **Francesco Guicciardini** (1482–1540), in his account of The Netherlands, published later in 1567. He referred to the merchants from Antwerp, who were accustomed to insuring their ships. The practice was introduced into England in the beginning of the 16th century. A French banker, **Lorenzo Tonti** (1620–1690), introduced the latest-surviver system of life insurance. **Nicholas Barbon** (1637–1698), an English physician, who played an important role in rebuilding London after its great fire in 1666, was the first to introduce insurance against the risk of fire. The first fire office for insurance was established in Paris in 1745. One of the earliest insurance societies for goods and household furniture, the Society of Clergy of Brandenburgh, was established in 1769. The earliest life insurance office in London, *The Amicable,* was founded in 1706. *Lloyd's,* the famous name in insurance, took its origin from a small coffee-house opened by Edward Lloyd, around 1689. His coffee-house became a popular haunt for ship merchants and traders, and Lloyd started *Lloyd's News,* which later became *Lloyd's List.* In 1691, he moved to Lombard Street, which was used as headquarters for London underwriting in the 18th century. In 1771, 79 leading underwriters formed an association which became the first committee of Lloyd's. The building of Lloyd's at Leadenhall Street was opened by King George V in 1828.

Integral   The term was first used by a Swiss mathematician of Dutch origin, **Jacques Bernoulli** (1654–1705), during his application of differential calculus to a problem in geometry. *See calculus.*

Integrated Circuit   The concept of the integrated circuit used in computers was first proposed in 1952 by an English engineer, **Geoffry W.A. Dummer** (b 1909).

Interference   A phenomenon fundamental to the wave theory of light, produced by passing light through two narrow slits. First observed by an Italian physicist, **Francesco Maria Grimaldi** (1618–1683) of Bologna, around 1638. An English physician and scientist, **Thomas Young** (1773–1829), rediscovered it in 1801.

Interferometer   An apparatus for studying the sources of electromagnetic radiation through interference patterns caused by two waves when they combine. Invented by two French physicists, **Charles Marie Paul Fabry** (1867–1945) of Marseilles, and **Alfred Perot** (1863–1925).

Intergral Calculus   *See calculus.*

Internal Combustion Engine   An engine capable of transforming chemical energy of fuel into mechanical energy, by controlled combustion of fuel inside the engine. In contrast the steam engine is an external combustion engine where fuel is burnt in a separate compartment. Both diesel and petrol engines employ internal combustion. A carriage with a two-cylinder, internal combustion, atmospheric gas engine was patented by Samuel Brown of London in 1826. In 1860, a Luxembourg-born French engineer, **Jean Joseph Etienne Lenoir** (1822–1900), built an engine for the first car with internal combustion. An engine consisting of a four-stroke cycle, induction, compression, power and exhaust was suggested by **Alphonse Beau de Rochas** (1815–1893) in 1862. A German engineer, **Nikolaus August Otto** (1832–1891), presented a monocylinder internal combustion four-stroke engine at the Paris Exhibition in 1878. In 1879, **Sir Dugald Clerk** (1854–1932) of England showed that the four-stroke could be reduced to a

two-stroke engine. **Gottlieb Daimler** (1834–1900) of Germany, developed an improved internal combustion engine and applied it to a bicycle with success in 1886. He built another engine in 1889 with double power which was later adapted to the motor car. In 1891, two Frenchmen, **René Panhard** (1841–1908) and Emile Levassor, built the first car with a chassis, having an internal combustion engine mounted to the front. A London engineer, **Sir Harry Ralph Ricardo** (1885–1974), designed a two-cylinder, two-stroke engine in 1905. Modern gas turbines and jet engines having internal combustion chambers were developed by an American aeronautical engineer, **Edward Story Taylor** (1903–1991). He published *The Internal Combustion Engine,* with C. Fayette Taylor, in 1936. The world's first gas turbine car, the Jet 1, was built by Rover, in 1950. In 1972, an Australian engineer, **Ralph Sarich** (b 1938) of Perth, built an orbital two-stroke reciprocating piston engine. *See diesel engines, gas engine.*

International Atomic Energy Agency (IAEA)   An agency of the United Nations with headquarters in Vienna established in 1957 to advise member countries in the development and appropriate use of nuclear power.

International Business Machines (IBM)   One of the leading companies in computer technology, founded by **Hermann Hollerith** (1860–1929) of Buffalo, New York, the inventor of the punched card technique for the US census. Hollerith established the Tabulating Machine Company in 1896, which later changed its name to International Business Machines. The IBM mark 7, a large electronic machine consisting of 800 cables, was built by an American mathematician, **Howard Hathaway Aikin** (1900–1973) of Hoboken, New Jersey in 1937. DOS, the first standard disk operating system for personal computers, was introduced by IBM in 1981. The first personal computer, PC-XT, with a built-in hard drive was produced by IBM in 1983. *See computers.*

Internet   A global network of computers started in the USA in the late 1960s for the military to preserve communication in case of nuclear attack. By connecting many computers through multiple pathways transmitting information was preserved even if parts of it were destroyed. It is now developed into a global communication system through telephone, radio, satellite links and fibre-optic cables. Electronic mail (e-mail) is one of its widest applications.

Intuitionism   A mathematical theory that propositions can be built up only from intuitive concepts that are easily recognized. Proposed by a Dutch mathematician, **Luitzen Egbertus Jan Brouwer** (1881–1966).

Invar An alloy of iron, nickel and a small amount of carbon. Owing to its very low coefficient of expansion it is used in the construction of precision instruments. It was invented and named by a Swiss physicist, **Charles Edouard Guillaume** (1861–1938), who was director of the Bureau International des Poids et Mesures at Sèvres. He was awarded the Nobel Prize for Physics in 1920.

Inverse Square Law Every particle of matter in the universe attracts every other particle with a force proportional to the product of their masses, and inversely proportional to the square of the distance between their centers of mass. Derived by **Sir Isaac Newton** (1642–1727) in his first book of *Philosophiae naturalis principia mathematica* (Mathematical Principles of Natural Philosophy) in 1685.

Invertebrates Animals without a backbone or notochord. **Aristotle** (384–322 BC), in his treatise *On the Generation of Animals*, referred to *inaima* (bloodless animals), a group similar to the current invertebrates. The first microscopic dissection of an invertebrate, a silkworm, was performed by the Italian microscopist, **Marcello Malpighi** (1628–1694), in 1669. **Jean Baptiste Antoine de Monet Chevalier de Lamarck** (1744–1829), in his seven-volume *Natural History of Invertebrate Animals* (1815–1822), made the clear distiction between vertebrates and invertebrates. A French zoologist, **Felix Dujardin** (1801–1860) from Tours, investigated protozoa and other invertebrates. An American zoologist, **Libbie Henrietta Hyman** (1888–1969), published six volumes of *The Invertebrates* (1940–1968). A London zoologist, **Sidnie Milana Manton** (1902–1979), made a detailed study, and introduced a new phylum, Uniraemia.

Iodine [Greek: *iodes*, violet] A non-metallic element of atomic number 53, first prepared in 1811 from seaweed, by **Bernard Courtois** (1777–1838), a manufacturer of niter.

Ion [Greek: *ienai*, go] An atom that is positively (cation) or negatively (anion) charged. *See electrolysis.*

Ionic Dissociation Theory *See dissociation.*

Ionium A parent element of radium and later known as thorium-203. Discovered by **Bertram Borden Boltwood** (1870–1927), an American chemist from Amhurst, Massachusetts, who was a pioneer in the study of isotopes.

Ionosphere or Heaviside layer. A conducting layer in the earth's upper atmosphere which accounts for electromagnetic waves being found so close to the earth's surface. First suggested in 1902 by a London physicist, **Oliver Heaviside** (1850–1925). An American engineer, **Arthur Edwin Kennelly** (1861–1939), who was professor of electrical engineering at Harvard (1902–1930), described it (Kennelly–Heaviside layer) in the same year. The Appleton layer, twice as high as the Heaviside layer, consisting of electrically charged particles in the upper atmosphere, was discovered by an English physicist, **Edward Victor Appleton** (1892–1965) from Bradford. This layer was found to play an essential role in wireless communication between distant stations, and in the development of radar. A Scottish physicist, **David Forbes Martyn** (b 1906), studied the reflection of radio waves and solar emission by the ionosphere.

Ipatieff, Vladimir Nikolayevich (1867–1952) *See petroleum.*

Iridium [Greek: *iris,* rainbow] A metallic element so named because its salts are multicolored. It was discovered in 1804 by an English chemist, **Smithson Tennant** (1761–1816) of Selby, Yorkshire.

Iron [Anglo-Saxon: *iren*] Meteorites and lodestone were the earliest sources of iron known to man around 4000 BC. They were thought to result from thunderbolts from the skies, and a reference to them is made in the holy writ of Joshua in 1400 BC. The dark reddish brown substance was recognized as a metal by the Egyptians in 4000 BC, although this idea became current only around 1350 BC. Iron objects were found in the tomb of Tutankhamun, who ruled around 1360 BC. Indians were experts at smelting iron in 950 BC. The Iron Age, which followed the Bronze Age, reached China around 600 BC. The Chinese perfected the method of making cast iron and built several enormous structures. A column made of 1325 tons of cast iron to commemorate the Chou Dynasty was built in AD 695 by the empress Wu Tse. Homer (*c.* 800 BC) wrote about the metal, and **Pliny the Elder** (AD 28–79) referred to the fatal use of iron weapons in wars, murders and robberies. Iron as a utility metal was known in Britain at least two centuries before the arrival of the Romans. Iron coins were introduced from Gaul, and Britons used iron bars as currency. Cast iron was made in Britain around AD 1300. The first industrial treatise on iron, *L'art de convertir le fer forgé en acier* (The art of converting iron into steel), was published in 1722 by **René Antoine Ferchault de Reaumer** (1683–1757). The symbol Fe, for ferrum in Latin, was assigned to the metal in 1826, by a Swedish physician and chemist, **Jons Jacob Berzelius** (1779–1848). A method of producing high-quality iron by using a reverberating furnace was invented in 1784 by a British engineer, **Henry Cort** (1749–1800) from Lancaster. In 1828, a Scottish engineer, **James Beaumont Nielson** (1792–1865) of Glasgow, invented the hot-blast, which revolutionized iron manufacture. *See Bessemer process, steel.*

Irrational Numbers A real number that cannot be represented as a fraction, or a number having no common measure, integral or functional. The Greek term *algos* for irrational numbers meant 'without a ratio'. **Abn Jafar Mohammed ibn Musa al-Khowarimi** (*c.* AD 825) referred to them as 'inaudible'. **Gerard of Cremona** (1147–1187) used the term *surd,* meaning deaf. **Pythagorus** (*c.* 580–500 BC) proved that the side and diagonal of a square are incommensurable. A Pythagorian, **Theodorus of Cyrene** (*c.* 400 BC), proved geometrically that roots of certain numbers are incommensurable with unity. **Euclid** (*c.* 300 BC), in his tenth book, dealt with certain irrational magnitudes.

Irrigation [Latin: *irrigo,* supply with fluid] *See agriculture, aqueduct, water pumps, water supply.*

St Isidore of Seville (AD 560–636) A Spanish-Roman encyclopedist and bishop of Seville in 600. He wrote *De natura rerum* (On the nature of things) and *Etymologies. See geography.*

ISIS An influential journal of biology and science founded in 1813 by a German naturalist, **Lorenz Oken** (1779–1851). He also initiated the first annual type of meeting for men of science in 1821. He proposed the vertebral theory of the skull in 1807 which was discredited by **Thomas Henry Huxley** (1825–1895) in 1858. His journal continued to publish important articles until 1848, when it ceased to exist. An international review on the history of science, ISIS, was founded by **George Alfred Leon Sarton** (1884–1956) in 1927. Sarton was a graduate from the University of Ghent and was appointed as professor of history of science at Harvard in 1940.

Isoelectric Point [Greek: *isos,* equal] It was first shown in 1899 that denatured egg albumen moved towards the cathode in acid solutions, and towards the anode in alkaline solutions. The pH value at which it did not move towards either of the electrodes was defined in 1910 as the isoelectric point, by a German-born US biochemist, **Leonor Michaelis** (1875–1949). W. B. Hardy in 1905 defined it as the pH at which the net positive and negative charge on a particle is zero. The isoelectric point was later found to be useful for the characterization, isolation and purification of proteins.

Isomerism [Greek: *isos,* equal + *meros,* part] In 1824, the two compounds silver fulminate and silver cyanate were first observed by **Justus von Liebig** (1803–1873) to have similar chemical composition, but different structure and properties. A German chemist, **Jons Jacob Berzelius**

(1779–1848), coined the term isomerism for this phenomenon. **Johannes Adolf Wislicenus** (1835–1902), a professor of chemistry at Leipzig (1885), independently studied the phenomenon. The study of isomerism was revived by a French-born Swiss chemist and Nobel Prize winner (1913), **Alfred Werner** (1866–1919). He proposed the modern theory of coordination bonds between molecules and published *Lehrbuch der Stereochemie* (1904).

Isomorphism [Greek: *isos,* equal + *morphe,* form] The existence of identical or similar crystalline forms in different chemical compounds. The phenomenon was discovered and named in 1819 by a German chemist, **Eilhardt Mitscherlich** (1794–1863).

Isotopes [Greek: *isos,* equal + *tropaos,* turn] A term coined in 1913 by **Frederick Soddy** (1877–1965), to denote the elements that have identical chemical qualities or atomic numbers, but different atomic weights. In the same year, **Kasimir Fajans** (1887–1975), a Polish chemist at the Technische Hochschule at Karlsruhe, proposed the same theory, independently of Soddy. The occurrence of isotopes of neon was first described by **Sir John Joseph Thomson** (1856–1940). His work was followed up by an English physicist, **Francis William Aston** (1877–1945) of Harbourne, Birmingham, who designed a mass spectrograph for the separation of isotopes, in 1924. The Nobel Prize for Chemistry in 1968 was awarded to a Norwegian-born American physical chemist, **Lars Onsager** (1903–1976), for his work on the theoretical basis for diffusion of isotopes. A Berlin-born US biochemist, **Rudolf Schoenheimer** (1898–1941), was the first to use isotopic tracers for studying biohemical processes, in 1935. A Hungarian chemist, **Georg Charles von Hevesy** (1885–1966), did further work on the use of isotopes for studying chemical reactions, for which he was awarded the Nobel Prize for Chemistry, in 1943.

Issigonis, Alec (1906–1988) *See car.*

Ivanovski, Dmitri Iosifovich (1864–1920) *See plant pathology, virus.*

Ives, Fredrick Eugene (1856–1937) *See cinema, color photography, photography.*

Ivory, Sir James (1765–1842) The son of a watchmaker from Dundee, Scotland who became the professor of mathematics at the Royal Military College, Great Marlow. He contributed over 15 papers on physical astronomy to the *Transactions of the Royal Society* of Edinburgh.

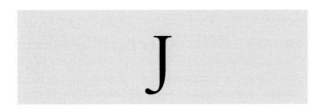

J

Jablochkoff, Pavel Nikolaivitch (1847–1894) *See arc light, electric lighting.*

Jackson, Benjamin Daydon (1846–1927) *See horticulture.*

Jacob, François (b 1920) *See genetic engineering.*

Jacobi, Carl Gustav Jacob (1804–1851) *See conical refraction.*

Jacquard System The use of punched cards in a loom for producing a complicated weaving pattern. First developed for making carpets, by a French engineer, **Joseph Marie Jacquard** (1752–1834) of Lyons. This was the first use of a computer concept in the weaving industry.

Jacquard, Joseph Marie (1752–1834) *See Jacquard system, textile industry.*

Jacuzzi A popular form of hydrotherapy, consisting of a pump, fixed in a bath, for producing a whirlpool effect, invented by and named after an Italian-born US inventor, **Candido Jacuzzi** (1903–1986).

Jacuzzi, Candido (1903–1986) *See jacuzzi.*

James, Charles (1880–1928) *See lutecia.*

Jansky Unit of radiation from outer space, used in radio astronomy, named after US engineer **Karl Guthe Jansky** (1905–1950)

Jansky, Karl Guthe (1905–1950) *See Jansky, radio waves, radioastronomy.*

Janssen, Pierre Jules César (1824–1907) *See celestial photography, helium, spectroscopy.*

Jardine, **Sir William** (1800–1874) *See scientific journals.*

Java Man The calvarium and femur of a primitive man (Java man) were discovered by **Marie Eugene François Thomas Dubois** (1858–1940), a surgeon in the Dutch army while he was stationed in Java in 1893. His finding was later acclaimed as the missing link in the evolution of man. Java man was later named *Pithecanthropus erectus*. The British anthropologist **Sir Arthur Keith** (1866–1955) estimated him to be 350 000 years old.

Jeans, Sir James Hopwood (1877–1946) A London physicist and professor of astronomy at the Royal Institution. He proposed the tidal theory for the origin of the planets and a theory for the development of spiral nebulae. He published *Dynamical Theory of Gases* (1904), *Problems of Cosmogeny and Stellar Dynamics* (1919), *Science and Music* (1938) and several other works. *See cosmology.*

Jeffreys, Alec John (b 1950) *See genetic fingerprinting.*

Jeffreys, Sir Harold (1891–1989) *See cosmology, earthquake.*

Jeffries, John (1744–1819) *See air balloon, channel flight.*

Jekyll, Gertrude (1843–1932) *See horticulture.*

Jensen, Johannes Hans Daniel (1907–1973) *See atomic nucleus.*

Jericho First known walled town, on the west bank of Jordan, around 9000 BC. Its inhabitants used sun-dried bricks held by mortar to build houses, and practiced farming. It was excavated in 1952 by an English archaeologist, **Dame Kathleen Mary Kenyon** (1906–1978), who published *Digging up Jericho* (1957).

Jessop, William (1745–1814) *See railway.*

Jet Engine An engine used for propelling an object in one direction by employing a jet, or stream of gases, which moves in the opposite direction. The principle is based on Sir Isaac Newton's third law of motion: 'To every action, there is an equal and opposite reaction'. The turbojet is the simplest form of gas turbine, used in aircraft well into the supersonic range. Jet propulsion in a steam boat was first attempted in 1787 by an American inventor, **James Rumsey** (1743– 1792). Pioneer work on supersonic projectiles and jets was carried out in 1887 by an Austrian physicist, **Ernst Mach** (1838–1916). The first jet-propelled aeroplane was built by **Henri Coanda** (1886–1972) of Romania, who later worked for the British & Colonial Aeroplane Company. The first practical jet engine was built and patented in 1930 by a British aeronautical engineer, **Frank Whittle** (1907–1996) of Coventry. His engine, successfully used in a Gloster aircraft in 1941, led to the world-wide use of jet engines in high-speed, high-altitude aircraft. The first turbojet engined flight was made in 1939 by a German, Erich Warsitz, in a Heinkel He-178. **Lawrence Dale Bell** (1895–1956), an aircraft designer from Indiana, produced the first jet-propelled aircraft in 1942, followed by the first manned aircraft to exceed the speed of sound in 1947. The first jet passenger airliner was built in 1949 by an English pioneer of aeronautics, **Geoffrey De Havilland** (1882–1965) from High Wycome. His company also developed the first series of fighter jets and bombers. A turbojet engine that passes all the air drawn in through the combustion chambers and expels it in a high-velocity jet was developed by an English engineer from Kent, **Stanley Hooker** (1907–1984). His engine, which was particularly efficient at high speeds, was incorporated into high-speed military aircrafts. Modern gas turbines, jet engines and internal combustion engines were developed by an American aeronautical engineer, **Edward Story Taylor** (1903–1991). He founded the Gas Turbine Laboratory at the Massachusetts Institute of Technology, in 1946.

Jet Plane   *See jet engine.*

Jobs, Steven (b 1955)   *See computers.*

Johannsen, Wilhelm Ludwig (1857–1927)   *See gene.*

Johanson, Donald Carl (b 1943)   *See hominids.*

Johanssen, Wilhelm Ludwig (1857–1927)   A Danish pioneer in experimental genetics. He was professor of botany at Copenhagen and published *Elemente der exacte Erblichkeit* (1909).

John of Halifax or **Johannes de Sacrobosco** (*c.* 1250)   *See astronomy, decimal notation.*

John of Pecham (*c.* 1230–1292)   A Franciscan monk at Oxford who became the Archbishop of Canterbury, in 1279. He published several scientific treatises, of which his *Perspectiva communis* is the best known.

John of Saxony (*c.* 1327–1355)   *See Alfonsine tables.*

Johnson, Leonard Clarence (1910–1990)   *See warplanes.*

Johnson, Eldridge R. (1866–1945)   *See gramophone, musical recording.*

Joliot, Irene née Curie (1897–1956)   *See radioactivity.*

Joliot, Jean Frédéric (1900–1958)   *See radioactivity.*

Joly, John (1857–1933)   *See petrology.*

Jones, Inigo (1572–1652)   *See architecture, British.*

Jones, Sir Harold Spencer (1890–1960)   *See Greenwich Observatory.*

Jones, William (1680–1749)   *See mathematical symbol, pi, shipping.*

Jordan, Marie Ennemond Camille (1838–1922)   *See group theory, topology.*

Jordanus of Nemore (*c.* 1230–1260)   A mathematician who taught at the University of Toulouse. He wrote a number of mathematical and other treatises.

Josephson, Brian David (b 1940)   *See superconductivity.*

Joule   An SI unit (Système International d'Unités) of energy, defined as the work done by a force, in moving its point of application through a distance of one meter. Named after a British physicist, **James Prescott Joule** (1818–1889) of Salford.

Joule, James Prescott (1818–1889)   A British natural philosopher from Salford. In 1840, he proposed (the Joule effect) that heat produced in a wire by an electric current is proportional to the resistance and square of the electric current. He demonstrated the conversion of work into heat in 1845 and calculated the average velocity of a gas molecule in 1848. His paper *On the Production of Heat by the Voltaic Electricity,* sent to the Royal Society in 1840 and published in the *Philosophical Magazine* (1841), contained the first suggestion of the mechanical equivalent of heat and work. *See electrical resistance, heat, Joule, Joule–Thomson effect, mechanical equivalent of heat, mechanical equivalent of work, tangent galvanometer, thermodynamics, velocity of gas molecules.*

Joule–Thomson Effect   The cooling or heating of a gas when passed through a porous plug under pressure. Named after **James Prescott Joule** (1818–1889) and **William Thomson** or **Lord Kelvin** (1824–1907). Thomson published *On the dynamical theory of heat* in 1851.

Journals   *See American scientific journals, scientific journals.*

Joy, Alfred Harrison (1882–1973)   An American astronomer from Greenville, Illinois who worked with **Walter Sydney Adams** (1876–1956) and **Milton Humason** (1891–1972) at Mount Wilson, to ascertain the spectral type and stellar distance of more than 5000 stars.

Julian Calendar   Every fourth year a leap year occurs, containing 366 days to account for overestimation of the sidereal year, or lunar year of 365¼ days, based on astronomy. First suggested by **Eratosthenes** (275–194 BC). Julius Caesar (102–44 BC) established the Julian calendar in consultation with an Alexandrian astronomer, **Sosigenes** (*c.* 100 BC) in 46 BC. It was replaced by the Gregorian calendar in 1582

Julian Day Count   Set in 1583 by **Joseph Justus Scaliger** (1540–1609) of Garonne, France. He took 1 January 4713 BC as the first day of the earth and named the calendar after his father, Julius Caesar Scaliger.

Jung, Joachim (1587–1657)   From Lübeck, was initially a physician who gave up his practice to study mathematics and botany. Although he did some important works in botany during the last 20 years of his life, while he was a director at a school in Hamburg, he failed to publish them. His

Doxoscopiae and *Isagoge phytoscopia* were published by one of his pupils after his death. Jung founded the *Societas Ereneutica,* one of the earliest scientific societies in Berlin. *See botanical classification, flower, leaves.*

Jupiter Fifth and largest major planet known to ancient astronomers. The four satellites of Jupiter were identified by **Galilei Galileo** (1564–1642) in 1610. The rotational speed of Jupiter was measured in 1665 by **Giovanni Domenico Cassini** (1625–1712) of Nice. In 1675, a Danish astronomer, **Olaus Roemer** (1644–1710), observed the different intervals between the eclipses of the moons of Jupiter in relation to the movement of the earth. A German astronomer, **Friedrich Wilhelm Bessel** (1784–1846), determined the mass of Jupiter, in 1842. The fifth satellite of Jupiter, Amalthea, was discovered in 1892 by **Edward Emerson Barnard** (1857–1923), an American astronomer from Nashville. Several moons of Jupiter, up to 13, had been discovered by 1974. They now number at least 16.

Jupiter Missile The first intermediate-range ballistic missile, launched by the United States in 1958.

Jurassic Period Middle Mesozoic period which lasted for 45 million years, around 208 to 146 million years ago, when dinosaurs were abundant. It was so named by a French geologist, **Alexandre Brongniart** (1770–1847), owing to the fact that limestone similar to that found in the Jura mountains started to be deposited during this geological age. **Alexander von Humboldt** (1769–1859) identified the period in 1799. An English geologist, **Sir Henry Thomas de la Beche** (1796–1855), gave an illustrative account of the Jurassic rocks of Dorset and Devon.

Jussieu, Antoine Laurent de (1748–1836) *See botany, taxonomy.*

Jussieu, Bernard de (1699–1777) *See taxonomy.*

Just, Ernest Everett (1833–1941) An American biologist from Charleston, South Carolina whose main research was on cell physiology and experimental embryology, including experimental parthenogenesis in marine eggs. He coauthored *General Cytology* (1924) and also published *Biology of the Cell Surface* (1939).

K

K'ung Fu-Tze or **Confucius** (552–479 BC) *See confucianism.*

Kaempfe, Hermann Anschutz (1872–1931) *See gyrostabilizer.*

Kamb, Walter Barclay (b 1931) *See glaciology.*

Kamen, Martin David (b 1913) *See photosynthesis.*

Kanada (*c.* 300 BC) *See atomic theory.*

Kane, Sir Robert John (1809–1890) *See radical.*

Kant, Immanuel (1724–1804) A German philosopher, born in Konigsberg, Prussia, where he became professor of logic and metaphysics, in 1770. His important works include *Kritik der reinen* (Critique of Pure Reason, 1781), *Kritik der Urteilskraft* (Critique of Judgement, 1790) and *Kritik der praktischen Vernuft* (Critique of Practical Reason, 1788). *See cosmology, evolution, geogeny.*

Kapitza, Pyotr Leonidovich (1894–1984) *See helium, radioastronomy.*

Kaplan, Viktor (1876–1934) *See hydroelectric schemes.*

Kapteyn, Jacobus Cornelius (1851–1922) *See galaxy.*

Karle, Jerome (b 1918) *See X-ray crystallography.*

Karman, Theodore von (1881–1963) *See aerodynamics.*

Karmann, Wilhelm (1914–1998) A German car designer who designed the first sports car for Volkswagen in 1955. His father, Wilhelm Karmann (d 1952), was a coachworks builder at Osnabrück, in 1874, and started making car bodies in 1902. Karmann Junior joined his father's firm in 1933.

Kastler, Alfred (1902–1984) *See laser, optical pumping.*

Kater, Henry (1777–1835) *See pendulum.*

Kay, John (1704–1780) *See textile industry.*

Keck Telescope World's largest optical telescope, owned by the California Institute of Technology and situated on Mauna Kea, Hawaii. It received its first images November 1990.

Keeler, James Edward (1857–1900) *See nebulae, Saturn.*

Keesome, Wilhelmus Henrikus (b 1876) *See helium.*

Keir, James (1735–1820) *See soda.*

Keith, Sir Arthur (1866–1955) *See Java man, Piltdown Man.*

Kekulé, von Stradonitz, Friedrich August (1829–1896) A German chemist, born in Darmstadt and educated at Giessen. He first suggested that molecules consist of atoms linked together by bonds, according to their valency. He proposed that carbon had a valency of 4 and that it could be linked in chains. In 1865 he demonstrated the 6-carbon ring structure for benzene. *See benzene, bonds, carbon, carbon cyclic ring, chemistry, valency.*

Kellner, Karl (1851–1905) *See Kellner process.*

Kellner Process Production of caustic soda from brine with the use of a mercury cathode. Patented in 1894 by **Karl Kellner** (1851–1905) of Vienna.

Kellogg, William (1852–1943) *See food industry.*

Kelly, William (1811–1888) *See Bessemer process, steel.*

Kendall, Henry Way (b 1926) *See quarks.*

Kennelly, Arthur Edwin (1861–1939) *See alternating current, ionosphere.*

Kennelly–Heaviside Layer *See ionosphere.*

Kent, William (1684–1748) *See architecture, British.*

Kenyon, Dame Kathleen Mary (1906–1978) *See Jericho.*

Kenyon, Joseph (1885–1961) *See stereochemistry.*

Kepler, Johannes (1571–1630) One of the greatest German astronomers, born in Weil near Stuttgart, where he underwent a childhood of poverty and ill health. He entered the University of Tübingen in 1589 and graduated in mathematics in 1594, before joining **Tycho Brahe** (1546–1601) at the castle of Benatsky in 1600. Kepler discovered the orbits of the planets to be perfect ellipses, with the sun at one focus, in 1604, and proposed two important laws related to orbital movement in astronomy. His important works include *Mysterium Cosmographicum* (1596), *Harmonices Mundi* (1619) and *Epitome Astronomiae Copernicanae* (1618–1621). He was one of the first to point out the role of the retina in vision in his *Dioptrice* (1611). *See astronomy, aurora borealis, celestial mechanics, comet, dioptrics, laws of planetary motion, optics, parallax, Rudolphine tables, supernova, telescope, tides, vision.*

Kepler's Laws *See laws of planetary motion.*

Kerr Effect or magneto-optic effect. Double refraction in certain media on the application of an electric field. Discovered in 1875 by a Scottish physicist, **John Kerr** (1824–1907) from Ardrossan, Ayrshire, who published *An Elementary Treatise on Rational Mechanics* (1867).

Kerr, John (1824–1907) *See Kerr effect.*

Kerr, Roy Patrick (b 1934) *See black hole.*

Kersey, John (1616–1702) *See umbrella.*

Ketone The term was introduced into chemistry in 1848 by a German chemist, **Leopold Gmelin** (1788–1853). His *Handbuch der anorganischen Chemie* (1811) was an early important work on organic chemistry.

Kew Gardens Known as the Royal Botanical Gardens at Kew, in London, opened in 1760. It changed from private to public ownership, owing to the efforts of **John Lindley** (1799–1865) from Norwich, who was professor of botany at University College, London, in 1840. In 1835, he prepared a report on Kew Gardens which saved it from extinction. The garden was developed and expanded under its first director, a botanist from Norwich, **Sir William Jackson Hooker** (1785–1865), over the next five years, and it had over six million species in its herbarium. The landmark pagoda in Kew Gardens was designed by a Scottish architect, **Sir William Chambers** (1726–1796).

Keyser, Hendrik de (1565–1621) *See architecture, European.*

Kharasch, Morris Selig (1895–1957) *See polymer.*

Khorana, Har Gobind (b 1922) *See artificial gene, genetic coding.*

Khurdadhbih, Abul Qasim ibn (c. 1100) *See roads.*

Kilburn, Tom (b 1921) *See computers.*

Kilby, Jack Saint Clair (b 1923) *See automation, calculating machine, computers.*

Kinematic Theory An alternative theory to Einstein's general theory of relativity, proposed in 1932 by an English physicist, **Edward Arthur Milne** (1896–1950) from Hull, Yorkshire. He was appointed as professor of mathematics at Oxford in 1928, and served as president of the Royal Astronomical Society from 1943 to 1945.

Kinematics The study of bodies in motion. *See motion.*

Kinetic Energy [Greek: *kinetikos*, pertaining to movement] The idea of continuous motion of all particles of matter was first proposed in 600 BC by a Greek philosopher, **Heraclitus of Ephesus**. The mechanical principles governing the motion of bodies were proposed by **Sir Isaac Newton** (1642–1727), in his work *Philosophiae Naturalis Principia Mathematica* (Mathematical Principles of Natural Philosophy). The term kinetic energy was coined by **Gustav Gaspard Coriolis** (1792–1843) of Paris, in his work *On the*

Calculation of Mechanical Action (1829). The conversion of kinetic energy into heat, and its reconversion into mechanical energy (later interpreted as conservation of energy), was demonstrated in 1842 by a German physician and physicist, **Julius Robert von Mayer** (1814–1878). A Scottish physicist, **John James Waterson** (1811–1883) of Edinburgh, submitted one of the first important papers on kinetic energy, to the Royal Society in 1845, but it went unheeded. It was discovered and published in 1892 by the English physicist, **Lord John William Strutt Rayleigh** (1842–1919). The formula $\frac{1}{2}mv^2$ for a mathematical expression of dynamics was introduced by **Gaspard Gustav Coriolis** (1792–1843). *See absolute zero, energy.*

Kinetic Theory of Gases A theory that attempts to explain the properties of gases on the basis of a vast number of molecules which move relative to each other. It was initiated by a Swiss physician and mathematician, **Daniel Bernoulli** (1700–1782) in his explanation of Boyle's law in his *Hydrodynamica* (1738). His work was revived by a Scottish engineer **John James Waterson** (1811–1883) from Edinburgh in 1845, and **Rudolf Julius Emmanuel Clausius** (1822–1888), a professor at Bonn in 1857. **James Clerk Maxwell's** (1831–1879) discovery of the law of distribution of velocities among gas molecules (1866) helped to advance the theory.

Kinetoscope An early device for movies. In 1889 **Thomas Alva Edison** (1847–1931) developed one with the use of Eastman's flexible film. It consisted of a four-foot high box with a peep hole through which the film could be viewed. Edison set up several coin-operated kinetoscope parlors in New York.

King, Gregory (1648–1712) *See vital statistics.*

Kipp's Apparatus Standard laboratory apparatus consisting of two glass vessels for continuous production of any gas. Named after its inventor, a Dutch chemist **Petrus Jacobus Kipp** (1808–1864) of Utrecht.

Kipp, Petrus Jacobus (1808–1864) *See Kipp's apparatus.*

Kipping, Frederick Stanley (1863–1949) *See polymer.*

Kircher, Athanasius (1601–1680) *See earthquake, geogeny, loudspeaker, microscope, volcanoes.*

Kirchhoff, Gottlieb Sigismond (1764–1833) *See starch.*

Kirchhoff, Gustav Robert (1824–1887) German physicist, born in Königsberg, who served as a professor at Heidelberg (1854–1875) and Berlin (1875–1886). He invented the spectroscope, with **Robert Wilhelm Bunsen** (1811–1899), in

1859. He was the first to measure electrical resistance in absolute terms, in 1849, and discovered the elements rubidium and cesium through spectral analysis, in 1860. *See absorption spectra, astronomy, cesium, electrical resistance, quantum theory, rubidium, spectroscopy.*

Kirkwood Gaps A consequence of perturbations caused by the planet Jupiter. Proposed in 1866 by an American astronomer, **Daniel Kirkwood** (1814–1895) of Hartford County, Maryland. He used the theory to explain the gaps in the rings of Saturn.

Kirkwood, Daniel (1814–1895) *See Kirkwood gaps.*

Kirwan, Richard (1733–1812) *See mineralogy.*

Kitaibel, Paul (1757–1817) *See tellurium.*

Kitchen Range *See cookers, pressure cooker, oven.*

Kite Invented by Lu Pan of China around 395 BC. The first treatise on kites in Europe was written in 1589 by **Giovanni Battista della Porta** (1535–1615), an Italian scientist from Naples. **Benjamin Franklin** (1706–1790) used it to prove that lightning is a form of electricity. In 1866, an American, **Mahlon Loomis** (1826–1886), observed the potential difference between two kites that were 14 miles apart, and obtained a patent for telegraphy without wires, in 1872. In 1901, the pioneer of wireless telegraphy, **Guglielmo Marchese Marconi** (1874–1937), used a kite to raise an aerial, for receiving messages from Cornwall to Newfoundland.

Kjeldahl Method Used for rapid estimation of nitrogen in organic chemistry, invented in 1883 by a Danish chemist, **Johan Gustav Christofer Thorsager Kjeldahl** (1849–1900). He used sulfuric acid for digestion, and estimated the ammonia produced.

Kjeldahl, Johan Gustav Christofer Thorsager (1849–1900) *See Kjeldahl method.*

Klaproth, Martin Heinrich (1743–1817) A German analytical chemist and the first professor of chemistry at the University of Berlin, founded in 1810. He discovered several new elements including zirconium, uranium, and chromium. *See cerium, chromium, strontium, tellurium, titanium, uranium.*

Klaus, Karl Karlovich (1796–1864) A Russian professor of chemistry at the University of Dorpat who discovered the rare element ruthenium.

Klebs, Theodor Albrecht Edwin (1834–1913) *See embedding.*

Klein Models Projective models for Euclidean, elliptic and hyperbolic geometries, developed by a German mathematician, **Christian Felix Klein** (1849–1925) from Düsseldorf. He founded the *Encyklopädie der Mathematischen Wissenschaften,* which was published in 23 volumes from 1890 to 1930.

Klein, Christian Felix (1849–1925) *See Klein models.*

Klein–Fock Equation *See Schrödinger equation.*

Kliegl Lights Brilliant carbon-arc lights used in early television and cinema, invented in 1911 by two German-born brothers John H. Kliegl (1869–1959) and Anton T. Kliegl (1872–1927).

Klingenstierna, Samuel (1698–1765) *See achromatic lens.*

Klitzing, Klaus von (b 1943) *See quantum hall effect.*

Klug, Sir Aaron (b 1926) A Lithuanian-born British molecular biologist who applied X-ray diffraction and electron microscopy to the study of biological macromolecules, for which he was awarded the Nobel Prize for Chemistry in 1982.

Knight, Thomas Andrew (1759–1838) *See hybridization, plant pathology, plant physiology.*

Knitting A method where only one thread is used with the help of a knitting needle to produce meshes resulting in a tissue resembling cloth. In the process of knitting stockings, meshes are produced without making knots. Woollen stockings were knitted in the 14th century and King Henry VIII during his reign from 1509 to 1547 wore woollen stockings made in England, and obtained his first silk stockings from Spain. Queen Elizabeth I was fond of silk stockings especially knitted for her by her silk-woman, Montague. The French had a Stocking Knitters' Guild, in 1527. The word knit was applied to stockings in 1530. In Germany the stocking-knitters were known as *hosenstriker* in the mid-16th century. The first stocking-loom, which could make rapid meshes of loops, was invented in 1589 by a clergyman, William Lee of Woodborough, Nottinghamshire. The knitting industry had become established in England by the end of the 16th century and Charles II (1630–1685) granted a charter to the Frame-work Knitters Society of London, in 1663. By 1670, there were about 700 stocking frames in England, and these increased to 14 000 by 1753. Stocking frames with rotary action were introduced in 1838, making hosiery manufacture an important industry. Over 3 million knitted stockings were produced annually in England by the mid-19th century.

Knitting Machine or stocking frame. Invented in 1589 by an English clergyman from Cambridge, William Lee. *See knitting.*

Knocking An effect in petrol engines caused by too-rapid burning of petrol in the engine cylinders. *See octane rating.*

Knopoff, Leon (b 1925) *See seismology.*

Knot Theory Originated with **Lord Kelvin**'s (1824–1907) suggestion that atoms are small loop-like vortices, in ether. The heavier atoms were supposed to contain more complex knots. After investigating the different ways in which a loop can be knotted, a Scottish mathematician **Peter Guthrie** (1831–1901), from Dalkeith, published a paper on the class-ification of knots, in 1876.

Kodachrome *See color photography.*

Koenig, Friedrich (1774–1833) *See newspapers, printing.*

Koenig, Karl Rudolph (1832–1901) *See acoustics.*

Kohlrausch, Friedreich Wilhelm (1840–1910) *See electrolysis.*

Kolbe, Adolf Wilhelm Hermann (1818–1884) *See acetic acid, organic chemistry, synthesis.*

Kolliker, Rudolph Albert von (1871–1905) *See cell division.*

Kolmogorov Equation A partial differential equation used widely in physics and chemistry, proposed by a Russian mathematician and professor at the Moscow State University, **Andrei Nikolaevich Kolmogorov** (1903–1987).

Kolmogorov, Andrei Nikolaevich (1903–1987) *See Kolmogorov equation.*

Kolreuter, Joseph Gottlieb (1733–1806) *See hybridization, pollination.*

Kopp, Hermann Franz Moritz (1817–1892) One of the founders of physical chemistry, with his work on molecular volumes, crystallography and dissociation. He was a hist-orian on chemistry and his *Geschichte der Chemie* in four volumes was published between 1843 and 1847.

Kornberg, Arthur (b 1918) *See deoxyribonucleic acid.*

Korolev, Seregi Pavlovich (1906–1966) *See space travel.*

Kossel, Walther (1888–1956) *See valency.*

Kovalevskaia, Sofya Vasilevna (1850–1891) A Moscow-born mathematician who became professor at Stockholm in 1889. Her main work was on partial differential equations and Abelian integrals, and in 1886 she won the *Prix Bordin*

of the French Academy of Sciences for a paper on the rotation of a rigid body about a point, a problem which the 18th-century mathematicians failed to solve.

Kratzer, Nicolas (1486–1550) *See sundial.*

Krebs Cycle Citric acid or tricarboxylic cycle, in the final stage of the biochemical breakdown of carbohydrates, dur-ing which energy is produced. Elucidated in 1937, by **Sir Hans Adolf Krebs** (1900–1982), while he was at Sheffield University.

Krebs, Nicholas or **Nicholas of Cusa** (b 1401) *See extra-terrestrial life, spectacles.*

Krebs, Sir Hans Adolf (1900–1982) *See Krebs cycle.*

Kronecker, Leopold (1823–1891) A German mathemati-cian who devised the Kronecker delta used in linear algebra. He attempted to unify all branches of mathematics – except geometry and mechanics – as parts of arithmetic. He also believed that whole numbers were sufficient for the study of mathematics.

Krupp, Alfred (1812–1887) *See firearms, railway.*

Krypton [Greek: *kryptos,* hidden] An inert gas, discovered in 1898 through spectroscopy by two London chemists, **Sir William Ramsay** (1852–1916) and **Morris William Travers** (1872–1961).

Kuhne, Willy (1821–1901) *See enzyme.*

Kuiper Band A number of bands due to the presence of methane in the spectra of Uranus and Neptune. First observed by a Dutch-born American astronomer, **Gerard Peter Kuiper** (1905–1973) around 1949. He also discov-ered the fifth moon of Uranus (1948) and the second moon of Neptune (1949). In 1951, Kenneth Edgeworth of England predicted this band or belt (Kuiper–Edgeworth belt) to be a source of short-period comets.

Kuiper, Gerard Peter (1905–1973) *See Kuiper band.*

Kuiper–Edgeworth Belt *See Kuiper band.*

Kummer, Ernst Eduard (1810–1893) Professor of mathe-matics at Breslau (1842–1855), whose main interest was number theory; he introduced the concept of ideal num-bers. *See Fermat's last theorem.*

Kundt, August Adolph Eduard Eberhard (1839–1894) *See dispersion of light, Kundt's tube.*

Kundt's Tube A simple device for measuring the velocity of sound in gases and solids. Invented in 1866 by a German physicist, **August Adolph Eduard Eberhard Kundt** (1839–1894).

Kurchatov, Igor Vasilevich (1903–1963) *See atomic power, nuclear fission, thermonuclear fusion.*

Kusch, Polykarp (1911–1993) *See Lamb, Willis Eugene; magnetic resonance imaging.*

Kyan, John Howard (1774–1850) An Irish inventor born in Dublin. In 1832, he patented a method for preserving wood, known as the kyanizing process. He was later involved in a scheme to filter the water supply to New York.

L

L'hospital, Marquis Antoine de (b 1661) *See calculus.*

Lacaille, Nicolaus Louis de (1713–1762) *See logarithms.*

Lacépède, Bernard de Laville (1756–1825) See *Buffon, George Louis Leclerc Compte de.*

Lacroix, François Antoine Alfred (1863–1948) *See volcanoes.*

Lagrange, Joseph Louis (1736–1813) *See acoustics, algebra, calculus, Fermat's last theorem.*

Laika The first animal, a dog, to travel in space for a sustained period. This was in the Russian space satellite, *Sputnik II.*

Laird, Macgregor (1808–1861) *See transatlantic voyage.*

Laithwaite, Eric Robert (1920–1997) *See linear induction motor.*

Lake Dwellings Structures erected by man on wooden poles driven into the ground, over lakes, in order to protect himself from wild animals and enemies. Built close to the end of the Stone Age in Europe. Remains have been found in Scandinavia, Germany, Switzerland and nothern Italy. Extensive surveys of these were carried out by G. Gams and R. Nordhagen, who published a classic work on the subject in 1923.

Lalande, Joseph Jerome Le François de (1732–1807) *See stars, Venus.*

Lamarck, Jean Baptiste Antoine de Monet, Chevalier de (1744–1829) A French evolutionist from Bazentin, in Picardy, who studied medicine in Paris before he took to botany and zoology. He proposed the term biology for the science of life. In his *Recherches sur l'Organisation des Corps Vivants* (1802) he suggested that function precedes and creates structure, and proposed the law of *use and disuse* related to adaptation. His *Philosophie Zoologique* (1809) contains his doctrine that great changes in the environment bring about changes in the habits of animals which could be inherited. He became blind in 1819 and completed *Histoire Naturelle des Animaux sans Vertèbres* through dictation to his daughter in 1822. *See adaptation, evolution, invertebrates.*

Lamb, Horace (1849–1934) *See hydrodynamics.*

Lamb, Hubert Horace (b 1913) *See weather forecast.*

Lamb Shift *See Lamb, Willis Eugene.*

Lamb, Willis Eugene (b 1913) An American physicist of Los Angeles, who described two possible energy states of hydrogen (Lamb shift) which led to the theory of quantum electrodynamics. In 1955 he shared the Nobel Prize for Physics with a German-born US physicist, **Polykarp Kusch** (1911–1993), who made a precise measurement of the electron's magnetic moment.

Lambert, Johann Heinrich (1728–1777) A German physicist who was the first to measure the intensity of light, in his *photometria* in 1760. *See galaxy, Milky Way, pi.*

Lamé Functions Mathematical functions to solve problems of temperature equilibrium in ellipsoids. Proposed by a French mathematician, **Gabriel Lamé** (1795–1870), who was a professor of physics at the École Polytechnique, Paris.

Lamé, Gabriel (1795–1870) *See Lamé functions.*

Lamont, Johan von (1805–1879) *See Uranus.*

Lamp Whale-oil lamps with asbestos wicks were used by the Chinese during the reign of King Chao of Yen, around 600 BC. Christians of Egypt used butter instead of oil to burn their lamps in the 3rd century. **Hero of Alexandria** (*c.* AD 100) invented a lamp that pushed the wick up by an ingenious mechanism, using a toothed wheel and a bar. The first large-scale illumination using large lamps with candles and metal reflectors was in Paris in 1667. The oil lantern was developed in 1744, and the standard oil lamp with a circular wick and glass chimney was invented by a Swiss chemist, **Aimé Argand** (1755–1803), in 1782. A mantle or woven net impregnated with thorium and cerium (Welsbach Mantle), which gave a white incandescence when heated, was invented in 1885 by an Austrian chemist, **Carl Auer von Welsbach** (1858–1929). *See Davy's lamp, Dobereiner lamp, electric light bulb, gas lighting.*

Lamy, Claude Auguste (1820–1873) *See thallium.*

Lanchester, Frederick William (1868–1948) *See airplane, car, warplanes.*

Land, Edwin Herbert (1909–1991) *See polaroid camera.*

Landau, Lev Davidovich (1908–1968) *See helium.*

Landberg, Helmut Eric (1906–1985) *See climatology, weather forecast.*

Landé Splitting Factor Ratio of an elementary magnetic moment to its causative angular momentum, used in quantum physics. Proposed in 1923 by a German-born US physicist, **Alfred Landé** (1888–1975).

Landé, Alfred (1888–1975) *See Landé splitting factor.*

Landolt, Hans Heinrich (1831–1910) *See conservation of mass.*

Langen, Eugen (1833–1895) *See Daimler, Gottlib; gas engine.*

Langevin, Paul (1872–1946) *See emulsification, magnetic theory, valency.*

Langley, Samuel Pierpont (1834–1906) *See aerodynamics, bolometer, radiometer (2).*

Langmuir, Irving (1881–1957) *See electric light bulb, surface chemistry.*

Lankester, Edwin Ray (1847–1929) A London zoologist who was instrumental in founding the Marine Biological Association in 1884. He was appointed as Linacre professor of comparative anatomy at Oxford in 1891, and became the director of the British Museum of Natural History in 1898.

Lannard-Jones, Sir John Edward (b 1894) *See surface chemistry.*

Lanston, Tolbert (1844–1913) *See typography.*

Lanthanum [Greek: *lanthaneo*, escape notice] An element with an atomic number of 57. Discovered in 1839 by a Swedish chemist, **Carl Gustav Mosander** (1797–1858).

Laplace, Pierre Simon Marquis de (1749–1827) A French mathematician and astronomer from Normandy. He published *Mécanique céleste* (1799–1825), *Système du monde* (1796) and several other important works. *See black hole, calorimeter, cosmology, Laplace theorem, nebular hypothesis, Saturn, velocity of sound, vital statistics.*

Laplace Theorem Any determinant is equal to the sum of all the minors, formed from any selected set of its rows, each minor being described by its algebraic complement. Proposed by a French mathematician, **Pierre Simon Marquis de Laplace** (1749–1827) from Normandy.

Lapworth, Arthur (1872–1941) A Scottish chemist from Galashiels and son of **Charles Lapworth** (1842–1920). He was appointed as the professor of organic chemistry at Manchester in 1913. *See organic chemistry.*

Lapworth, Charles (1842–1920) *See Ordovician.*

Lardner, Dionysius (1793–1859) A prolific Irish scientific writer from Dublin, and a professor of astronomy at University College, London. He edited *Lardner's Cabinet Cyclopedia* (1829–1849) in 133 volumes, and several other encyclopedic works.

Large Electron Positron Collider (LEP) World's largest particle accelerator, in operation since 1989 at the CERN laboratories near Geneva in Switzerland.

Larmor, Sir Joseph (1857–1942) *See Larmor precession.*

Larmor Precession Precessive motion of the orbit of a charged particle in a magnetic field. Described by an Irish physicist, **Sir Joseph Larmor** (1857–1942), who was professor of natural philosophy at Queen's College, Galway. He was knighted in 1909.

Lartet, Edouard Arman Isidore Hippolyte (1801–1871) *See prehistory.*

Laser Acronym for **L**ight **A**mplification by **S**timulated **E**lectromagnetic **R**adiation. First described in 1958 by an American physicist, **Arthur Leonard Schawlow** (1921–1999) of Mount Vernon, New York. The concept of the emission of radiation, stimulated by photons, was first proposed in 1917 by **Albert Einstein** (1879–1955). His theory was developed in 1951 into microwave amplification with the use of stimulated electromagnetic radiation (MASER), by an American physicist and Nobel laureate, **Charles Hard Townes** (b 1915) of Greenville, South Carolina, who produced the first practical maser in 1953. His device was modified and improved to work continuously, rather than intermittently, by a Dutch-born American physicist, **Nicolaas Bloembergen** (b 1920). He shared the Nobel Prize for Physics, for this work with Schawlow and a Swedish physicist **Kai Manne Börje Siegbahn** (b 1918), in 1981. The use of semiconductors in lasers was proposed by a Russian physicist, **Nikolay Gennadiyevich Basov** (b 1922), in 1955. The optical maser, or the laser suggested by Townes and Schawlow, was first built in 1960, by an American physicist, **Theodore Harold Maiman** (b 1927) of Los Angeles, at the Hughes Research Laboratories, in California. The gas laser was invented at the Bell Laboratories by Ali Javan and his team in 1961. The injection laser was developed by several groups of workers in 1962. Further work was done by a German-born French scientist, **Alfred Kastler** (1902–1984), who was awarded the Nobel Prize for Physics in 1966. Laser beams are the brightest artificial source of light, and are used in astronomy and other fields. *See optical pumping.*

Laser Mass Spectroscopy A forensic technique where a laser beam is used for scanning minute sample of evidence. The technique was first used in France 1993 to convict a mass murderer.

Lassell, William (1799–1880) *See Hyperion, Neptune, Uranus.*

Latent Heat [Greek: *latens*, hidden] The amount of heat needed to change the state of a substance from solid to liquid (or liquid to vapor) without changing its temperature. Discovered in 1762 by **Joseph Black** (1728–1799), a Scottish physician and professor of chemistry at Glasgow. A standard method of determining the latent heat of steam was invented by the French chemist and politician, **Pierre Eugène Marcellin Berthelot** (1827–1907). The latent heat of ice was calculated in 1772 by a German-born Swedish physicist, **Johan Carl Wilcke** (1732–1796).

Latham, John (1740–1837) *See ornithology.*

Lathe A machine for turning wood, ivory or metal known to the ancients. Talus is credited with its invention, by a Greek historian, **Diodorus Siculus** (d *c.* 20 BC). **Pliny the Elder** (AD 28–79) ascribed it to **Theodorus of Samos** (*c.* 530 BC). **Jacques Besson** (1535–1575), a French mathematician and inventor, described a screw-cutting lathe. The first screw-cutting lathe that incorporated a toolpost with a longitudinal movement was invented by a Parisian clock maker, **Antoine Thiout** (1692–1767), around 1741. **Jacques de Vaucanson** (1709–1782) of Grenoble, France built the first metal lathe, with a carriage that moved parallel to the axis of the centers. The modern lathe was invented in 1778 by an English iron-master, **John Wilkinson** (1728–1808) of Clifton, Cumberland. The slide rest for the lathe, which allowed the operator to use the lathe without holding the metal-cutting instruments in his hands, was invented in 1797 by an English engineer, **Henry Maudslay** (1771–1831) of Woolwich. One of his apprentices, **Sir Joseph Whitworth** (1803–1887) from Stockport, invented several devices, including a screw-measuring machine or bench micrometer and a screw-cutting lathe.

Latimer, Louis Howard (1848–1928) *See electric light bulb.*

Latour, Carl Gustav Patrick de (1845–1913) *See dairy industry.*

Latreille, Pierre Andrezac (1762–1833) *See entomology.*

Latrobe, Benjamin Henry (1764–1820) *See architecture, British.*

Lauchen, Georg Joachim von (1514–1576) *See trigonometry.*

Laue, Max Theodor Felix von (1879–1960) *See X-ray crystallography, X-rays.*

Laurent, Auguste (1807–1853) *See organic chemistry.*

Lauste, Eugene Augustin (1857–1935) *See cinema.*

Laval, Carl Gustav Patrick de (1845–1913) *See marine engineering, steamships, turbines.*

Laveran, Charles Louis Alphonse (1845–1922) *See parasitism.*

Lavoisier, Antoine Laurent (1743–1794) A French chemist in Paris, who established the study of chemistry on modern lines. He defined an element as 'a substance that cannot be split up into simpler form by any means', and investigated dephlogisticated air, previously described in 1774 by **Joseph Priestley** (1733–1804) of Leeds. He described the properties of hydrogen, nitrogen and oxygen in the air, explained fermentation on a chemical basis and identified carbon as a distinct element. His *Traité Elementaire de chimie* was published in 1789. Lavoisier and **Pierre Simon Marquis de Laplace** (1749–1827) were the first to prove that respiration is a process of combustion. Lavoisier was an advisory member of 'Ferme-General' which collected taxes from the people before the revolution. He was guillotined during the revolution for his involvement with the Ferme and other government affairs. *See acids, air, biochemistry, calorimeter, carbon, chemistry, conservation of mass, diamond, fermentology, hydrogen, nitrogen, oxygen, quantitative chemistry.*

Law of Attraction and Repulsion Relates to the forces between electrically charged bodies. Proposed in 1785 by **Charles Augustus Coulomb** (1736–1806). *See Coulomb's law.*

Law of Chemical Equilibrium When the temperature is raised, the reaction that is favored is that which takes place with absorption of heat. Lowering the temperature favors the reaction, which releases heat. Proposed in 1884 by a professor of chemistry at the University of Paris, **Henry Louis le Chatelier** (1850–1936). He made important contributions to metallurgy and became professor of industrial chemistry at the same institute, in 1887.

Law of Combination of Gases The ratio of combination of hydrogen and oxygen was determined in 1805 by a French chemist, **Joseph Louis Gay-Lussac** (1778–1850) and a German scientist, **Alexander von Humboldt** (1769–1859). The concept that gases combine with one another by volume in the ratio of whole numbers, and generally in small whole numbers, was proposed by Gay-Lussac, in 1808. He also discovered that the volume of a product, if gaseous, bears a simple ratio to the volume of the reacting gases.

Law of Comparison Used for calculating the force required to tow an object against the retarding wave raised by its own progress through the liquid. Discovered by an English civil engineer, **William Froude** (1810–1879) from Devon.

Law of Conservation of Mass *See conservation of mass.*

Law of Conservation of Momentum First suggested in 1668 by an English mathematician, **John Wallis** (1616–1703) from Ashford, Kent.

Law of Constant Composition In 1799, the French chemist **Claude Louis Comte de Berthollet** (1748–1822), proposed that the composition of a compound may vary. This was disputed by another French chemist, **Joseph Louis Proust** (1754–1826), who proved that no matter how or where a compound was prepared, its composition remained definite and constant.

Law of Crystallization *See crystallization.*

Law of Diffusion of Gases *See Graham, Thomas.*

Law of Dilution *See physical chemistry.*

Law of Distribution of Velocities *See kinetic theory of gases.*

Law of Electrolysis The amount of substance decomposed by electric current is proportional to the time of passage and the strength of the current. Proposed by **Michael Faraday** (1791–1867), in 1833.

Law of Equipartition of Energy *See Boltzmann, Ludwig.*

Law of Equivalent Proportions Discovered by a German chemist, **Jeremias Benjamin Richter** (1762–1807) of Silesia. He was a pupil of **Immanuel Kant** (1724–1804) at Konigsberg.

Law of Expansion of Gases *See Charles, Jaques Alexandre César.*

Law of Gravitation The astronomer **Johannes Kepler** (1571–1630) discovered three laws relating to the motion of the planets, which formed the basis for **Sir Isaac Newton's** discovery. In 1670 Newton elucidated the law of gravitation, which gave a physical meaning to Kepler's three laws, and published his findings in 1687.

Law of Inverse Square *See inverse square law.*

Law of Large Numbers A statistical principle when dealing with large numbers. Proposed in 1837 by a French physicist and astronomer, **Siméon Denis Poisson** (1781–1840).

Law of Magnetic Force *See magnetic theory.*

Law of Mass Action The speed of a reaction is proportional to the product of the concentrations of the reacting substances. In 1777, a German metallurgist, **Carl Friedrich Wenzel** (1740–1793) of Dresden, Saxony, first observed that the rate of solution of a metal was proportional to the concentration of the acid, thus forecasting the law of mass action. The law was proposed in 1864 by two Norwegian professors of chemistry at the University of Christiana (Oslo), **Cato Maximillian Guldberg** (1836–1902) and **Peter Waage** (1833–1900).

Law of Multiple Proportions *See atomic structure.*

Law of Octaves *See periodic law.*

Law of Partial Pressures *See Dalton, John.*

Law of Quadratic Reciprocity A theorem dealing with prime numbers, related to any two odd primes, first proposed in 1785 by a French mathematician, **Adrien-Marie Legendre** (1752–1833) of Toulouse. His classic treatise *Essai sur la théorie des nombres* (1798) contains his discovery. His other widely known work *Éléments de géometrie* was published earlier, in 1794. The law was discovered independently by **Carl Friedrich Gauss** (1777–1855) of Brunswick, who proved it in 1796. His disciple, **Henry John Stephen Smith** (1826–1883) of Dublin, specialized in the theory of numbers and published *On the Orders and Genera of Ternary Quadratic Forms* (1867).

Law of Refraction The Greek mathematician **Euclid** (*c.* 300 BC), in his *Optics,* observed that rays of light travelled in a straight line. One of the first recorded experiments was carried out by **Ptolemy of Alexandria** (*c.* AD 127–151), who came to the conclusion that the angle of incidence is proportional to the angle of refraction, for a given pair of media. The Arab mathematician **Alhazen or Ibn Al-Haitham** (AD 965–1038) of Basra, made experimental determination of refractive indices. The law of refraction that states that the ratio of the sines of the angles of the incident and refracted rays to the normal is a constant was discovered in 1624 by Snellius or **Willebrord Snell** (1591–1626), a professor of mathematics at Leyden. His work was first made known by **Christian Huygens** (1629–1695) in his *Dioptrica* in 1703.

Law of Universal Gravitation Discovered by **Sir Isaac Newton** (1642–1727) in 1665. It offered the explanation for Kepler's laws of planetary motion. *See gravity.*

Law of Use and Disuse The first suggestion that organs develop through exercise, and weaken when not used, was made by **Epicurus** of Samos (342–271 BC) around 300 BC. The modern theory that animals strengthen some organs by use, and weaken others by disuse, and pass on these acquired characteristics to the offspring, was proposed in 1809 by **Antoine de Monet Chevalier de Lamarck** (1744–1829), a French evolutionist from Bazentin, in Picardy. *See Lamarck, Antoine de Monet Chevalier de.*

Lawes, Sir John Bennet (1814–1900) *See agriculture.*

Lawrence, Ernest Orlando (1901–1958) *See cyclotron, lawrencium.*

Lawrence, John Hundale (1904–1991) A physician and brother of **Ernest Orlando Lawrence** (1901–1958), the inventor of the cyclotron. In 1936, he established the world's first facility for nuclear medicine, the Donner Laboratory, at the University of California, Berkeley, and studied the effects of radiation on humans.

Lawrence, Sir William (1783–1867) *See biology.*

Lawrencium An element with atomic number 13, synthesized in 1961, at the Lawrence Radiation Laboratory in California by Albert Ghiorso, Almon E. Larsh and Robert Latimer. It is named after **Ernest Orlando Lawrence** (1901–1958) of Canton, South Dakota, who developed the cyclotron.

Laws, Richard Maitland (b 1926) *See marine biology.*

Laws of Electrolysis Enunciated by **Michael Faraday** (1791–1867). The first law states that when an electrolyte is decomposed by the electric current, the amount of decomposition is proportional to the quantitiy of electricity which flows through the solution. The second law states that when the same amount of electricity is passed though the solutions of different electrolytes, the weights of ions discharged are in the ratio of their chemical equivalents.

Laws of Impact *See impact.*

Laws of Motion *See motion.*

Laws of Planetary Motion Three laws, proposed by a German astronomer, **Johannes Kepler** (1571–1630), in 1609. The first stated that each planet moves in an elliptical orbit. The second law stated that the line joining the orbit to the sun sweeps out equal areas, in equal times. He announced a third law, in 1618, that the cube of the distances of a planet from the sun is proportional to the square of the time required by it to complete one orbit.

Laws of Thermodynamics *See heat, thermodynamics.*

Layard, Henry Austen (1817–1894) *See Babylon, bell, convex lens, Nineveh.*

Le Bel, Joseph Achille (1847–1930) *See stereochemistry.*

Lead Chamber Process A method used for the manufacture of sulfuric acid, invented in 1746 by **John Roebuck** (1718–1794), a physician from Sheffield, and **Samuel Garbett** (1717–1805). Roebuck later established a large lead chamber works at Prestonpans, near Edinburgh.

Lead Known to the Hebrews and Egyptians as early as 4000 BC; a lead figure from 3800 BC is in the British Museum. The hanging garden of Babylon had pans made of lead, and lead pipes have been found in the ruins of Rome and Pompeii. **Theophrastus** (373–287 BC) described the preparation of lead oxide by treating lead with vinegar, in 300 BC.

Lead Tetrachloride First prepared in 1850 by an Italian chemist, **Ascanio Sobrero** (1812–1888).

Leakey, Louis Seymour Bazett (1903–1972) *See Homo habilis, hominids, Zinjanthropus.*

Leakey, Mary Douglas (1913–1997) A London archaeologist whose excavations with her husband in Africa greatly contributed to knowledge of the origin of early humans. Their first important finding was the remains of a 1.7 million-year-old primitive ape, at Rusinga, in Lake Victoria, in 1948. *See hominids, Zinjanthropus.*

Leakey, Richard Erskin (b 1944) *See hominids.*

Lear, William Powell (1902–1978) *See car radio.*

Leaves The morphology of leaves as the basis of the classification of plants was used by **Lobelius** or **Matthias de l'Obel** (1538–1616) of The Netherlands, a botanist at the botanical garden of Queen Elizabeth I, in England. The terms simple, compound, pinnate and digitate to describe various forms of leaves were coined by a botanist from Lübeck, **Joachim Jung** (1587–1657). In 1667, **John Ray** (1628–1705), an English biologist from Essex, classified plants into monocots and dicots on the basis of the number of their seed leaves.

Leavitt, Henrietta Swan (1868–1921) *See astrophysics, Magellanic clouds, variable star.*

Leavitt's Period-Luminosity Law *See variable star.*

Lebedev, Pyotr Nicolayevich (1866–1912) *See Maxwell, James Clerk, radiation pressure.*

Lebesgue Integral A new approach to the theory of measure and integration, which later proved important to curve rectification, trigonometric series and the development of measure theory. It was introduced by a French mathematician, **Henri Léon Lebesgue** (1875–1941) of Beauvais. A Hungarian mathematician, **Frigyes Riesz** (1880–1956) developed a new approach to the Lebesgue integral and wrote a textbook on functional analysis in 1952.

Lebesgue, Henri Léon (1875–1941)   *See Lebesgue integral.*

Leblanc Process The first simple and cheap commercial method of producing soda or sodium bicarbonate from salt and sulfuric acid. Invented in 1791 by a French physician and industrial chemist, **Nicolas Leblanc** (1742–1806). An English industrial chemist, **William Gossage** (1799–1877) of Lincolnshire, invented the towers for the system, which prevented the release of its toxic unwanted product, hydrochloric acid, into the atmosphere. His invention led to the Alkali Act (1863) in England, which required manufacturers to ensure absorption of 95% of the hydrochloric acid released in industry. The Leblanc process was superseded by the ammonia-soda process (Solvay process), devised in 1866 by a Belgian industrial chemist, **Ernest Solvay** (1838–1922).

Leblanc, Nicolas (1742–1806)   *See Leblanc process.*

Lebon, Phillipe (1767–1804)   *See gas lighting.*

Leclanché Cell   *See zinc carbon cell.*

Leclanché, Georges (1839–1882)   *See zinc carbon cell.*

Lécluse, Charles de (1525–1609)   *See botany, mycology.*

Leder, Phillip (b 1934)   *See genetic coding.*

Lederberg, Joshua (b 1925)   *See genetic engineering.*

Lederman, Leon Max (b 1922)   *See neutrino.*

Lee, James Paris (1831–1904)   *See firearms.*

Lee, Tsung Dao (b 1926)   *See parity.*

Leeuwenhoek, Anthoni van (1632–1723)   *See crystallography, fermentology, microscope, parasitism, protozoa, staining, starch.*

Lefschetz, Solomon (1884–1972)   *See topology.*

Legendre Polynomials Offer solutions to second-order differential equations, later found to be important in applied mathematics. Proposed in 1783 by a French mathematician, **Adrien-Marie Legendre** (1752–1833) of Paris.

Legendre, Adrien-Marie (1752–1833)   *See law of quadratic reciprocity, Legendre polynomials, prime number.*

Lehn, Jean Marie (b 1939)   *See cell membrane.*

Leibniz, Gottfried Wilhelm (1646–1716)   *See aneroid barometer, calculating machine, calculus, coordinate, geogeny.*

Leicester, Thomas William Coke, Earl of (1752–1842)   *See animal husbandry.*

Leith, Emmett Norman (b 1927)   *See hologram.*

Lemaître, Henri George (1894–1966)   *See Big Bang theory.*

Lemery, Nicolas (1645–1715)   *See chemistry.*

Lemonnier, Pierre Charles (1715–1799)   *See Uranus.*

Lenard, Phillip Anton Eduard (1862–1947)   *See cathode rays.*

Lennard-Jones, Sir John Edward (1894–1954)   *See molecular orbital theory.*

Lenoir, Jean Joseph Etienne (1822–1900)   *See car, internal combustion engine, motor boat.*

Lenormand, Louis Sebastian (1757–1839)   *See parachute.*

Lenotre, André (1613–1700)   *See horticulture.*

Lenz, Heinrich Friedrich Emil (1804–1865)   *See Lenz's law.*

Lenz's Law The direction of a current that is induced by an electromagnetic force always opposes the direction of the force that produces it. A fundamental law in electromagnetism proposed in 1833 by a Russian-born German physicist, **Heinrich Friedrich Emil Lenz** (1804–1865).

Leonov, Aleksey Arkhipovich (b 1934)   *See astronauts.*

Lepsius, Karl Richard (1810–1884)   *See paleography.*

Le Roy, Pierre (1717–1785)   *See escapement.*

Le Roy, Julian (1686–1759) A clockmaker and father of **Pierre Le Roy** (1717–1785). He invented a bimetallic device to compensate for heat in chronometers.

Lescot, Pierre (1510–1578)   *See architecture, European.*

Leslie, Sir John (1766–1832)   *See aethrioscope, food industry, thermometer.*

Lesseps, Ferdinand Vicomte de (1805–1894)   *See canals.*

Leucippus (*c.* 500 BC) of Elea.   *See Abdera, atomic structure.*

Leupold, Jacob (b 1674)   *See machine, mechanical engineering.*

Levan, Albert (b 1905) *See chromosomes.*

Levene, Phoebus Aaron Theodore (1869–1940) *See deoxyribonucleic acid (DNA).*

Lever A rigid beam with a fulcrum to enable the force applied at one end to be transmitted to a point on the other side of the fulcrum. First studied by a Greek philosopher, **Strato of Lampsacus** (Turkey), around 330 BC. **Archimedes** (278–212 BC) demonstrated its principle by pulling a large ship onto land by himself. He developed the theory of the lever in his two books *On the Equilibrium of Planes*. **Jordanus Nemorarius** (*c.* 1200) proposed the law of the lever in his *Mechanica* in AD 1220.

Leverhulme, William Hesketh Lever (1851–1925) *See soap.*

Leverrier, Urbain Jean Joseph (1811–1877) *See Mercury (planet), Neptune.*

Levi-Civita, Tullio (1873–1941) *See calculus.*

Levinstein, Ivan (1845–1916) *See dyes.*

Lewis, Gilbert Newton (1875–1946) *See acid–base theory, deuterium, dissociation, photons, valency.*

Lewis, John Robert (b 1924) *See marine biology.*

Lewis, Paul (d 1759) *See textile industry.*

Leybourn, William (d 1696) *See surveying.*

Leyden Jar An early form of electrical capacitor, invented in 1746 by a Dutch physicist, **Pieter van Musschenbroek** (1692–1761) of Leyden. It was improved by a French Abbé, **Jean Antoine Nollet** (1700–1770), a professor of physics at the Collège de Navarre in Paris.

Li Ch'un (*c.* 600 BC) *See bridges.*

Libavius, Andreas or **Libau** (1540–1616) *See chemistry, distillation.*

Libby, Williard Frank (1908–1980) *See carbon dating.*

Libraries [Latin: *liber,* book] The earliest known collection of archives, in the form of clay tablets, was held by King Ashurbanipal (668–628 BC). The Alexandrian museum and library was established by Ptolemy I Soter (d 283 BC) around 284 BC, but it finally came to an end in the late 3rd century AD. It had four departments: literature, mathematics, astronomy and medicine, and was the largest in the world with over 400 000 volumes or rolls. The library at Pergamum in Asia Minor, established by King Eumenes II around 200 BC, had to resort to a different writing material, parchment, since Ptolemy V around 190 BC blocked the supply of papyrus from Egypt to this rival library. The earliest known public library was that in Athens, founded by Pisistratus in 540 BC. The Vatican Library was founded by Pope Nicholas V in 1447. Around this period the books were so valuable that they had to be chained to the shelves in the monastic libraries. Some of the monarchs had to obtain books on loan from these libraries. Harvard University library was formed in 1638. The libraries in Great Britain were formed in the following order: St Andrews (1411), Glasgow University (1473), Royal College of Physicians (1518), Bodleian, Oxford (1598), Royal Society (1667) and Radcliffe, Oxford (1714). Presently the largest one, the United States Library of Congress in Washington DC, was founded in 1800. The New York Public Library was established in 1895.

Lichtenstein, Martin Hinrich Carl (1780–1857) *See zoology.*

Lie Groups Transformation groups that provide the means to deduce, from the structure, the type of auxiliary equations needed for integration. Devised by a Norwegian mathematician, **Marius Sophus Lie** (1842–1899). He became professor of mathematics at the Christiana University, Oslo, in 1872 and published *Theorie der Transformationsgruppe* (1888–1893) and several other important works. A Russian mathematician, **Izrail Moiseyevich Gelfand** (b 1913), worked on the representation theory of Lie groups which later became relevant to quantum mechanics. Lie's work was reformulated by a French mathematician, **Elie Joseph Cartan** (1969–1951), who created the theory of Lie groups which is now considered fundamental to particle physics.

Lie, Marius Sophus (1842–1899) *See Lie groups.*

Liebermann, Theodore (1842–1914) *See dyes.*

Liebig, Justus von (1803–1873) A German chemist who is regarded as the father of industrial chemistry. He was apprenticed as an apothecary at the age of 16, before he entered Bonn University. After graduation, he served as an assistant at **Joseph Gay-Lussac's** (1778–1850) laboratory in Paris, at the age of 19. His first achievement was the discovery of the structure of fulminic acid. At 23 years, he was made professor of chemistry at Giessen, which under his direction became one of the greatest schools of chemistry in the world. Much of the early development in biochemistry was based on his books, *Chemistry in its Application to Agriculture and Physiology* (1840), and *Organic Chemistry in its Application to Physiology and Pathology* (1842). *See aldehyde, biochemistry, chemistry, fertilizers, pyridine, silver plating.*

Light Dispersion *See dispersion of light.*

Light The wave theory of light was first suggested by an Italian physicist, **Francesco Maria Grimaldi** (1618–1683) of Bologna, who described it in his *Physicomathesis de lumine* (1665). **Robert Hooke** (1635–1703) independently suggested it in England in the same year. **Sir Isaac Newton's** (1642–1727) corpuscular theory, and **Christian Huygens'** (1629–1695) undulatory or wave theory, were proposed towards the end of the 17th century, and Newton's theory came to be more accepted. The experimental evidence for the wave theory was provided independently by an English physician **Thomas Young** (1773–1829), and a French physicist **Jean Augustine Fresnel** (1788–1827). An important treatise on light, which differentiated between red and violet rays, was written by Young in 1802. *See absorption spectra, diffraction of light, dispersion of light, velocity of light.*

Lighthill, James (b 1924) British mathematician who pioneered the application of mathematics to high-speed aerodynamics and jet propulsion.

Lighthouses The first lighthouse, with a beacon, was installed in 1611 at Tour de Condonan at the mouth of the Garonne River, in France. A concrete lighthouse with mortar that sets under water was designed by an English engineer, **John Smeaton** (1724–1792) from Austhorpe, near Leeds. In 1819, a French physicist, **Jean Augustin Fresnel** (1788–1827) from Normandy, replaced the lighthouse reflectors with a system of lenses. His device, known as the lenticular apparatus, substituted refraction totally or partially with reflection. In the 18th century, a French engineer, Teluère, substituted parabolic mirrors for spherical ones, and invented the revolving light. A lighthouse of this nature was erected at Dieppe in 1784. **Robert Stevenson** (1772–1850) of Glasgow built 23 lighthouses in Scotland, and invented a system of flashing lights for the lighthouse on the Bell Rock, off Arbroath. The polyzonal lenses for lighthouses were invented in 1835 by an English physicist, **Sir David Brewster** (1781–1868). The Foreland lighthouse, in Kent, was the first to be equipped with an electric arc light, in 1858. Automatic acetylene lighting with light-controlled valves for unmanned lighthouses was invented by a Swedish engineer, **Nils Gustav Dalen** (1869–1937), who was awarded the Nobel Prize for Physics for his work in 1912.

Lightning An Italian scientist, **Giambatista Beccaria** (1716–1781), was one of the first to study atmosphoric electricity and lightning. His work *Dell' Elettricismo Artificiale e Naturale* was reviewed by the American statesman and scientist, **Benjamin Franklin** (1706–1790), who in 1747

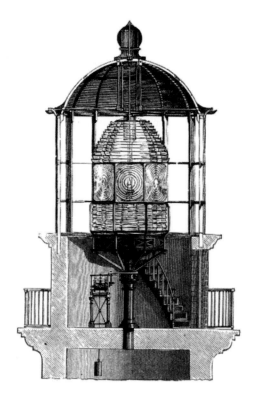

Figure 50 Fresnel's lenticular apparatus. Guillemin, Amédée. *The Applications of Physical Forces*. London: Macmillan and Co, 1877

discovered that a conductor can draw off electric charge from a charged body. This led to his invention of the lightning rod, in 1752. He used a kite to prove that lightning is a form of electricity. A surgeon at St Bartholomew's Hospital in London, John Freke, was the first in England to establish the association between lightning and electricity, in 1746. The causes of lightning were investigated by an English meteorologist, **Sir George Clark Simpson** (1878–1965) of Derby. Modern study of lightning flashes has revealed them to be a fourth stage of matter or state of ionized gases, known as plasma.

Light-Quantum Hypothesis The wave theory of light or energy, fundamental to quantum theory, was proposed in 1817 by an English physician, **Thomas Young** (1773–1829) who observed that light particles could behave like corpuscles and waves at the same time. An American physicist, **Gordon Hull** (1870–1956) developed the light-quantum hypothesis, which interprets light as a momentum bearing stream particles, similar to concentrations of energy or quanta. *See quantum theory.*

Lilienthal, Otto (1848–1896) *See airplane.*

Limelight Intense incandescent white light produced by heating lime with an oxyhydrogen flame, invented by **Goldsworthy Gurney** (1793–1875) from Treator, Cornwall, Great Britain. A Scottish statesman and inventor, **Thomas Drummond** (1794–1840), developed it and it bears his name.

Lindbergh, Charles Augustus (1902–1974) *See transatlantic flight.*

Lindblad, Bertil (1895–1965) *See galaxy.*

Linde, Karl von (1842–1934) *See oxygen, refrigerator.*

Lindemann, Carl Louis Ferdinand (1852–1939) *See pi.*

Lindley, John (1799–1865) *See Kew Gardens.*

Linear Induction Motor Production of continuous oscillation with the use of two linear motors, arranged back to back, without any switching device. First suggested in 1895, and developed by an English electrical engineer, **Eric Robert Laithwaite** (1920–1997) from Atherton, Yorkshire. It was used in the development of high-speed railways and other forms of transport.

Linnaeus, Carolus (1707–1778) A Swedish botanist (Carl von Linné) who travelled widely studying plants. He introduced the binomial system of classification of plants and animals to include the genus and species as names. Higher classifications of genera included classes and orders. This is the basis of modern taxonomy. Linnaeus described 11 800 species. His works include *Systema Naturae* (1735), *Fundamenta Botanica* (1736), *Genera Plantarum* (1737) and *Classes Plantarum* (1738).

Linnean Society A botanical society founded in 1788 and named after the Swedish botanist, **Carolus Linnaeus** (1707–1778). **James Edward Smith** (1759–1828) of Norwich was one of its founder members and first president. The society started publishing its *Transactions* in 1791. **George Bentham** (1800–1884), a British botanist from Devon, served as president of the Society from 1863 to 1874.

Linnett, John Wilfred (1913–1975) English chemist from Coventry whose work on explosion limits on the reaction between carbon monoxide, hydrogen, and oxygen, led to the study of atomic reactions on surfaces of metal alloys. In 1960 he proposed a modification to the octet rule concerning valency electrons.

Linoleum [Latin: *linum, flax + oleum,* oil] A floor material with a coat of oxidized oil, invented in 1860 by an English inventor, Frederick Walton.

Linotype Printing A type of printing with a lines of types, similar to the function of a large typewritter, which speeded up typesetting and revolutionized the printing industry. It was invented in 1884 by a German-born American inventor, **Ottomar Mergenthaler** (1854–1899), who emigrated to America around 1872. His linotype was first used in 1886 for printing the *New York Tribune.*

Liouville Theorem Complex function on the plane which is not a constant and must become infinite. Proposed by a French mathematician, **Joseph Liouville** (1809–1882).

Liouville, Joseph (1809–1882) *See Liouville theorem, scientific journals.*

Lipmann, Fritz (1899–1986) A German-born US biochemist who studied the mechanism of cell energy and pointed out the crucial role played by energy-rich phosphate molecule adenosine triphosphate (ATP). He shared the Nobel Prize for Physiology or Medicine in 1953 with Hans Krebs.

Lippershey, Hans (1571–1619) *See compound microscope, spectacles, telescope.*

Lippincott, Joshua Ballinger (1813–1886) *See bookshops.*

Lippmann, Gabriel Jonas (1845–1921) *See capillary electrometer, color photography.*

Lipschitz Algebra Complex system of number theory developed by a German mathematician Rudolf Otto Sigismund Lipschitz (1832–1903). He did extensive studies on Fourier series, differential equations and calculus of variations, and published *Grundlagen der Analysis* (1877–80).

Lipscomb, William Nunn (b 1919) *See boron.*

Liquefaction of Gases The first attempt at this was made independently by two English scientists, **Thomas Northmore** (1766–1851) and **Michael Faraday** (1791–1867). The method was refined by **Thomas Andrews** (1813–1885), a professor of chemistry, in Belfast. A French physicist, **Louis Paul Cailletet** (1832–1913) from Châtillon-sur-Seine, was the first to liquefy oxygen, hydrogen and nitrogen, in 1877. **Sir James Dewar** (1843–1923), of the Royal Institution in London, devised a method to liquefy large quantities of air and oxygen.

Lissajous Figures Obtained as a resultant of two simple harmonic motions at right angles to one another, and used for the visual demonstration of vibrations that produce sound waves. Devised by a French physicist, **Jules Antoine Lissajous** (1822–1880) from Versailles, who served as professor of physics at the Lycée Saint-Louis.

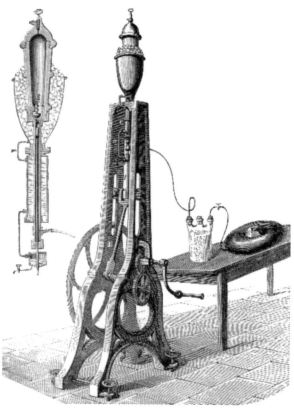

Figure 51 A mid-19th century apparatus for liquefaction of gases. Atkinson, E. *Elementary Treatise on Physics*. London: Longmans, Green, and Co, 1872

Lissajous, Jules Antoine (1822–1880) *See acoustics, Lissajous figures*.

Lister, Joseph Jackson (1786–1869) *See achromatic lens*.

Lister, Lord Joseph (1827–1912) The initiator of antisepsis in surgery and son of **Joseph Jackson Lister** (1786–1869).

Lister, Martin (1638–1712) *See fossils, geological map*.

Lister, Samuel Cunliffe (1815–1906) *See air brake, textile industry*.

Lithium [Greek: *lithos,* stone] Its compounds were discovered in 1818 by a Swedish chemist, **Johan August Arfwedson** (1792–1841) of Stockholm. A German chemist, **Leopold Gmelin** (1788–1853), observed its characteristic red flame in the same year. The metal was discovered later by **Sir Humphry Davy** (1778–1829). **Robert Bunsen** (1811–1899) obtained it in a metallic state through electrolysis, in 1855.

Lithography [Greek: *lithos,* stone + *graphein,* to write] The art of engraving on stone was invented in 1795 by a Bavarian

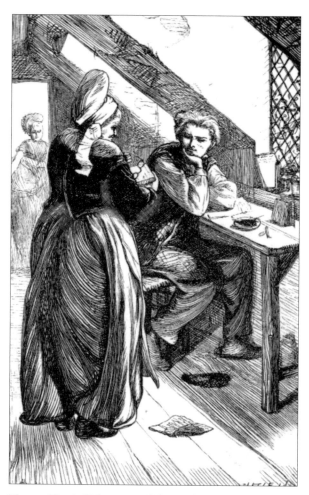

Figure 52 A 19th century lithograph. Temple, Ralph and Chandos. *Invention and Discovery*. London: Hodder and Stoughton, 1893

printer and playwright, **Alois Sennefelder** (1771–1834), born in Prague. He observed the effect of drawing with chalk on a wet stone, and made his discovery. His first printed work was some pieces of music, in 1796. After obtaining a patent in 1799, he failed to establish a trade in London, but was successful in Vienna in 1800. In 1806 Professor Mittner in Munich used a lithographic technique to multiply the copies of his work, for his pupils. Lithography was introduced into England in 1795 and was made a success by **Rudolph Ackermann** (1764–1834), who came from Saxony, during the French revolution and established a print shop in London.

Llewellyn, Dalziel (1887–1966) A London chemist who discovered the process of decarboxylation of quinaldinic acid by aldehydes and ketones.

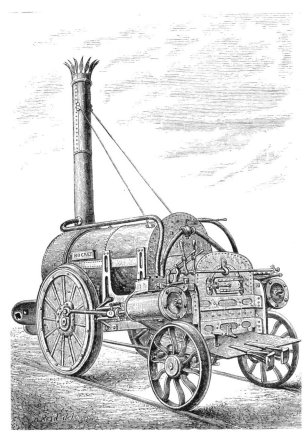

Figure 53 The *Rocket*. Guillemin, Amédée. *The Applications of Physical Forces*. London: Macmillan and Co, 1877

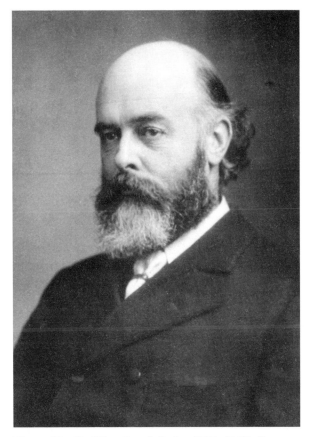

Figure 54 Sir Oliver Joseph Lodge (1851–1940). Courtesy of the National Library of Medicine

Lliboutry, Louis Antonin François (b 1922)   *See glaciology, tectonic theory.*

Lloyd, Humphrey (1800–1881)   An Irish scientist at Trinity College, Dublin, who discovered a method of producing interference fringes with a single mirror.

Lobachevskian Geometry   *See non-Euclidean geometry.*

Lobaschevsky, Nikolai Ivanovich (1793–1856)   *See hyperbolic geometry.*

Lobelius or **Matthias de l'Obel** (1538–1616)   *See botany, dicotyledon, monocotyledon.*

Lock   A Greek sculptor, **Theodorus** (*c.* 530 BC) from the island of Samos is credited with the invention of smelting metals for the purpose of making objects such as locks and keys. An effective lock was patented in 1784 by a London engineer and cabinet maker, **Joseph Bramah** (1748–1814) from Stainborough, Yorkshire, and it remained unpicked until 1851. Several improved locks in London were patented by an English locksmith, **Charles Chubb** (1777–1846). His

son **John Chubb** (1816–1872) took out further patents. **Linus Yale** (1821–1868) of Salisbury, New York, invented several types of lock including a small cylinder device, known by his name.

Locke, John (1632–1704)   *See perception.*

Locke, Joseph (1805–1860)   *See railway.*

Locks   *See canals.*

Lockyer, Sir Norman Joseph (1836–1920)   *See astrophysics, helium, scientific journals.*

Locomotive   A Cornish engineer, **George Trevithick** (1771–1833), built the first steam locomotive that ran on an iron plateway, and he demonstrated it at Coalbrookdale, Shropshire, in 1803. In 1829, **George Stephenson** (1781–1848) of Newcastle demonstrated his steam locomotive, the *Rocket,* which reached a speed of 30 miles an hour. Following Stephenson's improvement of the steam engine, steam locomotives became established around the country in England and in the rest of Europe around 1835. **Timothy**

Hackworth (1786–1850) of Northumberland, a rival locomotive engineer to Stephenson, built several locomotives including the *Royal George* and *Sans Pareil*. A Scottish engineer, **Patrick Stirling** (1820–1895) of Kilmarnock, together with his brother **James Stirling** (1835–1917) and cousin **Archibald Sturrock** (1816–1919), built several locomotives. His *Stirling Single* in 1870 was known for its power and speed. **Peter Cooper** (1791–1883), an inventor and philanthropist from New York, built the first locomotive engine in America, in Baltimore, in 1830. **Robert Livingston Stevens** (1787–1856) of Hoboken, New Jersey, was the first to use anthracite coal for a locomotive. An American industrialist and locomotive engineer, **Matthias William Baldwin** (1795–1866) from Elizabethtown, New Jersey, started manufacturing steam engines in 1827, and built his first locomotive *Old Ironsides,* in 1832. By 1861, he had built over 1000 locomotives at his factory, which became the world's largest producer of locomotives. An English-born Australian industrialist, **Thomas Sutcliffe Mort** (1816–1878), built the first Australian locomotive at his factory in 1870. In 1869, an American engineer, **George Westinghouse** (1846–1914) of New York, invented air brakes, a device which allowed a locomotive safely to apply uniform and simultaneous brakes to all carriages. An electric locomotive was developed in 1883 by a German-born British engineer, **Karl Wilhelm Siemens**, later **Sir Charles William Siemens** (1823–1883). Early diesel locomotives were built in Germany in 1912. An English engineer, **William Arthur Stanier** (1876–1965) of Swindon, designed many successful locomotives from 1932 to 1942. In 1938, **Sir Herbert Nigel Gresley** (1876–1941), of Edinburgh, built a high-speed steam locomotive that achieved a record speed of 126 miles per hour.

Lodestone *See iron, magnet, physics.*

Lodge, Sir Oliver Joseph (1851–1940) The first professor of physics at Liverpool, who applied the coherer to the production of wireless telegraphy. In 1894, he demonstrated to the British Royal Society that messages could be sent and received without wires. *See ether, electromagnetic theory.*

Loeb, Jacques (1859–1924) A biologist from Germany who graduated from Strasburg in 1884. He emigrated to America in 1891, and served as the head of experimental biology at the Rockefeller Institute for Medical Research from 1910 to 1924.

Logan, William Edmund (1798–1875) *See paleozoic period.*

Logarithms A German monk, **Michael Stifel** (1487–1567), in his *Arithmetica Integra* (1544), compared geometric and arithmetic progressions. This work contained the elements of logarithms, invented later by a Scottish mathematician **John Napier** (1550–1617). In 1594, Napier used logarithms for the purpose of simplifying calculations and published *Mirifici Logarithmorum Canonis Descriptio* (Description of the marvellous Canon of Logarithms) in 1614. His method was completed in 1616 by **Henry Briggs** (1561–1631) of Oxford, whose common logarithms were based on the power of 10. **Joost Bürgi** (1552–1632) of Switzerland independently discovered logarithms in 1620. A table of logarithms to seven places of decimals of sines and tangents of angles, was introduced by an English mathematician and astronomer, **Edmund Gunter** (1581–1626) of Hertfordshire, in the same year. A French mathematician and astronomer, **Nicolaus Louis de Lacaille** (1713–1762) published a table of logarithms in 1760.

Lomonosov, Mikhail Vasilievich (1711–1765) *See earth, glass, Venus.*

London Mathematical Society Founded in 1865 with an English mathematician **Augustus De Morgan** (1806–1871) as its first president.

London, Fritz Wolfgang (1900–1954) *See superconductivity.*

London, Heinz (1907–1970) *See superconductivity.*

London Equation *See superconductivity.*

Londsdale, William (1794–1871) *See Silurian period.*

Longomontanus, Christian Sörensen (1562–1647) *See observatories.*

Longuet-Higgins, Christopher (b 1923) *See molecular orbital theory, polymer.*

Lonsdale, Dame Kathleen (1903–1971) An Irish X-ray crystallographer from Droichead Nua, County Kildare who worked with **William Henry Bragg** (1862–1942) at University College, London. She was one of the first to determine the structures of organic molecules. *See X-ray crystallography.*

Loomis, Mahlon (1826–1886) *See kite, wireless telegraphy.*

Lorentz, Hendrik Antoon (1853–1928) *See dispersion of light, Lorentz–Lorenz formula, Zeeman effect.*

Lorentz–Lorenz Formula The mathematical relationship between the refractive index and the density of a medium. Independently published by a Danish mathematician, **Ludwig Valentin Lorenz** (1829–1891) in 1869, and a Dutch physicist, **Hendrik Antoon Lorentz** (1853–1928) of Leyden.

Lorenz, Konrad Zacharias (1903–1989) A physician, zoologist and pioneer in the study of ethology. He was the son of an eminent orthopedic surgeon, Adolf Lorenz (1854–1946) of Vienna, and took his doctorates in medicine and zoology respectively in 1928 and 1933. He published his first paper *Observations on Jackdaws* in 1927. *See ethology.*

Lorenz, Ludwig Valentin (1829–1891) *See dispersion of light, Lorentz–Lorenz formula.*

Loschmidt Number The number of molecules estimated in a given volume of gas at zero degrees Celsius and atmospheric pressure. Proposed in 1865 by an Austrian chemist, **Johann Joseph Loschmidt** (1821–1895).

Loschmidt, Johann Joseph (1821–1895) *See Loschmidt number.*

Lotze, Rudolf Herman (1817–1881) A German physician of Saxony, and one of the founders of physiological psychology. He opposed the popular theory of vitalism.

Loudon, John Claudius (1783–1843) *See horticulture.*

Loudspeaker or speaking trumpet. An instrument by which the voice can be heard at a much greater distance than normal. The manuscript *De Secretis ad Alexandrum Magnum* by **Aristotle** (384–322 BC), describes in detail a large horn used for this purpose by **Alexander's** (355–323 BC) army. The Grecians used a wind instrument with amplified bellowing sound to frighten away wild animals. An Englishman, **Samuel Moreland** (1625–1696), invented a loudspeaker, and made several experiments on the speaking trumpet before publishing a paper in 1671. The Jesuit priest **Athanasius Kircher** (1601–1680) of Geysen, who made an extensive study of the loudspeaker, also claimed priority for its invention. A modern form was invented by Horace Short of England in 1900.

Love, Augustus Edward Hough (1863–1940) *See elasticity.*

Lovelace, Countess Augusta Ada (1815–1852) *See Ada.*

Lovell, Sir Alfred Charles Bernard (b 1913) An English radio astronomer who applied the science of radar to the study of astronomy. In 1950, he discovered that galactic radio sources emitted at a constant wavelength and the fluctuations recorded on the earth's surface were a result of these radio waves crossing the ionosphere. He published *Radio Astronomy* (1951) and *The Exploration of Outer Space* (1961). *See radar.*

Lovelock, James Ephraim (b 1919) *See Gaia hypothesis.*

Low, William (1818–1886) *See Channel tunnel.*

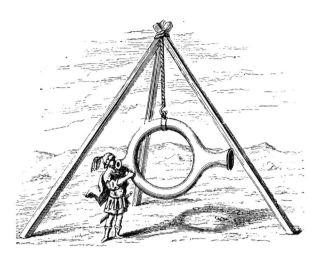

Figure 55 Alexander's trumpet. Guillemin, Amédée. *The Applications of Physical Forces.* London: Macmillan and Co, 1877

Lowell, Francis Cabot (1775–1817) An American industrialist who was mainly responsible for introducing new British textile technology to America. He established the Boston Manufacturing Company, a mechanized textile mill at Waltham, Massachusetts.

Lowell Observatory US astronomical observatory founded in 1896 by **Percival Lowell** (1855–1916) at Flagstaff, Arizona.

Lowell, Percival (1855–1916) *See Lowell Observatory, Mars, Pluto.*

Lowig, Carl (1803–1890) *See bromine.*

Lowontin, Richard Charles (b 1929) *See electrophoresis.*

Lowry, Thomas Martin (1874–1936) An English chemist from Bradford who experimentally confirmed the equation related to optical rotatory power and wavelength. His work confirmed that optical activity depends on the wavelength of light. He published *Historical Introduction to Chemistry*.

Lubbock, Sir John (1834–1913) or Lord Avebury. Born in London, and as a politician, he was responsible for the introduction of bank holidays in 1871, and the Shop Hours Act of 1889. He was also the president of the Anthropological Institute and in 1865 proposed the use of the terms Paleolithic (Old Stone Age) and Neolithic (New Stone Age), based on rough and smooth stone implements. He was elevated to the peerage in 1900, and he published several works on geology and ethnology. His *Prehistoric Times* on the study of ancient customs and manners is a well-known work. His work on entomology *Ants, Bees, and Wasps* was published in 1882.

A Dictionary of the History of Science

Lucretius (98–55 BC) *See atomic structure, evolution, magnet.*

Lumière, Auguste Marie Louis (1862–1954) *See cinema.*

Lumière, Louis Jean (1864–1948) *See cinema.*

Lummer, Otto Richard (1860–1925) *See black body radiation.*

Luneburg Lens Used in microwave antennae, invented by a German-born US physicist and optical scientist, **Rudolf Karl Luneberg** (1903–1949).

Luneburg, Rudolf Karl (1903–1949) *See Luneburg lens.*

Lutecia A rare earth, and source of the element, lutecium, named after the ancient Paris. It was discovered by a US chemist, **Charles James** (1880–1928), who was born in Northampton, England, and educated at University College London. He emigrated to America and became professor of chemistry at University of New Hampshire. However, a French professor of chemistry at the Sorbonne, **Georges Urbain** (1872–1938) published his results in 1907, before James, and was credited with the discovery.

Lwoff, André Michel (1902–1994) *See genetic engineering.*

Lyceum A school established by **Aristotle** (384–322 BC) in 336 BC. It was called, the peripatetic school (Greek: *peri,* around + *pateo,* walk) as the pupils were taught while they walked about its neighbourhood. It was closed by Emperor Justinian (AD 483–565) in AD 529.

Lyell, Sir Charles (1797–1875) *See Eocene Period, Miocene Period, Pliocene Period.*

Lyman, Theodore (1874–1954) A physicist of Boston, Massachusetts, and a pioneer in ultraviolet spectroscopy. He discovered the fundamental series of spectral lines for hydrogen, which is named after him. He served as professor of mathematics and natural philosophy at Harvard from 1921 to 1926.

Lyot, Bernard Ferdinand (1897–1952) A French astronomer who improved the coronograph and made it possible to observe the sun's corona in daylight rather than only during eclipses. His coronagraph permitted the observation of continuous changes in the corona making it possible for the corona to be filmed.

Lysenko, Trofim Denisovich (1898–1976) *See vernalization.*

Lysosome A cell organelle involved in intracellular digestion. Discovered by a British-born Belgian biochemist, **Christian René de Duve** (b 1917), who was awarded the Nobel Prize in Physiology or Medicine in 1974.

Lyttleton, Raymond Arthur (1911–1995) An English astronomer from Birmingham who studied stellar evolution and in 1959 with Hermann Bondi proposed the electrostatic theory of the expanding universe.

M

Macadamizing A method of preparing a road surface, with a firm base of large stones, and a layer of small stones with gravel on top, so as to give a convex shape for draining off water. Invented by a Scottish civil engineer, **John Loudon McAdam** (1756–1836) from Ayr, who was a pioneer in Britain on road construction, and published *Remarks on the Present System of Road Making* (1816).

MacCready, Paul (b 1925) *See solar energy.*

Macculloch, John (1773–1835) *See petrology.*

Mach Number The velocity of a body in a medium, relative to the velocity of sound in the same medium. An important concept in the study of projectiles and speed of aircrafts, proposed by an Austrian physicist, **Ernst Mach** (1838–1916), who was appointed professor of experimental physics at the University of Prague in 1867. It was introduced as a practical scale for the speed of aircraft by Professor Ackeret of Switzerland.

Mach, Ernst (1838–1916) *See Mach number, supersonic flight.*

Machine Defined in 1724 by **Jacob Leupold** (b 1674) of Planitz, Germany, as an artificial arrangement by means of which we are able to perform a beneficial movement, that is, to move something with economy of time and energy, which would not be possible in any other manner. *See machine tools, mechanical engineering.*

Machine Gun *See firearms.*

Machine Tools A Parisian clock and instrument maker, **Antoine Thiout** (1692–1767), was a pioneer in the field, who developed the earliest fusee engines. He invented the first screw-cutting lathe, which incorporated a toolpost with a longitudinal movement, around 1741. The modern lathe was invented in 1778 by an English iron-master, **John Wilkinson** (1728–1808) of Clifton, Cumberland. The first practical machine tools were produced by a London engineer, **Henry Maudslay** (1771–1831) of Woolwich around 1792. He invented the slide rest for the lathe, which allowed the operator to use the lathe without holding the metal-cutting instruments in his hands. One of his apprentices **Sir Joseph Whitworth** (1803–1887), from Stockport, invented several devices including a screw-measuring machine or bench micrometer, and a screw-cutting lathe.

Joseph Clement (1779–1844) built several planing machines, from 1817 to 1820. A Manchester boiler-maker, William Fairbairn, invented a riveting machine in 1838. The first steam-operated riveting machine was built by **François Cavé** (b 1794) of France. A leading British tool manufacturer, **Richard Roberts** (1789–1864) from Wales, invented several machines, including one for punching holes in steel plates, and a planing machine. In France, a mechanic and instrument maker, **Henri Prudence Gambey** (1787–1847), constructed lathes with toolposts, allowing movement across and along the bed controlled by micrometer screws. He is known for his several other advanced machine tools. *See lathe.*

Macintosh, Charles (1766–1843) *See bleaching powder, Macintosh cloth.*

Macintosh Cloth Waterproof cloth made out of rubber, invented by a Scottish industrial chemist, **Charles Macintosh** (1766–1843) of Glasgow, who patented the process in 1823. He started making it on a commercial basis with **Thomas Hancock** (1786–1865) of Manchester. Some historians have credited the Edinburgh surgeon **James Syme** (1799–1870) with the invention of waterproof cloth.

Maclaurin, Colin (1698–1746) A Scottish mathematician who developed Newton's work on fluxions and wrote an original work *A Treatise on Fluxions* (1742) and *Geometrica Organica* (1720). He became one of the youngest professors in Britain at Marischal College, Aberdeen, at the age of 19.

Macleod, John James Rickard (1876–1935) *See insulin.*

Maclure, William (1763–1840) *See geological map.*

Macmillan, Kirkpatrick (1813–1878) *See bicycle, tricycle.*

Macquer, Pierre Joseph (1718–1784) *See chemistry, porcelain.*

Macquorn, William John (1820–1872) *See potential energy.*

Macrobius, Ambrosius Aurel (c. AD 400) *See tides.*

Mädler, Johann Heinrich (1794–1874) *See Mars.*

Magellan, Ferdinand (1480–1522) A Portuguese navigator and explorer who was the first to sail around the world.

Magellanic Clouds Two relatively small nebular star clusters having a diameter of 25 000 light years, which lie at a distance of 170 000 light years, and separate from the Milky Way. They were discovered in 1921 and studied by an American astronomer, Henrietta Swan Leavitt (1868–1921) of Lancaster, Massachusetts at the Harvard Observatory. See galaxy.

Magendie, François (1783–1855) *See nutrition.*

Magnesium An earth metal discovered by an English chemist, **Sir Humphry Davy** (1778–1829), and named after the town of *Magnesia*, in Thessaly.

Magnet The magnetic properties of lodestone and amber were known to the ancients including the Greek philosopher, **Thales** (640–546 BC), around 600 BC. According to the Roman poet and philosopher **Lucretius** (98–55 BC), the magnet derives its name from its presence in the earth material, magnesia, found near Macedonia. According to **Pliny the Elder** (AD 28–79), a physician and poet **Nicander** (*c.* 140 BC) believed that it was named after a man, *Magnes*, who first observed it in Mount Ida. One of the first scientific treatises on the subject was written by a 13th century French scholar, **Peter Peregrinus** (b *c.* 1220) who described a simple compass consisting of a piece of magnetized iron on a floating wooden block in his *Epistola de Magnete* (1269). He introduced the term poles for the ends of a natural magnet. *See dip.*

Magnetic Dip *See compass, dip.*

Magnetic Needle An English scholar, **Alexander Neckham** (1157–1217) of St Albans, was the first in Europe to describe the use of a magnetic needle by sailors, in his *De Naturis rerum* and *De utensilibus*. The first Arabic treatise on the magnetic needle, as a ship's compass, was written by **Baylak al-Qibaji** (*c.* 1350) of Cairo. The tendency of the magnetic needle not only to turn towards the north but also to swing down from the horizontal was first observed in Europe by a London navigator and naval instrument maker, **Robert Norman** (1550–1600). His experiments were the first step towards the idea of a magnetic field, and he published *The Newe Attractive shewing The Nature Propertie and manifold vertures of the Loadstone with the Declination of the Needle*. The variation of the compass needle with time and place was described by **Henry Gellibrand** (1597–1636) in his treatise *A Discourse Mathematical on the Variation of the Magnetic Needle, together with its admirable Diminution lately discovered* (1635). In 1819, a Danish physicist, **Hans Christian Oersted** (1777–1851), demonstrated that a magnetic needle could be deflected by an electric current, and that its movements depended on the direction of the current.

Magnetic Poles The magnetic poles refer to positions towards which the needle of a magnetic compass will point. They differ from the geographical poles by angle of declination or magnetic variation, which varies at different points of the earth's surface and at different times. A teacher of navigation in London, Henry Bond, in his book *Longitude*

Found (1676), assumed that there were two magnetic poles, distinct from the geographical poles. A Scottish naval officer and polar explorer, **Sir James Clark Ross** (1800–1862) and his uncle **Sir John Ross** (1777–1856) located the magnetic north pole in 1831. A Yorkshire-born geologist in Australia, **Sir Douglas Mawson** (1882–1958), who joined the scientific staff of **Sir Ernest Henry Shackleton's** (1874–1922) Antarctic expedition in 1907, mapped the position of the south magnetic pole. A Norwegian explorer **Roald Engelbrecht Gravning Amundsen** (1872–1928) located the magnetic north pole. *See North Pole, South Pole.*

Magnetic Recording Involves the application of electrical impulses, which correspond to the sounds to be recorded on a magnetized metallic base. A prototype, using a steel wire, was invented in 1898 by a Danish electrical engineer, **Valdemar Poulsen** (1869–1942). Research into the magnetic properties of ferrimagnetic materials by a French physicist, **Louis Eugène Félix Néel** (b 1904), led to the coating of magnetic tapes. In 1970, he shared the Nobel Prize for physics with a Swedish physicist, **Hannes Olof Gösta Alfvén** (1908–1995). An American inventor, J.A. O'Neill, improved the magnetic recording wire by replacing it with diamagnetic ribbon, in 1927. Fritz Pfleumer of Germany discovered the method of coating strips of paper with magnetic materials, in 1928. Cellulose acetate tape started to be used in Germany around 1930. The compact cassette was invented at the Philips company in the Netherlands in 1963. A method for eliminating background sounds during magnetic recording was invented in 1967 by **Raymond M. Dolby** (b 1933). *See dictaphone, musical recording, tape recorder.*

Magnetic Resonance Imaging (MRI) A resonance method for precisely measuring magnetic moments, for the study of fundamental particles or atomic nuclei. It was developed by the Austrian-American physicist **Isidor Isaac Rabi** (1898–1988) and a German-American physicist **Polykarp Kusch** (1911–1993), in 1937. Kusch shared the Nobel Prize for physics for this work with **Willis Eugene Lamb** (b 1913), in 1955. The magnetic imaging was demonstrated independently in 1946 by a Zurich-born American physicist, **Felix Bloch** (1905–1983), a professor at Stanford University, and **Edward Mills Purcell** (1912–1997) of Illinois, who shared the Nobel Prize for physics in 1952. A Los Angeles chemist, **John D. Roberts** (b 1918), developed nuclear magnetic resonance (NMR) spectroscopy for the study of organic molecules. MRI continued to be used for over 40 years to study molecular structure in organic chemistry, until a Swedish physicist, Erik Odeblad, applied it to the study of living tissues, around 1960. An English chemist, **Sir Rex Edward Richards** (b 1922), later vice-chancellor of Oxford

University, made a significant contribution to the development of the NMR scan, as a diagnostic technique in medicine, in the late 1960s. A German chemist, **Heinrich Nöth** (b 1928) of Munich, developed NMR spectroscopy for analyzing inorganic material. High-resolution nuclear magnetic imaging spectroscopy was refined by a Swiss professor **Richard Robert Ernst** (b 1933), who was awarded the Nobel Prize for chemistry in 1991.

Magnetic Storm A disturbance in the earth's normal pattern of magnetism due to solar activity, related to sunspots. An English physical chemist from Lancashire, **Sydney Chapman** (1888–1979), proposed the first satisfactory theory for magnetic storms.

Magnetic Theory The French physicist **André Marie Ampère** (1775–1836) believed that magnetization was due to molecular currents in the particles of magnetizable material. A Norwegian naturalist, **Kristoph Hansteen** (1784–1883), investigated terrestrial magnetism and proposed a law of magnetic force, in 1821. A German physicist, **Wilhelm Eduard Weber** (1804–1891) from Wittenberg, suggested a similar theory. A French physicist, **Paul Langevin** (1872–1946) of Paris, applied the electron theory to magnetic phenomena, and deduced an important formula related to paramagnetic movement of molecules, in 1905. *See hysteresis.*

Magnetohydrodynamics Study of plasmas or ionized gases in a magnetic field. Developed by a Swedish astrophysicist, **Hannes Olof Gösta Alfvén** (1908–1995), who was awarded the Nobel Prize for physics in 1970. *See plasma physics.*

Magnetosphere A zone of high levels of radiation (Van Allen Belts) caused by trapped charged particles surrounding the earth. Discovered by an American physicist, **James Alfred Van Allen** (b 1914), who was professor of physics at the University of Iowa.

Magnetron A thermionic valve for generating high ultra-frequency oscillations of electromagnetic waves, used in the development of radar. *See radar.*

Magnus Effect The swerving of a golf or tennis ball when hit, due to the sideways force. Discovered and described by a German physicist, **Heinrich Gustav Magnus** (1802–1870), who became professor of technology and physics at the University of Berlin in 1845. He made his discovery in 1853 during his investigation of the flow of air over rotating cylinders for aerodynamic studies.

Magnus, Heinrich Gustav (1802–1870) *See Magnus effect.*

Mahavira (AD 850) *See mathematics.*

Maiden, Joseph Henry (1859–1925) A London botanist who in 1880 emigrated to Australia, where he became the first curator of the Sydney Technological Museum, in 1881. He served as Director of the Sydney Botanical Gardens (1896–1924), and published several important books on the flora of Australia.

Maillet, Benoit de (1656–1738) *See evolution.*

Maiman, Theodore Harold (b 1927) *See laser.*

Malinowski, Bronislaw Kasper (1884–1942) A social anthropologist who was professor at London University (1927) and Yale (1939). He published *Sex and Repression in Savage Society* (1927) and *The Sexual Life of Savages in N.W. Melanesia* (1929).

Malpighi, Marcello (1628–1694) *See cell, invertebrates, mycology, nitrogen fixing bacteria, plant physiology.*

Malthus, Thomas Robert (1766–1834) *See evolution.*

Malus Law *See polarization.*

Malus, Étienne Louis (1775–1812) *See polarization.*

Management Important concepts such as searching, finding, selecting, and assembling, in scientific management and efficiency, were proposed and studied by an American engineer, **Frank Bunker Gilbreth** (1868–1924). He started his career as a bricklayer and studied the basic elements in manual labor, with his wife **Lilian Evelyn Gilbreth** née **Molder** (1879–1972). An American engineer, **Frederick Winslow Taylor** (1856–1915), introduced time and motion study as an aid to efficient management and published *The Principles of Scientific Management and Shop Management* (1903).

Mandelbrot Set Constructed from simple mapping, by marking dots on a complex plane. Proposed by a Polish-born US mathematician, **Benoit Mandelbrot** (b 1924).

Mandelbrot, Benoit (b 1924) *See fractal, Mandelbrot set.*

Manganese Its oxide was known to the Romans who used it for decolorizing glass. A Swedish chemist and mineralogist, **Johan Gottlieb Gahn** (1745–1818), discovered metallic manganese in 1774. It derives its name from the town of *Magnesia* in Thessaly.

Manhattan Project War-time project for developing the atom bomb. *See atomic bomb, chain reaction.*

Mannesman Method A method of making a seamless steel tube, invented by a German steel industrialist, **Renihard**

Mannesman (1856–1922). It was demonstrated at the Chicago World Exhibition in 1893.

Mannesman, Renihard (1856–1922) *See Mannesman method.*

Mantell, Gideon Algernon (1790–1852) *See dinosaurs.*

Manton, Sidnie Milana (1902–1979) *See invertebrates.*

Manutius Aldus (d 1516) *See typography.*

Map *See atlas, cartography, geography, globe.*

Marcellus, Claudius (d 209 BC) *See military engineering.*

Marci, J.M. (1595–1667) *See dispersion of light.*

Marconi, Guglielmo Marchese (1874–1937) *See broadcasting, radar, radio waves, wireless telegraphy.*

Marcov Numbers A series of random variables in mathematics, named after the Russian mathematician, **Andrei Andreevich Markov** (1856–1922). He was appointed professor of mathematics at the University of St Petersburg in 1893 and published *Probability Calculus* (1900).

Marcus, Rudolph Arthur (b 1923) *See Marcus theory.*

Marcus Theory Related to electron transfer in reactions involving ions or molecules in solution. Developed by a Canadian physicist, **Rudolph Arthur Marcus** (b 1923). He was awarded the Nobel Prize for chemistry in 1992, for his work on oxidation and reduction reactions.

Margarine [Latin: *magarita*, a pearl] The French government offered a prize for a satisfactory substitute for butter, and this was won by **Hippolyte Mège Mouriès** (1817–1880), who invented the margarine in 1869. In 1872, F. Boudet made the product palatable and patented a process for emulsifying it with skim milk and water. His product, when chilled with ice-cold water, gave a pearly texture, hence its name.

Marggrafe, Andreas Sigismond (1709–1782) *See aluminum, beet sugar.*

Marignac, Jean Charles Gallisard de (1817–1894) *See gadolinium, ozone, yttrium.*

Marilaun, Anton Joseph Kerner von (1831–1898) *See ecology.*

Marine Archaeology Established as a science by an American, **Peter Throckmorton** (1928–1990). In 1960, he discovered the oldest wreck in the world dating back to 1200 BC, in the Mediterranean Sea. In 1975, he explored the Aegean Sea and discovered a sunken cargo ship of the Bronze Age. He published *The Lost Ships* (1964) and *Shipwrecks and Archaeology: The Unharvested Sea* (1970).

Marine Biology Two of the earliest works, *The Natural History of Strange Marine Fish* (1551) and *On Aquatic Life* (1553), were published by **Pierre Belon** (1517–1574), who dissected several marine animals such as dolphins, whales and fishes. The book of a French naturalist and physician, **Guillaume Rondelet** (1507–1566), the *Book of Marine Fish*, appeared in 1554 in Lyons, and a Latin version of it, *The Complete History of Fish*, was published in 1558. The term aquarium was coined by an English naturalist, **Phillip Henry Gosse** (1810–1988) from Worcester, whose special interest was coastal marine biology in Jamaica. He published *History of British Sea-anemones and Corals* (1860), *Manual of Marine Zoology* (1855–1856) and several books on natural history. Another British naturalist, from the Isle of Man, **Edward Forbes** (1815–1854), made a study of depth-related communities in the sea, and laid the foundation for marine biogeography and ecology. **Michel Sars** (1805–1869) of Norway is regarded as one of the founders of marine biology; he used a deep-sea dredge to collect his specimens and described many previously unknown larvae. **Victor Hensen** (1835–1924) of Kiel established *oceanic bionomics* or the study of the economics of the life of the ocean, and in 1888 coined the term *plankton* [Greek: *planketon*, drifting], to denote the floating life forms in the ocean. The world's first marine research institute, the Statione Zoologica in Naples, was founded in 1873 by a Polish-born German zoologist, **Anton Dohrn** (1840–1909). It focused its research on the embryology and physiology of marine animals. One of the naturalists on the Challenger expedition (1872–1876), a Canadian-born US marine biologist **Sir John Murray** (1841–1914), collected marine animals from all parts of world, and published *On the Structure and Origin of Coral Reefs and Islands* (1880). A London zoologist, **Edwin Ray Lankester** (1847–1929) was instrumental in founding the Marine Biological Association, in 1884. A Danish fisheries biologist, **Ernst Johannes Schmidt** (1877–1933), made an extensive study of the migration and distribution of the eel. **Gunnar Axel Thorson** (1906–1971) of Copenhagen did important research on marine invertebrates and published an influential monograph in 1946. A London marine biologist, **Raymond John Heaphy Beverton** (b 1922), who was professor of fisheries ecology (1984–1987) at the University of Wales Institute of Science and Technology, studied the life history of fishes, and the effects of overfishing. He researched on how to increase the population of fish and published *On the Dynamics of Exploited Fish Populations* (1957). An important book on marine ecology, *Ecology of*

Rocky Shores (1964), was published by an English marine biologist at Leeds University, **John Robert Lewis** (b 1924). **Howard Lawrence Sanders** (b 1921) of Newark, New Jersey, studied quantitative samples of organisms from the deep sea which revolutionized marine biology. He also described several previously unknown species. A population study of large mammals – seals and whales – was carried out by an English Antarctic scientist, **Richard Maitland Laws** (b 1926) of Northumberland, who was director of the Life Sciences Division of the British Antarctic Survey from 1973 to 1987. An English marine biologist, **Sir Eric James Denton** (b 1923), studied the visual and acoustic physiology of fish and made other several important contributions. In 1989, he was awarded the first award in the field of marine biology, the International Biology Prize, in Japan. *See oceanography.*

Marine Chronometer The first practical marine chronometer was invented by a London instrument maker, **John Harrison** (1692–1776) from Foulby, Yorkshire. His device won the British Board of Longitude Prize for finding a practical way for identifying longitude in the sea. A London horologist, **John Arnold** (1736–1799), improved it to its modern form. A Swiss clockmaker, **Ferdinand Berthoud** (1727–1807), improved the spring-driven marine chronometer, and constructed about 70 of them.

Marine Engineering A branch of engineering devoted to propulsive forces and mechanical devices for marine vessels. Sailing ships were used in Mesopotamia (now Iraq) around 5000 BC, and Minoan craftsmen around 2200 BC were skilled at ship building. A London engineer, **Sir Charles Algernon Parsons** (1854–1931), developed a steam turbine in 1884, and patented a turbo-generator for a ship in 1894. His first such ship, the *Turbinia,* was launched in 1897. High-efficiency steam turbines, using convergent and divergent nozzles, were developed by a Swedish engineer, **Carl Gustav Patrick de Laval** (1845–1913). He also invented a high-speed turbine to drive the propellor for marine use. An English engineer, **William Froude** (1810–1879), one of the pioneers in the field of modern marine engineering, studied the forces of water in relation to the stablility and speed of ships, and invented a hydraulic dynameter for measuring the output of marine engines, in 1877. The gyrostabilizer, a device to counteract a ship's roll and stabilize it, was developed by an American electrical engineer, **Elmer Ambrose Sperry** (1860–1930) of Cortland county, New York. **Hermann Anschutz Kaempfe** (1872–1931) of Germany independently developed a gyro mechanism, which he fitted to the German ship *Deutschland,* in 1908. The marine diesel engine which worked on the principle of internal combustion was introduced in 1911. *See boats, sailing ships, shipping, ships, steamships.*

Mariotte, Edmé (1620–1684) A French priest from Burgundy at the Cloister of Saint Martin, Dijon. He moved to Paris in 1670 and carried out some important experiments related to hydromechanics, vision and sap pressure in plants. He was one of the founder members of the Académie des Sciences. The blind spot of the retina was discovered by him in 1668. He independently discovered Boyle's law, which is known as Mariotte's law in France. *See Académie Royale des Sciences, hydrodynamics, hydrostatics, impact, plant physiology, structural engineering, vision.*

Marius, Simon (1573–1624) *See Andromeda nebula, sunspots.*

Markov Chains Sequences of mutually dependent variables in probability theory. Proposed by a Russian mathematician and a professor at St Petersburg, **Andrei Andereevich Markov** (1856–1922).

Markov, Andrei Andereevich (1856–1922) *See Markov chains.*

Marryat, Frederick (1792–1848) *See flag signalling.*

Mars Fourth planet from the sun, known to ancient astronomers. The surface features of the planet were first observed in 1659 by **Christian Huygens** (1629–1695). The distance from earth to Mars was calculated in 1671 by the professor of astronomy at the University of Bologna, **Giovanni Domenico Cassini** (1625–1712) of Nice. The first map of Mars was produced in 1840 by a German astronomer, **Johann Heinrich Mädler** (1794–1874). The two satellites of Mars (Deimos and Phobos) were discovered in 1877 by an American astronomer from Connecticut, **Asaph Hall** (1829–1907). A detailed study of the surface terrain of Mars was carried out by an Italian astronomer, **Giovanni Virginio Schiaparelli** (1835–1910) who discovered the 'canals' of Mars in 1877. An American astronomer and mathematician, **Percival Lowell** (1855–1916) of Boston, Massachusetts, made important observations on Mars and produced the first high-quality photographs of the planet in 1895. He published *Mars and its Canals* (1906) and *Mars as the Abode of Life* (1910). Several workers, including **Frank Washington Very** (1852–1927) of Salem, Massachusetts, showed the presence of oxygen and water vapor in the Martian atmosphere. An American astronomer and director of the Lick Observatory in California, **William Wallace Campbell** (1862–1938) from Ohio, demonstrated these to be of insufficient quantity, and his findings were subsequently confirmed by several space probes. He also made a detailed study of stellar radial velocities with **Heber Doust**

Curtis (1872–1942), in 1902. The American space probe Mariner 9 was the first probe successfully to orbit Mars, in 1971, and it safely returned to the earth with 7329 photographs of Mars. The Soviet space probe Mars 3 landed on Mars in the same year.

Marsh Test A standard test for arsenic, where it is reduced to arsine by the action of zinc and sulfuric acid in a heated glass tube, leaving behind a soluble product in sodium hypochlorite. Devised in 1836 by an English chemist, **James Marsh** (1789–1846).

Marsh, Charles Othniel (1831–1899) *See dinosaurs.*

Marsh, James (1789–1846) *See Marsh test.*

Marshall, Sir John Hubert (1876–1958) *See Indus Valley civilization.*

Marsigli, Louis Ferdinand (1658–1730) *See oceanography.*

Martin, Archer John Porter (b 1910) *See chromatography.*

Martin, James (1893–1981) *See ejection seat.*

Martin, John (1789–1819) *See dinosaurs.*

Martin, Pierre Emile (1824–1915) *See steel.*

Martyn, David Forbes (b 1906) *See ionosphere, radioastronomy.*

Martyn, Thomas (1735–1825) A professor of botany at Cambridge who held the post for 63 years until his death.

Maser The concept of the emission of radiation stimulated by photons was first proposed in 1917 by **Albert Einstein** (1879–1955). His theory was developed in 1951 into **m**icrowave **a**mplification with the use of **s**timulated **e**lectromagnetic **r**adiation (maser) by an American physicist and Nobel laureate, **Charles Hard Townes** (b 1915) of Greenville, South Carolina. In 1964 he shared the Nobel Prize for physics with two Russian scientists, **Nikolay Gennadiyevich Basov** (b 1922) and **Aleksandr Mikaylovich Prokhorov** (b 1916), who independently invented the maser in 1955. The technique was later developed into the laser (**l**ight **a**mplification by **s**timulated **e**lectromagnetic **r**adiation).

Maskelyne, Nevil (1732–1811) *See earth density, Greenwich observatory, shipping.*

Mason, Josiah (1795–1881) *See pen.*

Mason, Sir Basil John (b 1923) *See clouds.*

Mass Media *See broadcasting, newspapers, radio, television.*

Mass Spectrograph An instrument for determining the mass of individual atoms by means of positive ray analysis. Invented in 1919 by an English physicist, **Francis William Aston** (1877–1945) of Harbourne, Birmingham. He was awarded the Nobel Prize for Chemistry for his work on isotopes, in 1922. A machine that focused beams of varying velocity was developed by **Arthur Dempster** (1886–1950). A double focusing model was invented in 1936 by an American physicist, **Kenneth Tompkins Bainbridge** (1904–1996) from Cooperstown, New York, who was professor of physics at the Harvard University.

Mästlin, Michael (1550–1631) A German astronomer who promoted Copernicus' theory that the earth orbits the Sun. One of his pupils was German mathematician Johannes Kepler. Mästlin published an *Epitome of Astronomy* in 1582.

Masurium An element discovered by two German chemists, **Walter Karl Friedrich Noddack** (1893–1960) and his wife **Ida Eva Noddack** (b 1896) of Berlin. Its existence was doubted until 1937, when an Italian physicist, **Emilio Segre** (1905–1989), demonstrated it and named it technetium.

Matches These were used by the Chinese for lighting fire around AD 577. A tinderbox system of flint and steel was in use up to 1805. Chemical matches made of brimstone and asbestos mixed with oil of vitriol were invented by Chancel of Paris in 1805. In 1815 he used a mixture of potassium chlorate and sugar. The friction match, consisting of antimony, potassium chlorate, gum and sulfur, was invented in 1827 by **John Walker** (1781–1859), a chemist from Stockton-on-Tees, England. Also known as the Lucifer match, it was invented independently by a Scottish inventor, **Sir Isaac Holden** (1807–1897) from Renfrewshire. The first phosphorus matches were invented in 1830 by a Frenchman, Sauria. The industrially hazardous yellow phosphorus was used until the much safer red phosphorus or the safety match was invented by an Austrian chemist, **Anton Schrotter** (1802–1875). He also demonstrated red phosphorus to be an allotrope. Red phosphorus was manufactured by an English chemist from Oxfordshire, **Arthur Albright** (1811–1900), at Birmingham in 1845.

Mathematical Logic The use of mathematical symbolism (symbolic logic) to express logical relations, developed by an English mathematician, **George Boole** (1816–1864). He was professor of mathematics at Cork and published several papers including *Mathematical Analysis of Logic* (1847) and *Laws of Thought* (1854). The Venn diagram, used in logical teaching of elementary mathematics, was devised by a British logician and clergyman, **John Venn** (1834–1923) of Drypool, Hull. His published works include *The Logic of*

Chance (1866), *Symbolic Logic* (1881) and *The Principles of Empirical Logic* (1889). An Italian mathematician and professor of infinitesimal calculus at Turin, **Giuseppe Peano** (1858–1932), invented a system of mathematical symbolism which formed the basis for further work by other mathematicians. Two British mathematicians and philosophers, **Bertrand Arthur William Russell** (1872–1970) of Monmouthshire, and **Alfred North Whitehead** (1861–1947) of Ramsgate, Kent, published *Principia Mathematica* (1910) which treated logic as the basis of mathematics, and became an important landmark. **Ludwig Friedrich Gottlob Frege** (1848–1925) of Wismar is regarded as the founder of modern mathematical logic in Germany. He published *Die Grundlagen der Arithmetik* (1884), *Die Grundgesetze der Arithmetik* (1903) and several other works.

Mathematical Problems   These have existed since ancient times in an effort to link theory to reality and practicality. The Ahmes papyrus (1650 BC) refers to several, including one related to the numbering of cattle, and another on the adulteration of wine in a barrel, with water. An Athenian philosopher, Metrodorus, compiled a series of new and old problems around AD 310. His *Greek Anthology* contains problems such as draining and filling a cistern, and the proportion of various metals in constructing a crown.

Mathematical Symbols   Signs for addition (+) and subtraction (–) are found in the work of Johannes Widman, published in Germany in 1489. They were incorporated into algebraic expression by G. Vander Hoecke of Antwerp in 1514. An English book, *Whetstone of Witte* (1557) by a mathematician and physician, **Robert Recorde** (1510–1558) from Tenby, Pembroke, included the equals sign (=). The symbol for multiplication (×) was introduced by **William Oughtred** (1575–1660), a clergyman from Eton in his *Clavis Mathematica* (The Key to Mathematics) published in 1631. The symbol for division (÷) was used by a Swiss mathematician, **Johann Heinrich Rahn** (d 1676), in his *Teutsche Algebra* (1659), and it was introduced into England by **John Pell** (1610–1685) from Sussex. The sign π for the ratio of the circumference to the diameter of a circle was introduced in 1706 by a London mathematician, **William Jones** (1680–1749) from Anglesey. The greater than (>) and less than (<) signs were introduced by **Thomas Harriot** (1560–1621), a mathematician from Oxford. The symbol for the square root ($\sqrt{}$) was introduced by a German mathematician, **Christoff Rudolf** (b 1500) in 1525. The symbol for infinity (∞) was introduced by one of the founders of the Royal Society, **John Wallis** (1616–1703) in his *Arithmetica Infinitorum* (1655). The first use of the radical sign with indices such as 2 for a square root and 3 for a cube root was

used by a French mathematician, **Nicolas Chuquet** (1445–1500) in his treatise *Tripartie en la Science des Nombers*. Parentheses were first used by a Dutch mathematician, **Albert Girard** (1595–1632) in his book on algebra published in 1629.

Mathematics   [Greek: *mathematikos*]   The Chaldeans who ruled Babylonia from 606 to 539 BC applied mathematics to astronomy. They divided the Zodiac into 12 parts and the celestial equator into 360 degrees. The oldest existing mathematical manuscript, by Ahmes of Egypt in 1650 BC, which is partly a copy from an earlier manuscript, was brought to London around the middle of the 19th century by a Scottish Egyptologist, **Alexander Henry Rhind** (1833–1863), and became known as the Rhind's papyrus. It is now exhibited at the British Museum in London. **Thales** (640–546 BC), a merchant from the city of Miletus in Asia Minor, was one of the first to devote his time to the study of mathematics. He measured the height of a pyramid by its shadow and developed geometry. His pupil **Pythagoras** (*c.* 580–500 BC) from the island of Samos introduced geometry as an essential science. Other notable ancient mathematicians include **Euclid** (*c.* 300 BC), **Eratosthenes** (274–194 BC), **Hippocrates of Chios** (430 BC) and **Archimedes** (278– 212 BC). Four of the important Hindu mathematicians were **Aryabhata** (AD 475–550) of Benares, **Brahmagupta** (*c.* AD 598–660) of Ujjain, **Mahavira** (AD 850) of Mysore and **Bhaskara** (AD 1114–1185) of Ujjain. The University of Paris in 1336 declared that no student could graduate unless he had attended lectures in mathematics. In Britain the first books on mathematics, *Whetstone of Witte, The Ground of Arte* and *Pathwaie to Knowledge*, were published by an English mathematician and physician, **Robert Recorde** (1510–1558) from Tenby, Pembroke. Other early English mathematicians include **Thomas Harriot** (1560–1621), who contributed to algebra, **Henry Briggs** (1561–1631) and **John Napier** (1550–1617), who invented the logarithms, and **William Oughtred** (1575–1660), who invented the slide rule. The first substantial book on the history of mathematics, *Histoire des Mathematiques*, was published in 1758 by a Frenchman from Lyons, **Jean Étienne Montucula** (1725–1799). A Dutch mathematician, **Thomas Jan Stieltjes** (1856–1894), studied most of the problems in mathematical analysis up to his time and came to be regarded as the founder of analytical theory. The *Principia Mathematica* (1910) in three volumes by the British mathematicians and philosophers, **Bertrand Arthur William Russell** (1872–1970) of Monmouthshire, and **Alfred North Whitehead** (1861–1947) of Ramsgate, Kent, was an important landmark, in treating logic as the basis of mathematics. *See accountancy, algebra, arithmetic, calculus, geometry, numbers.*

Matrix Mechanics [Latin: *matrix*, source] Mathematical description of subatomic phenomenona which treats certain characteristics of particles as being matrices. Classical mechanics was interpreted on the basis of matrix mechanics by a German physicist, **Max Born** (1882–1970) and his pupil, **Werner Karl Heisenberg** (1901–1976) of Würzburg, in 1925. Heisenberg was awarded the Nobel Prize for physics for his work on quantum mechanics, in 1932. An Austrian–Swiss physicist, **Wolfgang Pauli** (1900–1958), was the first to apply matrices to the spin of the electron in the hydrogen atom. He was awarded the Nobel Prize for physics for his work on atomic physics, in 1945. A Hungarian-born US physicist, **Johann Von Neumann** (1903–1957), showed that the matrix mechanics developed by Born and Heisenberg, was equivalent to the wave mechanics of **Erwin Schrödinger** (1887–1961), and published *The Mathematical Foundations of Quantum Mechanics* (1932). In 1926 an American mathematician **Carl Eckart** (1902–1971), demonstrated a similar relationship between matrix mechanics and wave mechanics. *See quantum mechanics.*

Mats The oldest known woven mats are from Beida (presently Jordan) dating back to 6000 BC. *See weaving.*

Matthias, Bernard Teo (b 1918) *See superconductivity.*

Mattioli, Pietro Andrea (1501–1577) *See botany.*

Mauchly, John William (1907–1980) *See computers.*

Maudslay, Henry (1771–1831) *See lathe, machine tools.*

Maunder, Edward Walter (1851–1928) *See British Astronomical Association, sunspots.*

Maupertuis, Pierre-Louis Moreau de (1698–1759) *See quantum mechanics.*

Maurice, Paul Adrien (1902–1984) *See boson.*

Maurolico, Francesco (1494–1575) *See optics.*

Maury, Antonia Caetana de Paiva Pereira (1866–1952) A US radioastronomer who was the first to calculate the 104-day period of the star *Mizar*. In 1896 after examining nearly 5000 photographs of 700 bright stars in the northern sky she published her new classification scheme for spectral lines.

Maury, Matthew Fontaine (1806–1873) *See meteorology, oceanography.*

Mawson, Sir Douglas (1882–1958) *See magnetic poles, South Pole.*

Maxim, Sir Hiram Stevens (1840–1916) *See Maxim machine gun.*

Maxim Machine Gun Invented in 1883 by **Sir Hiram Stevens Maxim** (1840–1916), an American inventor from Sangersville, Maine. He emigrated to England in 1881.

Maxwell, James Clerk (1831–1879) The first Cavendish professor of experimental physics at University of Cambridge, was born in Edinburgh and educated at the university there. He published a paper on oval curves at the age of 15, and was appointed professor of natural philosophy at Marischal College, Aberdeen, in 1856. He believed that all electromagnetic phenomena consisted of matter and motion, and they came within the scope of Newtonian mechanics. He calculated the forces in an electrostatic field, defined the coefficient of electrical elasticity of a medium, proposed the displacement hypothesis of electricity and formulated the electromagnetic theory of light. His theory that light should exert a pressure on the surface on which it falls was experimentally proved by **Pyotr Nicolayevich Lebedev** (1866–1912) in 1899. The mechanism of dispersion of light was first suggested by Maxwell in 1869, and color photography was invented by him in 1861. Some of his important publications include *Theory of Heat* (1871), *Treatise on Electricity and Magnetism* (1873) and *Matter and Motion* (1877). *See wireless telegraphy.*

Maxwell–Boltzmann Distribution An equation in physics describing the distribution of velocities among the molecules of a gas. Derived independently by **James Clerk Maxwell** (1831–1879) and **Ludwig Boltzmann** (1844–1906).

Mayall, Nicholas Ulrich (b 1906) *See galaxy.*

Maybach, Wilhelm (1846–1929) *See car, motorcycle.*

Mayer, Christian (1719–1783) An Austrian astronomer and Jesuit priest who was the first to study and catalogue double stars. He measured the degree of the meridian, based on his work conducted in Paris and observed the transits of Venus in 1761 and 1769 in Russia at the invitation of Catherine II.

Mayer, Johann Tobias (1723–1762) *See cartography.*

Mayer, Julius Robert von (1814–1878) *See heat, kinetic energy, thermodynamics.*

Maynard Smith, John (b 1920) *See games theory.*

Mayow, John (1640–1679) *See air, atmosphere, oxygen.*

Mayr, Ernst Walter (b 1904) A German-born US zoologist and historian of biology. He published *Systematics and the Origin of Species* (1942), *The Growth of Biology Thought* (1982) and several other books on evolution and biology.

McAdam, John Loudon (1756–1836) *See macadamizing, roads.*

McBain, James William (1882–1953) *See soap.*

McClung, Clarence Ervin (1870–1946) *See chromosomes.*

McCollum, Elmer Verner (1879–1967) *See vitamins.*

McCormick, Cyrus Hall (1809–1884) *See agricultural instruments.*

McCrea, Sir William Hunter (b 1904) *See cosmic dynamics.*

McDonnell, James Smith (1899–1980) *See airplane.*

McKenzie, Dan Peter (b 1942) *See tectonic theory.*

McLennan, John Cunningham (1867–1935) *See helium.*

McMillan, Erward Mattison (1907–1991) *See americium, neptunium, plutonium.*

McNaught, William (1813–1881) *See steam engine.*

Measures *See units and measures.*

Mechanical Engineering [Greek: *mechano*, machine] Application of science to machines. One of the first known mechanical devices, the *dalu*, which is a water-raising device, was used by the Sumerians in lower Iraq in 3500 BC. The Archimedian screw used for raising water was invented by **Archimedes** (287–212 BC) during his visit to Egypt around 250 BC. His device has been in continual use in Egypt since then. He also demonstrated the principle behind the lever. **Pappus of Alexandria** (AD 300), described mechanics as a means of impelling bodies to change their position, contrary to their nature. **Hero of Alexandria** (*c.* AD 100) who is regarded as the father of mechanical engineering, described five simple machines, the wheel and the axle, the lever, a system of pulleys, the wedge and the screw. The first systematic work on mechanical engineering, entitled *Theatrum machinarum generale* (General theory of machines), was published by **Jacob Leupold** (b 1674) of Planitz, Germany in 1723. **Georgius Agricola** (1494–1555) described five types of hauling machines. An Italian engineer, **Agostino Ramelli** (*c.* 1531–1600), described hundreds of machines such as screw jacks, saw mills, pumps and grinding mills in his *Diversi et Artificiose Machine* published in Paris in 1588. **Jacques Besson** (1535–1575), a French

mathematician and inventor, described several mechanical devices including screw-cutting lathes in his *Théatre des Instruments et Méchaniques* (1578). **Christopher Polhem** (1661–1751) of Gotland, Sweden, is regarded as the father of Swedish mechanics. He used water power to operate grooved machines, shearing machines and several other mechanical devices for metal fabrication. A Scottish engineer, **James Nasmyth** (1808–1890), invented a steam pile-driver, a steam hammer and a hydraulic machine, and published *Remarks on Tools and Machinery* (1858). The first machine tools were produced by a London engineer, **Henry Maudslay** (1771–1831) of Woolwich, around 1792. His screw-cutting lathe was improved by **Richard Roberts** (1789–1864) of Montgomeryshire, Wales. The strength of materials in construction and metal strain were studied by an English engineer, **Eaton Hodgkinson** (1789–1861) of Anderton, Cheshire, who published *Experimental Researches on the Strength and the other Properties of Cast Iron* (1840). He was appointed professor of mechanical principles of engineering at University College London in 1847.

Mechanical Equivalent of Heat Its first determination, corresponding to a rise of temperature of 1 degree Fahrenheit of 1 pound of water, for the expenditure of 838 foot pounds of work, was made by **James Prescott Joule** (1818–1889), who published his method in his paper *On the calorific effects of magneto-electricity on the mechanical value of heat* (1843). A Danish physicist, **Ludvig August Colding** (1815–1888), independently measured it in the same year.

Mechanical Equivalent of Work The first suggestion of the mechanical equivalence of heat and work is found in the paper *On the Production of Heat by the Voltaic Electricity* sent in 1840 to the Royal Society by **James Prescott Joule** (1818–1889), and published in the *Philosophical Magazine* (1841).

Mechanical Tools *See mechanical engineering.*

Meer, Simon van der (b 1925) *See antiproton, boson.*

Meikle, Andrew (1719–1811) *See agricultural instruments, windmill.*

Meikle, James (*c.* 1690–1717) *See agricultural instruments.*

Meinesz, Felix Andries Vening (1887–1966) *See oceanography, submarines.*

Meiosis [Greek: *meiosis*, diminution] A process of reduction division in sex cells, at maturation, by means of which each daughter cell receives half the number of chromosomes found in the somatic cell. In 1885, a German professor of zoology at the University of Freiburg, **August Friedrich Leopold Weismann** (1834–1914) of Frankfurt, distinguished between body cells and germ cells, and postulated that some form of reduction must occur in the germ cells during division to prevent the genetic material from doubling. This process was first observed by a Belgian cytologist, **Edouard Joseph Louis-Marie van Beneden** (1846–1910) in 1887. The mechanism by which the nucleus divides twice but the chromosomes only once was described in 1905 by J.B. Farmer (1865–1944) and J.E. Moore (b 1892).

Meitner, Lise (1878–1968) *See atomic bomb, atomic energy, protactinium.*

Mellanby, Sir Edward (1884–1955) *See vitamins.*

Melloni, Macedonio (1798–1854) *See radiometer (2).*

Melvill, Thomas (1726–1753) *See absorption spectra, spectroscopy.*

Menaechmus (375–325 BC) *See analytical geometry, conics.*

Mendel, Gregor Johann (1822–1884) The founder of genetics, born near Udrau, a remote village in Moravia. He worked on hybridization of pea plants, while he was a monk at an Augustinian monastery at Brünn, growing about 30 000 plants which he artificially fertilized to study the inheritance of specific characteristics. He studied science in Vienna and returned to his monastery, to become an Abbot in 1868. As a lone worker he acquired his own microscope and worked laboriously, publishing his epoch-making work enunciating the laws of genetics. His laws of segregation and independent assortment were published in 1865. They went unheeded until a Dutch physiologist and genetist, **Hugo Marie de Vries** (1848–1935) and C. Correns recognized their significance, in 1900. The geneticist **William Bateson** (1861–1926) revived Mendel's work in his *Mendel's Principles of Heredity* (1902).

Mendeleev, Dmitri Ivanovich (1834–1907) Russian chemist, born in Tobolsk, Siberia. He was the 14th and youngest child of a schoolteacher. After his father lost his job because of blindness, his mother set up a glass workshop and worked single-handedly to support the family and educate her children. He studied at the local school and went to University of St Petersburg at the age of 16, and later studied at the University of Heidelberg. He became a professor at St Petersburg Technical Institute in 1863, and at University of St Petersburg in 1866. He published *Principles of chemistry* (1869), containing the periodic law, which he refined over the next 20 years. This was initially received with some scepticism but, as more elements that fitted his table were discovered, it became accepted. He recognized that some

elements still had to be discovered, and left gaps in his table for the predicted elements. *See periodic table.*

Mendelevium An element with atomic number 101, named after the Russian chemist, **Dmitri Ivanovich Mendeleev** (1834–1907) who proposed the periodic law. It was synthesized in 1955 by an American physicist, **Glenn Theodore Seaborg** (b 1912) and his team at Berkeley.

Menelaus (*c.* AD 100) *See trigonometry.*

Mengoli, Pietro (1626–1682) An Italian professor of mathematics at the University of Bologna who proposed a series for logarithms and gave a definition of the definite integral.

Mensuration Study of various properties of conic sections, established by **Archimedes** (287–212 BC) around 218 BC. A theorem related to mensuration of solid bodies proposed by **Bonaventura Cavalieri** (1598–1647) bears his name. The first German mathematical text *A Treatise on Mensuration*, in German, was published by a mathematician and engraver, **Albert Durer** (1471–1528) of Nuremberg, in 1525.

Menten, Maud Lenore (1879–1960) *See Michaelis–Menten equation.*

Menzel, Donald Howard (1901–1976) A US physicist and astronomer from Florence, Colorado who worked at the Harvard University Observatory from 1932 until his retirement in 1971. He constructed a coronagraph there which was the beginning of the High Altitude Observatory for solar physics research. He revolutionized solar astronomy through his research on the spectrum of the solar chromosphere, and applied atomic physics to astronomy.

Mercator, Gerardus (1512–1594) *See atlas, cartography, globe.*

Mercer, John (1791–1866) *See dyes, Mercerizing, textile industry.*

Mercerizing A process by which cotton is given a silky luster. Invented by an English dye chemist, **John Mercer** (1791–1866) of Blackburn, Lancashire. He also devised a method for photographic printing on fabrics.

Mercury (Metal) First mentioned by **Aristotle** (384–322 BC) who used the term *argyros chytos* meaning liquid silver. **Pliny the Elder** (AD 28–79) described the metal. The alchemists symbolized it with the planet Mercury. **Evangelista Torricelli** (1608–1647) used it first for constructing a barometer. **Gabriel Daniel Fahrenheit** (1686–1736) used it for the thermometer in 1720. *See quicksilver.*

Mercury (Planet) One of the nine major planets of the Solar system. Its transit across the face of the sun was first observed in 1631 by a French astronomer, **Pierre Gassendi** (1592–1655). An American professor of mathematics and natural philosophy at Harvard, **John Winthrop** (1714–1779) observed the transit of Mercury in 1740. Another French astronomer, **Urbain Jean Joseph Leverrier** (1811–1877) of Normandy, made his observations on the transit in 1845.

Mergenthaler, Ottomar (1854–1899) *See linotype printing.*

Meridian Circle of constant longitude passing through a given place and the terrestrial poles. The Ancient astronomer, **Hipparchus** (190–120 BC) set his prime meridian in Rhodes and made his observations. **Ptolemy** of Alexandria (*c.* AD 127–151) adopted the Fortunate Isles or the Canaries as the meridian. King Phillip II of Spain set the city of Toledo as the prime meridian in 1573. A French astronomer and mathematician, **Pierre Bouguer** (1698–1758), gave a measure of the length of a degree of a meridian in his *La figure de la terre déterminée* (1749). A French mathematician, **Jean Charles Borda** (1733–1799), designed his own instruments to measure an arc of a meridian. A French astronomer, **Jean Picard** (1620–1682), made the first accurate measurement of a degree of the meridian in France and deduced a value for the size of the earth. **Jean Baptiste Joseph Delambre** (1749–1822), a French mathematician and astronomer, gave a detailed account of his measurement of the meridian arc from Dunkirk to Barcelona in 1792 to 1799.

Merrett, Christopher (1614–1695) An English physician and naturalist who was one of the original members of the Royal Society. He published a work on British flora and fossils *Pinax rerum Naturalium Britannicarum, continens Vegetalia, Animalia, et Fossilia* (1667).

Merrifield, Bruce (b 1921) An American biochemist from Texas who was awarded the Nobel Prize for chemistry in 1984, for his work on the laboratory synthesis of proteins.

Mersenne, Marin (1588–1648) *See acoustics, number theory, velocity of sound.*

Meselson, Matthew Stanley (b 1930) *See genetic engineering.*

Meson The existence of an intermediate atomic nuclear particle, capable of becoming a neutron or a proton, was proposed by a Japanese physicist, **Hideki Yukawa** (1907–1981), in his attempt to explain the stability of the nucleus despite the positive charge on the protons. Yukawa was the first Japanese to receive a Nobel Prize (for physics), in 1949. The meson was demonstrated by an English physicist, **Cecil Frank Powell** (1903–1969) of Tonbridge, Kent, who was awarded the Nobel Prize for physics in 1950, for his discovery.

Mesopotamia [Greek: *mesos,* middle + *potamus,* river] Southwest Asia between the rivers Tigris and Eupharates (now Iraq) and the cradle of civilization around 4000 BC. The first system of writing was developed here by the Sumerians around 3000 BC. Sargon of Akkad produced the first map of Mesopotamia for the purposes of land taxation, in 2400 BC.

Mesozoic Period [Greek: *mesos,* intermediate + *zoe,* life] A transition period between the Paleozoic and Cainozoic eras, identified and named by the professor of geology at King's College, London, first, and later at Oxford, **John Phillips** (1800–1874) from Kent.

Messel, Rudolph (1848–1920) *See sulfuric acid.*

Messerschmitt, Wilhelm Emil (1898–1978) *See warplanes.*

Messier Catalog A list of nebulae and star clusters compiled in 1781 by a French astronomer, **Charles Messier** (1730–1817).

Messier, Charles (1730–1817) *See Messier catalog.*

Metabolism [Greek: *metabole,* change] A term coined by **Johann Fredrick Gmelin** (1748–1805), a physician from Tübingen, to denote the chemical transformations that food undergoes during the constructive (anabolic) and destructive (catabolic) processes concerned with nutrition. *See nutrition.*

Metallurgy Metals in their natural form were used as small jewels and tools 7000 years ago. Metallurgy came into existence with the discovery that metals could be made malleable, when heated. The Egyptians obtained their copper in large quantities from the Sinai peninsula around 3500 BC. **Theodorus** (*c.* 530 BC) from the Greek island of Samos is credited with the invention of metal smelting for the purpose of making objects such as locks and keys. Metallurgy was treated as a science in the 14th century, and the earliest book on the subject, entitled *Ein Nutzlich Bergbuchlein* (A useful Mining Booklet), was published anonymously in Germany in 1500. This was followed by another anonymous book, *Probierbuchlein* (Assaying Booklet), in 1510. The first important book on mining entitled *De la Pirotecnia* (1540) was published by an Italian, **Vanocchio Biringuccio** (1460–1538). An epoch-making work on mining was done by **Georgius Agricola** (1494–1555), a German physician from Glauchau in Saxony. He spent most of his career at

Joachimsthal in Bohemia, one of the greatest mining districts of Europe, from where he carried out pioneering work on metallurgy. His important illustrated work *De Re Metallica* was published in 12 volumes in Basel in 1556. The first treatise on mining and metallurgical chemistry, entitled *Bescherubung allerfurnemisten minerlischen Ertzt und Berkwerksarten* (1574), was written by **Lazarus Ercker** (1530–1593), a Bohemian metallurgist and superintendent of the mines of the Holy Roman Empire and Bohemia. **Leonardo da Vinci** (1452–1519) invented several mining devices. The gunpowder was first used for ground blasting by Casper Weinde from Schemnitz in 1627 and it was introduced for mining in Cornwall in 1689. An illustrated account of mining and smelting techniques *Regnum subterraneum* (1734) was published by a natural philosopher from Stockholm, **Emanuel Swedenborg** (1688–1772), who settled down in London in 1747. A safer method of mining by combining gunpowder with flax yarn, giving it a slow-burning fuse, was invented by **William Bickford** (1774–1834) of Cornwall. **Sir William Chandler Roberts-Austen** (1843–1902) of Kennington, a professor of metallurgy at the Royal School of Mines in London (1882), published *An Introduction to the Study of Metallurgy*. Earlier in 1875 he had studied metallurgy in relation to coining. A modern work on the subject, *Textbook of Metallography*, was published by a London metallurgist, **Cyril Henry Desch** (1874–1958).

Metals Six metals – gold, silver, copper, lead, tin and iron – were known before the Christian era. According to the Old Testament, gold, iron and brass were known before the Great Flood, and silver, lead and tin came later. Homer's (*c.* 800) writings show that he knew these metals. The alchemists during the Middle Ages attributed symbols of planetary bodies to the metals. They included: Sun for gold, Moon for silver, Venus for copper, Jupiter for tin, Saturn for lead and Mars for iron. *See metallurgy.*

Metamorphosis [Greek: *meta*, beyond + *morphe,* form] The term was first used in entomology to denote the changes of the embryo during the process of its development into an adult, by a London naturalist, **Thomas Moufet** (1553–1604), in his *Theatre of Insects* (1590).

Metaphase [Greek: *meta*, after + *phasis*, appearance] A stage in mitotic cell division, described and named by a German botanist and professor at Bonn, **Eduard Adolf Strasburger** (1844–1912) in 1884. He published *Cell Formation and Cell Division* in 1875.

Metaphysics [Greek: *meta*, after + *phusis,* nature] The science of abstract reasoning began with the essays of **Aristotle** (384–322 BC). **Andronicus of Rhodes**, a Greek philosopher who lived around 58 BC, introduced the term *metaphysics* to denote the science of thought and influences unseen, incapable of direct recognition by the senses. One of the earliest books on ethics, dealing with metaphysics and psychology, was written by **Baruch Spinoza** (1632–1677), a Dutch philosopher of Jewish descent in Amsterdam, and published after his death, in 1677. The International Institute of Metaphysics in Paris was founded by Charles Richet and Joseph Tessier of France in 1919.

Metcalf, John (1717–1810) A pioneer of modern roads in Great Britain who established highways in Yorkshire, Lancashire and Derbyshire in 1750. His work was followed by **Thomas Telford** (1757–1834) who built many important bridges and further roads. *See roads.*

Metchnikoff, Elie (1845–1916) Russian zoologist who discovered phagocytosis, and phagocytes in the blood. He shared the Nobel Prize with **Paul Ehrlich** in 1908. *See Ehrlich, Paul.*

Meteorites *See meteors.*

Meteorology [Greek: *meteor*, high in the air + *logos*, discourse] Study of motions and phenomena of the atmosphere mainly for the purpose of weather forecasting. **Aristotle** (384–322 BC) in his first three books of *Meteorologica* dealt with phenomena above the earth, such as rain, snow, comets, thunder and lightning. His physical geography included oceans, rivers and earthquakes. **Robert Hooke** (1635–1703) constructed a hygroscope out of the bristle from the husk of a wild oat, and used it for measuring moisture in the air. He also built a wind-gauge for measuring the direction and strength of the wind. In 1679 he completed a weather instrument that could record pressure, wind, humidity and rainfall. The first map of the winds on the earth's surface was published by **Edmund Halley** (1656–1742) in 1686. One of the earliest English treatises on hurricanes and the wind entitled *A Discourse concerning the Origine and the Properties of Wind* was published by Ralph Bohun in 1671. A system of weather reporting was devised by an American physicist, **Joseph Henry** (1797–1878), at the Smithsonian Institution. The German naturalist **Friedrich Heinrich Alexander von Humboldt** (1769–1859) studied the nature of tropical storms. A Jesuit priest, **Pietro Angelo Secchi** (1818–1878), constructed a meteorograph for recording various weather conditions. The Beaufort scale used for classification and description of wind force was proposed in 1805 by **Sir Francis Beaufort** (1774–1857), and it was revised and improved around 1921 by an English meteorologist from Derby, **Sir George Clark Simpson** (1878–1965). An Italian meteorologist and

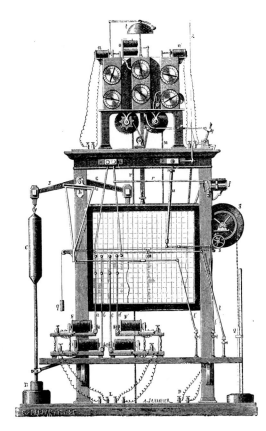

Figure 56   Secchi's meteorograph. Guillemin, Amédée. *The Applications of Physical Forces*. London: Macmillan and Co, 1877

professor at Naples, **Luigi Palmieri** (1807–1896), invented a rain gauge and several other meteorological instruments. An anemometer, an instrument for measuring the velocity of wind, was devised by an Irish astronomer, **John Thomas Romney Robinson** (1792–1882) of Dublin, in 1846. The science of ocean meteorology was founded by an American naval officer, **Matthew Fontaine Maury** (1806–1873) from Virginia, with his work on winds and currents of the ocean, in 1855. Important work in Scotland was done by a meteorologist from Kinross, **Alexander Buchan** (1829–1907) who published *Handy Book of Meteorology* (1867). A New York City meteorologist, **Cleveland Abbe** (1838–1916), was responsible for the introduction of the US system of standard time. **John Aitken** (1839–1919), a Scottish physicist from Falkirk, did extensive studies on climatology, dealing with atmospheric dust, dew and cyclones. His collected works were published posthumously in 1923. The Meterological Office was established in England in 1854, and **Robert Fitzroy** (1805–1865), the commander of the *Beagle* that carried **Charles Robert Darwin** (1809–1882), became its first director in 1855. **Sir William Napier Shaw** (1854–1945), who wrote *Life-History of Surface Air Currents*,

became a director there in 1905, and was made professor of meteorology at Imperial College, London, in 1920. His *Manual of Meteorology* (1919–1931) became a standard work. A London meteorologist and applied mathematician, **Sir Geoffrey Ingram Taylor** (1886–1975), in his work on dynamic meteorology, applied the knowledge of the turbulent motions of liquids to oceanography and meteorology. An American astronomer, **Walter Orr Roberts** (1915–1990), applied modern technology to the study of climate and founded the National Center for Atmospheric Research at the University of Colorado in 1960. A Dutch meteorologist, **Christoph Hendrik Diederik Buys Ballot** (1817–1890), founded the Royal Netherlands Meteorological Institute in 1854, and organized the first weather forecast and storm warnings, in 1860. **William Henry Dines** (1855–1927) of Oxshott, Surrey, in England, performed over 200 balloon ascents to study the relation between pressure and temperature and devised an anemometer (1901) and a radiometer (1920). He also gave an explanation for cyclonic circulation. An American meteorologist from San Francisco, **Jule Gregory Charney** (1917–1981), devised equations to predict the development of depressions. Supercomputers such as the Cray I, developed by **Seymour R. Cray** (1925–1996), came to be used for weather forecasting in the 1970s. A British meteorologist, **Sir John Theodore Houghton** (b 1931), designed selective radiometers that could detect the temperature structure of the atmosphere up to 50 miles, when flown on meteorological satellites. The first meteorological satellite, the Meteosat I, was launched in 1977 by the European Organization for the Exploitation of Meteorological Satellites. *See cyclone.*

Meteors   Light-phenomena caused by the entry of bodies (called meteorites or meteroids) into the earth's atmosphere. They were known as thunderbolts from the skies around 4000 BC and a reference to them was made in the Holy Writ of Joshua in 1400 BC. An English astrophysicist, **Alfred Charles Bernard Lovell** (b 1913) of Gloucestershire, used radar for the detection of meteors. Another British physicist, **James Stanley Hey** (b 1909), developed radar for studying meteors, and measured their velocity. The largest ever meteorite was found at Hoba West, near Grootfontein in South West Africa in 1920. It was estimated to weigh 59 tonnes and was 9 feet in length. The largest meteorite in any museum, at Hayden Planetarium, New York, was found in 1897, near Cape York, on the west coast of Greenland, by an American naval commander and explorer, **Robert Edwin Peary** (1856–1920) of Cresson Springs, Pennsylvania.

Meter The term for the SI unit of length was introduced by a French mathematician, **Jean Charles Borda** (1733–1799). It was initially defined as the distance between two points on a platinum rod at a specific temperature in the National Archives at Sèvres. An accurate measurement of a meter in terms of the wavelength of light was done by an American philosopher and scientist, **Charles Sanders Peirce** (1839–1914) of Cambridge, Massachusetts. Since 1983 it has been defined as the length of the path travelled by light in a vacuum during an interval of 1/299, 792, 458 of a second.

Metford, William Ellis (1824–1899) *See firearms.*

Metric System A French mathematician, **Jean Charles Borda** (1733–1799), played an important role in the introduction of metric system in France and he introduced the word, meter. In 1790 a committee appointed by the National Assembly in France, consisting of **Claude Louis Comte de Berthollet** (1748–1822), **Pierre Simon Laplace** (1749–1827) and others, devised a uniform system of measures. They defined a meter as the distance equal to a ten millionth part of the distance between the poles and the equator. The rest of the metric system was completed in 1799.

Meusnier, Jean Baptiste Marie (1754–1793) *See Meusnier theorem.*

Meusnier Theorem Relates to the center of gravity of any plane section. Proposed in 1777 by a French scientist, **Jean Baptiste Marie Meusnier** (1754–1793) of Paris.

Meyer, Julius Lothar von (1830–1895) *See atomic volume, periodic law, valency.*

Meyer, Viktor (1848–1897) *See stereochemistry, vapor density.*

Mezzotint Process A method of engraving where darker and lighter shades are produced by the difference in roughness of the plate. Invented in 1642 by a German military officer and engraver, **Ludwig von Siegen** (1609–1675), of Dutch origin. Only a few of his prints are extant.

Michaelis Constant *See isoelectric point.*

Michaelis, Leonor (1875–1949) *See isoelectric point, Michaelis–Menten equation.*

Michaelis–Menten Equation Relates enzyme concentration to the substrate concentration, giving half maximal velocity of the reaction. Derived in 1913 by a German-born US biochemist, **Leonor Michaelis** (1875–1949) and **Maud Lenore Menten** (1879–1960).

Michaux, François (1770–1852) *See forestry.*

Michel, Hartmut (b 1948) *See photosynthesis.*

Michell, John (1724–1793) *See Coulomb's law, earthquake, seismology, torsion balance.*

Michelson, Albert Abraham (1852–1931) The first American citizen to be awarded the Nobel Prize, in 1907. He was born in Strelno in Prussia, completed his higher education at the United States Naval Academy, Annapolis, and did postgraduate work in several European universities. After a short naval career he began his experiments on the velocity of light, in 1878, and was made professor of physics at Chicago in 1892. While working with **Edward William Morley** (1838–1923) of Newark, New Jersey, a professor of chemistry at Western Reserve University, Cleveland, he designed the famous Michelson–Morley experiment to study motion through the ether, in 1887. His work paved the way for **Albert Einstein's** theory of relativity. *See echelon grating, ether, Fitzgerald–Lorentz contraction, inferometer, relativity, spectroscopy.*

Michelson–Morley Experiment *See Michelson, Albert Abraham.*

Michie, Donald (b 1923) *See artificial intelligence.*

Microchip *See computers.*

Microcomputers *See computers.*

Microincineration A method used in the analysis of plant tissue, by calcination and reduction to ashes, losing all traces of organic matter with preservation of general structural characters. Invented in 1833 by a French chemist and physician, **François Vincent Raspail** (1794–1878).

Micrometeorite Particle below a certain size, incident on the earth's atmosphere, that, owing to its effective heat radiation, does not become molten. Described by an American astronomer, **Fred Lawrence Wheeler** (b 1906) of Iowa. An American cosmologist, **Howard Percy Robertson** (1903–1961), applied relativistic theory to the field, and in 1937 discovered the Poynting–Robertson effect of radiation pressure on micrometeorites.

Micrometer [Greek: *mikros*, small + *metron*, to measure] An instrument for measuring small angles in order to estimate distances and objects in astronomy and other sciences. It was invented by **William Gascoigne** (1612–1644) in 1640, and was effectively incorporated into the telescope by **Christian Huygens** (1629–1695) in 1658. The device was forgotten for the next ten years until Richard Townley revived it in 1667. Other models were invented independently by **Olaus Romer** (1672) and **Jean Picard** (1676). A French

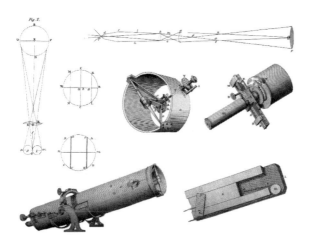

Figure 57 The micrometer and its principle. Partington F. Charles. *The British Encyclopaedia of the Arts and Sciences*. London: Orr & Smith, 1835

mathematician **Adrian Auzont** (1622–1691) wrote a treatise on the micrometer and its accuracy of measurements, which was published in 1693. He is supposed to have invented the instrument independently in 1667. The micrometer became a standard fitting to most astronomical telescopes around the mid-17th century.

Micron [Greek: *mikros,* small] Denoted by the Greek letter μ, it represents one millionth of a unit.

Microphone [Greek: *mikros,* small + *phone,* sound] A device that enabled the telephone to become a commercial success. It was invented in 1857 by **David Edward Hughes** (1831–1900) from a Welsh family in London. It became an integral part of **Alexander Graham Bell's** (1847–1922) telephone equipment in 1876. The term microphone for a sound magnifier was coined by **Sir Charles Wheatstone** (1801–1875), who invented one in 1860. **Thomas Alva Edison** (1847–1931) developed a carbon granule microphone. In 1947 Reg Moores of England devised the first radiomicrophone to be used as a bug, and it was later used at an ice show in the Brighton Stadium in 1949.

Microphotography [Greek: *mikros,* small + *phos,* light + *graphein,* to write] *See photomicrography.*

Microprocessor The first microprocessor, known as a chip, was introduced by the Intel company in 1971. The first small computer with a microprocessor, comparable to the size of a large television, was built by David Ahl in 1974.

Microprocessor *See computers.*

Microscope [Greek: *mikros,* small + *skopein,* view] The term was coined by **Johannes Faber** (1574–1629) of Bamberg, one of the original members of Accademia de Lincei. The identity of the inventor of the microscope has not been clearly established. **Cornelius Jacobson Drebbel** (1570–1633) of Holland, is said to have invented it in 1621. A Jesuit priest, **Athanasius Kircher** (1601–1680) of Geysen, used a primitive microscope of 32× magnification to view blood cells in 1658. The first description of a compound microscope was given by **Robert Hooke** (1635–1703) in 1667, and Eustachio Divini gave an account of his own compound microscope to the Royal Society, in 1668. A Dutch microscopist, **Anthoni van Leeuwenhoek** (1632–1723), ground his own lenses and constructed over 200 microscopes in the 17th century. He was the first to observe bacteria, spermatozoa and protozoa. Phillip Bonnai published an account of two compound microscopes in 1698. A French philosopher, Le Père Cherubin, was the first to view small objects under the microscope conjointly with both eyes, in 1677. The first complete history of early microscopes was given by **Johann Zahn** (1641–1707) in 1685. Benjamin Martin in England improved the microscope and sold pocket versions of it in 1740. Henry Baker of London improved the microscope in

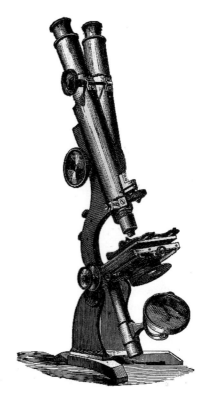

Figure 58 A mid-19th century binocular microscope. Hogg, Jabez. *The Microscope, Its History, Construction and Application.* London: George Routledge and Sons, 1887

1763, and recapitulated much of van Leeuwenhoek's work in his book *The Microscope made Easy* (1743). A diamond microscope was constructed in 1824 by Andrew Pritchard, who introduced 'test objects' to compare the quality of different microscopes. The Microscopical Society of London was established in 1839. An Italian astronomer, **Giovanni Battista Amici** (1786–1863) of Florence, constructed a reflecting microscope, and improved the achromatic objective of the microscope, in 1812. A spectrum microscope capable of detecting one millionth of a grain of blood was exhibited in 1865 by an English chemist and geologist, **Henry Clifton Sorby** (1826–1908) of Sheffield. A German physicist from Eisenach and a graduate of Göttingen University, **Ernest Abbe** (1840–1905), who was a partner of **Carl Zeiss** (1816–1888), modernized the microscope by adding the apochromatic objective and the oil immersion device in 1878. He added the sub-stage condenser in 1886, and improved the technique of phase contrast microscopy, in 1892. The modern phase contrast technique was introduced in 1935 by a Dutch physicist, **Frits Zernike** (1888–1966). The ultra-microscope capable of seeing particles below the usually visible wavelength of 400–700 μm was invented in 1903 by Siedentopf and **Richard Adolf Zsigmondy** (1866–1930). *See electron microscope, field-emission microscope.*

Microsoft Corporation   *See computers.*

Microtome [Greek: *mikros*, small + *tome*, cut] A section-cutting device for microscopic study of tissues. First used in 1770 by the English botanist, **John Hill** (1716–1775). The device was independently developed by **Gabriel Gustav Valentine** (1810–1883) and **Wilhelm His** (1831–1904), around 1866. Alexander Brandt devised one in 1870, and it was developed in 1880 by professor of Pathology at Heidelberg **Richard Thoma** (1847–1923). Automatic machines came into use after 1883.

Microwave Oven The idea of applying the principles of radar to cooking was patented in 1945 by a US inventor Percy LeBaron Spencer. The company, Raytheon, where he worked, manufactured the first model with a power of 1600 watts, for use in large institutional kitchens. Domestic microwave ovens were introduced by a subsidiary company of Raytheon in 1967.

Microwave Radiation   *See background radiation, cosmic rays.*

Midgley, Thomas (1889–1944)   *See food industry, octane rating, petroleum, refrigerator.*

Miescher, Friedrich (1844–1895)   *See deoxyribonucleic acid.*

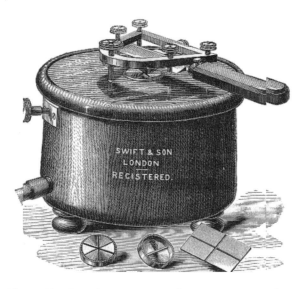

Figure 59   An early microtome and section-cutting machine. Hogg, Jabez. *The Microscope, Its History, Construction and Application*. London: George Routledge and Sons, 1887

Milankovitch Cycles Theoretical radiation curves of the past few hundred thousand years, used for comparison with observed climatic cycles. They are based on the concept that the amount of solar radiation received by the earth is a key to past climates. Proposed by a Yugoslav physicist, **Milutin Milankovitch** (1879–1958).

Milankovitch, Milutin (1879–1958)   *See Milankovitch cycles.*

Military Aircrafts   *See warplanes.*

Military Architecture Early castles were built on high ground or hills surrounded by bare land where enemies could be easily detected. Town castles relied more on high walls and moats. Stretegic points on the sea coast were chosen to ward off invasion by sea. An Italian mathematician, **Niccolò Fontana Tartaglia** (1499–1557) of Venice, in his *Quesite ed invenzioni diverse*, described gunpowder making and fortification. A French naval architect, **Nicolaus François Blondel** (1618–1686), fortified the channel ports of Dunkirk and Le Havre in the 1660s and established a naval base at Rochefort. **Bernard Forest de Bélidor** (1698–1761), a French engineer, published *Science des Ingénieurs* (1729–1749), which contained military designs including ballistics and fortifications. A London architect, **Sir Samuel Bentham** (1757–1831), improved British naval strength through his advanced naval architecture and designs for naval guns. *See military engineering.*

Military Engineering For nearly 4000 years, the bow and arrow, dagger, spear and sword remained as the main weapons.

Archimedes (287–212 BC) of Syracuse, a friend of king Hiero, is regarded as one of the first military engineers and he devised several weapons of warfare. The Greek historian and philosopher **Plutarch** (AD 46–120), in his biography of the Roman general **Claudius Marcellus** (d 209 BC) described a variety of devices invented by Archimedes to defend Syracuse against the general. The Greeks used a substance, known as Greek fire, which blazed when brought into contact with water. **Philo** of Byzantium (*c.* AD 200), in his work on mechanics *Belopoeica*, described the construction of artillery devices such as cannon, air pressure-operated guns and automatically loading guns. The principle of mechanical stone throwers was discussed by **Hero of Alexandria** (*c.* AD 100). His work contains a description of the construction of a *euthytonon,* a mechanical instrument for discharging arrows, and a *palintonon*, a device for projecting heavy stones. **Marcus Pollio Vitruvius** (*c.* AD 100) in his treatise *On Architecture* explained the principle behind catapults or *scorpiones*. War rockets propelled by gunpowder in China were described by Tseng Kung Liang in 1042. A German monk, **Berthholdus** or **Michael Bertholet Schwartz** (*c.* 1320), applied gunpowder to firearms. The principle of the crossbow was known to the ancient Egyptians, and were used in the Middle Ages. However, **Antonio Giambert da Sangallo** (1485–1546), of Florence, designed fortifications around Rome. Forts across the Venetian empire were built by **Michele Sanmichele** (1484–1559). An Italian mathematician, **Niccolò Fontana Tartaglia** (1499–1557) of Venice published a book on artillery science entitled *Nuova scienza* (1537). An Italian engineer, **Agostino Ramelli** (*c.* 1531–1600), while under the service of the Marquis of Marignano, specialized in the field and wrote on military bridges and ballistic engines. A French engineer, **Sebastian le Prestre de Vauban** (1633–1707), introduced the method of approach by parallels and built several fortresses along the French frontiers. He invented the socket bayonet in 1687. A Quaker mathematician and engineer to the East India Company, **Benjamin Robins** (1707–1751), wrote several treatises on projectiles and fortification, and published *New Principles of Gunnery* (1742). The first modern military rocket in Europe was developed in England by **William Congreve** (1772–1828), and it was used in 1806 by the Royal Navy against the French. A Belgian military engineer, **Henri Alexis Brialmont** (1821–1903), designed fortifications for Antwerp, Liège, Bucharest and other towns. A Scottish engineer, **Archibald Barr** (1855–1931) and an English physicist, **William Stroud** (1860–1938) were pioneers in naval range finding and they invented height finders for anti-aircraft guns. In 1931 they established the firm of Barr Stroud Ltd for making scientific instruments. The earliest anti-aircraft gun was used by the Prussians against French balloons, in 1870. The first tank, *Little Willie*, was constructed in September 1915. *See catapult, firearms, warplanes, warships.*

Military Ships   *See warships.*

Milk Industry   *See dairy industry.*

Milky Way   A spiral galaxy of 80 000 light years in diameter, which includes the Solar system. Out of the millions of galaxies it is one of the four galaxies visible to the naked eye from earth. The theory stating that the stars are contained in spherical giant clusters in the Milky Way was proposed in 1761 by a Swiss mathematician, **Johann Heinrich Lambert** (1728–1777). The first correct description of the shape of the Milky Way was given in 1785 by **Sir William Herschel** (1738–1822). The system of classification of the stars, depending on their spectra, was first proposed in 1867 by the Roman astronomer and priest **Pietro Angelo Secchi** (1818–1878). The first practical photographs of the Milky Way were taken by **Edward Emerson Barnard** (1857–1923) in 1895. In 1926, the Milky Way was discovered to be rotating. **Harlow Shapley** (1885–1972) of Nashville, Missouri, who was director of Harvard University Library (1921–1952), demonstrated that the Milky Way was much larger than had been supposed.

Miller, Dayton Clarence (1866–1941) *See acoustics, phonodeik.*

Miller, Hugh (1802–1856) A Scottish geologist from Cromarty who wrote *Footprints of the Creator* (1850), *The Testimony of the Rocks* (1857) and the *Sketchbook of Popular Geology*, which was published posthumously in 1857.

Miller Indices   A coordinate system of mapping the shapes and surfaces of crystals developed by Welsh crystallographer William Miller (1801–1880).

Miller, Stanley Lloyd (b 1930)   *See earth, geogeny.*

Millikan, Robert Andrews (1868–1953)   *See cloud chamber, cosmic rays, electric charge.*

Mills Cross Telescope   A radio telescope with two rows of aerials at right angles to each other, invented in 1953 by the Australian radio astronomer Bernard Mills (b 1920).

Mills, William Hobson (1873–1959) A London organic chemist and professor at Cambridge from 1912. His photographic emulsions prepared from cyanine dyestuffs were used by the military in World War I. His main work was on stereochemistry and the synthesis of cyanine dyes. *See stereochemistry.*

Milne, Edward Arthur (1896–1950) *See cosmic dynamics, earth, kinematic theory.*

Milne, John (1859–1913) *See earthquake, seismology.*

Milstar (Military Strategic and Tactical Relay) US communications satellite launched in 1994 to function in a nuclear war for broadcast orders to launch weapons.

Mimicry [Greek: *mimikos*, imitative] Deceptive resemblance of one species to another to promote survival. Described by an English botanist, **Henry Walter Bates** (1825–1892) from Leicester, who spent 11 years in Brazil studying plants and insects there, and published *Contributions to the Insect Fauna of the Amazon Valley* (1861). The theory that the mimicked species is unpalatable (Batesian mimicry) was proposed by **Fritz Muller** (1821–1891) of Germany.

Mimeograph [Greek: *mimeomai*, imitate + *graphein*, to write] An apparatus for holding stencils of written pages, from which many copies could be reproduced. *See copying.*

Mineralogy An epoch-making work on mining and mineralogy was produced by **Georgius Agricola** (1494–1555), a German physician from Glauchau in Saxony. He spent most of his career at Joachimsthal in Bohemia, one of the greatest mining districts of Europe. His important work *De Re Metallica* was published in 12 volumes in Basel in 1556. A Bohemian metallurgist, **Lazarus Ercker** (1530–1593) published *Beschreibung Allerfürnemisten mineralischen Ertzt und Berckwerksarten* (Description of leading ore processing and mining methods) in 1574. A German chemist, **Johann Joachim Becher** (1635–1682), proposed a classification of minerals in his *Physica Subterranea* (1669). A Swedish metallurgist, **Baron Axel Fredrik Cronstedt** (1722–1765) of Turinge, anonymously published an *Essay on New Mineralogy* (1758) in which he advocated the classification of minerals on the basis of their chemical composition. The first systematic English-language treatise on the subject, the *Elements of Mineralogy* (1784), was published by an Irish chemist and lawyer, **Richard Kirwan** (1733–1812). The Mohs scale for rating the hardness of substances in mineralogy was devised by a German chemist, **Friedrich Mohs** (1773–1839). A French chemist from Châtillon-sur-Loire, **César Antoine Becquerel** (1788–1878), was the first to use electrolysis as a means of isolating metals from their ores. A French mining engineer, **Gabriel Auguste Daubrée** (1814–1896), studied the permeability of rocks in relation to thermal waters and published over 300 papers on mineralogy and petrology.

Mining *See metallurgy.*

Minkowski, Rudolph Leo (1895–1976) *See radioastronomy.*

Minkowski Space A fourth mathematical axis in addition to three spatial dimensions, proposed by a Lithuanian mathematician, **Hermann Minkowski** (1864–1909), who was a teacher of **Albert Einstein** (1879–1955) at the Polytechnicum in Zurich.

Minkowski, Hermann (1864–1909) *See Minkowski space.*

Minoan Civilization The first European civilization, which began on the island of Crete 4500 years ago. Strange objects picked up by shepherds in Crete were first studied by Milchhoffer in 1883. An excavation was initiated by Halbherr in 1886 and further studies on the antiquities of Crete were carried out by **Sir Arthur John Evans** (1851–1941), the curator at the Ashmolean Museum in Oxford. His findings revealed a culture a few centuries older than the classical mainland Greek civilization. It started when the ancient Egyptians were supposed to have discovered the island. The lack of any evidence of Paleolithic culture on Crete confirms the fact that a previous civilization did not exist before the arrival of the Egyptians. The civilization of Crete overtook all the contemporary civilizations including those of mainland Greece and Egypt around 3000 to 2000 BC. The name Minoan for the civilization, given by Evans, follows the legendary stories of sea power held by Minos, the King of Crete, son of Jupiter and Europa, in 1406 BC. The sudden disappearance of Minoan civilization in 1400 BC is attributed to the eruption of the volcano Santorini.

Miocene Period [Greek: *mio*, less + *cene*, recent] A geological period in the earth's history 11 to 25 million years ago. It was identified and named in 1839 by a Scottish geologist, **Sir Charles Lyell** (1797–1875) from Kinnordy, Forfarshire.

Mirage An optical illusion by which inverted images of distant objects are seen as if below the ground or in the atmosphere. The effect is caused by refraction or bending of light as it passes through the hot air near the ground, so that it appears to come from the horizon. A French mathematican and physicist, **Gaspard Monge** (1746–1818), who accompanied Napoleon to Egypt, was the first to give a scientific explanation for it, based on the laws of optics.

Mises, Richard von (1883–1953) *See probability theory.*

Mitchell, Maria (1818–1889) An American astronomer who became the first female member of the American Academy of Arts and Sciences. She made a telescopic discovery of a comet in 1847.

Mitchell, Peter (1920–1992) An English chemist from Mitcham, London who was awarded the Nobel prize in 1978 for his work on the conservation of energy by plants during respiration and photosynthesis.

Mitchell, Reginald Joseph (1895–1937) *See warplanes.*

Mitchell, Sir Peter Chalmers (1864–1945) *See zoo.*

Mitochondrion [Greek: *mitos*, thread + *chondrion*, granule] A cell organelle identified and named by **Carl Benda** (1857–1933) of Germany, in 1898. A Belgian-born American biologist, **Albert Claude** (1898–1983), showed that mitochondria are the site of cellular respiration.

Mitosis [Greek: *mitos*, thread] The process of nuclear division involving the chromosomes in the cell was first observed in 1873 by a German cytologist, **Friedrich Anton Schneider** (1831–1890). It was named and described by a German biologist, **Walther Flemming** (1843–1905) of Sachenberg, in 1882. The different stages in mitosis – prophase, metaphase and anaphase – were described and named in 1884 by a German botanist and professor at Bonn, **Eduard Adolf Strasburger** (1844–1912).

Mitscherlich, Eilhardt (1794–1863) *See benzene, catalysis, isomorphism.*

Mivart, St George Jackson (1827–1900) *See vertebrates.*

Möbius Strip A one-sided surface constructed by half-twisting a rectangular strip and joining the ends together. Described by a German mathematician, **August Ferdinand Möbius** (1790–1868).

Möbius, August Ferdinand (1790–1868) *See barycentric calculus, Möbius strip.*

Mohists Named after their founder Mo Ti, who lived in China around 500 BC. Their thinking was based on fundamental scientific logic, although they had a bias towards physical sciences. Much of their work is preserved in *The Book of Master Chuang*. Their interest in defense and fortification led to some fundamental studies in mechanics.

Mohl, Hugo von (1805–1872) *See protoplasm.*

Mohorovicic Discontinuity A region of sudden change in the earth's crust, 3 to 4 miles below the basaltic crust. First described in 1909 by a Yugoslavian scientist **Andrija Mohorovicic** (1857–1936).

Mohorovicic, Andrija (1857–1936) *See Mohorovicic discontinuity.*

Mohs Scale A useful scale for rating the hardness of substances in mineralogy. devised by a German chemist, **Friedrich Mohs** (1773–1839), who published *The Natural History System of Mineralogy* (1821) and *Treatise on Mineralogy* (1825) in three volumes.

Mohs, Friedrich (1773–1839) *See mineralogy, Mohs scale.*

Moissan, Ferdinand Frederic Henri (1852–1907) *See artificial diamond, carborundum, electric furnace, fluorine.*

Moivre, Abraham de (1667–1754) *See De Moivre's equation, normal distribution curve, probability theory, trigonometry.*

de Moivre's Equation A formula for integers, proposed by a French mathematician, **Abraham de Moivre** (1667–1754) of Vitry, Champagne.

Molecular Beams The apparatus for analysis of light beams and study of free atoms was developed in 1929 by a German-born US physicist, **Otto Stern** (1888–1969) from Schrau, in Upper Silesia. His work led to a demonstration of the wave aspects of matter. He constructed the Stern–Gerlach apparatus for studying molecular beams with a German physicist, **Walther Gerlach** (1889–1979). Stern escaped from Nazi Germany to the United States in 1933, and was awarded the Nobel Prize for physics in 1943.

Molecular Clock A concept in molecular biology used for tracing human origins. It orginated from the assumption that a gene and its protein product in a sample of fossils shows evidence of mutation at a steady rate over a period of time. Discovered by an American biochemist, **Allan Charles Wilson** (1934–1991) and his colleague Vincent Sarich at the University of California, Berkeley. Wilson concluded from his DNA studies that modern humans originated in Africa about 200 000 years ago.

Molecular Orbital Theory Electronic energy states in relation to molecular structure and chemical bonding. Developed in the 1930s mainly by an American physicist, **Robert Sanderson Mulliken** (1896–1986) of Newburyport, Massachusetts, who was awarded the Nobel Prize for chemistry in 1966. It was developed by several other physicists including an English physicist from Lancashire, **Sir John Edward Lennard-Jones** (1894–1954). Another English physicist, **Charles Alfred Coulson** (1910–1974), the first professor of theoretical chemistry at Oxford, studied the application of molecular orbital theory to chemical bonds and published *Valence* (1952). Further work on the theory was done by **Christopher Longuet-Higgins** (b 1923) from Kent, who became professor of theoretical chemistry at Cambridge in 1954.

Molecule The smallest part of a chemical compound that still has all the properties of the compound. The term was first used by an Italian physicist, **Amedeo Avogadro** (1776–1856), to denote the smallest possible quantity of water. *See Avogadro's law.*

Molybdenum [Latin: *molybdaenia*, galena] A metallic element of atomic number 42, discovered in 1781 by a Swedish chemist, **Peter Jacob Hjelm** (1746–1813). He was a close friend and co-worker of **Carl Wilhelm Scheele** (1742–1786).

Momentum [Latin: *momentum*, motion] The mass of a body multiplied by its velocity. The law of conservation of momentum was first suggested in 1668 by an English mathematician, **John Wallis** (1616–1703) from Ashford, Kent.

Mond Process *See nickel.*

Mond, Ludwig (1839–1909) *See nickel.*

Monge, Gaspard (1746–1818) *See descriptive geometry, mirage.*

Monocotyledon A botanical term for a division of flowering plants (angiosperms) with a single-leafed seed, introduced in 1703 by **John Ray** (1628–1705), an English biologist from Essex. Classification based on single-leafed seeds (monocotyledons) and two-leafed seeds (dicotyledons) was proposed by **Lobelius** or **Matthias de l'Obel** (1538–1616) of the Netherlands in his *New Note-book of Plants*. A French botanist, **René Louiche Desfontaines** (1750–1833), described the differences between monocotyledons and dicotyledons in his *Mémoire sur l'Organisation des monocotylédones ou Plantes à une Feuille Séminare* (1796). An important study of the monocotyledon was done by a London botanist, **Agnes Arber** (1879–1960), who published *Monocotyledons* (1925) in which she explained the phyllode theory of the monocotyledonous leaf.

Monod, Jacques Lucien (1910–1976) *See genetic engineering.*

Monorail A system of transport where the vehicle is constrained to a single continuous, usually elevated, rail. The first one was built by a London engineer, Henry Robinson Palmer, who took out a patent for it in 1821. His monorail between the Royal Dock and the River Thames consisted of horse drawn carts on a rail fixed on elevated wooden planks. A modern system was invented by a German, **Fritz Bernhard Behr** (b 1842) of Berlin, who migrated to England in 1875. He exhibited a high-speed monorail train of 90 miles per hour at the exhibition in Berlin in 1897. A Swedish industrialist, **Axel Leonard Wenner-Green**

(1881–1961), developed it further. His system was installed in Japan between Tokyo and Haneda airport.

Monotype Used in printing, and invented in 1887 by an American, **Tolbert Lanston** (1844–1913) of Ohio.

Montgolfier, Jacques Étienne (1745–1799) *See air balloon, parachute.*

Montgolfier, Joseph Michel (1740–1810) *See air balloon.*

Montgomery, T.H. (1873–1912) *See chromosomes.*

Month The division of time into months by the ancients was based on various phases of the moon. The Greeks initially computed 12 months, each alternating with 30 and 29 days, in a year. As this fell short of the solar year, Cleostratus of Tenedos intercalated three months, with 30 days each. The Romans initially had 10 months, but later followed the Greeks and made it 12. **Geminus** (*c.* 300 BC), an astronomer and pupil of **Posidonius** of Alexandria (*c.* 400 BC), defined the month as the time from one full moon to the next full moon. The months of the year are named as follows: January after the god Janus, the god of beginnings; February after Februa, the Roman festival of purification; March after the god Mars; April after Aphrodite; May after the goddess Maia; June after the god Juno; July after Julius Caesar; August after the Emperor Augustus; September for *septem*, seven in Latin; October for *octo*, eight in Latin; November for *novem*, nine in Latin; December, for *decem*, ten in Latin.

Montucula, Jean Étienne (1725–1799) *See mathematics.*

Moon Clay tablets dating back to 2000 BC, discovered in the 19th century, revealed that the Babylonians were able to predict eclipses and the positions of the moon. A Greek philosopher, **Pytheas of Marseilles** (360–290 BC), interpreted the tides on the basis of moon and its phases. **Hipparchus of Bithynia** (190–120 BC) who is regarded as the father of observational astronomy, measured the motion of the sun and the moon. **Galilei Galileo** (1564–1642), one of the first to produce a telescope in astronomy, described the valleys on the moon. The first map of the side of the moon from the earth was given by a German astronomer, **Johannes Hevelius** (1611–1687) of Danzig, in his *Selenographia* (1647). A map of the moon was published by **Giovanni Domenico Cassini** (1625–1712) of Nice in 1679. The acceleration of the moon was discovered by the British astronomer, **Edmund Halley** (1656–1742), in 1720. A French novelist, **Jules Verne** (1828–1905) of Nantes, published *De la Terre à la Lune* (From the Earth to the Moon), the first fiction on space travel, in 1865. In 1878, a German astronomer, **Johann Friedrich Julius Schmidt** (1825–1884), published a map of the moon, consisting of 25 sheets. The historical landing on the moon was achieved by the American astronauts, **Neil Armstrong** (b 1930), **Edwin Eugene Aldrin** (b 1930) and **Michael Collins** (b 1930) in their *Apollo 11*, on 20 July 1969. Armstrong published *First on the Moon* in 1970.

Moore, Stanford (1913–1982)   *See chromatography, ribonucleic acid.*

Moore-Brabazon, John Theodore Cuthbert (1884–1964)   *See airplane.*

Moreland, Samuel (1625–1696)   *See loudspeaker.*

Morgan, Augustus de (1806–1871)   An English mathematician born in Madura, India. He published *Budget of Paradoxes* (1872), and a mathematical theorem is named after him.

Morgan, Garrett A. (1875–1963)   *See traffic signals.*

Morgan, Thomas Hunt (1866–1945)   *See genetics.*

Morgenstern, Oscar (1902–1977)   *See games theory.*

Morison, Robert (1620–1683)   *See botany.*

Morley, Edward William (1838–1923)   An American physicist from Newark, New Jersey, who conducted experiments with **Albert Abraham Michelson** (1852–1931), on ether-drift. *See ether, Fitzgerald–Lorentz contraction, water.*

Morphine   The first plant alkaloid, discovered in 1805 by a German apothecary and alkaloid chemist, **Friedrich Wilhelm Sertürner** (1783–1841). He demonstrated its salts, and in 1817 named it morpheum, after *Morpheus*, the Greek god of sleep. It was independently isolated by two French chemists **Bernard Courtois** (1777–1838) and **Baron Louis Bernand Guyton de Morveau** (1737–1816) of Dijon.

Morphology [Greek: *morphe*, form + *logos*, discourse] A term introduced into biology in 1817 by a German scientist and poet, **Johann Wolfgang von Goethe** (1749–1832), one of the pioneers in the study of evolution. He was the first since Aristotle to point out the uniformity of anatomical structures in animals.

Morris, Desmond John (b 1928)   *See ethology.*

Morse Code   A communication system in universal electric telegraphy in which the letters of the alphabet are represented by dots and dashes, produced by the making and breaking of an electric circuit. Invented by **Samuel Morse**

(1791–1872) of Charlestown, Massachusetts. Morse graduated from Yale in 1810 and started his experiments on telegraphy in 1814. He demonstrated his magnetic telegraph to Congress in 1837 and his system was officially established on an experimental basis between Baltimore and Washington in 1843. The first official message was sent in 1844. He developed the Morse code mainly for use with his telegraph. *See electric telegraphy.*

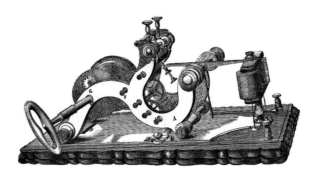

Figure 60   A common form of Morse telegraph used in America in the mid-19th century. Lardner, Dionysius. *Handbook of Natural Philosophy, Electricity, Magnetism, and Acoustics.* London: Walton and Maberly, 1856

Morse, Harmon Northup (1848–1920)   *See osmosis.*

Morse, Samuel (1791–1872)   *See Morse code.*

Mort, Thomas Sutcliffe (1816–1878)   *See food industry, locomotive.*

Morton, Thomas (1781–1832)   *See shipping.*

Morveau, Baron Louis Bernard Guyton de (1737–1816)   *See morphine.*

Mosander, Carl Gustav (1797–1858)   *See didumium, erbium, gadolinium, lanthanum, terbium, yttrium.*

Moseley, Henry Gwynn Jeffreys (1887–1915)   *See atomic number, Moseley's law, X-ray spectroscopy.*

Moseley, Henry Nottidge (1844–1891)   An English botanist, anatomist and astronomer from Wandsworth who observed the solar eclipse in Ceylon (Sri Lanka) in 1871. He was one of the founders of the Marine Biological Association, and became professor of human and comparative anatomy at Oxford in 1881.

Moseley's Law   Relating X-ray spectra and atomic number, proposed by an English physicist, **Henry Gwynn Jeffreys Moseley** (1887–1915) from Weymouth. He was the first to introduce X-ray spectroscopy for determination of the spectra of elements and predict their existence.

Moss   The first major botanical study of moss was done by a German botanist and artist, **Johann Jacob Dillen** (1687–1747). He published the first monograph on the subject, *Historia Muscorum* (1741), which gave detail illustrations of nearly 600 different species of moss. **Johannes Hedwig's** (1730–1799) *Species Muscotum*, published posthumously in 1801, was a starting point in the naming of the mosses.

Mössbauer Effect   Related to the recoil-free absorption of gamma radiation by the atomic nucleus, and it provided experimental verification of Einstein's theory of relativity. Descibed by a German physicist, **Rudolf Ludwig Mössbauer** (b 1929) who shared the Nobel Prize for physics (1961) with a New York physicist, **Robert Hofstadter** (1915–1990).

Mössbauer, Rudolf Ludwig (b 1929)   *See Mössbauer effect, quarks.*

Motion [Latin: *motio*, movement]   **Aristotle** (384–322 BC) in his work on dynamics dealt with the doctrine of natural or free motion, and unnatural or forced motion. An Augustinian monk, **Albert of Saxony** (*c.* 1316–1390), in the 14th century discussed the external and internal resistance to motion. He became the first rector of the University of Vienna in 1365, and was appointed bishop of Halberstadt in 1366. The factors controlling the motion of bodies were first studied by **Thomas Bradwardine** (*c.* 1290–1349) of Merton College, Oxford, who was later Archbishop of Canterbury for only a month before he succumbed to the Black Death. He completed his work *Tractatus de Proportionibus* in 1324. His mathematical theory of motion was advanced by **Nicole Oresme** (*c.* 1325–1382) of Normandy. The mechanisms of projectile motion were discussed and explained by **John Buridan** (*c.* 1300–1358) of Paris. Three mathematicians from Merton College, Oxford, **William Heytesbury** (1310–1380), **Richard Swineshead** (*c.* 1350) and **John Dumbleton** (*c.* 1340) developed the concept of acceleration and the theory related to the causes of motion. The study of motion was significantly advanced by **Galilei Galileo** (1564–1642) through his experiments on falling bodies through various inclinations, in 1604. An English physicist and mathematician, **George Atwood** (1746–1807), investigated the motion of falling objects with his 'fall machine' in 1837. The three important laws of motion were formulated by **Sir Isaac Newton** (1642–1727) in his *Principia*. Further study of the subject contributed to the development of the theory of relativity. The laws of motion were first applied to fluids in 1640 by **Evangelista Torricelli** (1608–1647). *See relativity.*

Motion Picture   *See cinema.*

Motor Boat   The first high-speed internal combustion engine was developed by **Gottlieb Daimler** (1834–1900), who fitted it to a boat for the first time, around 1886. A Luxembourg-born French engineer, **Jean Joseph Etienne Lenoir** (1822–1900) built an engine and used it for a boat in the same year.

Motorcar Industry   *See car, Chrysler, Walter Percy, Citroën, André Gustav, Daimler, Gottlib, Farina, Battista, Ferrari, Enzo, Ford, Henry, Holden, Sir Edward Wheewall, Peugeot, Rolls, Charles Stewart, Royce, Sir Frederick Henry.*

Motorcar   *See car, motorcar industry, motoring.*

Motorcycle   The first motorbike was built by **Gottlieb Daimler** (1834–1900), who installed one of his internal combustion engines into a wooden-frame bicycle, in 1885. It was first ridden by **Wilhelm Maybach** (1846–1929), and reached a top speed of 12 miles per hour. The first British motorcycles, the Holden flat-four, were built in 1898. The first factory for large-scale production of motorcycles was established in 1894 by Wilhelm Hildbrand and Alois Wolfmuller in Munich, Germany. They produced over 1000 machines in the first year. **Soichiro Honda** (1906–1992) of Japan started mass producing motorcycles in 1948.

Motoring   The 1861 Locomotive Act in England made taxes on steam-traction highway vehicles uniform with horse-drawn vehicles, and limited the speed of engined vehicles to 5 miles per hour in cities. The Red Flag Act in 1865 limited the speed further to 2 miles per hour in towns and villages and 4 miles per hour on the highways. Each engined vehicle had to be preceded by a person on foot carrying a red flag. The German engineer **Carl Friedrich Benz** (1844–1929) from Karlsruhe demonstrated the first petrol-driven car, a three-wheeler, in 1886. The world's first number or registration plates were introduced by the Parisian police in 1893. British motoring history started when Henry Hewetson drove his Benz Velo into London in 1894. Registration plates were introduced in Britain in 1903. The first number plate, A1, was obtained for his Napier model by an English politician, **John Francis Stanley Russell** (1865–1931), who was the brother of the philosopher **Bertrand Arthur William Russell** (1872–1970). The motor car company in the longest continuous production, the Morgan Motor Car Company of Malvern, was founded in 1910. *See car, parking meter, traffic signal.*

Mott, Sir Neville Francis (1905–1996) *See photography, van Vleck, John Hasbrouck.*

Mottelson, Benjamin Roy (b 1926) *See atomic structure.*

Moufet, Thomas (1553–1604) *See entomology, metamorphosis.*

Moulton, Forest (1872–1952) *See Chamberlin–Moulton hypothesis.*

Mount Palomar Observatory World's premier observatory in the 1950s at San Diego, California, completed in 1948.

Mount Stromlo Observatory Australian astronomical observatory established in 1923 in Canberra.

Mount Wilson Observatory Located in the mountains behind Pasadena, California, it was established in 1905 by the Carnegie Institution at the initiation of two American astronomers, **Walter Sydney Smith** (1876–1956) and **George Ellery Hale** (1868–1938). A 50-foot interferometer, used for directly measuring the diameters of stars at the observatory, was built by **Francis Gladheim Pease** (1881–1938), an astronomer and designer of optical instruments from Cambridge Massachusetts. Another American astronomer, **Walter Sydney Adams** (1876–1956), was mainly responsible for the design of the 5.08-meter telescope at the observatory.

Mouriès, Hippolyte Mège (1817–1880) *See margarine.*

Mouse A device used to control a pointer on a computer screen. It was invented in 1963 at the Stanford Research Institute, USA, by Douglas Engelbart, and was first made of wood. It was developed by the Xerox Corporation in the 1970s. The improved Microsoft mouse was introduced in 1983, and the Apple Macintosh mouse appeared in 1984.

Movable Type Printing First used in China around 1040 when Pi Sheng used type made from pottery. The Chinese invented wooden type 300 years later. Around 1450 **Johannes (Gensfleisch) Gutenberg** (1400–1468) of Mainz molded small pieces of lead alloy, one for each letter, and assembled them by hand to form words and sentences. *See Gutenberg Bible, printing.*

Moxon, Joseph (1627–1700) *See structural engineering.*

MS-DOS (Microsoft Disc Operating System) A widely used computer operating system first produced by the Microsoft Corporation in 1981.

Mudge, John (d 1793) *See reflecting telescope, watches.*

Mudge, Thomas (1715–1794) *See escapement.*

Mueller, Erwin Wilhelm (1911–1977) *See field-emission microscope, field-ion microscope.*

Muir, Thomas (1844–1934) A Scottish mathematician from Stonebrye, Lanarkshire whose main interest was determinants of which he published a five-volume treatise on their history in 1906–30. His other books include *A Treatise on the Theory of Determinants* (1882) and *The Theory of Determinants in its Historical Order of Development* (1890).

Mulder, Gerardus Johannes (1802–1880) *See nutrition, protein.*

Muller, Franz Joseph or **Baron von Reichenstein** (1740–1825) *See tellurium.*

Muller, Fritz (1821–1891) *See mimicry.*

Muller, Heinrich (1820–1864) *See fixatives.*

Muller, Hermann Joseph (1890–1967) *See mutation.*

Muller, Hermann Paul (1899–1965) *See textile chemistry.*

Muller, Johannes (1436–1476) *See scientific journals.*

Muller, Johannes Peter (1801–1858) *See scientific journals.*

Muller, Karl Alex (b 1927) *See superconductivity.*

Muller, Max (1823–1900) *See philology.*

Muller, Otto Frederick (1730–1784) *See diatoms.*

Mulliken, Robert Sanderson (1896–1986) *See molecular orbital theory.*

Mullis, Kary Banks (b 1944) *See polymerase chain reaction.*

Multiplication Tables of multiplication appeared in Mesopotamia around 1800 BC. The symbol for multiplication (×) was introduced by **William Oughtred** (1575–1660), a clergyman from Eton in his *Clavis Mathematica* (1631).

Munk, Walter Heinrich (b 1917) *See oceanography.*

Münster, Sebastian (1489–1552) *See geography.*

Muon An elementary atomic particle discovered in 1937 by the US physicists Jabez Curry Street (1906–1989) and Edward C. Stevenson.

Murchison, Roderick Impey (1792–1871) *See British Association for the Advancement of Science, Silurian period.*

Murdoch, William (1754–1839) A Scottish pioneer of gas lighting. He also invented an oscillating engine in 1785 and improved James Watt's steam engine. *See coal gas, gas lighting.*

Murray, Alexander (1775–1813) *See philology.*

Murray, Sir John (1841–1914) *See marine biology, oceanography.*

Museum The term museum was used by **Plato** (428–348 BC) for the temple of Muses in Athens. It later referred to schools of art and philosophy in ancient Greece, and the Alexandrian Museum (university) was founded in 331 BC. The term came into disuse and was revived in the 17th century to denote collections of natural curiosities. The earliest museum in England, the Tradescantianum, was established in Lambeth, London, by a gardener and botanist **John Tradescant** (1567–1637) and his son (1608–1662) with the same name. Their collection was acquired in 1694 by **Elias Ashmole** (1617–1692), who installed it in Oxford. The first scientific museum was established by the Royal Society, and a catalog of its collection was prepared by **Nehemiah Grew** (1641–1712) in 1681. This collection was transferred to the British Museum in 1781. **Sir Hans Sloane's** (1660–1753) vast collection was acquired by the British Museum in 1759. The largest museum in the world, the US Smithsonian Institution, was founded in 1846, and it contains nearly 140 million items. The American Museum of Natural History was founded in New York in 1869. The British Museum in London was founded in 1753 and opened to the public in 1759.

Mushet, Robert Forester (1811–1891) *See Bessemer process.*

Mushett, James (1793–1886) *See soda.*

Music [Greek: *mousike*] *See acoustics, music printing, musical instruments, musical recording, musical theory.*

Music Printing One of the earliest pieces of printed music in England, a church service book with musical notation, was printed in 1560 by a London printer, **John Day** (1522–1584).

Musical Instruments Flutes made of perforated bones have been found in Paleolithic sites dating back to 25 000 BC, in Hungary and Moldova. Yellow bells hung in Chinese temples around 3000 BC had a recognizable standard musical tone. A French-born British musical instrument maker, **Arnold Dometsch** (1858–1940), revived and restored many early musical instruments, and made the first modern recorder in 1919. *See accordion, automatic musical instruments, barrel organ, flute, gramophone, musical synthesizer, piano.*

Musical Recording The microphone was invented in 1857 by **David Edward Hughes** (1830–1900) from a Welsh family, in London. **Eldridge R. Johnson** (1866–1945) founded the Victor Talking Machine Company, a forerun-ner of the modern recording studio. The Italian operatic tenor, **Enrico Caruso** (1873–1921) of Naples, started making recordings of his performances in Milan in 1902. Leopold Stokowski (1882–1977), a London-born American conductor of Polish origin, had his performance recorded in 1917 by the Victor Recording Studio. The invention of the triode valve by **Lee de Forest** (1873–1961), in 1907, led to the development of the amplifier. The electromagnetic disk cutter for producing records was developed around 1920. AEG Telefunken of Germany developed the tape recorder around 1935. A British record producer, **John Culshaw** (1924–1980) developed new recording techniques and introduced echo chambers and the speeding and slowing of tapes to achieve effects not possible in live performances. The stereophonic sound system was introduced in 1933 by a British company, EMI. *See gramophone, video tapes.*

Musical Synthesizer An electronic instrument for making sound from analog or digital electrical signals. The first one was designed in 1955 by an American engineer, **Harry Ferdinand** (1901–1982) of Mount Pleasant, Iowa. It was named by an American inventor, Robert Moog (in collaboration with the music composers Harry Deutsch and Walter Carlos). He invented a more advanced synthesizer in 1964.

Musical Theory The Greek philosopher **Pythagoras** (*c.* 580–500 BC) from the island of Samos discovered the numerical ratio of sounds that are consonant with one another. In his work he also described octaves and semitones and investigated them on the basis of the length and thickness of strings. His discovery was described by a Roman philosopher, **Anicus Manlius Severinus Boethius** (AD 480–524) in his *De Institutione Musica*. **Eudoxus** (400–360 BC) and **Archytas of Tarentum** (428–347 BC) held the view that the doctrine of consonances depended on numbers, and they established the proportionality of pitch to vibrational frequency. According to **Theon of Smyrna** (*c.* AD 250), the early Pythagorean scholars, Larsus of Hermione and **Hippasus of Metapontium** (*c.* 450 BC) were the first to suggest that higher pitched sounds are more quickly propagated than lower sounds. Another Pythagorean philosopher, **Philolaus** (*c.* 450 BC), explained the five full tones and two semitones of the octave. Important work on harmonics including scales, intervals and notes is found in *Elements of Harmonics* by Aristoxenus of Tarentum, a pupil of Aristotle. *See acoustics.*

Musschenbroek, Pieter van (1692–1761) *See Leyden jar.*

Mutation [Latin: *mutare*, to change] A sudden and spontaneous change in the hereditary material. Described in

Oenothera (evening primrose) and named by a Dutch physiologist and genetist, **Hugo Marie de Vries** (1848–1935), while he was professor of botany at Amsterdam, in 1890. His work *Die Mutationstheorie* was published in 1901. An American biologist, **Hermann Joseph Muller** (1890–1967), studied the mutation of genes exposed to X-rays, for which he was awarded the Nobel Prize for Medicine or Physiology in 1946. He published *A phenotypic classification of mutations* (1933) and several other papers on the subject. The importance of mutation in the alteration of species was shown by an American biologist, **William Ernest Castle** (1867–1962) of Ohio, who was professor of genetics at Harvard from 1908 to 1936. A German-born British geneticist, **Charlotte Auerbach** (1899–1994), discovered chemical mutagenesis during her study on the effects of mustard gas on *Drosophila*.

Muybridge, Eadweard (1830–1904) *See zoopraxiscope.*

Mycenae A city in Peloponnesus, and the center of the first Greek civilization, around 1900 BC. It was excavated in 1876 by a German archaeologist, **Heinrich Schliemann** (1822–1890).

Mycology [Greek: *mykes*, fungus + *logos*, discourse] Study of fungi. In 1583 **Andrea Caesalpino** (1525–1603) of Italy considered fungi to be an intermediate between plants and animals. **Robert Hooke** (1635–1703) examined them under the microscope and described the yeast in 1680. A French botanist, **Carus Clusius** or **Charles de Lécluse**

(1525–1609), produced an illustrated work on fungi. **Marcello Malpighi** (1628–1694) studied the molds on fruits, cheese and wood in 1679. The first modern book on the subject, *Synopsis Fungorum* (1801), was published by a South African botanist, **Christian Hendrik** (1761–1836). The sexual process in fungi was discovered in 1818 by **Christian Gottfried Ehrenberg** (1795–1876) of Germany. Fungi became important as a medicinal source for many antibiotics, and in fermentation. Two French brothers and mycologists, **Louis René Tulasne** (1815–1885) and **Charles Tulasne** (1816–1884) studied the structure and development of fungi and published an illustrated work *Selecta Fungorum Carpologia* (1861–1865). Modern systematic mycology was founded by a Swedish botanist **Elias Magnus Fries** (1794–1878) who published *Systema mycologium* (1821–1830) in three volumes. His work is regarded as the starting point in fungal nomenclature. An Italian-born British agricultural scientist, **Guido Pontecorvo** (1907–1993), described the parasexual cycle in fungi, in 1950. He became professor of genetics at the University of Glasgow in 1956.

Mycorrhiza [Greek: *mykes*, fungus + *rhizon*, root] A group of fungi associated with the roots of higher plants. They facilitate the absorption of nutrients. Described and named by a German botanist, **Albert Bernhard Frank** (1839–1900).

Mylne, Robert (1734–1811) *See bridges.*

N

Nägeli, Carl Wilhelm von (1817–1891) *See phloem, pollination.*

Nagell, Trygve (b 1895) A Norwegian mathematician from Oslo who made important contributions to abstract algebra and number theory. He was professor at Uppsala, Sweden, from 1931 to 1962.

Namias, Jerome (b 1910) *See weather forecast.*

Nanotechnology Building of devices on one millionth of a scale. Micromachines, gears smaller in diameter than a human hair, have been made at the AT&T Bell laboratories in New Jersey, USA. The idea of manipulating material on a nanometer scale was first suggested by US physicist **Richard Phillips Feynman** (1918–1988) in 1959.

Nansen, Fridtjof (1861–1930) *See wind.*

Napier, John (1550–1617) Scottish inventor of logarithms, born at Merchiston Castle, near Edinburgh and educated at St Andrew's University. In his search for a shorter and simpler method of calculation he came up with the table of logarithms. His work on the subject entitled *Mirifici Logarithmorum Canonis Descriptio* (Description of the marvellous Canon of Logarithms) was published in 1614. He invented the calculating apparatus known as Napier's bones which he published in his *Rabdologiae* (1617).

Napier, Robert (1791–1876) *See warships.*

Napier's Rods or bones. A simple device to facilitate multiplication, designed by **John Napier** (1550–1617). He described his method in his *Rabdologiae, seu numerationis per virgulas, libri duo, Edinburgi* published in 1617. Some copies of Napier's tables, made of wood and sometimes out of paper, have survived.

NASA [National Aeronautics and Space Administration] A US government body set up in 1958 for crewed and uncrewed space flights. The Space Center at Houston, Texas and the Space Center at Cape Canaveral, Florida operate under it.

Nash, John (1752–1835) *See architecture, British, town planning.*

Nasmyth, James (1808–1890) *See mechanical engineering, steam hammer.*

Nathans, Daniel (b 1928) *See deoxyribonucleic acid.*

National Academy of Sciences *See academy.*

National Physical Laboratory (NPL) A research establishment under the control of the Department of Industry, set up in 1900 at Teddington, England. The first digital computer known as the ACE (Automatic Computing Engine) started being built there in 1944 and was completed in 1950.

Natta, Giulio (1903–1979) *See polymer.*

Natural Environment Research Council (NERC) A British organization for promoting research in earth sciences in order to protect the environment, established by royal charter in 1965. It comprises of several research bodies including British Geological Survey, Institute of Oceanographic Sciences, Institute of Terrestrial Ecology and Scottish Marine Biological Association.

Natural Numbers Refers to whole numbers used in counting and comprises all the positive integers, including zero. *See number theory.*

Natural Selection A concept based on the survival of the fittest. *See evolution.*

Naudin, Charles (1815–1899) *See hybridization.*

Nautilus The World's first atomic powered submarine launched at Groton, Connecticut on 21 January 1954. *See submarines.*

Navier, Claude Louis Marie Henri (1785–1836) *See bridges, elasticity.*

Navigation *See shipping, ships.*

Neanderthal Man or *Homo sapiens neanderthalensis.* Appeared about 100 000 years ago and became extinct with the emergence of modern man, around 35 000 years ago. Skeletal remains of this primitive man from the Paleolithic period, including a skull, were found in 1858 at a limestone cave at Neanderthal, near Düsseldorf, and described by **Hermann Schaafhausen** (1816–1893). Neanderthal man was followed by Cro-Magnon man or *Homo sapiens*, who had facial and other body features of modern man. The first complete Neanderthal skeleton was assembled by **Marcellin Boule** (1861–1942), a professor at the Natural History Museum in Paris, who published *Les Hommes Fossiles* (1921). *See Homo sapiens, Stone Age.*

Nebulae [Latin: *nebula*, mist] Objects in the sky which appear as hazy patches of light, first studied in detail by **Sir William Herschel** (1738–1822). The first telescopic study of a spiral nebula was carried out in 1850 by an Irish astronomer, **William Parsons, Lord Rosse** (1800–1867) of Birr Castle, County Offaly. He built one of the largest telescopes in the world with a metal reflector, which he used for his observations in astronomy. In 1862, the London astronomer **Sir William Huggins** (1824–1910) distinguished the two types of nebula, one with a greenish appearance from luminous gases, and the other which resembled the spectrum of light from the Milky Way. An American astronomer, **James Edward Keeler** (1857–1900), made a photographic discovery of over 120 000 nebulae and published *Spectroscopic Observations of Nebulae* (1894).

Nebular Hypothesis That the solar system had evolved from a condensing cloud of gas. Proposed by a French mathematician, **Pierre Simon Marquis de Laplace** (1749–1827) from Normandy, in his *Exposition du système du monde* (1796).

Neckham, Alexander (1157–1217) *See magnetic needle, shipping, vision.*

Néel, **Louis Eugène Félix** (b 1904) A French physicist from Lyons who served as professor of physics at Strasbourg from 1937 to 1940. He predicted the phenomenon of ferromagnetism which was confirmed in 1949. He shared the Nobel Prize for physics in 1970, for this work with a Swedish physicist, **Hannes Olof Gösta Alfvén** (1908–1995). *See magnetic recording, plasma physics.*

Negative Numbers A Hindu mathematician from Ujjain, **Brahmagupta** (*c.* 598–660), was the first to assign the rules for negative numbers. Arab mathematicians followed the use of negative numbers proposed by the Hindus. In 1225 an Italian mathematician, **Leonardo Fibonacci** (*c.* 1172–1250) of Pisa, proposed the concept of using negative numbers in the case of a man's debt. **Johann Hudde** (1633–1704), the burgomaster of Amsterdam, in his treatise in 1659 took the important step of using the same number with a positive or negative value.

Nemesis Theory Proposed in 1984 to explain the presence of a layer of iridium (an element found in comets and meteorites) in rocks dating from the end of dinosaur times. It suggests that a sister star to the Sun caused the extinction of the dinosaurs and other groups of animals, and is likely to recur every 26 million years.

Nemorarius, Jordanus (*c.* 1200) *See lever.*

Neodymium A metallic element with an atomic number of 60 obtained from didymium and named by Austrian chemist **Carl Auer von Welsbach** (1858–1929) in 1885.

Neolithic Age *See Stone Age.*

Neon Lighting [Greek: *neos*, new] Incandescent light used in signs by a French physicist, **Georges Claude** (1870–1960) of Paris.

Neptune [Latin: *Neptune*, god of the sea] Eighth major planet from the sun, independently predicted in 1846 by an English astronomer, **John Couch Adams** (1819–1892) of Launceston, Cornwall, and a French astronomer, **Urbain Jean Joseph Leverrier** (1811–1877) of Normandy. An English astronomer **James Challis** (1803–1882) observed it, in 1846, without realizing its significance. It was discovered by a German astronomer, **Johann Gottfried Galle** (1812–1910), in Berlin later in the same year. An American mathematician, **Benjamin Peirce** (1809–1880) of Salem, Massachusetts, wrote on the discovery of Neptune in 1848. An English astronomer from Bolton, **William Lassell** (1799–1880), discovered the first satellite of Neptune later in the same year. The Voyager imaging team discovered six new satellites in 1989.

Neptunium The first element (element 93) to be made synthetically in 1940, through the bombarding of uranium with electrons, by two American atomic scientists, **Erward Mattison McMillan** (1907–1991) of Redondo Beach, California and **Philip Hauge Abelson** (b 1913) of Tacoma, Washington. It was the first element heavier than uranium to be found.

Nernst, **Walther Hermann** (1864–1941) *See calorimeter, electric lighting, physical chemistry, specific heat, valency.*

Neugbauer, Gerald (b 1932) *See radioastronomy.*

Neumann, Balthaser (1687–1753) *See architecture, European.*

Neumann, Johann von (1903–1957) *See computers, games theory.*

Neuron [Greek: *neuron*, nerve] A term for the conducting cell of the nervous system, introduced by a German histologist, **Wilhelm Waldeyer-Hartz** (1836–1921), who was professor of Anatomy at several universities including Breslau, Strasbourg and Berlin.

Neutrino A hypothetical particle in atomic physics with no charge and zero mass at rest, responsible for apparent violation of energy and momentum during beta decay. It was proposed in 1930 by a Swiss physicist, **Wolfgang Pauli**

(1900–1958), named neutrino by **Enrico Fermi** (1901–1954) in 1934, and demonstrated in 1956 by two American physicists, **Clyde Lorrain Cowan** (1919–1974) of Detroit and **Frederick Reines** (1918–1998) of New Jersey. An American chemist, **Raymond Davis** (b 1914), devised the first experiment to detect neutrinos emitted from the core of the sun. In 1960, a New York physicist, **Melvin Schwartz** (b 1932), proposed an experiment for establishing that two kinds of neutrino existed. This was proved by another New York physicist, **Leon Max Lederman** (b 1922) and a German-born US physicist, **Jack Steinberger** (b 1921), in 1962. Lederman, Schwartz and Steinberger shared the Nobel Prize for physics for their work, in 1988.

Neutron [Latin: *neuter,* impartial] An elementary particle similar to a proton but with no charge on it. It serves as a building unit for all atomic nuclei. Proposed by **Lord Ernest Rutherford** (1871–1937) in 1920. It was demonstrated and given its present name by **Sir James Chadwick** (1891–1974) in 1932.

New York Mathematical Society After its founding in 1888 it changed its name to the American Mathematical Society, in 1894.

Newbery, John (1713–1767) *See bookshops.*

Newcomb, Simon (1835–1909) A Canadian mathematician and astronomer from Nova Scotia. He was one of the founder members of the American Astronomical Society and served as its first president from 1899 to 1905. He established a universal standard system for astronomical constants and edited the American *Nautical Almanac.*

Newcomen, Thomas (1663–1729) An English blacksmith from Dartmouth, Devon, who invented the first practical steam engine for pumping water from mines. His engine, set up at Dudley Castle in Wolverhampton in 1712, was the first to use a piston and cylinder mechanism. *See steam engine.*

Newlands, John Alexander Reina (1837–1898) *See atomic weight, periodic law.*

Newman, Max H.A. (1897–1985) *See computers.*

News Agency *See Reuter, Baron de.*

Newspapers They were first printed in the area that is now modern Beijing, China in AD 748. The first gazette or newspaper in Europe under the name *Mercure Françoise* was started in 1635 by a French physician, **Theophrastus Renaudot** (1583–1653) of Lundun, and it lasted for eight years. The oldest surviving news material is a news pamphlet published in Cologne, Germany, in 1470. The oldest news-

paper in the world, *Post och Inrikes Tisningar,* was published by the Royal Swedish Academy of Letters, in 1645. The earliest commercial newspaper *Haarlems Dagblad/Oprechte Haarlemsche Courant* was first published in Haarlem, the Netherlands in 1656. The earliest paper in England, *'Worcester Post Man,* founded in 1690, later changed its name to *Berrow's Worcester Journal,* and has appeared weekly since June 1709. The English adventurer **Daniel Defoe** (1660–1731) in 1704 founded a newspaper *The Review,* which appeared thrice weekly up to 1713. The oldest Sunday newspaper since 1791 is *The Observer.* The first daily newspaper in England, the *Daily Courant,* was started in London in 1702. An English journalist, **John Edward Taylor** (1791–1884) of Ilminster, founded the *Manchester Guardian* in 1821. In 1785, **John Walter** (1739–1812) of London, who was initially a coal merchant and underwriter, founded *The Daily Universal Register,* which became *The Times* in 1788. A steam-driven cylinder press, invented by a German printer, **Friedrich Koenig** (1774–1833) from Eisleben, was first used to print *The Times* in 1814. A New York industrialist **Richard March Hoe** (1812–1886) produced a printing machine used for printing the *Public Ledger* in 1846. **Robert Hoe** (1839–1909) and **William Bullock** (1813–1867) of Philadelphia devised a machine that folded the newspapers. From 1856 to 1862 several British newspapers acquired the Hoe machines. An Australian, **John Fairfax** (1804–1877), born in Warwick, England, founded the *Sydney Herald* (1841) which in 1842 became *The Sydney Morning Herald.* He was the first to use steam printing for newspapers in Australia, in 1853. **Robert Clyde Packer** (1879–1934) of Sydney founded the *Daily Guardian* in Australia. His son **Sir Frank Hewson Packer** (1906–1974), established the *Daily Telegraph.* The *Illustrated London News* was founded in 1842 by **Herbert Ingram** (1811–1860) of Boston, Lincolnshire. The Hungarian-born US founder of the annual Pulitzer prize for literature, drama and music, **Joseph Pulitzer** (1847–1911) established the *New York World* in 1883. **James Edmund Scripps** (1835–1906) from London was a pioneer of newspapers in America, and he founded the *Detroit Evening News.* The *Le Petit Journal* was the first to reach a circulation of a million, in 1886. The *Daily Mail* in England reached this figure in 1900. The *News of the World* was first published in 1843, and reached sales of one million in 1905. The American newspaper magnate, **William Randolph Hearst** (1863–1951), revolutionized newspaper publishing with the introduction of banner headlines, lavish illustrations and other methods. He acquired the *New York Morning Journal* in 1895, and launched the *Evening Journal* in 1896.

Newsreel   The first newsreel in France was made in 1909 by **Charles Pathé** (1863–1957). He also introduced the first newsreel into Britain.

Newton, Alfred (1829–1907)   *See zoology.*

Newton, Sir Isaac (1642–1727)   One of the greatest English scientists, from Woolsthorpe, Lincolnshire. His epoch-making contributions include the formulation of the binomial theorem, laws of motion, calculus and general theory of gravitation. He was educated at Grantham and entered Trinity College, Cambridge in 1660. He developed his binomial theorem at the age of 24, three years before he became a professor at Cambridge. His work on mechanical principles and the motions of bodies, *Philosophiae naturalis principia mathematica* (Mathematical Principles of Natural Philosophy) in three books was edited and published at the expense of his friend **Edmund Halley** (1656–1742) in 1687. The first book, finished in 1685, contained the derivation of the inverse square law. The second book, written in 1686, discussed motion in a resisting medium. In book three, he applied the law of gravitation to the motion of planets. *See absorption spectra, astronomy, binomial theorem, calculus, celestial mechanics, cosmic dynamics, geogeny, gravity, hydrostatics, physics, rainbow, relativity, Royal Society of London, sextant, space travel, thermometer, velocity of sound.*

Nicander (*c.* 140 BC)   *See magnet.*

Nichols, Ernest Fox (1869–1924)   *See radiation pressure.*

Nicholson's Hydrometer   An instrument to determine the specific gravities of solids as well as those of liquids. Invented by a London physicist, **William Nicholson** (1753–1815) from Portsmouth.

Nicholson, William (1753–1815)   *See electrolysis, Nicholson's hydrometer, voltaic pile, water.*

Nicholson, Max (b 1904)   *See ornithology.*

Nickel   Derived from the term, *kupfernickel* [German: *kupfer*, copper + *nickel*, refractory person]. Used by German copper miners to refer to the mineral that appeared like copper, did not yield any copper. It was discovered in 1751 by a Swedish metallurgist, **Baron Axel Fredrik Cronstedt** (1722–1765) of Turinge. The Mond process for extracting nickel from nickel carbonyl was invented by a German-born English industrial chemist, **Ludwig Mond** (1839–1909). He founded the chemical company that later became Imperial Chemical Industries.

Nicol Prism   A refractive device for demonstrating the polarization of light, made of a long crystal of Iceland spar, split into two equal parts and rejoined with Canada balsam. Invented in 1828 by a Scottish physicist, **William Nicol** (1768–1851), who was a professor of physics at Edinburgh, where **James Clerk Maxwell** (1831–1879) was his pupil.

Nicol, William (1768–1851)   *See Nicol prism, stereochemistry.*

Nicomachus of Gerasa (*c.* AD 100)   A Greek mathematician whose extant works include *Introduction to Arithmetic* and *Manual of Harmomy. See perfect number.*

Nicot, Jean (1530–1600)   *See nicotine.*

Nicotine   A plant alkaloid obtained from *Nicotiana tabacum*, and named after **Jean Nicot** (1530–1600), the French ambassador to Portugal, who brought the seeds to France for medical use, around 1560. The first pure form was prepared by Reimann and Posselt, in 1828. A Swiss chemist, **Amè Pictet** (1857–1937) of Geneva, synthesized it in 1903.

Nielson, James Beaumont (1792–1865)   *See iron.*

Niepce, Joseph Nicephore (1765–1833)   *See camera.*

Nieuwland, Julius Arthur (1878–1936)   *See acetylene, artificial rubber, polymer.*

Nineveh   An ancient city excavated in 1849 at Nimrud, in Iraq, by an English archaeologist, **Henry Austen Layard** (1817–1894).

Niobium   A metallic element of atomic number 42, discovered in 1801 by Charles Hatchett.

Nipkow Disk   A mechanical scanning device used in early television. It was invented by a German engineer, **Paul Nipkow** (1860–1940), and consisted of a revolving disk with a spiral pattern of apertures. It was superseded by electronic scanning.

Nipkow, Paul (1860–1940)   *See Nipkow disk, television.*

Nirenberg, Marshall Warren (b 1927)   *See genetic coding.*

Nitric Acid   A Persian chemist, **Geber** or **Abu Musa Jabir ibn Hayyan** (b AD 721), is credited with the discovery. It was prepared under the name aqua fortis by an alchemist, Raymond Lully in 1287. A German alchemist, **John Rudolph Glauber** (1604–1668), described its preparation obtained by heating saltpeter with sulfuric acid. An economic way of producing it from nitrogen and oxygen in the air was described by a Norwegian physicist, **Kristian Olaf Bernhard Birkeland** (1867–1917), who was professor of physics at the University of Kristiana. A cheap commercial process of producing nitric acid, using hydroelectricity, was developed by a Norwegian industrial chemist, **Samuel Eyde** (1866–1940).

Nitrogen [Greek: *nitron*, soda + *genos,* descent] The gas remaining in the air after complete combustion was demonstrated in 1772 by **Daniel Rutherford** (1749–1819), a pupil of **Joseph Black** (1728–1799), in Edinburgh. **Henry Cavendish** (1731–1810) independently discovered it in the same year. It was first called azote [Greek: *a*, without + *zoe*, life] by **Antoine Laurent Lavoisier** (1743–1794). Its present name was suggested in 1790 by a French chemist, **Jean Antoine Claude Chanteloup Chaptal** (1756–1832). Two Polish chemists, **Karol Stanislov Olszevski** (1846–1915) and **Zygmunt Florenty von Wroblewski** (1845–1888) liquefied nitrogen on a large scale, in 1883.

Nitrogen-Fixing Bacteria The nodules later found to contain these bacteria were first observed in leguminous plants by **Marcello Malpighi** (1628–1694) in 1686. The phenomenon of nitrogen fixation was described in 1837 by **Jean Baptiste Joseph Dieudonné Boussingault** (1802–1887). **Pierre Eugène Marcelin Berthelot** (1827–1907) of Paris in 1886 showed that nitrogen fixation was due to certain bacteria. A German botanist, **Hermann Helriegel** (1831–1895) observed the fixation of nitrogen from the air by some leguminous plants in the same year. The presence of nitrogen-fixing bacteria in the roots of certain legumes was demonstrated by **Sir Joseph Henry Gilbert** (1817–1901) at Rothamsted in England in 1893. The mechanism of nitrogen fixation was worked out by a Finnish biochemist, **Artturi Ilmari Virtanen** (1895–1973) of Helsinki. For his work on nutrition and the development of food resources, he was awarded the Nobel Prize for chemistry, in 1945.

Nitrous Oxide Discovered in 1772 by a British chemist, **Joseph Priestley** (1733–1804). In 1798 a French chemist, **Claude Louis Berthollet** (1748–1822), by heating ammonium nitrate, obtained it in a pure state. Its inhalational effects were studied by **Sir Humphry Davy** (1778–1829).

Nobel Prize The inventor of dynamite, **Alfred Bernhard Nobel** (1833–1896) of Stockholm, Sweden, after settling in Paris during his later life, left his vast fortune of 33 000 000 crowns to establish a trust for awarding annual prizes in chemistry, physics, medicine, literature and peace. The first series of Nobel Prizes were awarded in 1901. A sixth prize in economics was established in 1969 in his honor.

Nobel, Alfred Bernhard (1833–1896) *See dynamite, explosives, Nobel Prize.*

Nobelium A transuranic element of atomic number 102, discovered in 1957 at the Nobel Institute for Physics, Stockholm.

Nobili, Leopoldo (1784–1835) *See radiation of heat, radiometer (2), thermocouple, thermopile.*

Noble Gases A family of extremely unreactive elements or gases found at the far right of the periodic table. They have a stable arrangment of electrons in their outermost shell. *See argon, crypton, helium, neon, xenon.*

Noble Metals Those which are not attacked by acids or do not corrode. *See gold, silver, platinum.*

Noddack, Ida Eva (b 1896) *See masurium, rhenium.*

Noddack, Walter Karl Friedrich (1893–1960) *See masurium, rhenium.*

Noether Conditions Related to the theorem of algebraic curves. Proposed in 1873 by a German mathematician, **Max Noether** (1844–1921) of Manheim. He published a work on algebraic curves in 1882.

Noether, Amalie (1882–1935) *See Noetherian rings.*

Noether, Max (1844–1921) *See Noetherian conditions, Noetherian rings.*

Noetherian Rings A mathematical concept related to the neutral setting for problems in algebraic geometry and number theory. Proposed by **Amalie Noether** (1882–1935), a German mathematician and daughter of **Max Noether** (1844–1921).

Nollet, Jean Antoine (1700–1770) *See electrometer, Leyden jar, osmosis.*

Non-Euclidean Geometry A study of figures and shapes in curved space where Euclid's postulates may not apply. Initiated by Girolamo Saccheri in 1773 and developed by a Russian professor of mathematics at Kazan University, **Nikolai Lobachevski** (1792–1856), who published the first paper on the subject in 1829. A Hungarian mathematician **Janos Bolyai** (1802–1860), and **Carl Friedrich Gauss** (1777–1855) of Brunswick, independently developed non-Euclidean geometry, around 1840. The branch was further developed by a Scottish mathematician, **Duncan Maclaren Young Sommerville** (1879–1934), born in Rajasthan, India. He published four textbooks on the subject including *Elements of non-Euclidean Geometry.*

Nordenskiöld, Nils Adolf (1832–1901) *See cartography.*

Norfolk System A four-course system of crop rotation. Wheat or oats were cultivated in the first year, followed by oats or barley in the second year, clover or swedes in the third and turnips in the fourth year. *See agronomy.*

Normal Distribution Curve [Latin: *norma*, rule] A symmetrically bell-shaped curved fundamental to probability theory, devised in 1721 by a French mathematician, **Abraham de Moivre** (1667–1754) of Vitry, Champagne. He came to England in 1686 and published *The Doctrine of Chances* (1718), based on probability theory and a normal distribution curve in 1733. His fundamental law on complex numbers is known as the de Moivre theorem.

Norman, Robert (1550–1600) *See dip.*

Norrish, Ronald George Reyford (1897–1978) *See flash photolysis, photochemistry.*

North Pole One of the two diametrically opposite points (geographic poles) at which the earth's axis cuts the earth's surface. It is covered by the Arctic Ocean. The region was reached by English explorers, Sir Hugh Willoughby (1553), John Davis (1587) and Dutch explorers Willem Barents (1595) and Ian Cornelisz Ryp (1596). In 1607 Henry Hudson of Britain, with the company of Hopewell, reached 80.38°N. In 1806 **William Scoresby** (1789–1857), with a ship's company, reached 81.50°N, off Svalbard. Two arctic explorers, a physician, **Frederick Albert Cook** (1865–1940) of Calicoon Depot, New York State, and an American naval commander, **Robert Edwin Peary** (1856–1920) of Cresson Springs, Pennsylvania, made independent claims of reaching the North Pole (90°) first in 1909, although their claims lacked conclusive proof. Two American aviators **Floyd Bennett** (1890–1928) of Warrensburg, New York, and **Richard Evelyn Byrd** (1888–1957) of Winchester, Virginia, made the first flight over the North Pole in 1926. Another American explorer, from Chicago, **Lincoln Ellsworth** (1880–1951), with **Roald Engelbrecht Gravning Amundsen** (1872–1928), flew over the North Pole in his airship *Norge* in the same year. In 1937, Ivan Papanin of Russia landed at 89.43°N by aircraft from Zemlya Frantsa-Iosefa, and established the first Arctic Ocean drift station. A Russian team led by Pavel Afanasyevich set foot on the North Pole after flying there in 1948. An American, Ralph Plaisted and his team reached the North Pole by surface travel for the first time on 19 April 1968. A Japanese explorer, **Naomi Uemura** (1941–1984) was the first single person on an expedition to reach the North Pole, in May 1978.

North, John Dudley (1893–1968) *See cybernetics.*

Northmore, Thomas (1766–1851) *See liquefaction of gases.*

Northrop, John Howard (1891–1987) An American biochemist from Yonkers, New York, who did pioneering work on enzymes and published *Crystalline Enzymes* (1939). He shared the Nobel Prize for chemistry in 1946, with **Wendell Meredith Stanley** (1904–1971) and **James Batcheller Sumner** (1887–1955), for their work on purification of enzymes,.

Norton, Thomas (*c.* 1480) *See alchemy.*

Nöth, Heinrich (b 1928) *See magnetic resonance imaging.*

Noyce, Robert Norton (1927–1990) *See computers.*

Nuclear Bomb *See atomic bomb, H bomb.*

Nuclear Energy Energy released as a result of changes, either fusion or fission, in the nucleus of an atom. *See atomic bomb, atomic power, nuclear fission, nuclear fusion.*

Nuclear Fission [Latin: *fissura*, cleft] A process opposite to nuclear fusion, where a heavier nucleus such as that of uranium breaks up into lighter nuclei, releasing a large amount of energy. In 1938, a German physicist, **Otto Hahn** (1879–1968) and **Fritz Strassmann** (1902–1980) observed the products resulting from bombardment of uranium with neutrons. The uranium atom during the process split into two parts of comparable mass with the release of an enormous amount of energy. This phenomenon, named fission by Hahn, formed the basis for the development of the atomic bomb used on Japan during the Second World War. Hahn was awarded the Nobel Prize in Chemistry for this work, in 1944. Uranium-235 fission by slow neutrons was observed in 1940 by a group of American physicists including **John Ray Dunning** (1907–1975) from Shelby, Nebraska, German-born **Aristid V. Grosse** (b 1905) and their co-workers. A Soviet physicist, **Igor Vasilevich Kurchatov** (1903–1963) was instrumental in achieving Russia's first nuclear fission in 1949. *See atomic bomb, nuclear fusion.*

Nuclear Fusion The first nuclear fusion (creation of atoms of a heavier element – tritium – by fusing the elements of a lighter one – deuterium) was performed by three English physicists, **Lord Ernest Rutherford** (1871–1937), **I.M. Hunter** (1915–1975) and Australian-born **Sir Mark Laurence Elwin Oliphant** (1901–2000) in 1934. A Czech-born British chemist, **Martin Fleischmann** (b 1927), proposed an electrolytic method for nuclear fusion in 1989. *See thermonuclear fusion.*

Nuclear Particles *See atomic structure, electron, meson, plasma physics, proton.*

Nuclear Power *See atomic power.*

Nuclear Reactor The world's first nuclear reactor was demonstrated by an Italian, **Enrico Fermi** (1901–1954) and his colleagues at Chicago University on 2 December 1942. The world's largest nuclear reactor, at Ignalina Station in Lithuania, USSR, started operating to its full capacity in 1984. *See atomic bomb, atomic power.*

Nuclear Magnetic Resonance (NMR) *See magnetic resonance imaging.*

Nuclear Ships *See atomic ships.*

Nuclear Theory *See atomic theory.*

Nucleus Discovered in plant cells and named by a Scottish botanist and physician, **Robert Brown** (1773–1858) of Montrose. *See cell.*

Nuffield, William Richard Morris, Lord (1877–1963) *See car.*

Number Theory An abstract study of the structure of number systems and the properties of positive integers. **Diophantus** of Alexandria in the 3rd century proposed a theory of numbers. **Pythagoras** (*c.* 580–500 BC) commenced his theory of arithmetic by dividing all numbers into odd and even. He called the odd numbers *gnomons*. Fermat's theory of numbers (every natural number is the sum of at most three triangular numbers) was proposed in 1636 by a French mathematician, **Pierre de Fermat** (1601–1665) of Mountauban, in his letter to a Franciscan friar and mathematician, **Marin Mersenne** (1588–1648) of Paris. A German mathematician, **Peter Gustav Lejeune Dirichlet** (1805–1859), applied analytical techniques to develop the theory of numbers. A system of irrational numbers which became fundamental to the theory of numbers was proposed by a German mathematician, **Julius Wilhelm Richard Dedekind** (1831–1916). An Irish mathematician and Savillian professor of mathematics at Oxford (1860), **Henry John Stephen Smith** (1826–1883), was an authority on number theory during this period. An American mathematician, **Leonard Eugene Dickson** (1874–1957) of Iowa, published a monumental three-volume work *History of the Theory of Numbers* (1919–1923). *See negative numbers.*

Numbers Counting probably began long before written language or symbolism. The natural counting machine, the hand, gave rise to the system of numbers based on five, ten or twenty. A wolf bone of paleolithic times, with cuts arranged in groups of five, found in central Europe, suggests that man knew how to count more than 25 000 years ago. The Greek historian, **Herodotus** (485–425 BC) men-

tioned the use by Darius of knots, for counting the days. The Greeks developed a method based on the letters of the alphabet, around 450 BC. **Archimedes** (287–212 BC) proposed a system for counting infinite numbers in a pamphlet to the Gelon, the king of Syracuse. His work contained the elements of modern logarithms. Knotted cords of various colors were used by the Peruvians to construct a device called a *quipu* (knot) to count various commodities. They had officers in each town, known as *quipucamayocuna* (knot-officers), to tie and interpret the *quipu*. The Romans drove a nail for each year into the temple of Minerva. Their system, inherited from the Etruscans, provided a symbol for each number which could be used in an additive or subtractive form to represent numbers (V = 5, IV = 4 and VI = 6). The Babylonians derived their system, based on 60, from the division of a circle or a year. According to Moritz Cantor, a historian on mathematics, the Babylonians discovered the use of zero around 1700 BC. Their system led to the present system of 60 minutes to an hour and 60 times 6 degrees in a circle. The Egyptian hieroglyphic numerals in 3300 BC were based on symbols for 1, 10, 100, 1000 and 10 000. The Greeks represented the numbers with their 24-letter Greek alphabet. The Mayans in Meso-America developed a system based on 20, around 200 BC. The Hindu system was developed, probably in the 2nd century, from a base of nine numbers, each being given a symbol. The word *sifr* was used for the sign 0 by the Arabs. The word million was first used by Marco Polo (1254–1324) in the 13th century. The tombstone of the Indian war chief of the Wabojeeg who died in Lake Superior in 1793 has strokes inscribed to count the number of war parties led by him. Sticks made of willow (tally-sticks) were used by the British exchequer for counting money. Each of these sticks had notches of various sizes to account for pounds, shillings and other amounts. A great number of these tally-sticks were destroyed by the fire in the House of Commons in 1834.

Nuñez, Pedro (1492–1577) *See Vernier scale.*

Nutation [Latin: *nuto*, nod] Slight recurrent oscillation of the axis of the earth caused by a changing gravitational effect of the moon. Discovered in 1748 by **James Bradley** (1693–1762) from Sherbourne, Gloucestershire. He discovered the phenomenon of aberration of light in 1729, and succeeded **Edmund Halley** (1656–1742) as Astronomer Royal in 1742. A London astronomer and the tenth Astronomer Royal, **Sir Harold Spencer Jones** (1890–1960), determined the constant of nutation. *See equinox.*

Nutrition [Latin: *nutrio*, nourish] Athenaeus of Greece recorded the conversation about food and drink of a company of gentlemen in his *The Deipnosophists* (dinnertable philosophers) written around AD 200. According to **Diodorus Siculus** (d *c.* 20 BC), the Egyptians in the 1st century BC knew about diseases caused by overeating, and employed emetics and aperients to prevent them. The first experiments on nutrition were performed by **Erasistratus** (310–250 BC), who placed fowls in a jar and weighed them and their excreta before and after feeding. The Roman physician **Galen** (AD 130–200) studied the digestion in hogs and came to the conclusion that food was resolved into particles small enough to be absorbed, in the stomach. **Leonardo da Vinci** (1452–1519) compared nutrition to the burning of a candle flame that is fed by the liquor of the candle. **Sanctorius** (1561–1636), a professor at Padua, carried out the first systematic studies on metabolism. A French chemist and physician, **Antoine François Fourcroy** (1755–1809), investigated animal products on the basis of their nitrogen content and laid the foundation for the study of proteins. The Italian biologist **Lazzaro Spallanzani** (1729–1799) studied digestion by enclosing food in small cages tied to a string and withdrawing them after they had been in the stomach for some time. The nutritive effects of three types of food – proteins, carbohydrates and fats – were studied by a French physician, **François Magendie** (1783–1855). In 1822 an American surgeon, **William Beaumont** (1785–1853), studied the secretions and the process of digestion in the stomach, by withdrawing samples via a traumatic gastric fistula in a patient. The importance of protein in nutrition was first emphasized in 1838 by **Gerardus Johannes Mulder** (1802–1880), a Dutch chemist in Utrecht. **Charles Jacques Bouchard** (1837–1915), a French physician whose main interest was nutrition, published *Maladies par Raletissement de la Nutrition* (1882). **Russel Henry Chittenden** (1856–1943), an American physiologist from New Haven, Connecticut, is considered to be the founder of physiological chemistry and nutrition in America. His works include *Physiological Economy in Nutrition* (1905) and *Nutrition of Man* (1907). The concept of essential or accessory food factors, later known as vitamins, was proposed by **Sir Fredrick Gowland Hopkins** (1851–1947) in 1906. An American biochemist, **Henry Clapp Sherman** (1875–1955), who became professor of nutritional chemistry at the University of Columbia, published an important work *Chemistry of Food and Nutrition* (1911). The importance of trace elements in the diet of higher animals was established by **Thomas Burr Osborne** (1859–1929) and Lafayette Benedict Mendel in 1919. *See vitamins.*

Nuttall, Thomas (1786–1859) *See ornithology.*

Nye, John Frederick (b 1923) *See glaciology.*

Nyholm, Sir Ronald Sydney (1917–1971) *See valency.*

Nylon *See polymer, textile industry.*

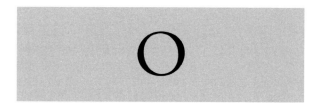

Oannes Babylonian god of mathematics and learning who is supposed to have risen from the Erythrean sea and had the body of a fish combined with a human head. He instructed men in the knowledge of writing and other sciences.

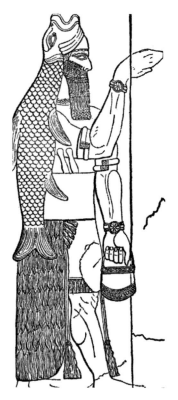

Figure 61 Oannes, the Egyptian god of mathematics. Rolt-Wheeler, Francis. *The Science-History of the Universe, Mathematics*. London: The Waverley Book Company Limited, 1911

Oatley, Sir Charles (1904–1996) *See electron microscope.*

Oberth, Herman Julius (1894–1990) *See rocket.*

Observatories [Latin: *observo*, watch] A term for laboratories used for observations in astronomy and meteorology. Evidence suggests that the megalithic structure in England, Stonehenge, built around 2800 BC, may have been an astronomical observatory. A scientist and philosopher, **Eudoxus** (400–360 BC), established a school and an astronomical observatory in Cnidos. The oldest surviving observatory building is that used by **Andronicus of Cyrrus** in

Athens around 100 BC. The remains of a Mayan observatory is found at Chichen Itza, in Mexico. One of the first astronomical observatories during the Middle Ages was built in 1259 at Maragha (now Iran) by Nasir al-Din al Tusi. The Aztecs built the El Caracol Observatory in Mexico. A ruler of Turkestan, **Ulugh-Beg** (1394–1449), established an observatory at Samarkand in 1424 which held astronomical instruments including a giant 132-foot quadrant. The first astronomical observatory in Europe was established in 1471 by a German astronomer, **Regiomontanus** (1436–1476) from Konigsberg, at Nuremberg. King Frederick II (1534–1588) of Denmark built an observatory for **Tycho Brahe** (1546–1601) in 1580. King Christian IV (1577–1648) of Denmark, the son of Frederick II, established a permanent observatory for Tycho Brahe's assistant, **Christian Sörensen Longomontanus** (1562–1647) in Copenhagen, in 1637. The Paris Observatory was established as part of the Académie des Sciences in 1667 and its building was completed in 1672. The Greenwich Observatory for meteorology and astronomy in London was founded in 1675 on the summit of Flamsteed hill, by King Charles II (1630–1685), at the initiation of **Sir Christopher Wren** (1632–1723) and Sir Jonas Moore. **John Flamsteed** (1646–1719) became its first Astronomer Royal in 1675. The Radcliffe Observatory in Oxford was founded in 1771 by the Savillian professor of astronomy, Hornsby, and named after the physician **John Radcliffe** (1650–1714). Jan Singh's observatory in Delhi, dating from 1719, took the form of a giant celestial staircase. The Harvard College Observatory, the first official astronomical observatory in America, was founded in 1839, with **William Cranch Bond** (1789–1859) of Portland, Maine, as its first director. The first astrophysical observatory in Europe was founded in Potsdam in Germany in 1874. The Mount Wilson Observatory located in the mountains behind Pasadena, California, was established in 1905 by the Carnegie Institution at the initiation of two American astronomers, **Walter Sydney Smith** (1876–1956) and **George Ellery Hale** (1868–1938). The first orbiting Solar observatory was launched in 1967. *See Yerkes Observatory.*

Ocean Meteorology *See oceanography.*

Oceanography [Greek: *okeanos*, sea + *graphein*, to write] **Crates of Mallus** (*c.* 200 BC) proposed that two oceans divided the inhabited portion of the world into land masses. In 79 BC, **Posidonus of Apamea**, by studying the motions of the moon, forecast the tides. A Latin writer, **Ambrosius Aurel Macrobius** (*c.* AD 400), wrote on tides and oceans. In 1666 **Robert Hooke** (1635–1703) devised an ingenious instrument, consisting of a ball of light wood and a stone, for estimating the depth of the sea without using a line. He

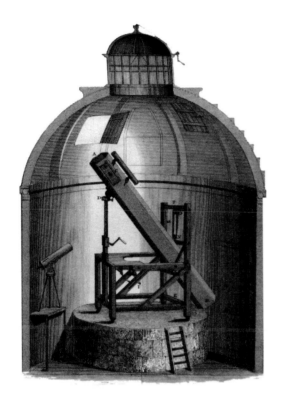

Figure 62   An early 18th century observatory. Partington, F. Charles. *The British Encyclopaedia of the Arts and Sciences*. London: Orr & Smith, 1835

also invented an apparatus for obtaining samples of water from any desired depth of the sea. The first treatise on oceanography *Histoire physique de la mer* (1725) was written by an Italian writer and marshal in the army, **Louis Ferdinand Marsigli** (1658–1730) of Bologna. The idea of geochemical balance was proposed by a Danish oceanographer, **Johan Georg Forschammer** (1794–1865) in his work *On the Components of Sea-water* (1859). An early monograph on oceanography, *The Natural History of European Seas*, written by a Scottish naturalist, **Edward Forbes** (1815–1854) was published posthumously in the same year. Forbes studied medicine at Edinburgh University where he later became a professor of natural history. He was appointed professor of botany at King's College, London in 1843. Another important work, *Physical Geography of the Sea* (1855), was published by an American naval officer, **Matthew Fontaine Maury** (1806–1873). His work on winds and currents of the ocean, founded the science of ocean meteorology. The method of deep-sea dredging which revealed the existence of many forms of life at the bottom of the ocean was introduced by a Scottish zoologist, **Sir Charles Wyville Thomson** (1830–1882), in 1868. The *Challenger*, one of the

first ships of the British Admiralty to be assigned to conduct an oceanic exploration, set sail in 1872. It contained six naturalists under Thompson and became the first steamship to cross the Antarctic Circle. It had sounding, dredging and other appliances for studying deep water and brought back a vast collection of specimens. **Jean Louis Rodolphi Agassiz** (1807–1873) founded the first American seaside laboratory on Penikese Island, in Buzzards Bay off Cape Cod, Massachusetts, in 1873. His son **Alexander Emmanuel Agassiz** (1835–1910), developed a steel wire rope for dredging and deep soundings. **Victor Hensen** (1835–1924) of Kiel, laid the foundation for *oceanic bionomics* or the study of the economics of the life of the ocean, and coined the term plankton [Greek: *planketon*, drifting], to denote the floating life forms on the ocean, in 1888. The first reliable map of the surface salinity and temperature of the ocean was produced by a Scottish oceanographer, **John Young Buchanan** (1844–1925) of Glasgow. A Swedish professor of chemistry at Stockholm, **Swen Otto Pettersson** (1848–1941), developed a method for determining dissolved gases in seawater and made several other contributions. **George Howard Darwin** (1845–1912), a grandson of Charles Darwin, did important work on the tides and their effects on the solar system, and published a treatise *The Tides* (1898). The variation of velocity of water in the ocean in relation to depth (Ekman Spiral) was shown by a Swedish oceanographer, **Vagn Walfrid Ekman** (1874–1954). An introductory book to the subject, *The Ocean* (1913), was published by a Canadian-born US marine biologist, **Sir John Murray** (1841–1914). Extensive study of the biology and distribution of fishes was carried out by a Danish biologist, **Ernst Johannes Schmidt** (1877–1933), who was vice-president of the International Council for the Investigation of the Sea. Gravitational studies in deep seas with the help of submarines were carried out by a Dutch geophysicist, **Felix Andries Vening Meinesz** (1887–1966). **Francis Parker Shepard** (1897–1985) of Massachusetts studied the sea-bed processes and published *Submarine Geology* (1948). Around 1940, **Harald Ulrik Sverdrup** (1888– 1957) of Oslo, Norway, made precise measurements of tides and wave heights, while he was director of the Scripps Institution of Oceanography in California. One of the first books to explore sea currents, *The Gulf Stream* (1947), was published by **Henry Melson Stommel** (1920–1992), a professor of oceanography at the Massachusetts Insitute of Technology. An American oceanographer of Chicago, **Wallace Broecker** (b 1931), made important studies of the chemical contents, temperatures and wind patterns of the oceans. An English geophysicist, **Sir Edward Crisp Bullard** (1907–1980), made the first reliable measurement of the heat flow through the oceanic crust, in 1940. An English oceanographer, **Sir George Edward Raven Deacon** (1906–1984), discovered a method of analyzing ocean waves, in 1944. An Austrian-born US oceanographer, **Walter Heinrich Munk** (b 1917), developed ocean acoustic tomography or three-dimensional modelling of the ocean temperature field which was later used to study global warming. A pioneer in the study of sea floor topography, **Bruce Charles Heezen** (1924–1977) of Iowa, using the echo-sounder, produced the first map of Atlantic fracture zones. Tectonic ocean mapping was also pioneered by a Dutch-born US geologist, **Tjeerd Hendrik van Andel** (b 1923), who contributed to the study of paleo-oceanography. *See marine biology, tides, undersea exploration.*

Ochoa, Severo (1905–1993) *See deoxyribonucleic acid.*

Ockham's Razor Entities should not be multiplied beyond necessity. An axiom proposed by an English philosopher, **William of Ockham** (1300–1349) of Ockham, Surrey. In modern terms, it means that when a phenomenon can be interpreted in several ways, its explanation lies in that which involves the least number of assumptions. Ockham wrote several works on logic while he was at Oxford and Avignon.

Octane Rating [Greek: *okta*, eight] A method of rating petrol quality for anti-knocking qualities. Initial investigations were begun on aviation fuel by **Sir Henry Thomas Tizard** (1885–1959) of Kent, in England, in 1920. The rating system was introduced by an American inventor, **Thomas Midgley** (1889–1944) of Beaver Falls, Pennsylvania. In 1921, he worked on the problem of knock in petrol engines, and found a method of overcoming it, by adding tetra-ethyl lead. A London engineer, **Sir Harry Ralph Ricardo** (1885–1974), contributed to the development of the octane rating system.

Odling, William (1829–1921) *See oxygen, ozone.*

Odometer [Greek: *hodos*, way + *metron*, to measure] Also was known as the pedometer, hodometer, perambulator, or way measurer. An instrument by which the steps of a person or revolutions made by a wheel of a carriage are counted. A hodometer for measuring distances was built by **Hero of Alexandria** (*c.* AD 100). The Roman architect, **Marcus Polio Vitruvius** (*c.* AD 100), in his tenth book described a machine that could be used for a carriage. John Fernal, the physician to Catherine of Medici (1513–1589), wife of Henry II, used the instrument in 1550 to measure a degree of a meridian between Paris and Amiens. An odometer was invented for the purpose of land surveying by Paul Pfinzing of Nuremberg in 1554. Augustus, the elector of Saxony,

employed a similar instrument, between 1553 and 1586, for measuring his territories. Emperor Rudolphus II, during his reign from 1576 to 1612, had two odometers capable of recording distances on paper. A description of one of these two instruments was given by De Boot in *Gemmarum et Lapidium Historia* (1647). A more advanced machine was constructed by an artist, **Hohlfeld** (1711–1771) from Hennerndorf, in the Saxony mountains. The principle of the odometer is used in the modern speedometer for automobiles and other vehicles.

Oersted The electromagnetic unit of magnetizing force named after the Danish physicist, **Hans Christian Oersted** (1777–1851), who is regarded as the father of electromagnetism. He became professor of physics at Copenhagen in 1806, and discovered the fundamental fact that a magnetic needle turns at right angles to an electric current. This principle was used in the development of the galvanometer.

Oersted, Hans Christian (1777–1851) *See aluminum, electricity, electric telegraphy, electromagnetic theory, galvanometer, magnetic needle, Oersted.*

Office Equipment *See computers, electric typewriter, electronic typewriter, facsimile machine, paper clip, pen, telephone, typewriter, writing devices, xerography, Xerox copier.*

Office Management *See accountancy, management.*

Ohm The SI unit (Système International d'Unités) of resistance in electricity, named after **Georg Simon Ohm** (1789–1854) of Erlangen, a German professor of physics at Nuremberg (1833–1849). He published the Ohm's law relating to voltage, current and electrical resistance in 1827, and later became professor of physics at the University of Munich in 1849.

Ohm, Georg Simon (1789–1854) *See acoustics, electrical resistance, ohm.*

Okazaki, Reiji (1930–1975) *See deoxyribonucleic acid.*

Oken, Lorenz (1779–1851) *See Isis.*

Olbers' Comet Discovered by **Heinrich Wilhelm Matthaus Olbers** (1758–1840) in 1815.

Olbers' Method Used for calculating the orbits of comets, devised by a German physician and astronomer, **Heinrich Wilhelm Matthaus Olbers** (1758–1840).

Olbers, Heinrich Wilhelm Matthaus (1758–1840) *See asteroids, Olbers' comet, Olbers' method.*

Oldenberg, Henry (1615–1667) *See scientific journals.*

Oldham, Richard Dixon (1858–1936) *See seismology.*

Olds, Ransom Eli (1864–1950) An American automobile manufacturer from Geneva, Ohio. In 1895 he produced a gas-powered vehicle and in 1899 founded the Olds Motor Vehicle Company which produced the popular Oldsmobiles in Detroit.

Oligocene Period [Greek: *oligos*, few + *cene*, recent] A geological period about 40 to 25 million years ago, which lasted for 15 million years. *See Tertiary Period.*

Oliphant, Sir Mark Laurence Elwin (1901–2000) An Australian nuclear physicist, born in Adelaide, who worked on the atomic bomb project at Los Alamos, in 1943. *See nuclear fusion, tritium.*

Olivetti, Adriano (1901–1960) *See typewriter.*

Olivetti, Camillo (1868–1943) *See typewriter.*

Olsen, Kenneth Harry (b 1926) *See computers.*

Olszevski, Karol Stanislov (1846–1915) *See nitrogen.*

Omar Khayam (1048–1142) A Persian poet, mathematician and philosopher who completed a seminal work of algebra at Samarkand and helped to build an observatory at Isfahan. He is better known for his poetical works, which were translated by Edward Fitzgerald and published as *The Rubaiyat of Omar Khayam* in 1859.

Omnibus [Latin: *omnibus*, for all] A common form of transport for several people with horse-ridden carriages was started by Pascal in 1662, and revived in 1828 by Stanislaus Baudry in Paris. Between 1828 and 1855, 20 different companies with a total of 40 omnibuses came to be established, and in 1855 they all merged to form the Compagnie Générales des Omnibus. The first omnibus from Paddington to the Bank of England in London was started by **George Shillibeer** (1797–1866) in 1825. It had about 12 passengers, attended by a footman or conductor, and was in operation until 1829. The first municipal motor omnibus service in the world was started in 1903 between Eastbourne railway station and Meads in East Sussex in England. *See coaches.*

Oncogenes Normal genes that regulate the normal growth and development of mammalian cells. Their abnormality may result in cancer. First noted in 1970 in a virus by Peter Duesberg Vogt. Further studies were done by an American molecular biologist, **John Michael Bishop** (b 1936), for which he was awarded the Nobel Prize in Medicine or Physiology in 1989.

Onnes, Heike Kamerlingh (1853–1926) *See helium, superconductivity.*

Onsager Law Also known as the fourth law of thermodynamics, proposed by a Norwegian-born US chemist, **Lars Onsager** (1903–1976). He was awarded the Nobel Prize in Chemistry in 1968, for his work on reversible reactions.

Onsager, Lars (1903–1976) *See isotopes, Onsager law.*

Oort Cloud A large reservoir of comets surrounding the solar system. It was predicted in 1832 by an Estonian astronomer, **Ernst Julius Opik** (1893–1985). A Dutch astronomer, **Jan Hendrik Oort** (1900–1992), discovered it as a source of long-period comets.

Oort, Jan Hendrik (1900–1992) *See Oort cloud.*

Oparin, Alexander Ivanovich (1894–1980) *See earth.*

Open Hearth Process *See steel.*

Opik, Ernst Julius (1893–1985) *See Oort cloud.*

Oppenheimer, Julius Robert (1904–1967) A New York physicist who served as director of the Los Alamos laboratory in New Mexico from 1943 to 1945. *See atomic bomb, plasma physics.*

Optical Pumping The use of the optical spectroscopic technique to investigate magnetic sublevels in particle physics. Study of resonance radiation by an American physicist, **Robert Williams Wood** (1868–1955) of Concord, Massachusetts, led to the development of the method by a French scientist, **Alfred Kastler** (1902–1984), who was awarded the Nobel Prize for physics, in 1966.

Optics [Greek: *opsis*, sight] The Arab mathematician **Alhazen or Ibn Al-Haitham** (AD 965–1038) of Basra, was the first to study the properties of light and the use of convex lenses. His work *Kitab Al-Manazir* (Book of Optics) which included refraction, reflection and the study of lenses, formed the basis for the invention of spectacles, the telescope and the microscope. The magnifying power of convex lenses and concave mirrors were described by **Lucius Annaeus Seneca** (d AD 65), around AD 50. The study of optics was introduced into Europe by **Vitello of Silesia** (Poland) (*c.* 1250), who wrote *Opticae Libridecem* (Ten books of Optics), around AD 1265. In 1210, a clergyman from Suffolk in England, **Robert Grosseteste** (1175–1253), who later became Bishop of Lincoln in 1235, studied light in detail and wrote on optics. Spectacles are said to have been invented by **Savinus Aramatus** of Pisa around 1300. The first application of the lens to the camera was made by a Venetian, Daniello Barbaro, in 1568. A landmark *Photisimi* *de lumine* (Light concerning light) was published in 1567 by a mathematician of Greek origin in Rome, **Francesco Maurolico** (1494–1575). It dealt with reflection, shadows, rainbows, the human eye and various kinds of spectacles. Experiments using various combinations of convex and concave lenses were described by **Giovanni Battista della Porta** (1535–1615) in his *De Refractione* (1593). The German astronomer, **Johannes Kepler** (1571–1630) of Wurtemberg, published *Dioptrice* (1611), and the law of refraction was discovered in 1624 by Snellius or **Willebrord Snell** (1591–1626), a professor of mathematics at Leyden. The process of vision was explained by **René Descartes** (1596–1650) in his *Dioptrique* (1637). The wave-like or periodic nature of light was suggested by an Italian physicist, **Francesco Maria Grimaldi** (1618–1663) of Bologna. A Scottish physicist, **Sir David Brewster** (1781–1868), commenced his researches in optics in 1814, and invented the kaleidoscope and lenticular stereoscope. *See microscope, telescope, vision.*

Optophone [Greek: *opsis*, sight + *phone*, sound]   A device by which blind people could read by ear, invented in 1912 by a London inventor, **Edmund Edward Fournier d'Albe** (1868–1933).

Ordovician   A geological stratum around 500 million years old, found between Cambrian and Silurian layers. In 1879, it was named after a celtic tribe, *Ordovices*, by a British geologist, **Charles Lapworth** (1842–1920) from Faringdon, who was professor of Geology at Birmingham.

Oresme, Nicole (*c.* 1325–1382)   *See motion.*

Organ   The son of an English organ-maker **Thomas Dallam** (*c.* 1599–1630), **Robert Dallam** (1602–1665) built the organs at St Paul's Cathedral, Jesus College at Cambridge, and Canterbury Cathedral. A French-born British organ builder, **René Harris** (1640–1715) built 39 organs for many important churches in England. *See barrel organ.*

Organic Chemistry [Greek: *organon*, instrument or tool] Chemistry of living matter. The synthesis of urea from potassium cyanate and ammonium sulfate by **Friedrich Wöhler** (1800–1882) in 1828, and of acetic acid in 1845 by **Adolf Wilhelm Hermann Kolbe** (1818–1884), brought down the barrier between organic chemistry and inorganic chemistry. **Pierre Eugène Marcellin Berthelot** (1827–1907), the first professor of organic chemistry at the Collège de France, produced benzene and naphthalene in 1851, and published *Organic Chemistry founded on Synthesis* (1860). In 1865, **August Kekulé** (1829–1896) defined it as the chemistry of carbon compounds in his book on organic chemistry,

published in 1860. A standard work on organic chemistry during this period, *Handbuch der Organischen Chemie* (1880), published by a German chemist, **Friedrich Konrad Beilstein** (1836–1906), contained a catalog of organic compounds. Organic reactions were independently explained on the basis of electronic theory by an English organic chemist, **Robert Robinson** (1886–1975) from Chesterfield, and a Scottish chemist, **Arthur Lapworth** (1872–1941) from Galashiels. Robinson was awarded the Nobel Prize for chemistry in 1947. A French chemist, **Auguste Laurent** (1807–1853), discovered anthracene in 1832, and proposed a new classification of organic compounds in 1837. He also developed the nuclear theory of organic radicals and his *méthode de chimie* was published posthumously in 1854. A German chemist, **Karl Graebe** (1841–1927) of Frankfurt-am-Main, introduced the terms ortho, meta and para for positions of substituents in aromatic compounds.

Origin of Species   *See evolution.*

Origin of the Universe   *See Big Bang theory, oscillating theory, Steady State theory.*

Ornithology [Greek: *ornis*, bird + *logos*, discourse]   The first printed monograph, containing a description of birds by **Aristotle** (384–322 BC) and **Pliny the Elder** (AD 28–79), was published in 1544 by an English naturalist from Cambridge, **William Turner** (1510–1568). One of the greatest treatises of the Middle Ages, including the habits, habitat, structure and classification of birds, was written by **Frederick II** (1197–1250) of Hohenstaufen, who was Holy Roman Emperor from 1220 to 1250. An early modern treatise on the subject entitled *Ornithology* (1599) was written by **Ulysses Aldrovandi** (1522–1605), professor of medicine and philosophy at Bologna. **Pierre Belon** (1517–1574), a medical graduate from Paris, wrote an important book *History of Birds*, which is one of the first books on comparative anatomy. An English naturalist and watercolor painter, **Elezar Albin** (d 1759), produced the first British book with colored plates of birds, *Natural History of British Birds* (1731–1738). A leading Dutch ornithologist from Amsterdam, **Coenraad Jacob Temminck** (1778–1858), published *Histoire Naturelle Générale des Pigeons et des Gallinacées* (1813–1815) in three volumes. A Scottish-born US ornithologist from Paisley, **Alexander Wilson** (1766–1813), was instrumental in publishing *American Ornithology* (1808–1814) in seven volumes. The eighth and ninth volumes were completed after his death. **John Latham** (1740–1837), a British physician from Dartford and an ornithologist, published a *General History of Birds* (1821–1828) in 11 volumes. A large folio of *Birds of America*

(1827–1838) was published by an American ornithologist in England, **John James Audubon** (1785–1851). It consisted of colored plates of 1065 birds in life size. **Thomas Nuttall** (1786–1859) from Yorkshire in England, while he was in America at Harvard, published *A Manual of the Ornithology of the United States and Canada* (1832). The first book containing life-size illustrations of British birds, entitled *Illustrations of British Ornithology* (1821–1834), was published by **Prideaux John Selby** (1788–1857) of Alnwick, Northumberland. Another English ornithologist, **John Gould** (1804–1881) from Lyme Regis, published *Birds of Europe* in five volumes (1832–1837), *Birds of Australia* in seven volumes (1840–1847), *Birds of Great Britain* in five volumes (1863–1873) and *Birds of Asia* (1849–1883). A book on *Ornithological Synonyms* (1855) was published by a zoologist, **Hugh Edwin Strickland** (1811–1853), a grandson of **Edmund Cartwright** (1743–1823), the inventor of the power loom. A Polish zoologist, **Ladislaus Taczanowski** (1819–1890), wrote *Birds of Poland* (1882) and *The Ornithology of Peru* (1884–1886). **Henry Seebohm** (1832–1895) of Yorkshire, published *A History of British Birds* (1883–1885), *Coloured Figures of Eggs of British Birds* (1896) and several other books on the subject. **Friedrich Hermann Otto Finsch** (1839–1917) of Germany, an expert on parrots, published *Die Papageien* in 1867. A London ornithologist, **Howard Saunders** (1835–1907), was an authority on gulls and he published *Illustrated Manual of British Birds* (1889). The American Ornithology Union was founded by **Barney Charles Cory** (1857–1921), the son of a millionaire from Boston. He published *Birds of the Bahamas* (1878), and *Birds of the Americas* (1918). The Ridgway color system for bird identification was invented by an American ornithologist, **Robert Ridgway** (1850–1929) of Mount Carmel, Illinois, who published several books on North American birds. An English ornithologist and one of the founders of the Oxford Ornithological Society in 1921, **Max Nicholson** (b 1904), published several books on the subject including *Birds in England* (1926) and *How Birds Live* (1927).

Orr, Lord John Boyd (1880–1971) *See animal husbandry.*

Ortel, Abraham or **Ortelius** (1527–1598) *See cartography.*

Osborne, Henry Fairfield (1857–1935) *See dinosaurs, vertebrates.*

Osborne, Thomas Burr (1859–1929) *See trace elements.*

Oscillating Theory An explanation for the origin of the universe. It claims that the universe from the Big Bang is expanding and will continue to do so for another 30 000 million years, after which time the gravitational attraction between galaxies will overcome centrifugal force to re-form into a primevial atom, which will again re-explode. The theory was revived in 1965 by an American astronomer, **Allan Rex Sandage** (b 1926) of Iowa. *See Big Bang theory, Steady State theory*.

Oscilloscope [Latin: *oscillare,* swing + Greek: *skopein,* to look] A cathode-ray tube for observation and recording of the variation of physical properties of matter over a time period. Invented in 1897 by a German physicist, **Karl Ferdinand Braun** (1850–1918).

Osmium [Greek: *osme,* smell] An element discovered in 1804 by an English chemist, **Smithson Tennant** (1761–1816) of Selby, Yorkshire. He became professor of chemistry at Cambridge, a year before his death in a riding accident.

Osmosis [Greek: *osmos,* impulse] The phenomenon was observed in 1748 by a French Abbé, **Jean Antoine Nollet** (1700–1770), professor of physics at the Collège de Navarre in Paris. He observed that water passed through a piece of pig's bladder into a solution of spirits and wines. A French physiologist in Paris, **René Joachim Henri Dutrochet** (1776–1847) from Poitou, showed that water from a weaker solution moved into a stronger solution through a membrane, and named the process osmosis in his *Nouvelles Recherches sur l'endosmose et l'exosmose* (1828). Diffusion across a membrane was attributed to osmotic pressure by **Thomas Graham** (1805–1869) in his paper *On Osmotic Force* in 1854. The semipermeability of the porous membrane involved in osmosis was demonstrated in 1867 by a plant physiologist **Moritz Traube** (1826–1894). A German botanist, **Wilhelm Friedrich Philipp Pfeffer** (1845–1920), demonstrated the process, using cane sugar solution in a vessel with semipermeable walls, and made the first quantitative measurement of osmotic pressure in 1877. He published a paper on the subject entitled *Osmotische Untersuchungen* in the same year, and served as professor of botany at Basel (1877), Tübingen (1878) and Leipzig (1887). Further work was done in 1877 by **Hugo Marie de Vries** (1848–1935) of Holland, and precise measurements were achieved in 1912 by **Harmon Northup Morse** (1848–1920) of America. Outstanding work on the osmotic pressure of proteins was done by **Søren Peter Lauritz Sørenson** (1868–1939) in 1917. Two English physiologists, **Hugh Davson** (b 1909) and **James Frederic Daniell** (1911–1984) studied the permeability of the cell membrane and published *Permeability of Natural Membranes* (1942).

Osmotic Pressure *See osmosis.*

Ostrovski, Yuri (1926–1992) *See hologram.*

Ostwald, Friedrich Wilhelm (1853–1932) A German professor of chemistry at Leipzig who proposed the law of dilution which bears his name. He invented a process for making nitric acid from ammonia, proposed a new theory of color, and defined a catalyst as an agent that accelerates the rate of a chemical reaction. His *Lehrbuch der allgemeinen Chemie* (1885) marked the beginning of physical chemistry, and he received the Nobel Prize for chemistry in 1909. *See catalysis, physical chemistry, valency.*

Otis, Elisha Graves (1811–1861) *See elevator.*

Otta, Gunner Elias (1897–1973) *See pollen analyis.*

Otto, Nikolaus August (1832–1891) *See gas engine, internal combustion engine.*

Oughtred, William (1575–1660) *See calculation, mathematical symbols, mathematics, multiplication, pi, slide rule.*

Oven Dutch ovens in the 16th century consisted of dome-shaped metal boxes with an open end that faced the fire. John Sibthorpe around 1630 in England invented an oven for use with coal. *See cookers.*

Owen, Robert Bowie (1870–1940) *See shipping.*

Owen, Sir Richard (1804–1892) An eminent British comparative anatomist and paleontologist from Lancaster who trained as a physician at Edinburgh and at St Bartholomew's Hospital. He served as the curator of the Royal College of Surgeons before he was appointed as the first director of the Natural History Department of the British Museum, in 1856. Owen was the first to describe the extinct bird *Archaeopteryx*. His treatise *Anatomy and Physiology of the Vertebrates* (1866–1868) was an important work based on his personal observations. *See ichthyology, paleontology, vertebrates.*

Oxygen [Greek: *oxys*, sour + *gennein*, to produce] Chemical union with a constituent of the atmosphere, when substances were burnt, was demonstrated by an English chemist, **John Mayow** (1640–1679). He called this atmospheric gas *igneo aereum* or *spiritus nitro-aerius*. His view on combustion was mostly rejected, and instead, an erroneous theory (when substances burn they use an essence within them called phlogiston), proposed by a German chemist **Georg Ernst Stahl** (1660–1734), became accepted. The phlogiston [Greek: *phlogistein*, to set on fire] theory was held for over 100, until **Joseph Priestley** (1733–1804), an English chemist, obtained pure oxygen by heating a metal oxide. He called the gas 'dephologisticated air' in 1774. Oxygen was discovered independently by a Swedish apothecary, **Carl Wilhelm Scheele** (1742–1786), in the same year. In 1775, **Antoine Laurent Lavoisier** (1743–1794) named the substance responsible for combustion the 'acidifying principle' in the belief that all acids contained oxygen. The atomic weight of oxygen was calculated at 32 by a London chemist and physician, **William Odling** (1829–1921), who became Fullerian professor of chemistry at the Royal Institution in 1867. The first commercial preparation of oxygen, using fractional distillation of air, was achieved by a German chemist, **Karl von Linde** (1842–1934), in 1895. In 1929, a Canadian-American chemist, **William François Giauque** (1895–1982) and Herrick Johnston examined the absorption bands of oxygen and came to the conclusion that it contained three isotopes of different atomic weights: 16, 17 and 18. This finding was later confirmed by mass spectrography.

Oxyhydrogen Blowpipe An early form of welding torch, invented in 1801 by an American professor of chemistry at the University of Pennsylvania, **Robert Hare** (1781–1858).

Ozone [Greek: *oze*, stench] Discovered and named by a German professor of chemistry and physics at Basel, **Christian Friedrich Schönbein** (1799–1868) in 1840. An Irish physical chemist, **Thomas Andrews** (1813–1885) and **Jean Charles Gallisard de Marignac** (1817–1894) independently demonstrated it to be an allotrope of oxygen. The presence of three oxygen atoms was suggested by an English chemist, **William Odling** (1829–1921) in 1861. The ozone layer in the upper atmosphere was discovered in 1913 by a French physicist, **Charles Marie Paul Fabry** (1867–1945).

Ozone Layer The part of the stratosphere at a height of nearly 14 miles in which the gas ozone is most concentrated. It shields the Earth from the harmful effects of solar ultraviolet radiation, but can be decomposed by complex chemical reactions involving chlorofluorocarbons (derivatives of methane and ethane). The ozone layer was discovered in 1913 by a French physicist, **Marie Paul Auguste Charles Fabry** (1867–1945). Concerns about holes in the ozone layer caused by pollution began in the 1980s, and in 1987 the Montreal Protocol was signed by 40 countries to limit the industrial use of chlorofluorocarbons (CFCs) and similar pollutants. The European Community meeting held in Brussels in 1989 agreed to cut CFC consumption as soon as possible, and end its use by the year 2000 – a goal which has not yet been achieved.

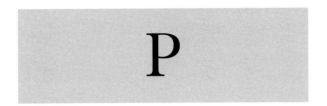

Pacioli, Lucas (1445–1510) *See calculation, probability theory.*

Packer, Robert Clyde (1879–1934) *See newspapers.*

Packer, Sir Frank Hewson (1906–1974) *See newspapers.*

Paleobotany *See paleophytology.*

Paleography [Greek: *paleo*, old + *graphein*, to write] Study of ancient writings. The German Egyptologist **Karl Richard Lepsius** (1810–1884) was a pioneer in the field who studied Etruscan, Egyptian and Oscan writings. His work formed the basis for modern philology. *See hieroglyphics, philology, pictogram, writing.*

Paleolithic Age [Greek: *paleo*, old + *lithos*, stone] *See Stone Age.*

Paleomagnetism [Greek: *paleo*, old] The study of magnetic properties of fossils and geological strata in relation to the formation of earth and its age, pioneered by an American physicist, **Allan Cox** (1927–1987) of Santa Ana, California. He collected samples from all over the world and studied their age and magnetism. He used his method to date the age of sea floors and to investigate plate tectonics. He published *Plate Tectonics and Geomagnetic Levels* (1973).

Paleontology [Greek: *palaios*, old + *onto* + beings + *logos*, discourse] A term first used by **Sir Richard Owen** (1804–1892) in 1838 to denote the study of the origin and development of life on earth. He published *Palaeontology* in 1860. The science started with studies of fossils by **Conrad Gesner** (1516–1565) in 1565, and **Georges Cuvier** (1769–1832) of Paris established it as a science around 1800. The Palaeontographical Society was founded in London in 1847, and it published important treatises on the earth's organic remains. **Karl Alfred von Zittel** (1839–1904) of Baden was a pioneer in the field and he published *Handbook of Palaeontology* (1876–1893) in five volumes and several other books on the subject. *See fossils.*

Paleophytology [Greek: *paleo*, old + *phuton*, plant + *logos*, discourse] A branch of paleontology that deals with fossil plants. Pioneer work was done by the British botanist **Robert Brown** (1773–1858), in 1851. Further contributions were made by a French paleobotanist, **Adolphe Theodore Brongniart** (1801–1876). **William Crawford Williamson** (1816–1895) of Owens College, Manchester, and his associate **Dunkinfield Henry Scott** (1854–1934) at the Jodrell Laboratory, Kew, studied coal in relation to plant fossils. Williamson published *Studies in Fossil Botany* in 1900. One of the early modern works on the subject *Fossil Botany* (1891) was published by Solms-Laubach of the University of Göttingen. Several books on the subject including *English Wealden Flora* (1894), *Jurassic Flora* (1900–1903) and *Plant Life through Ages* (1931) were published by an English botanist, **Sir Albert Charles Seward** (1863–1941) of Lancaster, who was professor of botany at Cambridge from 1906 to 1936. A Canadian geologist and authority on fossil plants, **Sir John William Dawson** (1820–1899), published *Origin of the World* (1877), *Fossil Men* (1878) and *Relics of Primevial Life* (1897).

Paleozoic Period [Greek: *paleo*, old + *zoe*, life] The era related to the lowest stratified layer of the earth containing the remains of the earliest forms of life dating back over 400 million years. It was identified and named by the British geologist, **Adam Sedgwick** (1785–1873). A Canadian geologist, **William Edmund Logan** (1798–1875) of Montreal, provided the first evidence for the existence of land animals in the upper Paleozoic era, in 1841.

Palladio, Andrea (1518–1590) *See architecture, Italian.*

Palladium An element similar to platinum discovered in 1803 by an English chemist from Norfolk, **William Hyde Wollaston** (1766–1822). It was named after a minor planet *pallas*, discovered in 1802.

Pallas, Peter Simon (1741–1811) *See taxonomy, zoogeography.*

Palmen, Erik Herbert (1898–1985) *See cyclone.*

Palmieri, Luigi (1807–1896) *See meteorology, seismology.*

Palmiter, Richard de Forest (b 1942) *See genetic engineering.*

Paneth, Frederick Adolph (1887–1958) *See artificial transmutation, petrology.*

Pangaea *See tectonic theory.*

Panhard, René (1841–1908) *See car.*

Paper Originated in China and was known to have been used as packing material and for clothing, rather than for writing, around 170 BC. They used hemp, cotton and the bark of trees for making paper. This form of paper started to be made in Samarkand in AD 800, and reached Cairo around the 10th century. In Europe, paper was first made out of cotton in 1100, and out of rags in 1300. The first paper mill was established in Nuremberg in 1391, and the first one in England was built at Dartford in 1494. Coarse white paper was produced for the first time by an Englishman of German origin, Sir John Speilman, at Dartford in 1590. Nicolaus Louis Robert of France developed an advanced paper-making machine in 1798. His patent was acquired by two brothers, the British papermakers **Henry Fourdrinier** (1766–1854) and **Sealy Fourdrinier** (d 1847), who started producing the first continuous paper of indefinite length in 1807. Their improved machine, developed in conjunction with **Bryan Donkin** (1768–1855) of Northumberland, was patented in 1806. By 1850, Donkin had made over 200 machines, revolutionizing the British paper and printing industry. The longest roll of paper, measuring 13 800 feet in length, was made at Derbyshire, England in 1830. *See writing materials.*

Paper Clip   The first metallic clip for attaching several sheets of paper together was invented by a Norwegian, Johann Valer, who patented his invention in Germany in 1900.

Paper Money   The forerunners to paper money were paper bank drafts first issued by the Chinese government in AD 812. The Chinese used movable print to produce paper money in Szechuan in 880. Colored paper money was introduced by the Chinese in 1101 mainly to overcome the problem of counterfeiting. The Ming Dynasty issued a large paper money measuring 32 centimeters in 1368. The world's earliest bank notes were issued in Stockholm, Sweden, in 1661. The Bank of England produced limited numbers of 1 million pound notes mainly for internal use before 1812. The English inventor **Joseph Bramah** (1748–1814) from Barnsley, Yorkshire invented an ingenious machine for printing bank notes in 1806. A German inventor, **Heinrich Wilhelm Dove** (1803–1979), invented a stereoscope for detecting forged bank notes.

Papin, Denis (1674–1712)   A French physician and physicist, born in Blois. He studied medicine at the University of Angers, and in 1680 came to England where he worked for a brief period with **Robert Boyle** (1627–1691). In 1681, he invented an apparatus called a steam digester, with a safety valve, which he used for dissolving bone and other products, under pressure. His principle was later applied to the development of the domestic pressure cooker. *See steam engine.*

Pappus of Alexandria (*c.* AD 300–350)   A Greek mathematician whose *Synagogue* has conveyed to us the works of Ptolemy, Euclid and Diodorus. His above work, known as the *Collection*, was written in eight parts, and apart from commentaries on previous mathematical works by others, it also contained elements of analytical and projective geometry. *See analytical geometry, geometry.*

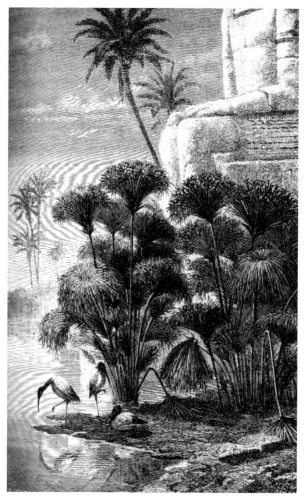

Figure 63   Egyptian papyrus plant in a 19th century landscape. Pouchet, F.A. *The Universe.* London: Blacke and Son, 1871

Papyrus   Used by the Egyptians for writing. A sheet is made by cutting lengthwise sections of the reed-like papyrus plant and joining them in two layers. Ancient institutions such as the Alexandrian Library had thousands of long sheets of papyrus or scrolls usually attached at each end to a wooden rod. The library at Pergamum in Asia Minor established around 200 BC had to resort to a different writing material, parchment, as Ptolemy V around 190 BC blocked the supply of papyrus from Egypt to this rival library established by King Eumenes II of Pergamum. *See Ahmes papyrus, writing.*

Paracelsus or **Theophrastus Bombastus von Hohenheim** (1493–1541)   *See alchemy, biochemistry, gas, hydrogen, quicksilver, zinc.*

Parachute [Latin: *prepare*, to make ready + French: *chute*, fall]   A device known to the ancient Chinese, and mentioned in Ssuma Chien's *Historical Records* written in 90 BC. The first workable parachute was described by **Leonardo da Vinci** (1452–1519) in 1480. **Louis Sebastian Lenormand** (1757–1839) was the first to try the parachute in Europe, in 1783. He used a quasi-parachute during his jump from a tower at Montpellier, France, in 1783. The first practical parachute was invented by a French balloonist, **Jean Pierre François Blanchard** (1753–1809) of Les Andeleys, who performed the first parachute jump from a balloon in 1793. Blanchard was subsequently killed during one of his parachute jumps from his balloon. **André Jacques Garnerin** (1769–1823) parachuted from an air balloon in Paris in 1797. He and his brother, **Jean Baptiste Olivier Garnerin** (1766–1849), made several improvements to the parachute. The French pioneer of the air balloon, **Jacques Étienne Montgolfier** (1745–1799), also designed a parachute. The first parachute descent from an aircraft was made in 1912, over Missouri.

Parallax Displacement of an object in optics or astronomy, caused by a change of the point of observation. A principle that is used for calculating astronomical distances. A German astronomer, **Friedrich Georg William Struve** (1793–1864) was the first to measure a stellar parallax. An English astronomer, **Jeremiah Horrocks** (1618–1641), made a new estimate of solar parallax, which had been previously measured by **Ptolemy of Alexandria** (*c.* AD 127–151), **Johannes Kepler** (1571–1630) and several others. **Giovanni Domenico Cassini** (1625–1712), professor of astronomy at the University of Bologna, collaborated with a French astronomer, **Jean Richer** (1630–1696), and reported a measurement of the sun's parallax corresponding to a distance of 87 000 000 miles.

Parasitism [Greek: *parasitos*, one who eats at another's expense + *logos*, discourse] The word parasite first appeared in English in relation to plants, in 1727. **Pliny, the Elder** (AD 28–79) recognized mistletoe as a parasitic plant. Intestinal worms were the first animal parasites to be identified by ancient physicians as a cause of disease. Examination of tissues from 3000-year-old Egyptian mummies have shown the presence of diseases caused by parasites such as *Trichinella spiralis* and *Schistosoma hematobium*. **Hippocrates** (*c.* 460–*c.* 377 BC) studied parasites and divided intestinal worms into round lumbricae (*Ascaris*) and broad lumbrici (*Taenia*). Intestinal worms resembling earthworms were described by **Paul of Aegina** (625–690). The first protozoan parasite to be observed, *Giardia lamblia*, was identified by **Antoni van Leeuwenhoek** (1632–1723), who noted it in his stools in 1681. The egg and the reproductive process of the roundworm was described in 1684 by **Francesco**

Redi (1626–1698) of Italy, who is regarded as the first parasitologist. In 1876, **Sir Joseph Bancroft** (1836–1894) discovered *Wuchereria bancrofti*, the cause of filariasis, in Brisbane, Australia. The protozoan *Plasmodium* which causes malaria was discovered in 1880 by a French parasitologist, **Charles Louis Alphonse Laveran** (1845–1922), while he was a professor of pathological anatomy at the University of Rome. Laveran received the Nobel Prize for Physiology or Medicine, for his work on malaria, in 1907. A French botanist, **G. Bonnier** (1853–1922) identified and described several parasitic plants in botany. **M. Clifford Dobell** (1886–1949), an eminent protozoologist, published the classic works *Amoeba living in Man* (1919), and *Intestinal Protozoa of Man* (1921).

Parchment *See writing materials.*

Parity A concept in particle physics. It refers to electromagnetic and strong nuclear forces which conserve a quantum property. Two Chinese-born US physicists, **Tsung Dao Lee** (b 1926) and **Chen Ning Yang** (b 1922) studied it in relation to weak interactions, in 1956, and they shared the Nobel Prize for physics in 1957. Another Chinese-born US physicist, **Chien Shiung Wu** (1912–1997) from Shanghai, confirmed their findings in the same year. She was appointed as a professor at Columbia University, New York, in 1957.

Parkes, Alexander (1813–1890) *See celluloid, electroplating, vulcanization.*

Parking Meter Invented by an American, Carlton C. Magee, and first installed in 1935 in Oaklahoma city. They were introduced into London in 1958. *See motoring.*

Parkinson, John (1567–1650) An English botanist from Nottinghamshire who proposed a classification of plants in his *Theatrum Botanicum* in 1640.

Parmenides of Elea (*c.* 500 BC) *See climatic zones, conservation of mass.*

Parsons, Sir Charles Algernon (1854–1931) *See steamships, turbine.*

Parsons, William, Lord Rosse (1800–1867) *See galaxy, nebulae, reflecting telescope.*

Parthenon The chief temple of Athens on the Acropolis, devoted to the cult of Athena Parthenos or 'the virgin'. The sculptor Phidias worked with the architects **Ictinus** (*c.* 500 BC) and **Callicrates** (*c.* 500 BC) to complete the temple in 438 BC.

Particle Accelerator A device for accelerating subatomic particles to high velocities. The Stanford Positron–Electron Accelerating Ring (SPEAR), an accelerator for colliding electrons and positrons at high energies, was developed by a New York physicist, **Burton Richter** (b 1931). In 1974, he used the device to discover a new atomic particle, for which he shared the Nobel Prize for physics in 1976 with another US physicist, **Samuel Chao Chung Ting** (b 1936), who independently devised the technique. Several different types of accelerators, including synchrotrons, linear accelerators and cyclotrons, have since been built in Europe and the USA. *See antiproton, boson, cyclotron.*

Particle Physics *See atomic structure, atomic theory, boson, cyclotron, electron, meson, particle accelerator, pion, plasma physics, positron, proton, psi.*

Partington, **James Riddick** (1886–1965) An English professor of chemistry at Queen Mary College, London University and science historian from Bolton, Lancashire. He published *Origins and Development of Applied Chemistry* (1935), *A Short History of chemistry* (1937) and *Advanced Treatise on Physical Chemistry* (1949–1954) in three-volumes.

Pascal Triangle An array of numbers that gives the coefficient of the exponents of $(a + b)^n$ where n is a positive integer. It was known to the Chinese around 1300 and is depicted in Chu Shih-Chieh's *Precious Mirror of the Four Elements* in 1303. The first print of it in Europe appeared in 1527 in the work of **Peter Apian** (1495–1552) who was professor of astronomy at the University of Ingolstadt, Germany. **Jacques Bernoulli** (1654–1705) referred to it a century later. **Blaise Pascal** (1623–1662) used the triangle to derive several important theorems.

Pascal, Blaise (1623–1662) *See Académie Royale des Sciences, calculating machine, Fermat's theory, Pascal triangle, Pascal's law, probability theory.*

Pascal's Law Pressure applied within a liquid is transmitted in all directions. It was discovered by a French mathematician and one of the founders of hydrodynamics, **Blaise Pascal** (1623–1662) of Paris. His work *Traité de l'équilibre des liqueurs* enunciating the above principle was posthumously published in 1633.

Paschen, Friedrich (1865–1947) *See Pauli's exclusion principle.*

Pasteur, Louis (1822–1895) A French chemist from Dôle who is regarded as the father of bacteriology and pasteurization. He started his study on fermentation in 1857, and showed the presence of living cells in fermentation around 1864, at a time when his findings were opposed by several prominent men who advocated the spontaneous generation theory. He was appointed professor of chemistry at the Sorbonne in 1867 where his work on tartaric acid led to the discovery of the existence of crystals in two mirror image forms. He postulated the 'germ theory' of disease and showed that the anthrax bacillus could be modified to confer immunity without producing disease. He used the Latin word *vacca*, meaning cow, and administrated the first rabies vaccine in 1885. He served as the first director of the Pasteur Institute in Paris, which was founded in 1888 with a public donation of 2.5 million francs.

Pasteurization Heat treatment of milk to destroy bacteria, invented by **Louis Pasteur** (1822–1895). *See dairy industry.*

Pathé, **Charles** (1863–1957) *See newsreel.*

Pattinson Process A method for desilverization of lead invented in 1829, by an English chemist, **Hugh Lee Pattinson** (1796–1858) of Alston, Cumberland.

Pattinson, Hugh Lee (1796–1858) *See Pattinson process.*

Paul of Aegina (625–690) *See parasitism.*

Paul Trap A device in the study of particle physics for observing and measuring electrons and ions. It was invented by a German physicist, **Wolfgang Paul** (1913–1993), who shared the Nobel Prize for physics for this work with a German-born American physicist, **Hans Georg Dehmelt** (b 1922) and another American physicist, **Norman Foster Ramsey** (b 1915), in 1989.

Paul, Wolfgang (1913–1993) *See Paul Trap.*

Pauli, Wolfgang (1900–1958) *See matrix mechanics, neutrino, Pauli's exclusion principle.*

Pauling, Linus Carl (1901–1994) An American molecular chemist from Portland, Oregon. In 1931 he used quantum mechanics to explain chemical bonding and the structure of molecules, and published *The Nature of the Chemical Bond* (1939). The three-dimensional spiral structure of proteins (alpha helix) was demonstrated by B.B. Corey and Linus Pauling in 1951. Pauling received two Nobel Prizes, one for chemistry in 1954, and another in 1962 for peace.

Pauli's Exclusion Principle A law of quantum theory which states that no two electrons in an uncharged atom can have the same set of quantum numbers. Originated from the transition principle discovered in 1912 by **Friedrich Paschen** (1865–1947) and **Ernst Back** (1881–1959), and proposed by an Austrian–Swiss physicist, **Wolfgang Pauli** (1900–1958), who was awarded the Nobel Prize for physics for his work, in 1945. *See matrix mechanics, quantum theory.*

Pavlov, Ivan Petrovich (1849–1936) *See digestion.*

Payen, Anselme (1795–1871) *See amylase, starch.*

Payne-Gaposchkin, Celia Helena (1900–1979) *See variable star.*

Peano, Giuseppe (1858–1932) *See mathematical logic.*

Pearson, Karl (1857–1936) *See statistics.*

Peary, Robert Edwin (1856–1920) *See meteors, North Pole.*

Pease, Francis Gladheim (1881–1938) *See Mount Wilson Observatory.*

Pedersen, Charles (1904–1990) *See cell membrane.*

Pedomorphosis [Greek: *paidos*, child + *morphe*, form + *osis*, condition] A process in which an organism retains its juvenile or larval traits into later life, often characterized by acceleration of sexual maturation relative to normal development and retardation of bodily development with respect to the onset of reproductive activity. This concept was developed by an English zoologist, **Walter Garstang** (1868–1949) from Blackburn. It was proposed as a factor in evolution by a London biologist, **Sir Gavin Rylands De Beer** (1899–1972).

Peebles, Phillips James Edwin (b 1935) *See Big Bang theory.*

Pei, Ieoh Meng (b 1917) *See architecture, American.*

Peierls, Sir Rudolf Ernst (1907–1995) *See diamagnetic.*

Peirce, Benjamin (1809–1880) *See Neptune.*

Peirce, Charles Sanders (1839–1914) Son of **Benjamin Peirce** (1809–1880) who devoted his life to the study of philosophy and logic. He is regarded as the founder of pragmatism. *See meter.*

Peking Man Human ancestor (*Homo erectus*) whose fossils in China were unearthed in 1922 by a Swedish archaeologist, **Johan Gunner Andersson** (1874–1960). A Canadian anatomist, **Davidson Black** (1884–1934) unearthed further remains while he was professor of anatomy at the Union Medical College, Peking (Beijing), in 1927.

Peligot, Eugene Melchior (1811–1890) *See uranium.*

Pell, John (1610–1685) An English mathematician from Southwick, Sussex, who became professor of mathematics at Amsterdam in 1643. He introduced the division sign (÷) into England.

Pelletier, Pierre (1788–1842) *See chlorophyll.*

Peltier Effect *See thermocouple.*

Peltier, Jean Charles Athanase (1785–1845) *See thermocouple.*

Pelton Wheel *See hydroelectric schemes.*

Pelton, Lester Allen (1829–1918) *See hydroelectric schemes.*

Pen The ancient Egyptians used a holder for their brushes for writing on sheets of papyrus and a palette for their ink. A goose feather (quill) was one of the earliest devices used for writing in Europe from the Middle Ages until around 1700. Steel nibs were invented in 1803, and they were commercially produced in Birmingham, England, around 1830. They were perfected by **Joseph Gillott** (1799–1873) of Sheffield and **Josiah Mason** (1795–1881) of Kidderminster. John Sheaffer in England invented a fountain pen in 1819. A fountain pen with a device for continuous flow of ink was patented in 1884 by Lewis Edson Waterman of New York City. The ink container for these pens initially had to be filled with an eye dropper. Self-filling pens came in the early 1900s. The ball point was first patented by an American, John J. Loud in 1888, but it failed to make a commercial success. The present ball-point pen was invented by a Hungarian journalist Laszlo Biro and his brother Georg Biro while they were in Argentina to escape from the Nazis in 1938. It was patented in Argentina and was first sold in Buenos Aires in 1945.

Pencil *See writing devices.*

Penck, Albrecht (1858–1945) *See glaciology.*

Pendulum [Latin: *pendere*, to hang] **Galilei Galileo** (1564–1642) of Pisa first observed the principle of the pendulum from the oscillations of a suspended lamp in the cathedral at Pisa in 1583. His observation that the oscillations were equal in time whatever their range, led to its use for measuring time. His work on the pendulum started towards the end of his life and he had to leave his project to his son Vincenzio and his pupil Viviani to complete. Vincenzio, although he made a drawing of his father's invention, he was not able to complete the project within his own lifetime. **Christian Huyghens** (1629–1693), a Dutch physicist from the Hague, while at the Accademia del Cimento, continued Galileo's work and invented a bifilar pendulum in 1656, and patented a pendulum clock in 1657. Huygens' description of the mechanism of the pendulum clock is found in his book *Horologium Oscillatorium* published in 1673. The mercurial pendulum, which eliminated the error due to the expansion of its metal rod, was invented in 1710 by **George Graham** (1673–1751). The ballistic pendulum was invented by a Quaker mathematician, **Benjamin Robins** (1707–1751) of Bath, in 1730. He became an engineer in the East India Company in 1749, and died in Madras, South India. An English physicist from Bristol, **Henry Kater** (1777–1835), developed a modern accurate pendulum for measuring seconds, and it formed the basis for a more accurate system of British weights and measures. *See clock.*

Pengelly, William (1812–1894) *See prehistory.*

Penney, Baron William George (1909–1991) *See atomic bomb, H bomb.*

Pennington, Mary Engle (1872–1952) *See dairy industry.*

Penny, Thomas (d 1519) *See entomology.*

Penny-Farthing *See bicycle.*

Penrose, Roger (b 1931) *See black hole.*

Pentium Computer microchip first produced by Intel in 1993. It was designed to take advantage of the PCI local bus architecture and increase the available bandwidth between devices.

Penzias, Arno Allan (b 1933) *See background radiation, Big Bang theory, cosmic rays, helium, radioastronomy.*

Perception In 1690, the English philosopher **John Locke** (1632–1704), from Somerset, argued that all knowledge of man came from experience and sensations only. A British philosopher, **George Berkeley** (1685–1753), developed the concept of space perception acquired through visual and tactile sensations from childhood. The role of the human senses in perception was first studied on an objective scientific basis by an American psychologist, **James Gibson** (1904–1979) from McConnelsville. His work led to the development of a new field, ecological optics.

Percer, Charles (1764–1838) *See architecture, European.*

Peregrinus of Maricourt, Peter (b c. 1220) *See compass (1), magnet.*

Perey, Marguerite Catherine (1909–1975) *See francium.*

Perfect Number A number that is equal to the sum of all its factors. **Euclid** (*c.* 300 BC) in his *Elements VII* defined it as that which is equal to its own parts. Four such numbers (6, 28, 496, 8128) were proposed by a Greek mathematician, **Nicomachus of Gerasa** in AD 100, and his work on arithmetic remained as a standard authority on the subject for nearly 1000 years. **Theon of Smyrna** (*c.* AD 250) wrote on over-perfect numbers whose sum of factors is greater than the whole number. A fifth perfect number (33 350 336)

was included by **Hudalrichus Regius** in his *Utriusque arithmetices* (1536). The sixth and seventh perfect numbers were discovered in 1603 by an Italian professor of mathematics at the University of Bologna, **Pietro Antoine Cataldi** (1548–1626).

Periodic Law Certain relationships between the atomic weights of certain analogous elements were observed in 1829 by **Johann Wolfgang Dobereiner** (1780–1849), a German professor of chemistry in Jena. He classified these elements into groups of triads. A French geologist, **Alexandre Emile de Bèguyer** (1819–1886), made a suggestion of periodicity of elements which went unnoticed. In 1864, a London chemist, **John Alexander Reina Newlands** (1837–1898), developed the law of octaves which stated that the properties of elements and their compounds were a periodic function of their atomic weight. His first paper on the subject was published in *Chemical News* in 1863. A professor of chemistry at the University of Petersburg, **Dmitri Ivanowitsch Mendeleev** (1834–1907) from Tobolsk, Siberia, developed the periodic law in 1868, which expressed the relation between general properties of elements and their atomic weights in a comprehensive manner. A physician and chemist, **Julius Lothar von Meyer** (1830–1895), proposed the same law independently in Germany in 1869.

Periodic Table *See atomic weight, Mendeleev, Dmitri Ivanovich, periodic law.*

Periscope Developed and perfected by **Sir Howard Grubb** (1844–1931) of Dublin, for use in submarines.

Perkin, Sir William Henry (1838–1907) *See aniline, dyes.*

Perkin, William Henry (1860–1929) Son of **Sir William Henry Perkin** (1838–1907) and professor of chemistry at Manchester (1892) and Oxford (1912). *See camphor.*

Perkins, Jacob (1766–1849) *See postal service.*

Permutation Variation of the order of a set of things. The term permutations was first used by a Swiss mathematician, **Jacques Bernoulli** (1654–1705) in his *Ars Conjectandi* published posthumously in 1713. Various permutations of a set of broken and straight lines in triads are found in the mystic trigrams of the ancient Chinese classic *I-ching*. A Roman philosopher, **Anicus Manlius Severinus Boethius** (AD 480–524), gave a rule for the number of combinations taken two at a time. A Hindu mathematician and astrologer from Ujjain, **Bhaskara** (AD 1114–1185), dealt with permutations in his treatise *Lilavati*. Around 1140, a Hebrew writer, Rabbi Ben Ezra, wrote on the subject. An Italian mathematician, **Niccolò Fontana Tartaglia** (1499–1557) of Venice, applied theory to the chances of throwing a dice. J. Buteo in 1559 discussed the number of combinations in a lock for a given number of movable cylinders.

Perot, Alfred (1863–1925)   *See interferometer.*

Perpetual Motion   A theory that a machine can operate indefinitely without an external power source. **Bhaskara** (AD 1114–1185), a Hindu mathematician and astrologer from Ujjain, was one of the first to postulate the perpetual motion of a machine, in 1150. This theory was disproved through the laws of thermodynamics and conservation of energy in the 18th century.

Perrault, Claude (1613–1688)   *See architecture, European.*

Perrelet, Abraham-Louis (1729–1826)   *See watches.*

Perrin, Jean Baptiste (1870–1942)   *See Brownian movement, cathode rays.*

Perronet, Jean Rodolphe (1708–1794)   *See bridges.*

Personal Computers   *See computers.*

Perspex   Trade name for partially transparent lightweight, tough plastic (polymethylmethacrylate) first produced in 1930.

Perthes, Jacques Boucher de (1788–1868)   A French archeologist from Rethel, who found evidence for early Stone Age or Paleolithic culture in Abbeville, France. His findings of stone instruments and the remains of extinct animals provided the first proof that humans existed over 20 000 years ago, at the time of the extinct species. His presentation to the Society of Emulation of Abbeville, in 1838, was published in 1847.

Perturbation   A transient gravitational effect caused by a body, on another body in space. *See Kirkwood Gaps.*

Peruzzi, Baldassare Tommaso (1481–1536)   *See architecture, Italian.*

Petit, Alexis Thérèse (1791–1820)   *See atomic heat, Dulong and Petit law, specific heat.*

Peto, Samuel Morton (1809–1889)   *See railway.*

Petrie, Sir Flinders (1853–1942)   *See Ur.*

Petrochemical Industry   *See petroleum.*

Petroleum [Greek: *petra*, rock + Latin: *oleum,* oil]   The earliest reference to American petroleum was made in 1640 by Albaro Barba who described its physical properties and called it Oyl of Peter. A professor of chemistry at Yale,

Benjamin Silliman Junior (1816–1885), showed that petroleum was a mixture of hydrocarbons, and could be separated by fractional distillation. The petroleum industry was launched by **Edwin Laurentine Drake** (1890–1880) of Greenville, New York, a pioneer prospector of oil in America. In 1859, he invented a tube to protect the drill hole down to the bed rock, and struck oil at a depth of 69 feet in Titusville, Pennsylvania. A useful catalytic hydrogenation reaction for converting coal into useful hydrocarbons such as gasoline and lubricating oil was devised by a German industrial chemist, **Friedrich Karl Rudolf Bergius** (1884–1949). He shared the Nobel Prize for chemistry for this work with **Carl Bosch** (1874–1940), in 1931. **Thomas Midgley** (1889–1944), an American inventor from Beaver Falls, Pennsylvania, devised the octane rating method for gasoline. An American chemist **David Talbot Day** (1859–1925) of East Rockport, Ohio made significant contributions and published *Handbook of the Petroleum Industry* (1922). A Russian chemist, **Vladimir Nikolayevich Ipatieff** (1867–1952), made fundamental contributions to the field with his discovery of several reactions that are now used in the petrochemical industry. He left Russia in 1930 and joined the Universal Oil Products Company of Chicago, where he worked for the rest of his life. He developed a process for manufacturing high-octane gasoline.

Petrology [Greek: *petra*, rock + *logos*, discourse]   Study of the origin and nature of rocks. A German physician and metallurgist, Johann Lehmann, in the Berezov mine at Ekaterinberg published a *History of Stratified Rocks* (1756). A German geologist born in Silesia, **Abraham Gottlob Werner** (1749–1817), was the first to classify rock formations on the basis of mineralogical structure. In his classification of rock layers into five groups, he disregarded their organic contents. The English geologist, **William Smith** (1769–1839), dated rocks by studying the fossils in them and published *Strata Indentified by Organised Fossils* (1816). Another pioneer in petrology, **John Macculloch** (1773–1835), published an important work *A Geological Classification of Rocks, with descriptive synopses of the species and varieties, comprising the Elements of Practical geology* (1821). An English chemist and geologist, **Henry Clifton Sorby** (1826–1908) of Sheffield, devised a method of preparing thin slices of rock for examination under the microscope. The method was developed by another English geologist from Birmingham, **William Johnson Sollas** (b 1849), who investigated the method of formation of igneous rocks. Determination of the age of radiactive rocks, through measurement of the percentage of the end product, lead, was carried out by an American geochemist, **William Francis Hillebrand**

(1853–1925). He became the chief chemist at the American Bureau of Standards in 1908. **John Joly** (1857–1933), an Irish physicist and geologist, studied the alpha particles emitted from zircon and allanite and arrived at a method of estimating the age of rocks. An English petrologist, **Alfred Harker** (1859–1939) of Kingston-upon-Hull, studied important aspects of igneous rocks in Scotland. Some of his published works include *The Tertiary Igneous Rocks of Skye* (1904), *Natural History of Igneous Rocks* (1909) and *Geology of the Small Isles of Invernesshire* (1908). In 1907, **Bertram Borden Boltwood** (1870–1927), an American chemist from Amhurst, Massachusetts, used the ratio of lead to uranium, for dating rocks. **Robert John Strutt Rayleigh** (1875–1947), an English physicist and son of **Lord John William Strutt Rayleigh** (1842–1919), carried out important studies on the radioactivity of rocks. An English geologist, **Arthur Holmes** (1890–1965), used radioactive end products for measuring the age of rocks, and published *Petrographic Methods and Calculations* in 1921. An Austrian-born British chemist, **Frederick Adolph Paneth** (1887–1958), determined the age of rocks by measuring the helium formed by the disintegration of radium, and applied it to the study of meteorites. A Canadian geochemist, **Norman Levi Bowen** (1887–1956) of Ontario, applied physical chemistry to petrology and published *The Evolution of Igneous Rocks* (1928). An English petrologist, **George Walter Tyrrell** (1883–1961) of Watford, made important contributions and published *Principles of Petrology* (1926) and several other books on the subject. The oldest known rock was discovered in 1984 by Samuel Bowring in Northwest Territories in Canada, and with the use of SHRIMP (Sensitive High-mass Resolution Ion Micro-Probe) it was demonstrated to be 3962 million years old.

Pettenkofer, Max von (1818–1901) *See calorimeter.*

Pettersson, Swen Otto (1848–1941) *See oceanography.*

Petty, William (1623–1687) *See copying, Royal Society of London, statistics.*

Peuerbach, Georg von (1423–1461) An Austrian mathematician who lectured in Vienna. He was court astrologer to the Hungarian king Ladisius V, and later to the Holy Roman Emperor. His translation of Ptolemy's *Almagest* was completed after his death by his pupil **Regiomontanus** (1436–1476). *See sines.*

Peugeot Car manufacturing firm in France founded in 1885 by Armand Peugeot (1849–1915). It initially began making bicycles and in 1889 Peugeot produced his first steam car.

In 1890 he developed his first petrol-driven car, with a Daimler engine.

Pewter An alloy of tin and lead, known to the Romans around AD 200. The London Guild of Pewtera was formed in 1300, and pewter vessels and plates became common in Europe after this period. Modern pewter contains mainly tin with some antimony and copper.

Pfeffer, Wilhelm Friedrich Philipp (1845–1920) *See osmosis.*

Pflucker, Julius (1801–1868) *See X-rays.*

Phanerozoic [Greek: *phanero* , visible] A geological period lasting over the most recent 570 million years. It includes the Palaeozoic, Mesozoic, and Cenozoic eras.

Phase Contrast Microscopy A method of increasing or decreasing contrast in images formed by the microscope. In 1892 **Ernest Abbe** (1840–1905) improved the technique of phase contrast microscopy by means of glass wedges placed in the back of the focal plane of the objective. It was further developed in 1934 by a Dutch physicist, **Frits Zernike** (1888–1966), who was awarded the Nobel Prize for physics in 1953, for his work.

Phase Rule *See Gibbs–Donnan equilibrium.*

Philips Dutch electrical and electronic manufacturing firm founded in 1891 under the name The Philips Bulb and Radio Works by an industrialist Anton Philips (1874–1951).

Phillips, John (1800–1874) *See Mesozoic period.*

Phillips, Peregrine (c. 1800–1831) *See sulfuric acid.*

Philo (c. 200 BC) A Byzantian scientist who first demonstrated that combustion brought about a change in air. He showed that contraction of air, in a globe, over water, occurred when a candle was burnt in it. *See catapult, military engineering.*

Philolaus (c. 450 BC) *See geogeny, musical theory.*

Philology [Greek: *philos*, friend + *logos*, discourse] Comparative study and origin of languages. An early work on Sanskrit and Indo-Germanic languages was published in 1808 by **Friedrich von Schlegel** (1772–1829) of Hanover. A Bavarian philologist, **Johann Kasper Zeuss** (1806–1856), is regarded as the founder of Celtic philology; he published *Grammatica Celtica*. **Max Muller** (1823–1900), a professor of comparative philology at Oxford, classified Latin and Greek under the Aryan group of languages, owing to their resemblence to Sanskrit, in his *Lectures on the Science of Language* (1861). **Horace Hayman Wilson** (1786–1860), an earlier professor of philology at Oxford, was one of the first to study Sanskrit in detail. He translated the RigVeda, the sacred hymns of the Hindus, and published a dictionary of Sanskrit in 1852. Muller's rival in America, **William Dwight Whitney** (1827–1894), who disputed some of the theories proposed by Muller, became professor of Sanskrit at Yale (1854) and published *Language and Study of Language* (1867), *Life and Growth of Language* (1876) and several other works. A Scottish philologist, **Alexander Murray** (1775–1813), wrote a *History of the European Languages* which was posthumously published in 1823.

Philoponus, Ionnes (*c.* AD 550)   Also known as **John the Grammerian** or **Ionnes Gramaticus.** A philosopher who wrote on science, mathematics and theology. He produced comments on eleven of the works of Aristotle, and one on the *Arithmetic* of Nicomachus.

Philosophy [Greek: *phileo*, to love + *sophia*, wisdom] **Thales** (640–546 BC) of Miletus is regarded as the father of philosophy. The term philosophy was first adopted by **Pythagoras** (*c.* 580–500 BC) who called himself a philosopher around 528 BC. Before his time, this subject was studied by people who called themselves *sages*. Thales was followed by **Aristotle** (384–322 BC) and **Plato** (428–348 BC). The first of the moral philosophers from the east was **Gaudama Siddartha Buddha** (568–488 BC), a Hindu prince from Benares in Nepal. He proposed the concept of *nirvana,* a complete withdrawal of interest from the external world to the inner-self in order to attain a tranquil state devoid of passion. During the 17th century, philosophy was classified into: moral or ethical and intellectual and natural (physical). Some of the eminent British philosophers include Roger Bacon, Sir Francis Bacon, John Locke and Herbert Spencer. A German philosopher and professor of Logic and Metaphysics, **Immanuel Kant** (1724–1804), published several important works on natural and ethical philosophy including *Kritik der reinen* (Critique of Pure Reason, 1781), *Kritik der Urteilskraft* (Critique of Judgement, 1790) and *Kritik der praktischen Vernuft* (Critique of Practical Reason, 1788).

Phloem   A tissue in plant stems containing sieve-tubes and vascular bundles, for transporting sap from the leaves to other parts of the plant. Identified by a Swiss botanist, **Carl Wilhelm von Nägeli** (1817–1891).

Phlogiston Theory [Greek: *phlogistein*, to set on fire]   Proposed in 1697 as a cause of burning and rusting, by **Georg Ernst Stahl** (1660–1734) of Germany. His theory was upheld for over a century until it was disproved with the discovery of oxygen in 1774 by a French chemist, **Antoine Laurent Lavoisier** (1743–1794). *See oxygen.*

Phonodeik   A mechanical device for photographically recording sound waves, invented by an American physicist, **Dayton Clarence Miller** (1866–1941) of Ohio.

Phonograph   Name given by **Thomas Alva Edison** (1847–1931) to his sound-recording apparatus. *See gramophone.*

Phosgene   Carbonyl chloride, first used as a chemical weapon by the Germans in 1915 during World War I.

Phosphorus [Greek: *phos*, light + *phereo*, I bear]   A non-metallic element discovered in 1669 by a German, Hennig Brand, a merchant of Hamburg, during his search for the philosopher's stone. In 1693, **Wilhelm Homberg** (1652–1715) of Batavia, obtained a form of it by heating sal ammoniac and lime. Johann Kunckel or Kungelius, a metallurgist to Charles II of Sweden, obtained it from urine in 1678. The English chemist **Robert Boyle** (1627–1691) independently obtained it from urine in 1680. A French chemistry student, Charles Sauria, first used phosphorus in the composition of matches, in 1830. The industrially hazardous yellow phosphorus was in use until an Austrian chemist, **Anton Schrotter** (1802–1875), discovered the much safer red phosphorus, and demonstrated it to be an allotrope. Red phosphorus started to be manufactured in Birmingham in 1845 by an English chemist from Oxfordshire, **Arthur Albright** (1811–1900). An English chemist and science historian from Manchester, **Sir Thomas Edward Thorpe** (1845–1925), was mainly responsible for replacing the yellow phosphorus with red phosphorus in the match industry.

Photochemistry [Greek: *phos*, light + *chymos*, juice]   Study of chemical reactions initiated by light. A Swedish chemist, **Carl Wilhelm Scheele** (1742–1786), discovered the action of light on silver salts – a finding used 50 years later in photography. A German physicist, **Johann Wilhelm Ritter** (1776–1810) from Silesia, studied the role of light in chemical reactions, around 1800. Pioneer work in modern photochemistry was carrried out by an English chemist, **Ronald George Reyford Norrish** (1897–1978) in 1923. He shared the Nobel Prize for chemistry in 1967 for his work on flash photolysis with the English chemist, **George Porter** (b 1920), and **Manfred Eigen** (b 1927) of Germany, who first studied fast reactions in liquids. *See flash photolysis.*

Photocopying   Invented in 1903 by an American office worker, G.C. Beidler, who patented it in 1906. A modern machine was invented in 1935 by another American, Chester Carlson. *See copying.*

Photoelectric Cell A device that produces an electrical output when exposed to light. Invented in 1896 by a German physicist, **Johann Phillip Julius Elster** (1854–1920) and his colleague **Hans Friedrich Geitel** (1855–1923), a professor at the Brunswick Technical Institute. It consisted of an electronic tube with a cathode, sensitive to light rays, which emitted electrons when hit by photons. The current generated by the device is proportional to the intensity of the light used. An American, Charles E. Fritts, has also been credited with the invention of the photoelectric cell, in 1883. The modern photoelectric cell was developed in 1954 by Chapin, Fuller and Peterson of the Bell Telephone Company. The priciple of electric photometry was used in astronomy by an American astronomer, **Joel Stebbins** (1878–1966) of Omaha, to study the light curves of stars. A German astronomer, **Paul Guthnick** (1879–1947), perfected the method of photoelectric photometry in astronomy.

Photoelectricity The production of electricity by certain materials when they are exposed to light. The phenomenon was first observed by a German physicist, **Heinrich Rudolf Hertz** (1857–1894), and investigated by W. Hallwachs of Dresden. **Albert Einstein** (1879–1955) proposed a theory in 1905. These light particles, later known as photons, proposed by Einstein to explain the photoelectric effect, were demonstrated by an American physicist, **Arthur Holly Compton** (1892–1962). Compton received the Nobel Prize for physics for his study of the particle nature of light, in 1927.

Photoengraving In 1841, the French physicist, **Armand Hippolyte Louis Fizeau** (1819–1896) tried to reproduce images on Daguerre plates by electroplating and was successful in transforming them into copper plate engravings. In 1853, a French chemist, **Joseph Nicephore Niepce** (1765–1833) used bitumen, benzene and sulfuric ether to make permanent prints on steel plates.

Photographic Photometry Substitution of a photographic plate instead of the eye-piece in a telescope, in order to measure various densities of objects with a photometer. A method first introduced into astronomy by a German astronomer, **Karl Schwarzschild** (1873–1916).

Photography [Greek: *phos,* light + *graphein,* to write] The action of light on chloride was first studied in 1777 by a Swedish apothecary and chemist, **Carl Wilhelm Scheele** (1742–1786). Thomas Wedgewood demonstrated the process and published *An Account of a method of paintings upon glass and of making profiles by the agency of light upon the silver nitrate* (1802). In 1839, **Louis Jacques Mande Daguerre** (1789–1851) of Cormeilles, near Lisieux, France, introduced a

method of using sodium thiosulfate solution to remove the unchanged silver iodide, in photographic development. Around the same time an English Victorian squire, **William Henry Fox Talbot** (1800–1877) from Melbury House in Evershot, Wiltshire, independently developed a similar process. He used a weak silver chloride solution and produced outlines of leaves and lace in 1834. In the following year he discovered the negative from which unlimited positives could be made. Talbot's method was more advanced than that of Daguerre, which required the laborious task of taking photographs each time a copy or positive was required. Both Daguerre's and Talbot's works contributed to the shortening of exposure time required for photographic impression, from a few hours to a few minutes. Talbot's *Pencil of Nature* (1844) was the first photographically illustrated book to be published. The first human portrait was taken by a professor of chemistry and later medicine in New York, **John William Draper** (1811–1882). An English portrait sculptor, **Frederick Scott Archer** (1813–1857) of Bishop's Stortford, Hertfordshire, used pyrogallic acid as a developer. He invented the collodion or wet plate process in photography. The photographs produced by this process were known as ambrotypes. In 1853 a French teacher, Adolphe Alexandre Martin, used the collodion process to produce positives on thin sheets of tin. His method, known, as tintype, was popular with travelling photographers. In 1871, an English physician, Richard Leach Maddox, invented the process using a dry plate coated with a gelatine emulsion of silver bromide. A carbon process of photographic printing was invented by an English physicist, **Sir Joseph Wilson Swan** (1828–1914) of Sunderland, in 1864. He also invented the dry plate in 1871 and bromide paper in 1879. An English chemist from Derby, **Sir William de Wiveleslie** (1844–1920), invented a new gelatine emulsion that made instant photography possible. **Fredrick Eugene Ives** (1856–1937), an American inventor from Connecticut, invented the half-tone process in 1878 and a more effective process in 1885. The first successful roll-film in photography was produced in 1884 by **George Eastman** (1854–1932), an inventor from Waterville, New York. The Kodak box camera was invented by him in 1888, and he made it possible for the camera to be loaded in daylight. He produced the Brownie camera in 1900. He established the Eastman Kodak Company in 1892. Nitrocellulose photographic film was invented in 1898 by an American clergyman, Hannibal Williston Goodwin, and Eastman introduced a similar method in 1889. Eastman's work with **Thomas Alva Edison** (1847–1931) contributed to the development of the moving picture industry. The electronic theory regarding the change in chemicals when a photo-

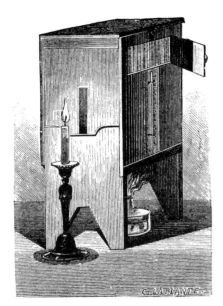

Figure 64 A mercury box for developing Daguerrotype. Guillemin, Amédée. *The Applications of Physical Forces*. London: Macmillan and Co, 1877

graphic film is exposed to light was postulated by an English physicist, **Sir Neville Francis Mott** (1905–1996) from Leeds. High-speed photography in America was developed by an electrical engineer, **Harold Eugene Edgerton** (1903–1990), who also invented momentary lighting used in flash photography. *See camera, celestial photography, color photography, microphotography, Polaroid camera.*

Photogravure A method of engraving on a photographically prepared plate with the use of ink. It was invented in 1852 by an English Victorian squire, **William Henry Fox Talbot** (1800–1877) from Melbury House in Evershot, Wiltshire. The method was perfected and made a commercial success by two brothers, Max and Louis Levy, in 1893. *See photoengraving.*

Photometry [Greek: *phos*, light + *metron*, to measure] The first attempt to quantify and compare the light from the sun, planets and stars was made in 1655 by a French physicist, **Adrian Auzont** (1622–1691). A French astronomer and mathematician, **Pierre Bouguer** (1698–1758), invented a heliometer in 1748 for measuring the light of the sun, and wrote *Traité d'optique sur la gradation de la lumière* which was published in 1760. *See electric photometry, photographic photometry.*

Photomicrography [Greek: *phos*, light + *mikros*, small + *graphein*, to write] The production of photographs on microscopic slides. The method was developed in 1840 by a London optician and instrument maker, **John Benjamin Dancer** (1812–1887).

Photons The light particles of an electromagnetic nature, later known as photons, were proposed by **Albert Einstein** (1879–1955) to explain photoelectric effect. His theory was confirmed by an American physicist, **Arthur Holly Compton** (1892–1962), who received the Nobel Prize for physics in 1927, for his study of the particle nature of light. The term photon was coined in 1926 by an American chemist and professor of chemistry at the University of California (1912), **Gilbert Newton Lewis** (1875–1946). An Italian-born US physicist at Cornell University, **Bruno Rossi** (1905–1994), identified photons.

Photosynthesis [Greek: *phos,* light + *synthesis*, putting together]. The English chemist and clergyman, **Joseph Priestley** (1733–1804) of Leeds, was the first to observe that plants were capable of using the carbon dioxide in the atmosphere and replacing it with oxygen. The use of carbon dioxide by plants in the daytime and its release during the night was observed by a Dutch plant physiologist, **Jan Ingenhousz** (1730–1799), who worked in England. His work *Experiments upon vegetables, discovering their great power of purifying the common air in the sunshine and of injuring it in the shade and at night* was published in 1779. A Swiss botanist, **Jean Senebier** (1742–1809) of Geneva, was one of the first to demonstrate the basic principle of photosynthesis, and he published *Action de la Lumière sur la Végétation* (1779) and

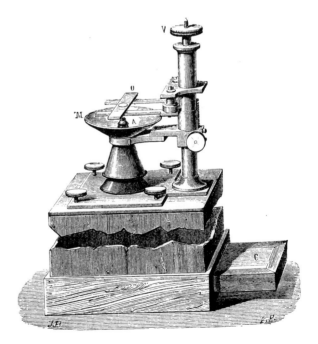

Figure 65 A mid-19th century photographic microscope Guillemin, Amédée. *The Applications of Physical Forces*. London: Macmillan and Co, 1877

Expériences sur l'Action de la Lumière Solaire dans la Végétation (1788). **Nicholas Theodore de Saussure** (1767–1845), a physician from Geneva, and a pioneer in the field of plant nutrition, was one of the first to demonstrate the role of carbon dioxide in photosynthesis. In 1860, a French agricultural chemist from Paris, **Jean Baptiste Joseph Dieudonné Boussingault** (1802–1887), demonstrated that the process starts as soon as a plant is exposed to sunlight and stops in the dark. **Julius von Sachs** (1832–1897), a professor at Würzberg, proposed that the green pigment was not diffusely present in the plant tissues, but was contained in special bodies. These bodies were identified and named as chloroplasts by **Andreas Franz Wilhelm Schimper** (1856–1901) of Basel, in 1883. **Johann Friedrich Wilhelm Adolf von Baeyer** (1835–1917), an organic chemist from Berlin, did further studies on the mechanism of photosynthesis. The green pigment that aided in photosynthesis was identified as chlorophyll by a German chemist **Richard Willstätter** (1872–1942) and his colleagues in 1913. He received the Nobel Prize for chemistry in 1915 for his work on plant pigments. The source of oxygen used in photosynthesis was proved to be from water, and not carbon dioxide, by a Canadian-born American biochemist, **Martin David Kamen** (b 1913). The carbon-14 isotope for investigating photosynthesis was introduced in 1945 by an American chemist of Russian origin, **Melvin Calvin** (1911–1997) of Minnesota. Paul was awarded the Nobel Prize for chemistry in 1961, for his work on the role of chlorophyll in photosynthesis. The mechanism of the conversion of light energy to chemical energy during photosynthesis was elucidated by a German biochemist, **Otto Heinrich Warburg** (1883–1970). He was awarded the Nobel Prize for Physioloy or Medicine, for his work on iron-containing cellular respiratory enzymes, in 1931. The energy transfer process involved in photosynthesis was worked out in 1985 by a German biochemist, **Hartmut Michel** (b 1948). For his discovery of the structure of the membrane protein, he shared the Nobel Prize for chemistry in 1985 with two other West German chemists, Johan Deisenhofer and Robert Huber. *See chlorophyll, chloroplasts, plant physiology.*

Physical Chemistry The *Physica Subterranea* (1669) by a German chemist, **Johann Joachim Becher** (1635–1682), was probably the first attempt to unify physics and chemistry. A graduate of Yale and later a professor there in 1871, **Josiah Willard Gibbs** (1839–1903) of New Haven, Connecticut, was one of the founders of the field. He applied the principles of thermodynamics to chemistry, and proposed the ionic theory of the Gibbs–Donnan equilibrium, related to chemical thermodynamics. **Jacobus Henricus**

van't Hoff (1852–1911) did early work on chemical kinetics. The Swedish physical chemist, **Svante August Arrhenius** (1859–1927), developed the theory of electrolytic dissociation. **Friedrich Wilhelm Ostwald** (1853–1932), a German professor of chemistry at Leipzig, applied physics to chemistry and published *Lehrbuch der allgemeinen Chemie* (1885). He proposed the law of dilution that bears his name, and defined a catalyst as an agent that accelerates the rate of a chemical reaction. A German physical chemist, **Walther Hermann Nernst** (1864–1941) from Briesen, West Prussia, is regarded as the co-founder of modern physical chemistry with Jacobus Henricus van't Hoff and Svante August Arrhenius. He developed the theory of electrode potential and the concept of the solubility product. Nernst was awarded the Nobel Prize for chemistry for his work on thermochemistry, in 1920. **Arthur Rudolf Hantzsch** (1857–1935) of Dresden, Saxony, was another pioneer in physical chemistry who studied the relation between chemical and physical properties of organic compounds. A Scottish chemist, **Sir James Walker** (1863–1935), who was professor of chemistry at Dundee (1894–1898) and Edinburgh (1908–1928), made several contributions to the study of ionization and amphoteric electrolytes, and published *Introduction to Physical Chemistry* (1899). An American physical chemist, **Louis Plack Hammet** (1894–1987), established the field of physical organic chemistry and published *Physical Organic Chemistry* (1940).

Physics [Greek: *phusis*, nature] The study and application of mechanisms that govern nature. Many of the phenomena of physics were considered to be supernatural by the ancients. **Aristotle** (384–322 BC) investigated the electrical nature of the torpedo fish, 2000 years before it was established as a form of animal electricity. He also distinquished between a mathematician and a physicist. The magnetic attraction of the lodestone, known to the ancients, was used in the construction of the compass needle, pivoted on a card or floated on water, in the 12th century. A Greek scientist, **Anaxagoras** (500–428 BC) of Ionia, attempted to explain rainbows on the basis of a natural phenomenon rather than a divine one. Using a prism and directing a single shaft of light towards it in an otherwise darkened room, **Sir Isaac Newton** (1642–1727) discovered that light is made up of numerous constituent parts (light spectrum) so characteristic of a rainbow. The electrical property of amber, when rubbed, was observed by the Greek philosopher **Thales** (640–546 BC), around 600 BC. An English physician, **William Gilbert** (1544–1603) of Colchester, demonstrated that apart from amber other materials also produced electricity, and published *De Magnete, Magneticisque Corporibus, te de Magno Magnette Tellure, Physiologia Nova* (1600), which established him as the initiator of the study of modern electricity. Although the power of steam was demonstrated by **Hero of Alexandria** around AD 100, its full potential was only realized in the 19th century with the invention of the steam engine. The discovery of the law of flotation by **Archimedes** (287–212 BC) established the basis of modern hydrodynamics and hydrostatistics. The theory of atoms proposed by **Democritus** (c. 460–c. 370 BC) and his master **Leucippus** at the school of Abdera (c. 500 BC) over 2000 years ago was revived on a modern basis by the English physicist, **Lord Ernest Rutherford** (1871–1937) and his theory of atomic structure formed the basis for development of atomic physics.

Pi   The ratio of the circumference to the diameter of a circle has been studied for a long time under the term quadrature of a circle. Its value was calculated by the ancient Chinese and Egyptians, Archimedes, Ptolemy, Vitruvius, Brahmagupta and Bhaskara. The symbol π was first used to denote the circumference of the circle by **William Oughtred** (1575–1660) of Eton, England, in his *Clavis Mathematicae* (1647). The numerical approximation of π correct to 35 decimal places (Ludolph's number) was found by a Dutch mathematician, **Ludolph van Ceulen** (1539–1610) in 1610. Its present sign (π) for the ratio of the circumference to the diameter was introduced by an English mathematician, William Jones (1680–1749) from Anglesey, in 1707. Its use in mathematics was popularized by a Swiss mathematician, **Leonhard Euler** (1707–1883) in 1737. In 1768 a Swiss mathematician, **Johann Heinrich Lambert** (1728–1777) of Mülhausen, proved that π is an irrational number. The value of π to 707 decimal places was calculated by W. Shanks in 1873. A German mathematician **Carl Louis Ferdinand Lindemann** (1852–1939), published a paper in 1882 on π as a transcendental number.

Piano   The oldest surviving piano, preserved in the Metropolitan Museum of Art, New York, was built in 1720 in Florence, Italy, by **Bartolommeo Christofori** (1655–1731) of Padua. A Scottish piano manufacturer, **John Broadwood** (1732–1812), established one of the early pianoforte houses in London in 1770. His grandson, **Henry Fowler Broadwood** (1811–1893) greatly improved the piano. A French pianoforte maker, **Sebastien Erard** (1752–1831) invented a piano with double escapement, and also built a harp with double pedals.

Piazzi, Giuseppe (1749–1826)   *See asteroids, Bode law.*

Picard Theorem   Related to the integral function of the complex variable, proposed and proved by a French mathematician, **Charles Emile Picard** (1856–1941) of Paris. He also made significant contributions to analytical geometry and published *Traité d'Analyse* (1891–1896) in three volumes.

Picard, Charles Emile (1856–1941)   *See Picard theorem.*

Picard, Jean (1620–1682)   *See meridian, micrometer.*

Piccard, Auguste Antoine (1884–1962)   *See air balloon, bathysphere, stratosphere, undersea exploration.*

Piccard, Jean Felix (1884–1963) Brother of **Auguste Antoine Piccard** (1884–1962), was born in Basel and became professor of aeronautical engineering at Minnesota University. He made important contributions to the study of the stratosphere.

Pickering, Edward Charles (1846–1919)   *See celestial photography.*

Pickering, William Hayward (b 1910)   *See rocket.*

Pickering, William Henry (1858–1938)   *See celestial photography, Saturn.*

Picric Acid [Greek: *picros,* bitter]   An explosive compound, first obtained in 1771 by an English chemist, **Peter Woulfe** (1727–1803). It was named on the basis of its bitter taste, by a French chemist, **John Baptiste André Dumas** (1800–1884), and was introduced as an explosive in France, in 1885.

Pictet, Amè (1857–1937)   *See nicotine.*

Pictet, Marc Auguste (1752–1825)   *See radiation of heat.*

Pictet, Raoul Pierre (1846–1929)   *See cascade process.*

Pictogram   An early form of writing, consisting of 2000 pictures and symbols, was used in Erech and Sumeria around 3500 BC. This was developed into hieroglyphics. *See hieroglyphics, paleography, philology, writing.*

Pierce, John Robinson (b 1910)   *See satellite.*

Pietro, Andrea de (1508–1590)   *See theater.*

Piezoelectric Effect   The property of some crystals to produce an electric potential when subjected to pressure. A phenomenon discovered by **Pierre Curie** (1859–1906) in 1880. W.A. Morrison of Bell Telephone Laboratories in the USA developed a clock in the 1920s, based on the electrical properties of a crystal of quartz. In this clock the crystal was made to oscillate at a rate of 100 000 times a second, bringing the accuracy of time within one second in three years.

Pilkington, Sir Lionel Alexander Bethune (1920–1995)   *See glass.*

Piltdown Man One of the greatest frauds in scientific history. A solicitor from Sussex, **Charles Dawson** (1864–1916), who had a special interest in paleontology, while walking on the common at Piltdown in 1911 obtained some fragments of a skull from workmen who found them while digging gravel. He presented his findings to **Arthur Smith Woodward** (1864–1944), keeper of the Geological Department of the Natural History Museum in London, who declared the fragment to be that of the earliest known ancestor of man. This finding was hailed as the missing link between man and ape. However, in 1952, further tests by Kenneth P. Oakley proved that the skull was that of a modern man and the jaw belonged to an orang-utan. Many eminent paleontologists, including **Sir Arthur Keith** (1866–1955) and Dawson, were suspected of being the perpetrators of the hoax. A canvass trunk later found under the roof of the Natural History Museum in the 1970s provided further clues to the Piltdown hoax. This trunk, which belonged to Martin Alister Campbell Hinton**,** the former curator of the zoology section of the museum who died in 1961, contained bones of animals stained with iron and manganese to make them look old, in the same proportion as those found in the Piltdown skull. It is believed that Hinton, who fell out with Woodward, perpetrated the hoax.

Pimental, George Claude (1922–1989) *See spectroscopy*.

Pinch Effect A phenomenon important to thermonuclear fusion. In 1946, J.A. Samson and R.E. Vollrath of University of Southern California, passed an electric current through a tube of gas and observed that the gas tended to form a narrow column without coming into contact with the walls of the container. This was explained on the basis of the electromagnetic force created by the current, which kept the gas particles together. This phenomenon, known as the pinch effect, provided a way of attaining very high temperatures during experiments on thermonuclear fusion.

Pinchbeck, Christopher (1670–1732) *See watches*.

Pinchbeck, Christopher (1710–1783) *See watches*.

Pion or pi-meson. A subatomic particle discovered in 1947 by an English chemist, **Cecil Frank Powell** (1903–1969) of Tonbridge, Kent. He was awarded the Nobel Prize for physics in 1950, for his discovery.

Pippard, Brian (b 1920) *See superconductivity*.

Pistols *See firearms*.

Pitch The Italian scientist **Galilei Galileo** (1564–1642) discovered that the pitch of a note depended on the number of vibrations in unit time. *See musical theory*.

Pithecanthropus [Greek: *pithecos*, ape] A name given in 1866 by **Ernst Heinrich Haeckel** (1834–1919), to a hypothetical missing link in the evolution of man. The teeth, calvarium and femur of a primitive man were discovered in Java by **Eugene Marie Dubois** (1858–1940), a Dutch physician and paleontologist from Eijsden. His finding gave rise to the speculation that Java or Eastern Asia was where man evolved, and not Africa, as suggested by Darwin. Dubois's finding was acclaimed as the missing link, and the primitive man to whom the fragments belonged was named *Pithecanthropus erectus*.

Pitiscus, Bartholomeus (1561–1613) *See decimal notation, trigonometry*.

Pitman, Benjamin (1822–1910) *See engraving, shorthand*.

Pitman, Sir Isaac (1813–1897) *See shorthand*.

Pitot Tube Used for measuring the relative velocity of a fluid at the orifice of a tube, invented by French engineer **Henri Pitot** (1695–1771) of Languedoc.

Pitot, Henri (1695–1771) *See Pitot tube*.

Pixie, Hippolyte (1808–1835) *See dynamo*.

Planck, Max Karl Ernst Ludwig (1858–1947) *See black body radiation, Planks' constant, quantum theory*.

Planck's Constant Fundamental unit of spin angular momentum denoted by the symbol h. Discovered by a German physicist, **Max Karl Ernst Ludwig Planck** (1858–1947) of Kiel. He served as professor of physics in Berlin and was awarded the Nobel Prize for physics in 1918 for his work on quantum theory.

Planes *See airplane, airlines, electric plane, seaplane, warplanes*.

Planetarium One of the first devices to demonstrate the different motions of celestial bodies was constructed by **Archimedes** (287–212 BC) of Syracuse. He used this sphere to demonstrate the movements of the sun, moon and five planets. A rotatable globe of nearly 4 tonnes was built by Andreas Busch in Denmark in 1660. The first modern planetarium was designed by Walther Bauersfelt, and it opened in Jena, Germany, in 1923.

Planets [Greek: *planetes*, wanderer] *See Earth, Jupiter, Mars, Mercury (planet), Neptune, Pluto, Saturn, Uranus, Venus*.

Plankton [Greek: *planketon*, drifting] A term independently coined in 1888 by a Swiss oceanographer **Alexander Emmanuel Agassiz** (1835–1910) and **Victor Hensen** (1835–1924), to denote the floating life forms found in the ocean. An automatic plankton recorder was invented by an

English professor of zoology at Oxford, **Alister Clavering Hardy** (1896–1985) from Nottingham, who received a knighthood in 1957. The value of specific types of plankton as indicators of different types of water was established by a British biologist, **Frederick Stratten Russell** (1897–1984) of Bridport, Dorset, who published *Eggs and Planktonic Stages of British Marine Fishes* (1976).

Plant Anatomy   One of the first English botanical works, *Anatomy of the Plants* (1682), was published by **Nehemiah Grew** (1641–1712). In this work, he described different types of tissues in plants and identified, for the first time, the male and female parts of flowering plants. A German botanist, **Heinrich Anton de Bary** (1831–1888), established some principal features and terminology in plant anatomy in his publication *Comparative Anatomy of Ferns and Phanerogams* (1877). The Jodrell Laboratory at Kew in London, for investigations into plant anatomy and physiology, was established in 1876 by **Sir Joseph Dalton Hooker** (1817–1911), an English botanist from Suffolk.

Plant Breeding   *See hybridization.*

Plant Classification   *See botanical classification.*

Plant Growth   Various aspects of plant growth were experimentally studied in 1724 by an English vicar at Teddington, **Stephen Hales** (1696–1761) from Bekesbourne, Kent. The effect of gravity on plant growth was demonstrated by J.B. Denis in 1672. Auxins [Greek: *auxein*, to increase], plant hormones that stimulate growth, were discovered and named by Kögl of Holland, in 1933. The first auxin to be identified was indoleacetic acid.

Plant Nutrition   A French chemist and botanist, **Henri Louis Duhamel** (1700–1782) of Paris, was one of the first to study the subject in detail. Studies on plant nutrition were carried out by a Swiss naturalist, **Charles Étienne Bonnet** (1720–1793), who published *Recherches sur l'usage des feuilles des plantes* in 1754. **Nicholas Theodore de Saussure** (1767–1845), a physician from Geneva, and a pioneer in the field of plant nutrition, was one of the first to demonstrate the role of carbon dioxide in photosynthesis. *See photosynthesis, plant physiology.*

Plant Pathology   The study of diseases in plants. **Theophrastus** (380–287 BC), the founder of botany, in his treatise *Historia Plantarum* described the diseased or abnormal appearance of plants caused by worms, excess sunlight and heavy rain. The bunt of wheat was investigated by M. du Tillet (1755) and B. Prevost (1807). Experimental work on the disease was done by a London botanist, **Thomas Andrew Knight** (1759–1838), in 1804. Plant pathology was

established as a science by a German botanist, **Heinrich Anton de Bary** (1831–1888), who worked out the life histories of certain pathogenic fungi. The first book on the subject, *Die Krankheiten der Kulturgewächse* by J. Kühn, was published in 1858. A Russian botanist, **Dmitri Iosifovich Ivanovski** (1864–1920), investigated the mosaic disease of the tobacco plant in 1892, and discovered that it was caused by particles (viruses) that passed through the bacterial filter.

Plant Physiology   The movement of sap in plants was first proposed in 1670 by the Italian microscopic anatomist and physician, **Marcello Malpighi** (1628–1694). The existence of this phenomenon was demonstrated by **Stephen Hales** (1696–1761), an English vicar at Teddington. He began his experimental studies on plant physiology in 1724, and demonstrated how water was drawn from the roots to the leaves, where it was lost by transpiration. He studied the various aspects of growth in plants and published *Vegetable Staticks* in 1738. A French priest from Burgundy, **Edmé Mariotte** (1620–1684), investigated sap pressure in plants and compared it to the circulating blood of animals, in 1676. In 1779, a Dutch physician, **Jan Ingenhousz** (1730–1799), demonstrated the two respiratory cycles in plants involving oxygen and carbon dioxide,. Soil as the source of nitrogen for plants

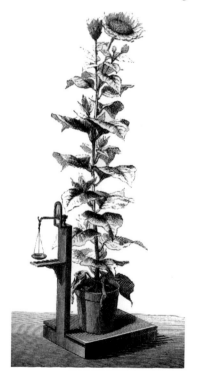

Figure 66   Experiments on plant physiology by Stephen Hales. Pouchet, F.A. *The Universe*. London: Blacke and Son, 1871

was demonstrated in 1840 by a French agricultural chemist from Paris, **Jean Baptiste Joseph Dieudonné Boussingault** (1802–1887). The direction of movement of plants (tropism) during germination was demonstrated by **Thomas Andrew Knight** (1759–1838). **Julius von Sachs** (1832–1897), a professor of botany at Würzburg, is regarded as the founder of modern plant physiology. He determined the mineral requirements of plants, studied the conversion of sugar into starch in chloroplasts and observed the effect of light and heat on plant growth. His *Lehrbuch der Botanik* (1868) was translated into English under the title of *Textbook of Botany* in 1875. The Jodrell Laboratory at Kew, for investigations into plant anatomy and physiology, was established in 1866 by **Sir Joseph Dalton Hooker** (1817–1911), an English botanist from Suffolk. A London botanist and physician, **Frederick Frost Blackman** (1866–1947), did fundamental research on plant respiration and published *Experimental Researches in Vegetable Assimilation* in 1895. *See chlorophyll, photosynthesis.*

Plante, Gaston (1834–1889) *See battery.*

Plaskett Twins Binary stars previously thought to be a single massive star. Discovered in 1922 by a Canadian astronomer, **John Stanley Plaskett** (1865–1941) from Woodstock, Ontario. During his work at the Dominion Observatory, Ottawa, he improved the spectrograph.

Plaskett, John Stanley (1865–1941) *See Plaskett's twins.*

Plasma Physics The study of constituent atoms, chiefly of gases, in a state of ionization. The ionized gas having an equal number of positively charged ions and free electrons is known as a plasma. It also has been referred to as the fourth stage of matter, and its existence was demonstrated in 1873 by a London molecular physicist and chemist, **Sir William Crookes** (1832–1919). Plasma physics was pioneered by a Swedish physicist, **Hannes Olof Gösta Alfvén** (1908–1995), who became professor of plasma physics at Stockholm, in 1964. He shared the Nobel Prize for physics in 1970, with the French physicist, **Louis Eugène Félix Néel** (b 1904). An American theoretical physicist, **David Joseph Bohm** (1917–1992), during his work with **Julius Robert Oppenheimer** (1904–1967) at the University of California at Berkeley, developed techniques to study and describe oscillations in plasmas. His work later led to the understanding of the behavior of electrons in metals. *See magnetohydrodynamics.*

Plastics *See cellophane, celluloid, polymer, polythene.*

Plate Tectonics *See tectonic theory.*

Plateau, Joseph Antoine Ferdinand (1801–1883) *See cinema, surface chemistry.*

Platinum In 1557, Justus Scaliger referred to a metal found in Colombia that could not be melted in a furnace. In 1735, Don Antonio de Ulloa, a Spanish naval officer, found the same mineral in Peru. In 1741, Charles Wood, an English metallurgist, sent an English chemist and physician, **William Brownrigg** (1711–1800) of Cumberland, to Cartagena in Colombia, to investigate this metal, known to the Spaniards as *Platina de Pinto*. Brownrigg presented his report to the Royal Society in 1750 and described it as a previously undescribed semi-metal. Around 1748, it had no commercial value, and the Spanish mined it in Peru to adulterate gold. The South American mines were later closed; trade in platinum was revived when Russia started exporting it in 1824. The catalytic properties of platinum were demonstrated in 1780 by a Bavarian chemist, **Johann Wolfgang Döbereiner** (1780–1849). An ingot of malleable platinum was produced by a French chemist from Charente, **François Chabaneau** (1754–1842), in 1783. It was produced in commercial quantities in 1855 by **Henri Étienne Sainte-Claire Deville** (1818–1881), a French chemist of West Indian origin.

Plato (428–348 BC) A philosopher and mathematician from a noble family in Athens who proposed the *Doctrine of Ideas,* and divided philosophy into three branches – ethics, physics and dialectics. His original name was Aristocles, but he received the name Plato because of his large shoulders. He met Socrates at the age of 20, and remained his pupil for eight years. Following the execution of Socrates in 399 BC, Plato travelled extensively before he retired in 387 BC to the groves of Academus near Athens, where he established his school. *See artificial transmutation, Atlantis, element, Euclid, museum, philosophy.*

Plato of Tivoli (*c.* AD 1120) *See cosine.*

Playfair, John (1748–1819) A Scottish geologist and mathematician from Forfarshire, who promoted **James Hutton's** (1726–1797) theory of the earth, and published *Illustrations to the Huttonian Theory* (1802) and *Elements of Geometry* (1795).

Pleistocene [Greek: *pleistos,* most + *cene,* recent] Early Quaternary period, which began 1.64 million years ago and ended 10 000 years ago.

Plesiosaurus [Greek: *pleistos,* most + *saurus,* lizard] The first fossil skeleton of a plesiosaurus was discovered in 1828 by an English paleontologist, **Mary Anning** (1799–1847) of Lyme Regis.

Plimsoll Line *See shipping.*

Plimsoll, Samuel (1824–1898) *See shipping.*

Pliny, Gaius Plinius Secundus, The Elder (AD 28–79) Roman naturalist and prolific writer who wrote an encyclopedia of natural history, *Historia Naturalis*, comprising 160 books, of which only 37 have survived. His work covering 20 000 subjects by Greek and Roman authors and scientists has provided a valuable insight into the culture and science during Roman and earlier Greek times. He was a military officer in Emperor Vespasian's army at the time of the eruption of Vesuvius, which destroyed Pompeii and took his life. The first translation of his work into Latin appeared in Venice in 1469, and an English translation was published in 1601. *See antimony, borax, butter, dairy industry, diamond, flint tools, glass, gold, gold gilding, lathe, magnet, mercury (metal), ornithology, soap, sodium, tides, wine.*

Pliocene Period [Greek: *pleo*, more + *cene*, recent] Fifth and last epoch of the Tertiary period of geological time, 5.2–1.64 million years ago, identified and named in 1839 by the eminent Scottish geologist, **Sir Charles Lyell** (1797–1875) from Kinnordy, Forfarshire. His published works include *Principles of Geology* (1830, 1832, 1833) in three volumes, *Elements of Geology* and *Geological Evidences of the Antiquity of Man* (1863). He was knighted in 1848, and made a baronet in 1864.

Plücker, Julius (1801–1868) *See analytical geometry, cathode rays, electron, Geissler tube.*

Plutarch (AD 46–120) *See military engineering, wine.*

Pluto The ninth and the smallest major planet of the sun. A Scottish physicist, **George Forbes** (1849–1936), predicted its existence in 1880. It was also predicted by an American astronomer and mathematician, **Percival Lowell** (1855–1916) of Boston, Massachusetts, and discovered in 1930 by an American astronomer, **Clyde William Tombaugh** (1906–1997) of Streator, Illinois, at the US Naval Observatory, Flagstaff, Arizona. Its companion, Charon, was discovered in the same observatory in 1978.

Plutonium An element with an atomic number of 94, discovered in 1940 by an American physicist, **Glenn Theodore Seaborg** (b 1912) through bombarding uranium with deuterons. He shared the Nobel Prize for chemistry in 1951 with another American atomic scientist, **Erward Mattison McMillan** (1907–1991) of Redondo Beach, California.

Pneumatic Drill Based on the principle of compressed air that releases bursts of impact. Invented in 1861 by a French engineer, Germain Sommeiller (1815–1871).

Pneumatic Tire *See tire.*

Pocket Calculator *See calculating machine.*

Pocket Watch *See watches.*

Poggendorff, Johann Christian (1796–1877) A German physicist and professor of physics at Berlin, who invented a device to magnify small deflections, which was used in mirror galvanometers and other instruments. His device consisted of a small suspended mirror that reflected a beam of light onto a scale. *See aldehyde, scientific journals.*

Pogson Scale A logarithmic system for assessing the brightness of stars, proposed by an English astronomer, **Norman Robert Pogson** (1829–1891) of Nottingham.

Pogson, Norman Robert (1829–1891) *See Pogson scale.*

Pohl, Frederik (b 1919) *See science fiction.*

Poincaré, Jules Henri (1854–1912) A French mathematician from Nancy who introduced automorphic functions in pure mathematics. His work on the dynamics of the electron contained many elements in common with Einstein's theory of relativity. His publications include *Leçons sur le calcul des probabilités* (1895), *Électricité et Optique* (1901) and *La Science et l'Hypothèse* (1906). His last theorem, left unproved when he died, was proved by an American mathematician, **George David Birkhoff** (1884–1944), who was a professor at Wisconsin (1902–1909), Princeton (1909–1912) and Harvard (1912–1939).

Poiseuille Law Relates the rate of flow of liquid through a tube to the pressure, temperature, diameter and length of the tube. Named after a French physiologist, **Jean Leonard Marie Poiseuille** (1799–1869).

Poiseuille, Jean Leonard Marie (1799–1869) *See Poiseuille law.*

Poisson Ratio Ratio between the lateral and longitudinal strain in a wire in the study of elasticity. Proposed by a French physicist and astronomer, **Siméon Denis Poisson** (1781–1840). He also proposed a two-fluid theory of electricity in 1812, and a theory of magnetism in 1824. His publications include *Mathematical Theory of Heat* (1835), *Treatise of Mechanics* (1833) and several other important works.

Poisson, Siméon Denis (1781–1840) *See elasticity, law of large numbers, Poisson ratio.*

Polanyi, John Charles (b 1929) A Berlin-born Canadian physical chemist, and son of **Michael Polanyi** (1891–1976). He shared the Nobel Prize for chemistry in 1971, for his work on chemical elementary processes, with an American physical chemist, **Dudley Robert Herschbach** (b 1932) of San Jose, California, and a Shanghai-born US physicist, **Tsung Dao Lee** (b 1926).

Polanyi, Michael (1891–1976) A British physicist born in Budapest, Hungary, where he graduated in medicine. After studying physical chemistry and electrochemistry in Berlin he left Nazi Germany and became professor of physical chemistry at Manchester University in England in 1933. He made significant contributions to the field of moleculer kinetics and the study of crystals.

Polar Light Another term for the aurora borealis or northern lights. *See aurora borealis.*

Polar Planimeter An instrument used to measure the area on a curved surface. Invented by a Swiss mathematical physicist and precision instrument maker, **Jakob Amsler-Laffon** (1823–1912).

Polarization A property of light discovered and named in 1808 by a French physicist, **Étienne Louis Malus** (1775–1812) of Paris. The law for polarized light, which states that the sum of intensities of the transmitted rays is equal to the intensity of the incident ray, is named after him. A polarization filter was constructed by **Dominique François Arago** (1786–1853) of France in 1810. The circular polarization of light was discovered in 1815 by a French physicist and professor of physics at the University of Paris, **Jean Baptiste Biot** (1774–1862). The explanation of polarization was given in 1816 by another French physicist, **Jean Augustine Fresnel** (1788–1827). A French physicist and physician, **Felix Savart** (1791–1841), invented a quartz plate (Savart's quartz plate) for studying the phenomenon.

Polarography An electrochemical method of chemical analysis, invented by a Czech chemist, **Jaroslav Heyrovsky** (1890–1967) of Prague. He was awarded the Nobel Prize for chemistry in 1959, for his above discovery.

Polaroid Camera A device capable of producing instantly developed photographs was invented by the Agfa photographic company in 1928. The method was revived and developed in 1947 by **Edwin Herbert Land** (1909–1991), an American inventor from Bridgeport, Connecticut. His one-step Polaroid camera developed pictures within the camera within one minute. He commercialized the method through his Polaroid Corporation, which he had previously established in 1937 for the production of Polaroid filters.

The Polaroid pictures initially appeared only in black and white, until 1963, when Land introduced a technique for producing colored pictures.

Polaroid Lenses Plastic light-polarizing material prepared by aligning and embedding submicroscopic crystals of iodoquinine sulfate in a synthetic sheet; used in sunglasses, cameras and three-dimensional movies. Invented in 1932 by an American physicist **Edwin Herbert Land** (1909–1991), who founded the Polaroid Corporation in 1937.

Polhem, Christopher (1661–1751) *See mechanical engineering.*

Pollen Analysis Botanical studies of pollen were done by a Swedish paleontologist, **Gunner Elias Otta** (1897–1973), who published *An Introduction to Pollen Analysis* in 1943. The study of pollen analysis in England was pioneered by **Sir Harry Godwin** (1901–1985) of Yorkshire, who also studied pollen zones based on the relative abundance of pollen of different tree species.

Pollination [Latin: *pollen*, fine flour] The first mention of gender in plants was made by a professor of botany at Tübingen, **Rudolph Jacob Camerarius** (1665–1721), in his *De sexu plantarum* (1694). Experimental work using animal pollinators was done in 1763 by **Joseph Gottlieb Kolreuter** (1733–1806), the director of the botanical gardens at Carlsruhe. A study of fertilization brought about by insects and wind, in plants, was carried out in 1793 by a German botanist, **Christian Conrad Sprengel** (1750–1816) of Brandenberg, who published *The Newly Revealed Mystery of Nature in the Structure and Fertilization of Flowers* (1793). Microscopic observations during pollination were made by **Giovanni Battista Amici** (1786–1863), in 1823. The first male elements of plants (in the fern) were discovered in 1884 by a Swiss botanist, **Carl Wilhelm von Nägeli** (1817–1891). The female elements were revealed by a German botanist, **Wilhelm Friedrich Benedikt Hofmeister** (1824–1877) of Leipzig, Saxony, who published *On the Embryology of Flowering Plants*, and held the professorial chairs at Heidelberg and Tübingen. A German botanist, **Carl Franz Joseph Erich Correns** (1864–1933), proved that sex in plants (*Bryonia*) is inherited in a Mendelian fashion. The first modern study of flowers pollinated by birds was done by an American geneticist, **Verne Edwin Grant** (b 1917) of San Francisco, who published *Flower Pollination in the Phlox Family* (1965) and *Hummingbirds and their Flowers* (1968).

Pollution *See ozone layer.*

Polonium A highly radioactive element discovered in 1893 by the French scientists **Antoine Henri Becquerel** (1852–1908) and **Marie Curie** (1867–1934). Marie Curie named the metal polonium, in honor of her country.

Polybius (204–122 BC) *See climatic zones, geography.*

Polymer [Greek: *polys*, many + *meros*, parts] A large molecule consisting of several thousands of repeating molecules, or monomers. In 1929, a Belgian-born American chemist, **Julius Arthur Nieuwland** (1878–1936), showed that acetylene could be polymerized to produce a rubber-like solid. Research on polymers leading to the discovery of new industrial materials was initiated by two chemists, **Karl Ziegler** (1898–1973) of Germany, and **Giulio Natta** (1903–1979) of the Milan Institute of Technology, Italy, who shared the Nobel Prize for chemistry in 1963. An American chemist, **Wallace Hume Carothers** (1896–1937) from Burlington, Iowa, developed commercial polymers and produced nylon and neoprene in 1931. His assistant, **Paul John Flory** (1910–1985) of Sterling, Illinois, while at Du Pont, Wilmington, did extensive studies on the properties of polymers in relation to kinetics and thermodynamics, for which he was awarded the Nobel Prize for chemistry in 1974. A revolution in polymer fabrics was brought about by the discovery of Terylene by **John Rex Whinfield** (1901–1966) of Sutton, Surrey. He first discovered in 1941 that a polymerized condensate of terephthalic acid and ethylene glycol could be drawn out as a fiber. The term silicones, for the entire class of oxygen-containing organosilicone polymers, was coined by an English physicist, **Frederick Stanley Kipping** (1863–1949) of Manchester, who conducted research on plastics while he was professor of chemistry at Nottingham. A theory on the thermodynamic properties of mixtures applicable to polymers was developed by an English theoretical chemist, **Christopher Longuet-Higgins** (b 1923) from Kent. In 1926 a German chemist, **Hermann Staudinger** (1881–1965), proposed that polymers were giant molecules held by simple chemical bonds, and put forward a principle for determining the high molecular weights of polymers, now known as Staudinger's law. Staudinger was awarded the Nobel Prize for chemistry for his work on polymers, in 1953. Polymerization mechanisms as a part of the American synthetic rubber program was studied by a US chemist from the Ukraine, **Morris Selig Kharasch** (1895–1957), in the early 1940s. Diffusion in polymers was studied with the use of tagged organic molecules by the London physicist, **David Tabor** (b 1913). An English physicist, **William Thomas Astbury** (1898–1961), did pioneering work on the application of X-rays for the analysis of polymers. A study on how the polymer chains

and their individual parts move was done by a French physicist, **Pierre-Gilles de Gennes** (b 1932). He was awarded the Nobel Prize for physics in 1991 for his explanation of how complex forms of matter such as liquid crystals and polymers behave during their transition from a state of order to a state of disorder.

Polymerase Chain Reaction This allows minute quantities of DNA to be copied several millions of times, in order to make a practical analysis of it. Discovered by an American biochemist, **Kary Banks Mullis** (b 1944) of North Carolina. In 1993 he shared the Nobel Prize for chemistry, for this work with a Canadian biochemist, **Michel Smith** (b 1932).

Polynomial An algebraic expression that has one or more variables, denoted by letters. *See Alexander polynomial, Legendre polynomial, polynomial equation.*

Polynomial Equation In 1823, a Norwegian mathematician, **Niels Henrik Abel** (1802–1829), proved that there is no algebraic formula for the solution of a general polynomial equation of the fifth degree. A French mathematician, **Jacques Charles François Strum** (1803–1855), proposed a theorem for dealing with real roots of a polynomial equation, which is named after him. *See Alexander polynomial theorem, Legendre polynomials.*

Polythene An artificial plastic invented in 1933 by R.O. Gibson and E.W. Fawcett of England.

Pompeii The ancient city of Campania in southern Italy, demolished by an earthquake in AD 63. It was rebuilt, but was destroyed again during the eruption of Versuvius in AD 79. The remains of Pompeii were discovered in 1594, and its first part was cleared in 1750. A layer-by-layer excavation, preserving the existing buildings, were carried out from 1860 to 1875 by an Italian archaeologist, **Gieuseppe Fiorelli** (1823–1896).

Poncelet, Jean Victor (1788–1867) *See projective geometry.*

Pond, John (1767–1836) *See Greenwich Observatory.*

Pons, Jean Louis (1761–1831) *See comet.*

Pontecorvo, Guido (1907–1993) *See mycology.*

Pontryagin, Lev Semyonovich (1908–1988) *See topology.*

Pope, William Jackson (1870–1939) *See stereochemistry.*

Popham, Sir Home Riggs (1762–1820) *See flag signalling.*

Popov, Alexander Stepanovich (1859–1905) *See aerial, broadcasting, radio, wireless telegraphy.*

Popper, Karl Raimund (1902–1994) A Vienna-born British scientific philosopher who proposed that science is not certain knowledge but a series of conjectures and refutations never reaching a definitive truth. He published *The Open Society and its Enemies* (1945), *The Logic of Scientific Discovery* (1935) and *Conjectures and Refutations* (1963).

Porcelain The art of making porcelain was first known to the Chinese, and it was probably brought to Europe by the Portuguese after their discovery of the East. Chinese porcelain reached its perfection during the time of the Ming dynasty (1368–1644). An English potter, John Dwight from Oxfordshire, patented a transparent earthware resembling porcelain, at his factory in Fulham, in 1671. The first porcelain was made in Europe at Meissen by **Johann Friedrich Böttger** (1682–1719) of Schleiz, in Reuss, and became known as Meissen or Dresden porcelain. The manufacture of porcelain at Meissen was under the direction of a Saxon mineralogist, **John Frederic Henckel** (1679–1744) from Freiberg, who published *Pyritologia*. In 1740, a French naturalist and metallurgist, **René Antoine Ferchault de Reaumer** (1683–1757), produced an opaque form of porcelain, which is known by his name. A French physician and chemist, **Pierre Joseph Macquer** (1718–1784), studied the effects of firing on hundreds of different kinds of clay, and became an adviser to the porcelain factory at Sèvres, in 1766. The discovery of Cornwall China-clay or kaolin near St Austell in 1756 by **William Cookworthy** (1705–1780) of Kingsbridge, Devon, increased the quality and production of porcelain in Britain. He later established a china factory near Plymouth. In 1800, **Josiah Spode** (1754–1827) of Stoke-on-Trent, in England, used a mixture of bone and felspar and made porcelain with a special shine and beauty. He was appointed potter to George III in 1806. Thenard blue, used for coloring porcelain, was discovered by a French chemist, **Louis Jacques Thenard** (1777–1857). An English china manufacturer, **Willliam Taylor Copeland** (1797–1868), invented a filter press for working clay.

Porsche, Ferdinand (1875–1951) *See car.*

Porta, Giovanni Battista della (1535–1615) An Italian scientist from Naples, who described the camera obscura in detail in 1585, and gave a description of an opera glass in 1590. He is regarded as the father of physiognomy, owing to his *De Humana Physiognomonia* published in 1586. *See camera, camera obscura, kite, optics, spectacles.*

Porter, Sir George (b 1920) *See flash photolysis.*

Portland Cement Derives its name from its resemblance to Portland stone used in the building industry. It was first produced from clay and limestone in 1824 by an English bricklayer, **Joseph Aspdin** (1779–1855) of Leeds. *See cement.*

Portrait Photography The first human portrait by light was taken by a professor of chemistry and later of medicine in New York, **John William Draper** (1811–1882). In 1851, an English portrait sculptor, **Frederick Scott Archer** (1813–1857) of Bishop's Stortford, Hertfordshire, with **Peter W. Fry** (d 1860) devised the first cheap form of photographic portraiture, which led to its common use.

Posidonius of Alexandria (*c.* 400 BC) An astronomer and engineer, who accompanied Alexander the Great (356–323 BC). He invented a revolving tower to help Alexander during his sieges. *See earth size.*

Posidonus of Apamea (*c.* 79 BC) *See oceanography, tides.*

Positron An elementary particle with one positive charge and the same mass as an electron. It confirmed the existence of antimatter predicted in 1930 by an English physicist, **Paul Adrien Maurice Dirac** (1902–1984) of Bristol, and it was discovered by an American physicist, **Carl David Anderson** (1905–1991), in 1932. For this work, Dirac shared the Nobel Prize for physics in 1933, with an Austrian physicist, **Erwin Schrödinger** (1887–1961). In 1932 an English physicist, **Patrick Maynard Stuart Blackett** (1897– 1974), independently discovered the positron with the use of **Charles Thompson Rees Wilson's** (1869–1959) cloud chamber. He was awarded the Nobel Prize for physics, for his work on atomic physics, in 1948.

Positron Microscope Uses positrons instead of electrons to produce images. The first image was produced by James Van House and Arthur Rich in 1988.

Positive Rays *See canal rays.*

Postal Service The first chief postmaster of England, Thomas Randolph, was appointed by Queen Elizabeth I in 1581, and the postal communication between various parts of England, Scotland and Ireland was established in 1635. Monsieur de Velayer of Paris, under a royal authority, established a private penny post in 1653. Around 1830, Charles Whiting and Charles Knight, in England, suggested a stamped wrapper for newspapers. A uniform rate of postage in England, prepaid by purchasing stamps, was advocated by **Sir Rowland Hill** (1795–1879) of Kidderminster, in his *Post-office Reform* in 1837. In 1839, the government issued a public invitation to artists, men of science and others to invent a stamped envelope that could not be forged. The prize sum of 200 GBP was won by an artist named Mulready, but his envelope fell into disuse. The penny post was introduced in the same year, and the first penny postage stamp in England was printed in 1840 by an engraver from America, **Jacob Perkins** (1766–1849), who migrated to England and established an engraving factory in 1818. Adhesive postage stamps were invented by a Scottish bookseller, **James Chalmers** (1782–1853), who campaigned for faster postal services, in 1825. In 1839, an American inventor, **James Bogardus** (1800–1874) of Catskill, New York, invented a method of engraving postage stamps that was adopted by the British government. Sir Rowland Hill established the bookpost and money order office in 1848. Henry Archer designed the process of printing stamps in perforated sheets so that they could be detached easily or folded and stored. His invention was purchased in 1852 by the British government for the sum of 4000 GBP.

Potassium [Dutch: *potasch*]   A metallic element discovered in 1807 by **Sir Humphry Davy** (1778–1829).

Potassium Chlorate   Used in fireworks, explosives, as a bleaching agent and disinfectant. It was isolated in 1786 by **Claude Louis Comte de Berthollet** (1748–1822).

Potential [Latin: *potens*, powerful]   A term introduced in 1828 by an English businessman and mathematician, **George Green** (1793–1841) of Nottingham, in his pamphlet *An essay on the application of mathematical analysis to the theories of electricity and magnetism*. This work contained a set of mathematical functions, named after him, and it provided a valuable technical tool for solving partial differential equations, which are difficult to solve by other methods.

Potential Energy [Latin: *potens*, powerful, Greek: *energos*, active]   The term was suggested by a Scottish scientist, **William John Macquorn** (1820–1872), to denote anything that was not energy, but could be potentially converted into energy.

Pouillet, Claude Servais Matthias (1790–1868)   *See chronoscope, tangent galvanometer.*

Poulsen, Valdemar (1869–1942)   *See tape recorder.*

Powell, Cecil Frank (1903–1969)   *See meson, pion.*

Powell, John Wesley (1834–1902)   *See geology.*

Power Loom   *See Cartwright, Edmund, textile industry.*

Poynting, John Henry (1852–1914)   English physicist, born in Monton, Lancashire, and educated at Cambridge. He was appointed professor of physics at Birmingham in 1880, and in 1884 proposed the Poynting factor in electromagnetic energy, following his deduction of **James Clerk Maxwell's**

(1831–1879) hypothesis. He wrote *A Textbook of Physics* (1899) with **John Joseph Thompson** (1856–1940), and also published *On the Mean Density of Earth* (1893), *The Earth* (1913) and a paper *On the Transfer of Energy in the Electromagnetic Field* (1884).

Prandtl, Ludwig (1875–1953)   *See aerodynamics.*

Praseodymium [Greek: *prasinos*, green + *didymos*, twin]   An element with an atomic number of 59, discovered in 1885 by **Carl Auer von Welsbach** (1858–1929).

Precambrian Period   A geological time, 4.6 billion to 570 million years ago. Around 1863 Sir A.C. Ramsay observed that the rocks which belonged to this age, before the Cambrian period, contained no fossils or any other evidence of life.

Preece, Sir William Henry (1834–1913)   *See railway signals, telephone exchange, wireless telegraphy.*

Pregl, Fritz (1869–1930)   *See quantitative chemistry.*

Prehistory [Latin: *prae*, before + Greek: *historeo*, learn by inquiry]   An era before history was written. It was classified into the Stone Age, Iron Age and Bronze Age and studied on the basis of weapons and tools by a Danish archaeologist and numismatist, **Christian Jörgensen Thomsen** (1788–1865). In 1859, a London naturalist and professor of geology at Oxford, **Sir Joseph Prestwich** (1812–1896), demonstrated that man coexisted with prehistoric animals, through his findings of stone implements and fossils of extinct animals in the same strata, in the Somme. Stone instruments, weapons and fossils of prehistroric animals were discovered around 1870 at Brixam Cave and Kent's Hole in Torquay, Devonshire, by a Cornish explorer, **William Pengelly** (1812–1894). The term prehistory was popularized by a Scottish archaeologist, **Sir Daniel Wilson** (1816–1892) of Edinburgh. In 1860, a French paleontologist, **Edouard Arman Isidore Hippolyte Lartet** (1801–1871), studied the prehistoric sites at Massat and Aurignac, provided further evidence for the existence of man at the time of extinct species. A Danish zoologist, **Johannes Lapetus Steenstrup** (1813–1897), studied Danish peat bogs in relation to prehistoric climatic conditions. An English archaeologist, **Sir John Evans** (1823–1908), published *Ancient Stone Implements, Weapons, and Ornaments of Great Britain*, in 1872. Prehistoric culture in China was unearthed in 1922 by a Swedish archaeologist, **Johan Gunner Andersson** (1874–1960). He found important fossils of *Homo erectus* known as Peking Man, amongst 800 000-year-old deposits and stone implements. He published *Children of the Yellow Earth: Studies in Prehistoric China*

(1934) and *Research into the Prehistory of China* (1943). Prehistoric development in Europe was studied by an Australian archaeologist, **Vere Gordon Childe** (1892–1957), who published *The Dawn of European Civilisation* (1925) and *The Danube in Prehistory* (1929). An American archaeologist, **William Henry Holmes** (1846–1933), studied prehistoric stone technology and ceramics and published *Handbook of American Aboriginal Antiquities* (1919). *See Stone Age.*

Prelog, Vladimir (1906–1998) A Swiss organic chemist who determined the structure of many alkaloids such as quinine and strychnine. He also studied the metabolic products of microorganisms and developed several antibiotics. He shared the Nobel Prize for chemistry in 1975, for his work on the stereochemistry of biochemical compounds, with a British chemist, **John Warcup Cornforth** (b 1917) of Sydney. *See stereochemistry.*

Pressure Cooker A steam digester with a safety valve to dissolve bone and other products under pressure was invented by the French physician and physicist from Blois, **Denis Papin** (1647–1712) in 1681. His principle was later applied to develop the present-day domestic pressure cooker.

Prestwich, Sir Joseph (1812–1896) *See Ice Age, prehistory, Quaternary Period.*

Prévost, Pierre (1751–1839) *See thermodynamics.*

Priestley, Joseph (1733–1804) An English clergyman and chemist from Fieldhead, near Leeds, who established the chemistry of gases as a science in England. He found the composition of ammonia in 1774, and muriatic acid in 1772. He invented the eudiometer to measure the quantity of oxygen in air, in 1772. His dissident views led him to emigrate to America in 1794, and he died in Northumberland, Pennsylvania. *See ammonia, chemistry, chlorophyll, earthquake, eudiometer, nitrous oxide, oxygen, photosynthesis, rubber, sulfurous acid.*

Prigogine, Ilya Vicomte (b 1917) *See thermodynamics.*

Prime Number Any positive integer, excluding 1, which has no integral factors other than itself and 1. **Eratosthenes** (274–194 BC) made a study of prime numbers and invented a device called a *sieve* for locating them. **Euclid** (*c.* 300 BC) defined the properties of prime numbers. A French mathematician, **Jacques Hadamard** (1865–1963), proved the definitive form of the prime number theorem, previously attempted by **Adrien-Marie Legendre** (1752–1833) and **Carl Friedrich Gauss** (1777–1855). It was proved in a weaker form by a Russian mathematician, **Pafnuty**

Lvovich Chebyshev (1821–1894). The largest prime number to be discovered in 1989 was with the help of the supercomputer Amdahl 1200, at Santa Clara, California. The highest prime number in 1994, consisting of 258 756 digits, was discovered by two computer scientists Paul Gage and David Slowinski, at Cray Research Inc., Minnesota.

Prince, **Louis Aimé Augustin Le** (1842–1890) *See cinema.*

Pringsheim, Ernst (1859–1917) *See Stefan law.*

Pringsheim, Nathaniel (1823–1894) *See algae.*

Printing The art of printing with a seal and a rotating cylinder seal was known to the ancient Romans and the Greeks. The Chinese used block printing in AD 868, and movable type was familiar to them long before it was introduced into Europe in the 15th century. They used the method to print books in 1050, and in 1107 introduced multicolored printed paper money to overcome counterfeiting. The first printed items in Europe, a set of playing cards, appeared in Germany in 1377. The first book printed with movable type is claimed by the Dutch to be that of **Laurens Janszoon Coster** (1370–1440) in 1430. It is alleged that some workmen stole the type from Coster and carried it to **Johannes (Gensfleisch) Gutenberg** (1400–1468) of Mainz, who then propagated movable type printing in Europe. Gutenberg worked at Strasbourg as a mechanic and goldsmith around 1434 before he formed a partnership for a printing press with **Johann Fust** (d 1466), in 1450. They printed the famous first full-length book, a Latin Bible, around 1456. Their partnership was dissolved after a legal battle, and Gutenberg acquired the press and managed it with the help of a skilled metal worker, **Peter Schoeffer** (1425–1502) from Darmstardt, until 1462. Gutenberg established another press in 1463, following which the knowledge and art of printing spread widely to Italy, Germany and other parts of Europe. Gutenberg, despite his pioneering works on printing, did not include his name or the mark of his press until the issue of the *Mainz Psalter* (1457). Strasbourg was one of the first places to transplant the art of printing from Mainz. Printing was set up in the city of Tours in 1469, and at Venice and Paris in 1469. The first book from the Sorbonne, the *Epistolae Gasparini Pergamensis*, was released by Gering's (d 1510) press in 1470. The first printer in England was **William Caxton** (1412–1492) from Kent, who spent some time during his youth in Europe and learnt printing while he was in Flanders. In 1471 he printed his first book on the history of Troy (*Recuyell of the Historyes of Troye*), which he translated from the French. He returned to England around 1472, and set up his press near Westminster Abbey, and printed the first three books in England, entitled *The Game* *and Playe of the Chesse* (1474), *A boke of the hoole Lyf of Jason* (1475) and *The Dictes and Notable Wyse Sayenges of the Phyloso- phers* (1477). The first printing press in Scotland was set up by **Walter Chepman** (1473–1538) of Edinburgh. In 1534, the Cambridge University Press received Royal Letters Patent to print and sell all manner of books, and has maintained a continuous history of publishing since 1584. The first book in Oxford was printed in 1478. The first book on typesetting and engraving, entitled *Manuel Typographique* (1764), was published by **Pierre Simon Fournier** (1712–1768) of France. The first printing press in the American colonies was set up at Cambridge in Massachusetts in 1638. The first two printed works from this press, *Fremman's Call* and *Almanac for New England*, were issued in 1639. The first printed American book was a New England version of Psalms in 300 pages, and regular printing of books began in Boston in 1676. Printing became known in Philadelphia in 1686, and in New York in 1693. In 1700, there were only four printing presses in the American colonies. A London aristocrat and scientist, **Charles Stanhope** (1753–1816), invented the first hand-operated printing press. One of the first rotary printing machines in England was patented in 1813 by two British engineers, **Bryan Donkin** (1768–1855) of Northumberland and **Richard Bacon** (1775–1844). The steam-driven cylinder press was invented in 1810 by **Friedrich Koenig** (1774–1833), a German printer from Eisleben, and it was improved by a London printer, **Augustus Applegarth** (1788–1871) in 1813. Applegarth built a vertical-drum rotary printing press for *The Times* newspaper in London. A London printer, **William Clowes** (1779–1847) and his son **William Clowes** (1807–1883) were the first to use steam-driven machines for regular printing in England. **William Haas** (d 1800), a letter-founder in Basel, invented a balance-press. The idea of stereo-typed plates in printing was put forward by **Tilloch Alexander** (1759–1829) of Glasgow, who moved to London in 1787 and purchased *The Star,* an evening paper, which he continued printing until 1825. The web printing press was invented in 1847 by a British-born New York industrialist, **Richard March Hoe** (1812–1886). He developed the rotary printing press, which was first used for the *Philadelphia Public Ledger* in 1846. His nephew, **Robert Hoe** (1839–1909), developed color printing. In 1865, **William Bullock** (1813–1867) of Philadelphia, introduced a rotary machine for printing on continuous paper. Printing is so advanced today that an electrosensitive system printer at the Lawrence Livermore Radiation Laboratory, in Livermore, California, is able to print over 700 000 words in 65 seconds. *See engraving, lithography, movable type printing, typography*.

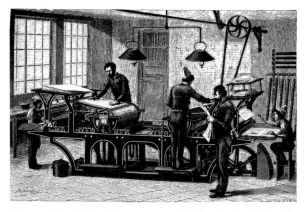

Figure 67 A French steam-press. Guillemin, Amédée. *The Applications of Physical Forces*. London: Macmillan and Co, 1877

Prism A block of transparent material, usually of glass, used for refracting light. *See dispersion of light, Nicol prism, rainbow, spectroscopy.*

Pritchard, Charles (1808–1893) An astronomer and Savillian professor at Oxford, who published a work on stellar photometry entitled *Uranometria Nova Oxoniensis* (1885).

Probability Theory The calculation of chance was first known to the Franciscan friar, **Lucas Pacioli** (1445–1510) of Tuscany, in 1494. An Italian, **Girolomo Cardan** (1501–1576) of Pavia, studied it in 1539, and **Niccolò Fontana Tartaglia** (1499–1557) investigated it in 1556. Basic laws of probability were proposed by **Blaise Pascal** (1623–1662) and **Pierre de Fermat** (1601–1665), in 1654. A Dutch mathematician and scientist, **Christian Huygens** (1629–1695), published a mathematical discussion of the chances of winning in certain games. A Swiss mathematician, **Jacques Bernoulli** (1654–1705), in his *Ars Conjectandi* published posthumously in 1713, treated the subject in detail and suggested that it could be applied to civil and economic affairs. A French mathematician, **Abraham de Moivre** (1667–1754) of Vitry, Champagne, published *Doctrine of Chances* (1718), based on probability theory. A French mathematician, **Pierre Simon Marquis de Laplace** (1749–1827) of Normandy, published an important treatise, *Théorie analytique des probabilités* in 1812. One of the first English books on the theory of probability was published by an American mathematician, **Julian Lowell Coolridge** (1873–1954) of Brookline, Massachusetts, in 1925. An Austrian mathematician, **Richard von Mises** (1883–1953), made significant contributions and published *Probability, Statistics and Truth* (1928). A Yugoslavian-born American mathematician, **William Feller** (1906–1970), who was professor of mathematics at Princeton University, popularized probability theory outside the field of mathematics, and published *Introduction to Probability Theory and its Applications* (1950).

Proctor, Richard Anthony (1837–1888) *See scientific journals.*

Projectiles *See ballistics, dynamics, supersonic flight.*

Projective Geometry The study of geometrical figures that remain unaltered, when drawn from various points. The basics were set out by an architect, **Gérard Desargues** (1593–1662), in 1639. A French mathematician, **Jean Victor Poncelet** (1788–1867), developed the subject as a new area of geometry and published *Traité des Propriétés Projectives des Figures* (1822). Another contributor to the subject, **Joseph Diez Gergonne** (1771–1859), developed the use of poles and polars. A Swiss mathematician, **Jakob Steiner** (1796–1863), is regarded as the founder of projective geometry, which was developed independently by a French mathematician, **Michel Chasles** (1793–1880), who published a classic paper *Aperçue historique sur l'origine et la développement des méthodes en géometrie* (1837).

Prokhorov, Aleksandr Mikaylovich (b 1916) *See maser.*

Prolog (Programming in Logic) High-level computer-programing language based on logic. It was invented in 1971 at the University of Marseille, France.

Promethium [Greek: *Prometheus*, a Titan who gave fire and the arts to man] An element with an atomic number of 61 in the periodic table predicted in 1902 by a Czech chemist, **Bohuslav Brauner** (1855–1935). It was discovered in 1947 by J.A. Marinsky and L.E. Glendenen at the Clinton National Laboratory, Oak Ridge, Tennessee.

Prophase [Greek: *pro*, before + *phasis*, appearance] A stage in mitotic cell division, described and named in 1884 by a German botanist and professor at Bonn, **Eduard Adolf Strasburger** (1844–1912).

Protactinium [Greek: *proteios*, first + Latin: *activus*, engaged in action] First in the series of radioactive elements, having an atomic number of 91. It was discovered independently in 1917 by an English physicist, **Frederick Soddy** (1877–1965), and two Germans **Otto Hahn** (1879–1968) and **Lise Meitner** (1878–1968).

Protein [Greek: *proteios*, first] A complex organic substance; a polymer of amino acids, acting as structural tissue and enzymes, first studied and named *proteine*, in 1838 by **Gerardus Johannes Mulder** (1802–1880), a Dutch chemist at Utrecht.

Proterozoic Second division of the Precambrian era lasting from about 3.5 billion to 570 million years ago.

Proton [Greek: *proteios*, first] A stable subatomic particle with unit positive charge and mass greater than that of an electron. It was discovered in 1914 by **Lord Ernest Rutherford** (1871–1937). The US physicist **Richard Phillips Feynman** (1918–1988) predicted that the proton and neutron are not elementary particles, and both these particles are now known to be composed of quarks.

Protoplasm [Greek: *proteios*, first + *plasmein*, to mold] Discovered in 1835 by a French zoologist, **Felix Dujardin** (1801–1860) from Tours, who named it sarcode. A French botanist, **C.F. Brisseau-Mirbel** (1776–1854), used the term cambium for the mucilaginous matter in the cell. The term protoplasm in cytology was introduced in 1839 by **Johannes Evangelista Purkinje** (1787–1869). **Hugo von Mohl** (1805–1872), a German professor of botany at Tübingen, independently used the term protoplasm in 1846. The alveolar or foam theory, explaining living protoplasm as a complex fluid of varying viscosity, was proposed in 1878 by a German professor at Heidelberg, **Otto Bütschli** (1848– 1920).

Protozoa [Greek: *proteios*, first + *zoon*, animal] A group of microscopic unicellular organisms established and named by a German zoologist, **Carl Theodor Ernst von Siebold** (1804–1885), in 1846. He was made professor of zoology, comparative anatomy and veterinary medicine at Erlanger in 1840, and published *Lehrbuch der vergleichen den Anatomie* with **Hermann Stannius** (1808–1883). The first protozoan parasite to be identified, *Giardia lamblia*, was identified under the microscope in 1681 by **Antoni van Leeuwenhoek** (1632–1723). **M. Clifford Dobell** (1886–1949), an eminent protozoologist, published the classics in the field *Amoeba living in Man* (1919) and *Intestinal Protozoa of Man* (1921).

Proust, Joseph Louis (1754–1826) *See atomic structure, law of constant composition.*

Proust Law *See law of constant composition.*

Prout, William (1785–1850) An English physician and chemist, born in Horton, Gloucestershire, who graduated in medicine from Edinburgh in 1811. He settled in London where he established his own chemical laboratory, in 1812. He was the first to demonstrate the presence of free hydrochloric acid in the stomach, in 1823. He proposed the law (Prout's law) which states that the relative atomic weights of all elements are multiples of the relative atomic weight of hydrogen. *See Bridgewater treatises.*

Prout's Law *See Prout, William.*

Psi A heavy elementary particle created and demonstrated by an American physicist, **Burton Richter** (b 1931).

Pterodactyl [Greek: *pteron*, feather + *daktylos*, finger] A fossil skeleton of the extinct species was found in Bavaria in 1788. **Friedrich Blumenbach** (1752–1840) of Göttingen, considered it to be a bird, in 1807. **Georges Cuvier** (1769–1832) identified it as a flying reptile in 1812, and gave it its present name. The first evidence for it in America was provided by an American paleontologist from Lockport, **Charles Othniel Marsh** (1831–1899).

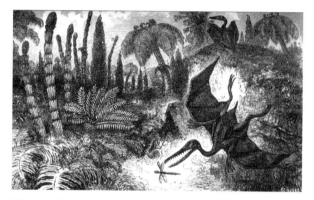

Figure 68 A 19th century imaginary landscape with pterodactyls. Pouchet, F.A. *The Universe*. London: Blacke and Son, 1871

Ptolemy of Alexandria (*c*. AD 127–145) A geographer and astronomer whose real name was Claudius. He was born in Ptolemais in Upper Egypt and came to spend most of his life in Alexandria. He wrote *Geographia* and *Mathematical Syntaxis*, known to the Arabs as *Almagest* [Arabic: *Al*, the + *majiste*, greatest]. The latter work in 13 books dealt with distances and time in astronomy, and trigonometry of celestial figures. His *Geography* consisted of eight books and it listed latitudes and longitudes of important places and included a map of the world. Ptolemy's system considered the earth as the center of the universe with heavenly bodies revolving around it. *See Almagest, astronomy, eclipse, geometry.*

Pugin, **August Welby Northmore** (1812–1852) *See architecture, British.*

Pulitzer, Joseph (1847–1911) *See newspapers.*

Pulley A simple machine with grooved wheel for lifting heavy objects. **Pythagoras** (*c*. 580–500 BC) invented a system of pulleys. The principle of the pulley was developed by **Archytas of Tarentum** (Italy) around 410 BC.

Pullman Sleeper A railway sleeping-car for comfortable travel was patented by an American inventor, **George Mortimer Pullman** (1831–1897) of Brocton, New York, in 1864. Pullman also introduced dining cars for trains, in 1868.

Pullman, George Mortimer (1831–1897) *See Pullman sleeper.*

Pulsar A source of radio emission in our galaxy that gives out radiation in intermittent pulses. Discovered in 1967 by two British astronomers **Antony Hewish** (b 1924) of Cornwall and **Chester Gordon Bell** (b 1934) of York. Hewish was awarded the Nobel Prize for physics in 1974, with another British astronomer **Martin Ryle** (1918–1984) of Brighton. Ryle pinpointed radio sources such as sunspots in 1946, and developed radio telescopes in Cambridge, where he became the first professor of radio astronomy in 1959. Other pulsating radio stars were discovered by a British astronomer, **Susan Jocelyn Burnell** née **Bell** (b 1943) of York in 1967. In 1968, an Austrian-born US astronomer, **Thomas Gold** (b 1920), suggested the currently accepted theory that pulsars are rapidly rotating neutron stars which produce beams of radio waves from their poles. An English astronomer from Roehampton, **Francis Graham Smith** (b 1923), proposed a mechanism for pulsars in 1970 and discovered that they emitted polarized radiation. An American physicist, **Joseph Hooton Taylor** (b 1941) of Philadelphia, and Russell Hulse discovered the first binary pulsar, for which they were jointly awarded the Nobel Prize for physics in 1993.

Punnett, Reginald Crundall (1875–1967) *See genetics.*

Poulsen, Valdemar (1869–1942) *See magnetic recording.*

Pupin, Michael Idvorsky (1858–1935) *See X-rays.*

Purcell, Edward Mills (1912–1997) *See magnetic resonance imaging, radioastronomy.*

Purkinje, Johannes Evangelista (1787–1869) *See fingerprints, protoplasm.*

Pye, John David (b 1932) *See echolocation.*

Pynson, Richard (d 1530) *See typography.*

Pyramid The stepped pyramid at Saqqara was built in 2780 BC by Imhotep, the principal officer of King Djoser of the third dynasty. The great pyramid at Giza was built by the Egyptian pharaoh, **Cheops** (*c*. 2600 BC), to serve as his tomb. Its construction shows that the Egyptians were experts in geometry, and it has a base that is perfectly square with the greatest deviation from a right angle of only 0.05%.

It was built with 2 300 000 blocks of stones, each weighing about 2.5 tonnes, a marvel by today's standards. The next largest pyramid in Egypt was built by his son and successor, Chephren. The Olmec pyramids in La Venta (Tabasco, Mexico) were built around 800 BC. The largest pyramid in the world, Quetzacòatl, in Choula de Rivadabia, south east of Mexico City, was built around AD 400.

Pyridine An organic compound discovered by a Scottish chemist from Leith, **Thomas Anderson** (1819–1874), who studied under **Justus von Liebig** (1803–1873) at Giessen. He succeeded **Thomas Thomson** (1773–1852) as Regius professor of chemistry at Glasgow in 1852. **Sir James Dewar** (1843–1923), a Scottish physicist from Kincardine-on-Forth, developed the theory of the pyridine ring.

Pyrometer [Greek: *pur,* fire + *metron*, to measure] Used for checking high temperatures in furnaces for making pottery. Invented in 1782 by the English potter, **Josiah Wedgwood** (1730–1795) of Staffordshire.

Pyrrole An organic compound obtained from coal tar by a German physician and chemist, **Friedlib Ferdinand Runge** (1795–1867). A Scottish chemist from Leith, **Thomas Anderson** (1819–1874), gave its current chemical formula.

Pythagoras (*c.* 580–500 BC) A Greek philosopher and mathematician, born in Samos, who settled in the Greek colony of Crotona, in southern Italy, where he established his famous school. He taught the doctrine of transmigration of souls from one body to another. He founded the study of geology with his observations on the physical changes in the land and its volcanic eruptions. He established the modern system of astronomy, improved geometry, and invented multiplication tables. His followers, known as Pythagoreans, made several significant contributions to mathematics.

Pytheas of Marseilles (360–290 BC) *See moon, tides.*

Pythagorean Society Founded by **Pythagoras** (*c.* 580–500 BC) of Samos, its members had a mystical belief in numbers, and explained the entire universe on the basis of numbers. An Athenian philosopher and nephew of Plato, **Speusippus** (407–339 BC), wrote on Pythagorean numbers; only one fragment of his writings is extant.

Pythagorean Theorem States that the sum of the squares on the sides of a right-angled triangle equals the square on the hypotenuse. It was known to the Babylonians and the Chinese before the time of **Pythagoras** (*c.* 580–500 BC). About 370 different proofs for it have been offered by various mathmaticians up to today.

Q

Quadrant [Latin: *quattuor*, four] A mathematical instrument in the form of a quarter of a circle introduced around 200 BC. Arabian astronomers had a quadrant of 21 feet radius, at the caliphate of Baghdad in AD 995. An Italian mathematician, **Leonardo Fibonacci** (*c.* 1172–1250) of Pisa, in his *Liber Quadratorum* (1220) dealt extensively on the use of the quadrant. A portable quadrant used by navigators was invented by the English mathematician, **Edmund Gunter** (1581–1626) of Herefordshire. A giant quadrant of 19 feet radius was constructed in 1569 by **Tycho Brahe** (1546–1601) for the Burgomaster of Augsburg. It turned in several planes around the vertical axis, and was capable of being projected on any celestial body. **John Hadley** (1682–1774), a London mathematician and astronomer, invented a reflecting quadrant in 1731.

Quadratic Equation A polynomial equation of the second degree in which the highest power is 2. It was known in Mesopotamia around 2000 BC. The Hindu mathematician, **Brahmagupta** (*c.* AD 598–660), solved the quadratic equation. The rules for the solution of the equations were given by an Islamic mathematician, **Alkarismi** or **Abu Jafar Mohammed ibn Musa Al-Khowarimi** in the 9th century. A complete generalization of quadratic forms (Hermitean forms) was given by a French mathematician, **Charles Hermite** (1822–1901) around 1850.

Qualitative Chemistry [Latin: *qualitas*, condition] Identification of chemical compounds or elements without taking into account their proportions. A German pioneer of analytical chemistry, **Karl Remigius Fresenius** (1818–1897), designed a systematic way of identifying compounds by precipitating various radicals through a series of precipitating reactions. His work, translated into English under the title *Elementary Instruction in Qualitative Analysis*, was published in 1841. *See analytical chemistry.*

Quantitative Chemistry [Latin: *quantus*, how many] Determination of the amount or proportion of one or more constituents. **Joseph Black** (1728–1799) and **Henry Cavendish** (1731–1810) used balances in the study of chemical processes. **Antoine Laurent Lavoisier** (1743–1794) established quantitative analysis as a branch of chemistry. A London chemist, **Sir Henry Enfield Roscoe** (1833–1915), carried out research on quantitative photo-

chemistry with **Robert Bunsen** (1811–1899). The field of quantitative organic microchemistry was developed by an Austrian physician and chemist, **Fritz Pregl** (1869–1930), who published *Die quantitative organische Mikroanlyse* (1917), and became the editor of the new journal *Mikrochemie*, in 1923. He was awarded the Nobel Prize for chemistry in 1923, for his work on organic microchemistry. Another Austrian chemist and colleague of Pregl, **F. Emich** (1860–1940) developed microchemical quantitative methods in inorganic chemistry.

Quantum The smallest part of the energy of electromagnetic radiation that can be converted to matter. *See quantum theory.*

Quantum Chromodynamics (QCD) A theory relating to strong forces between elementary particles (quarks), including the interaction of neutrons and protons in a nucleus. In quantum chromodynamics, quarks are considered to interact by exchanging particles called gluons, which carry the strong nuclear force and act to 'glue' quarks together. Mainly developed by a New York physicist, **Sheldon Lee Glashow** (b 1932), whose work gave an explanation for the forces that hold the elementary particles of matter together. He shared the Nobel Prize for physics in 1979, for his work on particle interaction with a Pakistani theoretical physicist, **Abdus Salam** (b 1926), and **Steven Weinberg** (b 1933) of New York.

Quantum Electrodynamics (QED) A theory which combines quantum theory and relativity, to describe the interaction of charged subatomic particles within electric and magnetic fields. Developed by a New York physicist, **Richard Phillips Feynman** (1918–1988). He shared the Nobel Prize in 1965, for developing the theory of quantum electrodynamics, with two other independent pioneers in the field, **Julian Schwinger** (1918–1994) of New York, and **Sin-Itero Tomanaga** (1906–1979) from Kyoto, Japan. A British physicist from Newcastle upon Tyne, **Peter Ware Higgs** (b 1929), further advanced the theory of particle interaction, based on their theory.

Quantum Hall Effect Related to two-dimensional electronic behavior, discovered in 1977 by a German physicist, **Klaus von Klitzing** (b 1943), who was awarded the Nobel Prize for physics in 1985.

Quantum Mechanics System of mechanics based on the concept of the quantum. Originated by an Irish mathematician, **Sir William Rowan Hamilton** (1805–1865), with his work on a new approach to dynamics. His concept was based on the generalization of the principle of least action (which stated that a mechanical system evolves in such a way that its action is as small as possible) proposed on a theoretical basis in 1744 by a French mathematician, **Pierre-Louis Moreau de Maupertuis** (1698–1759). Classical mechanics was interpreted on the basis of systematic quantum mechanics, and in terms of matrices (matrix mechanics), by a German physicist, **Max Born** (1882–1970) and his pupil, **Werner Karl Heisenberg** (1901–1976) of Würzburg, in 1925. Heisenberg was awarded the Nobel Prize for physics for his work in 1932. His concept was supported by the idea that particles can behave as waves (de Broglie waves), proposed by a French professor of physics, **Louis Victor Pierre Raymond de Broglie** (1892–1987), who was awarded the Nobel Prize for chemistry in 1936. The field of quantum mechanics was established on a scientific basis by an Austrian physicist, **Erwin Schrödinger** (1887–1961) in 1926. The work was further advanced by an American physicist, **David Joseph Bohm** (1917–1992), who published *Quantum Theory* in 1951. A German mathematician, **Hermann Weyl** (1885–1955), wrote on the relation between mathematics and quantum mechanics. A US physicist, **Hugo Everett** (1930–1982), formulated the relative state in quantum mechanics.

Quantum Optics Work on optical coherence by a US physicist, **Emil Wolf** (b 1922), laid the foundation for the field. A New York theoretical physicist, **Roy Jay Glauber** (b 1925), published two seminal papers in 1963 establishing it as a distinct science.

Quantum Physics A branch of physics dealing with the quantum nature of matter, energy and radiation. *See quantum mechanics, quantum optics, quantum theory.*

Quantum Theory The wave theory of light or energy, fundamental to quantum theory, was proposed in 1817 by an English physician, **Thomas Young** (1773–1829), who observed that light particles could behave like corpuscles and waves at the same time. As a result of experiments on thermodynamics carried out by **Gustav Robert Kirchhoff** (1824–1887) in 1859, a group of physicists – **Josef Stefan** (1835–1893), **Ludwig Boltzmann** (1844–1906) and **Max Karl Ernst Ludwig Planck** (1858–1947) – proposed the concept, in 1900, that radiation emissions came in indivisible units or *quanta*. This concept, applied to the law of thermodynamics and black body radiation, deviated from classical dynamic principles, and led to the theory that energy was released in abrupt installments or quanta. Planck's quantum theory formed the basis of **Albert Einstein's** work on the theory of light in 1905, leading to the theory of relativity. The experimental evidence for

Planck's quantum theory was provided by a German-born US scientist, **James Franck** (1882–1964), who shared the Nobel Prize for physics in 1925, for this work, with **Gustav Hertz** (1887–1975). The splitting of spectrum lines in a strong electrostatic field (Stark effect), which rendered support to Planck's theory, was proposed in 1913 by a German physicist, **Johannes Stark** (1874–1957), who was awarded the Nobel Prize for physics in 1919. Planck's quantum theory was applied to the study of subatomic physics by a Dutch physicist, **Niels Henrick David Bohr** (1885–1962) in 1913. The study of wave mechanics as a part of the quantum theory was proposed by an Austrian physicist, **Erwin Schrödinger** (1887–1961) in 1928. He shared the Nobel Prize for physics with **Paul Dirac** (1902–1984) and **Werner Heisenberg** (1901–1976) in 1933. The English physicist, **Lord Frederick Alexander Lindemann** or **Viscount Cherwell** (1886–1957) contributed to the field and published *The Physical Significance of Quantum Theory*. An American physicist, **David Joseph Bohm** (1917–1992) made a lifelong study of quantum mechanics and published an important work, *Quantum Theory*, in 1951. **Albert Einstein** (1879–1955) extended the theory to electromagnetic radiation, including light.

Quarks Set of particles that may be fundamental constituents of all forms of matter including protons and neutrons. Discovered by a New York physicist, **Robert Hofstadter** (1915–1990), who was appointed professor of physics at Stanford University in 1954. For his work, he shared the Nobel Prize for physics in 1961, with **Rudolf Ludwig Mössbauer** (b 1929). The quark theory was initiated by a New York theoretical physicist, **Murray Gell-Mann** (b 1929), who won the Nobel Prize for physics for his work on subatomic particles, in 1969. A similar theory was developed independently by a Moscow-born US physicist, **George Zweig** (b 1937). Three American physicists, **Jerome Isaac Friedman** (b 1928) of Chicago, **Richard Edward Taylor** (b 1929) from Alberta, Canada, and **Henry Way Kendall** (b 1926) of Boston, provided the conclusive evidence for quarks as real dynamic entities, for which they shared the Nobel Prize for physics in 1990.

Quartz The optical activity of the quartz crystal was discovered by **Dominique François Arago** (1786–1853) of France in 1811. *See piezoelectric effect. See quartz clock.*

Quartz Clock The property of some crystals to produce an electric potential when subjected to pressure was discovered by **Pierre Curie** (1859–1906) in 1880. In 1929 Warren Alvin Morrison of the Bell Telephone Laboratories in the USA developed a clock based on the electrical properties of a crystal of quartz. In this clock the crystal is made to oscillate at a rate of 100 000 times a second, thus recording time with an accuracy of one second in three years.

Quasars Objects appearing like stellar sources and travelling at immense speed away from the earth, emitting enormous amounts of radio energy. Quasar light shows a large red shift, indicating that the objects are very distant. An American astronomer, **Allan Rex Sandage** (b 1926) of Iowa, made the first optical identification of a quasar, in 1960. It was independently recognized in space by a Dutch-American astronomer, **Maarten Schmidt** (b 1929), in 1962. He also found that the number of quasars increases with the distance from the earth, which provided evidence for the Big Bang theory. An English astrophysicist, **Geoffrey Burbidge** (b 1925) of Chipping Norton, and his astronomer wife, **Elenor Margaret Burbidge** (b 1923), published an important work on quasars in 1967. The US astronomer, Alton Christian Arp (b 1927) proposed theories in the 1980s on the red shift of quasars. An English astronomer, **Alexander Boksenberg** (b 1936) studied the absorption lines in the spectra of quasars. This study, with his 'Image Photon Counting System' has contributed to the unraveling of the nature and evolution of the universe.

Quaternary Period A geological period that began with the recent Ice Age 1.64 million years ago, and is divided into Pleistocene and Eocene periods. **Sir Joseph Prestwich** (1812–1896), professor of geology at Oxford (1874–1888), who was an authority on the Quaternary period, published several papers on the subject.

Quaternions A concept of another dimension to algebra, which allowed the introduction of vectors into physical problems. Described by an Irish mathematician and professor of astronomy in Dublin, **Sir William Rowan Hamilton** (1805–1865).

Quetteville, **Gordon de** (b 1921) *See glaciology.*

Quicksilver Represented by the planet mercury and given its name. It was known in the 4th century BC, and was first used as medicine by a Swiss alchemist and physician, **Paracelsus** or **Theophrastus Bombastus von Hohenheim** (1493–1541), in the 16th century. *See mercury (metal).*

Quinoline Synthesized in 1880, by heating a mixture of aniline, nitrobenzene, glycerol and sulfuric acid, by an organic chemist of Prague, **Zdenko Hans Skraup** (1850–1910).

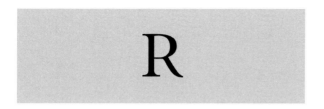

R

Rabi, Isidor Isaac (1898–1988) *See magnetic resonance imaging.*

Radar [**ra**dio **d**etection **a**nd **r**anging] A term coined by the American Navy, for a device that used microwaves to detect objects. It was developed from an observation in 1866 by a German physicist, **Heinrich Rudolf Hertz** (1857–1894), that electromagnetic waves could be deflected, refracted and reflected. The possibility of detecting a moving object by radio waves was suggested by **Nikola Tesla** (1856–1943) in 1900. In 1904, a German engineer, Christian Hülsmeyer, suggested a radio echo device similar to radar, but his suggestion went unheeded. The idea of radar was further developed by an Italian physicist, **Guglielmo Marchese Marconi** (1874–1937) of Bologna, in 1922. In 1926, by examining the behavior of long-distance radio waves, **Sir Edward Victor Appleton** (1892–1965), professor of experimental physics at King's College London (1924–1936), and later Jacksonian professor of natural philosophy (1936–1939) at Cambridge, demonstrated the existence of a reflecting or refracting layer, about 150 miles above the ground. The construction of radar later was based on this layer, which enabled radio waves to bend and pass round the earth. The first radar was built by a Scottish scientist, **Robert Alexander Watson-Watt** (1892–1973) of Brechin, Angus, who patented his radiolocator in 1919, and had perfected it by 1935. His radar was used by the British during the Second World War, and by 1939 most approaches to Britain were guarded by radiolocation stations. For his contribution, he was honored with a knighthood in 1942. In 1939, two British physicists, **Sir John Turton Randall** (1905–1994) and H.A.H. Boot started working on a multi-cavity magnetron valve, capable of operating on very short wavelengths. It rendered the reflections from the radar object more sharply defined and made the radar less heavy. It was perfected in 1949 by the Irish professor of electron physics at Birmingham, **James Sayers** (b 1912). The first use of radar imaging to measure the height and density of the earth's ionosphere was made by a Russian physicist, **Gregory Breit** (1899–1981). The radar guidance system for landing aircraft in poor weather conditions was invented by an American physicist, **Louis Walter Alvarez** (1911–1989). A diode with microwave frequencies for radar was developed in 1963 by a British physicist, John Gunn, at the IBM Research Center, New York State. Radar methods were used by an English electronics engineer, **Eric Eastwood** (1910–1981) of Lancashire, to study meteorological phenomena and the flight behavior of birds. In 1950, an English astrophysicist, **Sir Alfred Charles Bernard Lovell** (b 1913) of Gloucestershire, who worked on the use of radar in World War II, applied the device for detection of meteors and the study of galactic radio sources.

Radcliffe, John (1650–1714) *See observatories.*

Radiant Heat *See radiation of heat.*

Radiation of Heat The English scientist **Robert Hooke** (1635–1703) discovered that glass absorbed radiant heat. A theory of exchanges related to laws of radiation was proposed by a Swiss physician and physicist, **Pierre Prévost** (1751–1839) of Geneva. An apparatus for measuring radiation of heat, the thermopile, was invented by an Italian physicist, **Leopoldo Nobili** (1784–1835) and developed in 1850 by another Italian scientist, **Macedonio Melloni** (1798–1854) of Parma. A French chemist of Montpellier, **Jacques Etienne Berard** (1789–1869), showed that radiant heat, like light, could be polarized. A Swiss physicist, **Marc Auguste Pictet** (1752–1825) of Geneva, showed that radiant heat could be reflected like light in his *Essai sur le Feu* (1790). The polarization of radiant heat by tourmaline crystals was studied by a Scottish physicist from Edinburgh, **James David Forbes** (1809–1868). The measurement of loss of heat using a platinum wire was made by the Irish physicist **John Tyndall** (1820–1893). His work was advanced by a Viennese physicist, **Josef Stefan** (1835–1893), who proposed that the amount of energy radiated per second from a black body is proportional to the fourth power of the absolute temperature. In 1863, he became professor of physics at the University of Vienna and held the post for the rest of his life.

Radiation Pressure A consequence of electromagnetic theory, in which electromagnetic waves falling perpendicularly on a plane surface exert on it a pressure equal to the density of the electromagnetic energy per unit volume. Predicted by **James Clerk Maxwell** (1831–1879), and demonstrated independently by a Russian physicist, **Pyotr Nikolayevich Lebedev** (1866–1912) of Moscow, and an American physicist, **Ernest Fox Nichols** (1869–1924) of Kansas. An English physicist, **John Henry Poynting** (1852–1914) of Monton, Lancashire, devised a method of measuring it, in 1903. An American cosmologist, **Howard Percy Robertson** (1903–1961), applied relativistic theory to the field, and discovered the Poynting–Robertson effect of radiation pressure on micrometeorites, in 1937.

Radical The radical theory in chemistry was promoted by an Irish chemist, **Sir Robert John Kane** (1809–1890), who in 1833 proposed that alcohol and ether were components of the same radical. He became professor of chemistry in the Apothecaries Hall, Dublin, at the age of 22, and founded the *Dublin Journal of Medical and Chemical Science* which later became the *Irish Journal of Medical Science*. He was knighted in 1846. A German pioneer in analytical chemistry, **Karl Remigius Fresenius** (1818–1897), designed a systematic way of identifying compounds by precipitating various radicals through precipitating reactions.

Radio [Greek: *radio,* to emit, or Latin: *radius,* ray] Radio waves were discovered by a German physicist, **Heinrich Rudolf Hertz** (1857–1894) of Hamburg. They were first transmitted in 1897 over a distance of 5 kilometers, with the help of an antenna, by a Russian physicist, **Alexander Stepanovich Popov** (1859–1905). He was the first to use a suspended wire as an aerial. A physicist and pioneer in radio and wireless telegraphy, **Lee De Forest** (1873–1961) of Iowa, who is regarded as the father of radio in America, introduced the grid into the thermionic valve and patented over 300 other inventions. A radio-engineer from East Bolton, in Quebec, **Reginald Aubrey Fessenden** (1866–1932), patented over 500 inventions, and devised the first amplitude modulation in radio transmission with which he was able to broadcast the first American radio program from Brant Rock, Massachusetts, on the Christmas eve of 1906. In 1926, **Sir Edward Victor Appleton** (1892–1965), a Jacksonian professor at Cambridge, by examining the behavior of long-distance radio waves, showed that a reflecting or refracting layer existed about 150 miles above the ground. The construction of radar was later based on this discovery and it led to the establishment of the first radio link between England and Australia in 1918. The FM frequency modulation for radio was perfected in 1929 by an electrical engineer, **Edwin Howard Armstrong** (1890–1954) of New York. The first car radio, which worked on a car battery with an external aerial, was invented in 1932 by the German designer, Blaupunkt, and it was first fitted to an American Studebaker. Another early practical car radio was built by an American inventor, **William Powell Lear** (1902–1978) of Missouri. An American electrical engineer, **Harvey Fisher Schwarz** (1905–1988) of Edwardsville, Illinois, was the first to construct a domestic radio that used a screen-grid valve. He also developed a prototype radio navigation system that was used for the first time at the D-day landing during the invasion of Normandy, in 1944. The junction transistor that miniaturized circuits in radios was invented in 1947 by

William Bradford Shockley (1910–1989) of Bell Telephone Laboratories. *See broadcasting.*

Radio Telescope A large telescope in radioastronomy that works on the principle of collecting radio waves through an aerial, and bringing them to a focus at a point in front of the aerial. The British astronomer **Martin Ryle** (1918–1984) of Brighton, who pinpointed radio sources from sunspots, developed a radio telescope at Cambridge. In 1947, another English astronomer, **Sir Alfred Charles Bernard Lovell** (b 1913) and his colleagues built a large radio telescope, which paved the way for one of the important radio telescopes, the Jodrell Bank radio telescope, installed in Cheshire, England.

Radio Waves Waves of an electromagnetic nature, discovered by a German physicist, **Heinrich Rudolf Hertz** (1857–1894) of Hamburg. The practical implications of his discovery were developed by **Guglielmo Marchese Marconi** (1874–1937). Radio waves of cosmic origin were first detected in 1931 by an American radio engineer, **Karl Guthe Jansky** (1905–1950) from Oklahoma. His discovery laid the foundation for radio astronomy. The first radio map of the Milky Way was produced around 1940 by **Grote Reber** (b 1911) of Wheaton, Illinois. His device also recorded radio waves from the sun. *See radio, wireless telegraphy.*

Radioactive Decay *See radioactivity.*

Radioactivity In 1895, a French physicist in Paris, **Antoine Henri Becquerel** (1852–1908) discovered that certain substances, like uranium, emitted radiation similar to X-rays, and named the phenomenon radioactivity. In 1900 **Sir William Crookes** (1832–1919) noted the radioactive decay of uranium due to its copious emission of beta rays. In 1902, **Lord Ernest Rutherford** (1871–1937) and **Frederick Soddy** (1877–1965) proposed that radioactive elements made of complex particles underwent spontaneous changes or disintegration, with discharge of high velocity negatively charged electrons or beta rays, and positively charged particles or alpha rays. Radioactivity of thorium, uranium and other possible minerals in pitchblende was demonstrated in 1898 by **Marie Curie** (1867–1934) and **Pierre Curie** (1859–1906), for which they were awarded the Nobel Prize for physics, with Becquerel, in 1903. Another English physicist, **Sir James Chadwick,** (1891–1974), with Rutherford, published *Radiation from Radioactive Substances* (1930). In 1934, **Irene Joliot née Curie** (1897–1956), the daughter of Marie Curie, and her husband **Jean Frédéric Joliot** (1900–1958), made the first artificial radioactive isotope (of phosphorus) by bombarding aluminum with alpha particles, for which they were awarded the Nobel Prize for chemistry in 1935.

Radioastronomy The use of radiowaves and radar in astronomical observations was initiated in 1931 by two astronomers **Karl Guthe Jansky** (1905–1950) of Oklahoma, and **Grote Reber** (b 1911) of Wheaton, Illinois. Jansky discovered cosmic radio waves, and Reber mapped all the extraterrestrial sources of radio emission. The use of radar in radioastronomy was pioneered by an English physicist from the Lake District, **James Stanley Hey** (b 1909). A Scottish physicist, **David Forbes Martyn** (b 1906), made one of the first analyses of the temperature and constituents of the upper atmosphere through radiowave probing. The first extragalactic radio source was optically identified in 1951 by two German-born American pioneers in radioastronomy, **Rudolph Leo Minkowski** (1895–1976) and **Walter Baade** (1893–1960). In 1944, a Dutch astronomer, **Hendrik Christofel van de Hulst** (b 1918), suggested that interstellar hydrogen might be detected at radio wavelengths, and this was confirmed by **Edward Mills Purcell** (1912–1997) in 1951. A quasar, a radio source travelling at immense speed away from the earth, was first recognized in 1963 by a Dutch–American astronomer, **Maarten Schmidt** (b 1929). He found that the number of quasars increased with the distance from the earth, and his discovery provided evidence for the Big Bang theory. The existence of background microwave radiation as a result of the Big Bang, predicted previously by **Ralph Asher Alpher** (b 1921), was confirmed in 1964 by two American radioastronomers, **Arno Allan Penzias** (b 1933) of German origin, and **Robert Woodrow Wilson** (b 1936). Penzias and Wilson shared the Nobel Prize for physics, with **Pyotr Leonidovich Kapitza** (1894–1984), in 1978. The first extensive infrared map of the sky was achieved by a German-born US astronomer, **Gerald Neugbauer** (b 1932), in the 1960s. An American physicist, **Alan H. Barrett** (1927–1991), was the first to detect the presence of hydroxylions in interstellar space. This discovery of the first molecule in the Milky Way in radioastronomy led to the study of other molecules in the distant universe.

Radiocarbon Dating *See carbon dating.*

Radioglaciology *See glaciology.*

Radioisotope Studies A Berlin-born US biochemist, **Rudolf Schoenheimer** (1898–1941), was the first to use isotopic tracers for studying biohemical processes, in 1935. A Hungarian chemist, **Georg von Hevesy** (1885–1966), did further work on the use of isotopes in studying chemical reactions, for which he was awarded the Nobel Prize for

chemistry in 1943. An American microbiologist, **Irwin Clyde Gunsalus** (b 1912) of South Dakota, was one of the first to use radio-labelling for metabolic studies. By labelling glucose in bacteria, he studied the metabolic pathway of glucose.

Radiometer (1) A term used for an instrument consisting of vanes with shiny and blackened surfaces in a partly evacuated glass tube. The light falling on the device moves the molecules of air, which in turn move the vanes. It was invented by **Sir William Crookes** (1832–1919) and initially used as a curious exhibit. Martin Knudson developed the device into an absolute manometer and used it to measure very low pressures.

Radiometer (2) An apparatus for measuring the radiation of heat. Its prototype, the thermopile, was invented by an Italian professor of physics at Florence, **Leopoldo Nobili** (1784–1835) and developed in 1850 by another Italian scientist, **Macedonio Melloni** (1798–1854). An American physicist, **Samuel Pierpont Langley** (1834–1906) of Massachusetts, built a radiometer in 1878. A micro-radiometer consisting of a thermocouple and galvanometer was invented in 1888 by an English physicist, **Sir Charles Vernon Boys** (1855–1944). He used the instrument to measure the heat radiation from the moon and the planets. The theory involved in the radiometer was developed by a British physicist, **Osborne Reynolds** (1842–1912) from Belfast. Following his education at Cambridge, he became professor of engineering at Manchester in 1868.

Radon Radium emanation or a radioactive gas emitted by radium. It was discovered in 1900 by a German chemist, **Friedrich Ernst Dorn** (1848–1916). The English physicist **Sir William Ramsay** (1852–1916) isolated it and investigated its properties in 1908.

Raffles, Sir Thomas Stamford (1781–1826) *See flower, zoo.*

Rahn, Johann Heinrich (d 1676) *See mathematical symbols.*

Railway Wagons that ran on timber plates were used in 1550 in mining at Leberthal, Alsace. A similar method was used for transporting coal from 1603 to 1615 at Wollaton, near Nottingham, and at Broseley colliery in Shropshire in 1602. The first plateway to hold the wheels onto the plates was laid from Coalbrookdale to the Severn, by Richard Reynolds, in 1767. The first all-iron rail was laid around 1790. The fishbellied cast-iron rails were invented by an English engineer, **William Jessop** (1745–1814) from Devon. The first London plateway, with a wagon drawn by horses from Croydon to Wandsworth, was known as the Surrey Iron Railway, was established in 1802. **George**

Trevithick (1771–1833), a Cornish Engineer, built his first steam locomotive, which ran on an iron plateway, and demonstrated it at Coalbrookdale, Shropshire, in 1803. Wrought iron rails were introduced in 1810 at Rainhill, near Liverpool. The earliest commercially successful steam locomotive operated at Middleton Colliery Railway, Leeds, in 1812. In 1813, **William Hedley** (1779–1843) of Newburn, near Newcastle upon Tyne, improved Trevithick's locomotive, and demonstrated that metal wheels could grip onto metal rails. His locomotive was known as the *Puffing Billy*. The first railway for passengers in England ran from Shildon to Stockton, via Darlington, over a distance of 37 miles, in 1825. The first regular service was established in 1830 between Bogshole Farm and South Street in Whitstable, Yorkshire, over a distance of one mile. In 1829, **George Stephenson** (1781–1848) of Newcastle upon Tyne, demonstrated his locomotive, the *Rocket,* which reached a speed of 30 miles an hour. Following Stephenson's improvement of the steam engine, steam locomotives were established around Britain and Europe around 1835. His son **Robert Stephenson** (1803–1859) was a civil engineer and a pioneer in steam locomotives and built his first engine, the *Lancashire Witch*, in 1828. George Stephenson was also instrumental, with **Charles Blacker Vignoles** (1793–1875) of Woodbrook, County Wexford, in building the first railway in Ireland in 1932. **Joseph Locke** (1805–1860) from Yorkshire, was another English pioneer in railway engineering, who along with Stephenson and **Isambard Kingdom Brunel** (1806–1859) of Portsmouth, constructed most of the major railways in Britain. An English civil engineer, **Samuel Morton Peto** (1809–1889) of Woking, Surrey, was instrumental in laying railways in England, Norway, Russia and Algiers. The first seamless steel railway wheels were invented in 1852 by a German metallurgist, **Alfred Krupp** (1812–1887) of Essen. A British philosopher from Bristol, **John Herapath** (1790–1868), published an early journal *The Railway Magazine and Annals of Science* from 1836 to 1839. In 1844, a Belgian engineer, **Égide Walschaerts** (1820– 1901), improved Stephenson's radial valve gear, and patented it in other countries, where it became widely used for railway locomotives. It was adopted by the British Railway around 1878. The world's first railway station, the Liverpool Station at Greater Manchester, came into operation in 1830. **Williams Bridges Adams** (1797–1872), an English inventor from Madeley, Staffordshire, took out over 32 patents related to locomotives, carriages, roads and bridges. An English engineer, **John Urpeth Rastrick** (1780–1856), built the London & Brighton Railway, which opened in 1841. The fish-plate, which is widely used for joining rails, was invented by Adams in 1846. The first

locomotive in America was built in 1830 by Peter Cooper for the Baltimore & Ohio Railroad. A Scottish-born Canadian engineer and a pioneer of Canadian railways, **Sir Sanford Fleming** (1827–1915), directed the Canadian Pacific Railway from 1872 to 1880. The Central Pacific Railway (1869) and Southern Pacific Railway (1881) in America were pioneered by **Collis Porter Huntington** (1821–1900) of Harwinton, Connecticut. The world's largest railway station, the Grand Central Terminal at Park Avenue and 43nd Street, New York, was built in 1903–1913. *See air brakes, electric railway, locomotive, pullman sleeper, railway signals, steam engine, tram car, underground railways.*

Railway Signals The first was used around 1821 by a stationmaster on the Stockton and Darlington railway in England. He lit a candle at a window to stop the train. If it was unlit the train passed through, without stopping. A lantern by night, and a ball by day, was used on the British Great Western line. The semaphore signal was introduced in 1842. Electricity was first used to operate signals and points in 1884. A Welsh electrical engineer in Great Britain, **Sir William Henry Preece** (1834–1913), improved the system. An American engineer, **George Westinghouse** (1846–1914) of New York, developed an improved electrical light system for railway signals in America. The modern light signals were installed at Liverpool Overhead Railway in 1921. *See semaphore.*

Railway Timetable The first one was published in 1839 by a British printer and engraver George Bradshaw (1801–1853).

Rain Making *See artificial rain.*

Rain *See artificial rain, clouds.*

Rainbow A Greek scientist, **Anaxagoras** (500–428 BC) of Ionia, attempted to explain rainbows on the basis of a natural phenomenon, rather than a divine one. **Aristotle** (384–322 BC) proposed that the appearance of the rainbow was due to reflection from raindrops which formed a better mirror than mist. The English Franciscan monk, **Roger Bacon** (1214–1298) of Ilchester, gave a theory for the rainbow, and the German scholastic philosopher **Albertus Magnus** (c. 1192–1280) proposed that it was produced by the interaction of light with each drop of rain. A German Dominican priest, **Theodoric of Freiberg** (1250–1310), studied the phenomenon in relation to light and wrote *De iride* (On the Rainbow). The diagrams of his experiments are preserved in the Basel University Library. A clergyman from Sussex in England, **Robert Grosseteste** (1175–1253), experimented with lenses and explained the phenomenon on the basis of optics. An Islamic scientist and geographer, **al-Qazvini Zakaraya** (*c.* 1350), explained the rainbow on a scientific basis. In 1611, Antonio de Dominis, the Archbishop of Spalatro, suggested that the light reflected by raindrops was colored by traversing different thicknesses of water in the rainbow. **René Descartes** (1596–1650) gave an explanation for the rainbow, on the basis of physics, in his *Les météores* (1637). The riddle of the rainbow was solved by **Sir Isaac Newton** (1642–1727), when he made a small hole in the wall of a darkened room, to let in a ray of light along the path of a prism, which resulted in the production of intense colors as seen in a rainbow.

Rainwater, James Leo (1917–1986) *See atomic structure.*

RAM (**R**andom **A**ccess **M**emory) The first successful electrostatic random access memory (RAM) for digital computer, with the use of cathode-ray tubes, was built in 1946 by an electrical engineer, **Frederic Calland Williams** (1911–1977) of Cheshire. A chip with four times the memory of the earlier chips for computers was introduced by the IBM company in 1984.

Raman Effect *See Raman, Chandrasegar Venkata.*

Raman, Sir Chandrasekhara Venkata (1888–1970) An eminent Indian physicist, born in Trichinopoli and educated at Madras University. He was appointed as professor of physics at Calcutta in 1917, and in 1928 described the Raman effect, connected with the frequency of scattered light waves produced by the impact of waves on molecules. He founded the *Indian Journal of Physics* in 1926, and became the president of the Indian Science Congress in 1928. He was knighted in 1929 and was awarded the Nobel Prize for physics in 1930.

Ramanujan, Srinivasa (1887–1920) An Indian mathematical prodigy, born to a poor Brahmin family in Madras. He worked as a clerk and learnt mathematics from books (mainly *Synopsis of Pure Mathematics* by G.S. Carr), and sent 100 of his theorems to Cambridge, where they were studied by **Godfrey Harold Hardy** (1877–1947), who offered him a scholarship to Cambridge in 1914. Ramanujan published 25 mathematical papers over the next few years, and was made a fellow of the Royal Society in 1918. He died due to poor health within a year of his return to India.

Ramelli, Agostino (*c.* 1531–1600) *See mechanical engineering, military engineering.*

Ramsay, Sir William (1852–1916) A Scottish chemist born in Glasgow, where he studied classics, before he qualified in chemistry from Tübingen. In 1880 he was appointed

professor of chemistry at University College, Bristol, and moved to London in 1887. He was the first to realize the significance of **Henry Cavendish's** (1731–1810) experiments, which pointed to the presence of a gas other than nitrogen and oxygen in the air. Working on this hypothesis, Ramsay and **John William Strutt Rayleigh** (1842–1919) announced their discovery of argon in 1894. Ramsay also studied Brownian movement proposed by **Robert Brown** in 1827, and explained it on the basis of a collision between particles (pollen grains) and molecules of the liquid, in 1879. He served as professor of chemistry at University College London (1887–1912), and was awarded the Nobel Prize for chemistry in 1904. He published *Essays Biographical and Chemical* (1908), *The Gases of the Atmosphere and the History of Their Discovery* (1905) and several other works. *See argon, helium, krypton, radon, xenon.*

Ramsden, Jesse (1735–1800) An English mathematical instrument maker from Halifax, who introduced the equatorial mounting for telescopes. In 1785, he designed an instrument for accurately measuring the expansion of a metal bar. He constructed quadrants, circles and micrometers used in astronomy and an instrument for measuring the size of lenses. He invented a machine for producing electricity in 1768. *See automation, theodolite.*

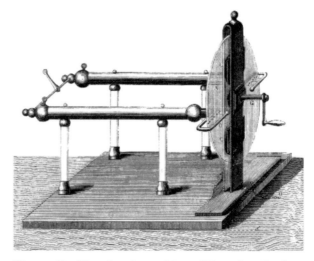

Figure 69 The electric machine of Ramsden. Lardner, Dionysius. *Handbook of Natural Philosophy, Electricity, Magnetism, and Acoustics.* London: Walton and Maberly, 1856

Ramsey, Norman Foster (b 1915) *See atomic clock, Paul Trap.*

Randall, Sir John Turton (1905–1994) *See radar.*

Rankine Cycle *See Rankine, William John Macquorn.*

Rankine, William John Macquorn (1820–1872) An engineer from Edinburgh who was elected to the chair of Engineering at Glasgow University in 1855. He improved the efficiency of the steam engine, and contributed to thermodynamics and the theory of elasticity. His description of the thermodynamic stages in the steam engine is called the Rankine cycle.

Ransome, Robert (1753–1830) *See agricultural instruments.*

Raoult Law Relates the vapor pressure of a solution to the number of molecules of the solute in it. Discovered in 1882 by a professor of chemistry at the University of Grenoble, **François Marie Raoult** (1830–1901).

Raoult, François Marie (1830–1901) *See freezing point, Raoult law.*

Raschig, Friedrich August (1863–1928) A German industrial chemist from Brandenburg who discovered nitramide and chloramine. He also developed new methods for producing phenol and hydrazine.

Raspail, François Vincent (1794–1878) *See frozen sections, histochemistry, microincineration.*

Rastrick, John Urpeth (1780–1856) *See railway.*

Rational Number Fraction Ratio of integral numbers. The theory of rational numbers is discussed in **Euclid's** (*c.* 300 BC) VII, VIII and IX books. A sequence of rational numbers that represent a definite symbolic form was proposed by a Swiss mathematician, **Jacques Bernoulli** (1654–1705) in his *Ars Conjectandi*, published posthumously in 1713.

Ray, John (1628–1705) An English biologist born to a blacksmith in Essex, and educated at Cambridge, before he took orders in the Church of England. He was one of the first to attempt the classification of the plant and animal kingdoms, and his system of zoology formed the basis for **Georges Cuvier's** (1769–1832) work. Ray's works include *Catalogus* (1697) of British plants, *Historia Piscium* (1686), and *Historia generalis plantarum* (1686–1704) in three volumes. His *Catalogus Plantarum Angliae* (1682) contained the principles of plant classification into cryptogams, monocotyledons and dicotyledons.

Rayleigh, Lord John William Strutt (1842–1919) An eminent British physicist born in Essex, who graduated from Trinity College, Cambridge, in 1861. He completed a classic work on the theory of sound in 1878. **William Ramsay** (1852–1916) and Rayleigh discovered the new inert gas helium in 1894. Rayleigh received the Nobel Prize for physics in 1904, for his work on gas density and the discovery of argon. *See acoustics, argon, kinetic energy, surface chemistry.*

Rayleigh, Robert John Strutt (1875–1947) *See petrology.*

Rayon *See artificial silk, textile chemistry.*

Razor *See safety razor.*

Read, Albert Cusion (1887–1967) *See transatlantic flight.*

Reaumer, René Antoine Ferchault de (1683–1757) *See entomology, iron, porcelain.*

Reber, Grote (b 1911) *See radioastronomy.*

Recapitulation Theory A concept that an embryo retraces the steps taken by its ancestors through evolution. First advocated by **Ernst Heinrich Haeckel** (1834–1919) in 1866, and supported by a Swiss-American naturalist and glaciologist, **Jean Louis Rodolph Agassiz** (1807–1873). A detailed criticism of this theory was given in 1930 by a London zoologist, **Sir Gavin Rylands de Beer** (1899–1972), who published *Introduction to Experimental Embryology* (1926).

Recorde, Robert (*c.* 1510–1558) *See algebra, calculation, early printed science books, mathematical symbols.*

Records *See gramophone, musical recording.*

Red Shift Lengthening of the wavelengths of light from a celestial object as a result of the object's motion away from earth. It is an example of the Doppler effect. *See expanding universe, galaxy, quasars.*

Redfield, William (1789–1857) *See American Association for the Advancement of Science, storms.*

Redi, Francesco (1626–1698) An Italian physician and naturalist from Arezzo who is regarded as the father of parasitology. He disproved the theory of spontaneous generation of maggots, in 1668. *See parasitism.*

Redman, Roderick Oliver (1905–1975) *See Hertzsprung–Russell diagram.*

Reflecting Telescope Uses mirrors to magnify and focus an image onto the eyepiece. It overcomes the spherical aberration caused by a normal telescope. The first one used in astronomy was invented by **James Gregory** (1638–1675), a mathematician from Aberdeen, and he announced his invention in his *Optica Promota* (1662). Another reflecting telescope was built by **Sir Isaac Newton** (1642–1727) in the same year, and he used it to observe the satellites of Jupiter and the phases of Venus. In 1672 a French physician,

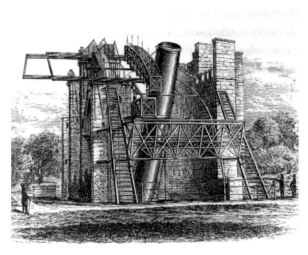

Figure 70   Rosse's giant metal reflecting telescope. Pouchet, F.A. *The Universe*. London: Blacke and Son, 1871

N. **Cassegrain** (1650–1675), devised a large reflecting telescope, and several of the world's largest telescopes came to be built on his principle. **John Hadley** (1682–1774), a London mathematician and astronomer, developed the reflecting telescope in 1731. **John Mudge** (d 1793), a physician and mechanic of Plymouth, improved the reflecting telescope in 1793. The first ever observation of a spiral galaxy was made in 1845 by an Irish astronomer, **William Parsons, Lord Rosse** (1800–1867), with his giant metal-mirror reflecting telescope. An Estonian optical instrument maker, **Bernhard Voldemar Schmidt** (1879–1935), eliminated the optical distortion or spherical aberration by bringing the entire image into single focus, with the use of a special lens and a spherical mirror. *See telescope.*

Refraction   Bending or deflection of light rays as they pass from one medium to another of greater or lesser density. Work on molecular refraction of liquids was done by two London physical chemists, **Thomas Pelham Dale** (1821–1892) and **John Hall Gladstone** (1827–1902), and they proposed the law which stated that the refractive index of a transparent gas is proportional to the density of the gas. **Paul Drude** (1863–1906), professor of physics at Leipzig (1894) and Giessen (1900), did work on refraction and measured the refractive index of metallic sodium, the smallest known. *See conical refraction, law of refraction, optics, Snell's law, spectacles.*

Refractive Index   When a ray of light passes from one medium to another, the sine of the angle of incidence divided by the sine of the angle of refraction remains a constant, which is known as refractive index. It was discov-

ered in 1624 by **Willebrord Snell** (1591–1626), professor of mathematics at Leyden. *See law of refraction.*

Refrigerator   The method of lowering the temperature with the use of ammonia was invented by **Michael Faraday** (1791–1867) in the 1820s. The first vapor-compression refrigerator was invented in 1834 by Jacob Perkins of Massachusetts, in America. James Harrison of Australia built one in 1850. A French chemist in Paris, **Eugene Anatole Demarcay** (1852–1903), designed a machine that achieved low temperatures by compressing gases and allowing them to expand, and his invention formed the basis for the production of refrigerators. The era of modern refrigeration began with the invention of the compression method, with the use of ammonia, by a French engineer, Ferdinand Carre, in 1857. Freon, as a non-toxic and non-flammable agent for domestic refrigerators, was introduced around 1923 by an American scientist, **Thomas Midgley** (1889–1944) of Beaver Falls, Pennsylvania. A German refrigeration engineer, **Karl von Linde** (1842–1934) from Bavaria, made many important contributions to the development of the refrigeration industry and took out several patents. **Sir Edward John Lees Hallstrom** (1886–1970) of Coonamble, New South Wales, was a pioneer of refrigeration in Australia. He made ice chests and wooden cabinets for refrigerators, before he started designing his own refrigeration units.

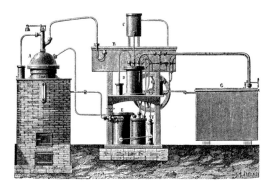

Figure 71   Ferdinand Carre's apparatus for making artificial ice. Guillemin, Amédée. *The Applications of Physical Forces*. London: Macmillan and Co, 1877

Regener, Erich Rudolph Alexander (1881–1955)   *See cosmic rays.*

Regiomontanus (1436–1476)   *See observatories, sines, tangent, trigonometry.*

Regnault, Henri Victor (1810–1878)   *See Boyle's law, hypsometer, respiratory quotient.*

Reich, Ferdinand (1799–1882) *See indium.*

Reichenbach, Georg Friedrich von (1772–1826) A German instrument maker who, in 1804, established a factory in Munich for making precision surveying and astronomical instruments. He designed a rifled cannon for the Bavarian army.

Reines, Frederick (1918–1998) *See neutrino.*

Reinhold, Arnold William (1843–1921) *See surface chemistry.*

Relativity Physicists up to the end of the 19th century believed that motion of all bodies was governed by **Sir Isaac Newton's** (1642–1727) laws of motion. An invisible hypothetical substance or medium in space, ether, through which light travelled in waves, was proposed by an English physician, **Thomas Young** (1773–1829) in 1803. In 1888, **Albert Abraham Michelson** (1852–1931) and **Edward William Morley** (1838–1923) made an attempt to determine the velocity of the earth, by measuring the velocity of light in relation to ether. Their work showed that the velocity of light was the same in all directions and was independent of the motion of the earth. In 1905, **Albert Einstein** (1879–1955) discarded the ether medium in his calculations and came to the conclusion that speed can only be measured in relation to another object. His general theory of relativity, based on the assumption that the laws of physics would also be the same in systems that were accelerating relative to each other, was published in 1916. In his work he concluded that the effects of gravity and acceleration were equivalent. In 1919, an English astronomer and professor at Cambridge, **Sir Arthur Stanley Eddington** (1882–1944), gave the first experimental proof of Einstein's general theory of relativity. He showed that stars whose light passed close to the sun appeared to be displaced by a minute amount which corresponded to the value calculated by Einstein.

Remak, Robert (1815–1865) *See fixatives.*

Remington, Philo (1816–1889) *See firearms, typewriter.*

Remote Control The use of radio for the remote control of machines was pioneered by a German engineer, **Anton Flettner** (b 1885), who invented a remote controlled tank in 1915.

Remsen, Ira (1846–1927) *See saccharin.*

Renaudot, Theophrastus (1583–1653) *See newspapers.*

Rennie, John (1761–1821) *See bridges, canals.*

Rennie, Sir John (1794–1874) *See bridges, warships.*

Rensch, Bernhard (b 1900) *See ethology.*

Renwick, James (1790–1863) An American naturalist and philosopher from Liverpool, in England, who became professor of natural philosophy and experimental chemistry at Columbia College in 1820. He published a *Treatise on Steam Engine* (1830).

Renwick, James (1818–1895) Son of **James Renwick** (1790–1863) and an architect who designed St Patrick's Cathedral, in New York, the State Bank of New York and the Smithsonian Institution.

Repsold, Johann Georg (1770–1830) *See heliometer.*

Reproduction *See fertilization, pollination.*

Respiratory Quotient The volume of carbon dioxide expired, divided by the volume of oxygen consumed. First determined in 1849 by a German-born French scientist, **Henri Victor Regnault** (1810–1878). He was made professor of chemistry at the Collège de France in 1840. He discovered carbon tetrachloride.

Retrosynthesis [Latin: *retro*, back + Greek: *synthesis*, putting together] A method of building more complex molecules from smaller, simpler and more readily available molecules. Developed by **Elias James Corey** (b 1928) in the 1960s, and used extensively in the chemical and pharmaceutical industries.

Reuter, Baron de (1821–1899) The founder of the telegraphic agency for collecting news was born in Cassel in Germany, and emigrated to England in 1851, where he established a telegraphic business for conveying private messages between England and continental Europe. In 1858, he persuaded several newspapers to use his agency, which he developed into the Reuters company for collection and transmission of news.

Reuters *See Reuter, Baron de.*

Revelle, Roger Randall Dougan (1909–1991) *See global warming.*

Reynold's Number A dimensionless ratio related to the dynamic state of fluid, named after the Belfast-born British physicist, **Osborne Reynolds** (1842–1912).

Reynolds, Osborne (1842–1912) *See hydrodynamics, radiometer (2), Reynold's number.*

Rhenium An element with an atomic number of 75, discovered in 1925 by two German chemists, **Walter Karl Friedrich Noddack** (1893–1960) and his wife **Ida Eva Noddack** (b 1896), of Berlin. It is named after the river Rhine.

Rheticus, Georg Joachim or **G.J. von Lauchen** (1514–1576) *See trigonometry.*

Rhijn, Pieter Johannes van (b 1886) *See galaxy.*

Rhind Papyrus *See Ahmes papyrus.*

Rhind, Alexander Henry (1833–1863) *See Ahmes papyrus, mathematics.*

Rhodium [Greek: *rhodon*, red] An element similar to platinum with an atomic number 45, discovered 1803 by an English chemist from Norfolk, **Hyde William Wollaston** (1766–1822).

Ribbing Machine Used for the manufacture of stockings, this was invented in 1758 by **Jedediah Strutt** (1726–1797) of Derbyshire, England.

Ribonucleic Acid (RNA) Transfer RNA, which plays an important role in intracellular protein synthesis, was first isolated by a Boston biochemist, **Mahlon Bush Hoagland** (b 1921), in the late 1950s. An American biochemist, **Boehmer Christian Anfinsen** (1916–1995), did research on the structure and shape of the ribonuclease enzyme, for which he shared the Nobel Prize for chemistry in 1972, with two other American biochemists, **Stanford Moore** (1913–1982) of Chicago, and **William Howard Stein** (1911–1980), of New York. The *reverse transcriptase* enzyme capable of transcribing RNA into DNA was discovered by an American microbiologist, **David Baltimore** (b 1938) of New York, in 1970, and his finding formed the basis for the manipulation of the genetic code. In 1983, a Canadian biologist, **Sidney Altman** (b 1939), discovered that an RNA component of ribonuclease alone catalyzes the maturation of transfer RNA. In 1989 he shared the Nobel Prize for chemistry for his work with an American molecular biologist **Thomas Cech** (b 1947) of Chicago, who discovered the property of RNA of acting as a biological catalyst. **Phillip Allen Sharp** (b 1944) of Kentucky developed a method known as S1 nuclease mapping for detecting the size of unknown RNA molecules. He shared the Nobel Prize for Medicine or Physiology in 1993 with a British physiologist, **Richard Roberts** (b 1943).

Ricardo, Sir Harry Ralph (1885–1974) *See internal combustion engine, octane rating.*

Riccati Equation A type of differential equation proposed in 1676 by an Italian mathematician, **Count Jacopo Francesco Riccati** (1676–1754) of Venice. His works were published posthumously in 1758.

Riccati, Count Jacopo Francesco (1676–1754) *See Bernoulli, Daniel, Riccati equation.*

Ricci Calculus A system of absolute differential calculus devised around 1890 by an Italian mathematician, **Gregorio Ricci-Curbastro** (1853–1925) while he was professor of mathematical physics at Padua.

Ricci-Curbastro, Gregorio (1853–1925) *See calculus, Ricci calculus.*

Richard of Wallingford (*c.* 1292–1336) An English engineer, clergyman, astronomer and mathematician from Wallingford, in Berkshire, who studied at Oxford from 1318 to 1327. He constructed one of the first mechanical astronomical clocks and published a work on trigonometry, *Quadripartitium* (1320).

Richards, Sir Rex Edward (b 1922) *See magnetic resonance imaging.*

Richards, Theodore William (1868–1928) *See atomic weight.*

Richardson, Lewis Fry (1881–1953) *See weather forecast.*

Richardson, Sir Owen Willans (1879–1959) *See thermionics.*

Richer, Jean (1630–1696) *See parallax.*

Richter Scale Measurement of an earthquake on a scale of 1 to 9 where an increase of one unit corresponds to 30 times the seismic energy. Invented in 1932 by an American seismologist, **Charles Francis Richter** (1900–1985) of Hamilton, Ohio, and a German-born American geophysicist, **Beno Gutenberg** (1889–1960) from Darmstadt. Gutenberg made the first correct determination of the earth's core in 1914.

Richter, Burton (b 1931) *See particle accelerator, psi.*

Richter, Charles Francis (1900–1985) *See Richter scale, seismology.*

Richter, Hieronymus Theodor (1824–1898) *See indium.*

Richter, Jeremias Benjamin (1762–1807) *See law of equivalent proportions.*

Rickover, Hyman George (1900–1986) *See atomic ships, submarines.*

Ride, Sally Kristen (b 1951) *See astronauts.*

Ridgway, Robert (1850–1929) *See ornithology.*

Riemann Geometry A system of non-Euclidean geometry developed in 1854 by a German mathematician, **Georg Friedrich Bernhard Riemann** (1826–1866). His classic work *On the Hypothesis which forms the foundation of Geometry* was published in 1867.

Riemann, Georg Friedrich Bernhard (1826–1866) *See hyperbolic geometry, Riemann geometry, Riemann integral, Riemann zeta function.*

Riemann Integral A new system for integral in the trigonometric series, proposed by **Georg Friedrich Bernhard Riemann** (1826–1866).

Riemann Zeta Function Fundamental to the study of the distribution of prime numbers, based on a hypothesis proposed by a German mathematician, **Georg Friedrich Bernhard Riemann** (1826–1866). The conditions under which the zeta function is zero is described in the Bohr–Landau theorem proposed in 1914 by a Danish mathematician, **Harold August Bohr** (1887–1951) of Copenhagen, and Edmund Landau.

Riemer, Pieter de (1760–1831) *See frozen sections.*

Riese, Adam (1489–1559) *See accountancy, early printed science books.*

Riesz, Frigyes (1880–1956) *See Lebesgue integral.*

Righi, Augusto (1850–1920) *See wireless telegraphy.*

Río, Andrés Manuel del (1764–1849) *See vanadium.*

Ritter, Johann Wilhelm (1776–1810) *See accumulator, battery, photochemistry, ultraviolet rays.*

Rivaz, Peter Joseph (1711–1772) *See watches.*

Rivers Some of the important ancient civilizations were built around rivers. Southwest Asia between the rivers Tigris and Euphrates, known as Mesopotamia [Greek: *mesos,* middle + *potamus,* river], became the cradle of civilization around 4000 BC. A Jesuit priest, **Athanasius Kircher** (1601–1680) of Geysen in his *Subterranean World* (1665) considered the sea as the only source of water for rivers. An Italian naturalist and professor of medicine at Padua, **Antonio Vallisneri** (1661–1730), suggested rain as the main source of water for rivers. An American geologist, **William Morris Davis** (1850–1935), defined the role of rivers in the production of landscape.

Riveting Machine *See machine tools.*

Roads As early as 3000 BC the towns around the Tigris and Euphrates in Mesopotamia had metalled roads. They were surfaced with bitumen, which was rediscovered for modern road surfacing in the 19th century. Around AD 1380, the Yuan Dynasty in China improved roads and built new ones. The oldest known trackway in England, made from felled trees, in the Somerset area, dates back to 4000 BC. A prehistoric road made of wooden logs at Corlea, in Ireland, has been carbon dated at 2500 BC. The Romans made roads to suit the climate, availability of materials and the nature of traffic. In forest areas they used tree trunks, and in towns, stone flags. One of the earliest treatises on roads, the *Book of Roads and Provinces,* in Arabic, was written by **Abul Qasim ibn Khurdadhbih** (*c.* 1100) of Persian descent, who was chief officer of information in the city of al-Jibal in Tigris. Up to the 17th century most roads used in Europe were remains of Roman roads consisting of rough tracks. Around 1765, an English engineer, **John Metcalf** (1717–1810), known as Blind Jack of Knaresborough, built over 185 miles of roads linked by bridges in Lancashire and Yorkshire. The first Turnpike Act for roads in Britain was passed in 1663, and it was extended to the whole country in 1767. This led to the collection of toll money meant for road building and maintenance. A French engineer, **Pierre Marie Jerome Tresaguet** (1716–1796), was one of the first to build modern roads that could stand the weather and traffic. He dug out the roadways, and built the roads on a solid foundation of layers of stones, with a smooth surface. His first major road was laid from Paris to the Spanish border. A Scottish engineer, **Thomas Telford** (1757–1834) from Westkirk, Dumfries, modernized the old Roman roads in Britain in a similar manner. **Richard Lovell Edgeworth** (1744–1817) of Bath, Somerset, in England, proposed an advanced method of road building, in 1813. A method of preparing the road surface by raising it above a firm base of large stones, onto which small stones with gravel were applied, so as to give a convex shape for draining off water, was invented by a Scottish civil engineer, **John Loudon McAdam** (1756–1836) from Ayr, who wrote several books on construction of roads. Road building in Australia was pioneered by **William Cox** (1764–1837) from Dorset in Britain, who built roads in the Blue Mountains and other parts of New South Wales. **Fritz Todt** (1891–1942), a German inspector of roads during Hitler's regime, was responsible for the construction of *Reichsautobahnen* or the German highways.

Robert de Ketene (*c.* AD 1143) *See university gown.*

Robert of Chester (*c.* AD 1200) *See alchemy, trigonometry.*

Roberts, John D. (b 1918) *See magnetic resonance imaging.*

Roberts, Richard (1789–1864) *See machine tools, textile industry.*

Roberts, Richard (b 1943) *See ribonucleic acid.*

Roberts, Walter Orr (1915–1990) *See meteorology.*

Roberts-Austen, Sir William Chandler (1843–1902) A London metallurgist who was a professor at the Royal School of Mines, where he designed an automatic pyrometer for high temperatures. The iron-carbide solution (austenite) formed during the process of cooling steel is named after him. *See metallurgy.*

Robertson, Howard Percy (1903–1961) *See micrometeorite.*

Robertson, Robert (1869–1949) *See explosives.*

Roberval, Gilles Personne de (1602–1675) A French professor of mathematics in Paris who introduced the method of indivisibles for quadranture of surfaces, and also wrote a treatise on mechanics.

Robins, Benjamin (1707–1751) *See ballistics, military engineering, pendulum.*

Robinson, John Thomas Romney (1792–1882) *See anemometer, wind.*

Robinson, Robert (1886–1975) *See organic chemistry.*

Robinson, William (1838–1935) *See horticulture.*

Robiquet, Jean-Pierre (1780–1840) *See dyes.*

Rochas, Alphouse Beau de (1815–1893) *See internal combustion engine.*

Rockefeller Foundation Founded in 1913 with funds provided by the oil magnate **John Davison Rockefeller** (1839–1937), the founder of the Standard Oil Company (1870), in Cleveland, Ohio. He gave over 500 million dollars to medical research, universities and Baptist churches, for promoting the well-being of mankind. One of his sons, John Davison Rockefeller III (1906–1978), became chairman of the foundation in 1952.

Rockefeller, John Davison (1839–1937) *See Rockefeller Foundation.*

Rocket War rockets propelled by chemicals were described by Tseng Kuang Liang of China in 1042. Early forms were used for the first time in Europe at the battle of Chioggia between the Genoese and Venetians in 1380. Rockets were revived in 1803 as destructive war implements by lieutenant-colonel **Sir William Bart Congreve** (1772–1828) of England, and used during the war in Bologne in 1806 to set the town on fire. The first suggestion that liquid-fueled rockets could be used to propel vehicles in space was made in 1895 by a Russian physicist, **Konstantin Tsiolkovsky** (1857–1935). The first liquid-propelled rocket was launched in 1926 by an American physicist, **Robert Hutchings Goddard** (1882–1945) of Worcester, Massachusetts. Goddard built the first instrument-carrying rocket used for flight observations, in 1929. The tube-launched rocket, the bazooka, was invented in 1918 by Robert Goddard. In 1935 he constructed the first rocket to exceed the speed of sound. A Hungarian-born German astronomer, **Herman Julius Oberth** (1894–1990), published *Rocket to Interplanetary Space* (1923), and played an important role in developing space rockets in the USA. A German engineer, **Walter Robert Dornberger** (1895–1980), set up an experimental rocket station at Kummersdorf, and launched a 650-pound thrust motor in 1932. His V-2 rockets with warheads were launched against England. He later emigrated to America and became a consultant to the air force there. A liquid-fuel rocket reaching a height of 2.4 kilometres was developed in 1934 by a German engineer, **Wernher von Braun** (1912–1977). He founded a society for space travel, and a rocket-launching site, near Berlin, in 1930. He also developed the V-2 rockets that were used against the British in the Second World War. He was made a US citizen in 1955, and became a pioneer in space travel there. He developed the *Saturn V* rocket for the *Apollo II* moon landing in 1969. The first telemetry system used in rockets for space exploration was developed by a New Zealand-born US physicist and space scientist, **William Hayward Pickering** (b 1910). In 1949, **Samuel Kurtz Hoffman** (b 1902), professor of aeronautical engineering at Pennsylvania State University, started developing powerful rockets. By 1960 he had improved the thrust of the engine from 75 000 pounds to 1.5 million pounds, and Hoffman's engines were used in 1969 for the journey to the moon.

Rocks *See petrology.*

Roe, Alliot Verdon (1877–1958) *See airplane.*

Roebling, John Augustus (1806–1869) *See suspension bridges.*

Roebling, Washington Augustus (1837–1926) *See suspension bridges.*

Roebuck, John (1718–1794) *See lead chamber process.*

Roemer, Olaus (1644–1710) *See Jupiter, thermometer, velocity of light.*

Rohrer, Heinrich (b 1933) *See electron microscope.*

Rolle, Michel (1652–1719) *See Rolle's theorem.*

Rolle's Theorem Dealing with the position of the roots of an equation in algebra, this was proposed in 1689 by a French mathematician, **Michel Rolle** (1652–1719) of Paris.

Rolls, Charles Stewart (1877–1910) An English motor car manufacturer who, in 1902, founded C.S. Rolls & Co, which made his first car in 1904. He went into partnership in 1906 with **Sir Frederick Henry Royce** (1863–1933) and established Rolls-Royce Ltd, which made motor cars and airplane engines. *See car, Channel flight.*

Romanus, Aegidius (*c.* 1245–1316) *See embryology.*

Romé de L'isle, Jean Baptiste Louis (1736–1790) *See crystallography.*

Romer, Alfred Sherwood (1894–1973) *See vertebrates.*

Romer, Olaus (1644–1710) A Danish astronomer from Jutland who was educated in Copenhagen. He invented the transit circle, a complicated instrument designed to measure the time of transit across the meridian. He calculated the speed of light through space with an impressive accuracy, for the first time from astronomical observations, in 1695.

Ronalds, Sir Francis (1788–1873) *See electric telegraphy.*

Rondelet, Guillaume (1507–1566) *See ichthyology.*

Röntgen, Wilhelm Conrad (1845–1923) *See X-rays.*

Rooke, Laurence (1622–1662) *See Royal Society of London.*

Roots An account of morphological appearances of different kinds of roots, their pattern of growth and structure, was given by **Theophrastus** (380–287 BC) from the Greek island of Lesbos, in his treatise *History of Plants.* A French botanist, **D. Dodart** (1634–1707), studied the effect of gravity on roots. **Stephen Hales** (1696–1761), an English vicar at Teddington, began his experimental studies on plant physiology in 1724, and showed that water was drawn from the roots to the leaves, where it was lost by transpiration. The presence of nitrogen-fixing bacteria in the roots of certain legumes was demonstrated by **Sir Joseph Henry Gilbert** (1817–1901) at Rothamsted, in England, in 1893.

Roozeboom, Hendrik Willem Bakhuis (1856–1907) *Gibbs–Donnan equilibrium.*

Roscoe, Sir Henry Enfield (1833–1915) *See actinometer, quantitative chemistry, vanadium.*

Rosing, Boris (d 1918) *See cathode ray tube, television.*

Ross, Sir James Clark (1800–1862) *See magnetic poles, volcanic eruptions.*

Ross, Sir John (1777–1856) *See magnetic poles.*

Rossby, Carl Gustav Arvid (1898–1957) *See weather forecast.*

Rossby Waves *See weather forecast.*

Rosse, William Parsons, Lord (1800–1867) *See galaxy, nebulae, reflecting telescope.*

Rosetta Stone An ancient Egyptian stone with three different scripts inscribed on it. Discovered by Napoleon's soldiers while they were digging near the Rosetta branch of the Nile in 1799. It was brought to England in 1802 and was placed in the British Museum. **Jean François Champollion** (1790–1832) of France, used the inscriptions of three different kinds (Greek, Demotic or enchorial, and hieroglyphic) found on the stone, as a key to decipher Egyptian hieroglyphics.

Rossi, Bruno (1905–1994) An Italian physicist from Venice who did pioneering work on cosmic rays and published *Rayons Cosmiques* (1935). He described the showers caused by primary radiation in the atmosphere, which collided with oxygen, nitrogen and other atoms. He invented a circuit that is named after him. He became professor of physics at Cornell University in 1940. *See photons.*

Rotary Engine An internal combustion rotary engine, which has an approximately triangular rotor, driven in an elliptical combustion chamber containing an air-fuel mixture. It produces more power for its weight than diesel and standard petrol engines. It was developed in 1953 by a German engineer, **Felix Wankel** (1902–1988) from Luhran, in conjunction with the German company N.S.U.

Rothlisberger, Hans (b 1923) *See glaciology.*

Rouelle, Guillaume François (1703–1770) A French chemist from Caen who first differentiated between acidic, basic and neutral salts. His brother **Hilare Martin Rouelle** (1718–1779), discovered urea in urine.

Rouelle, Hilare Martin (1718–1779) *See Rouelle, Guillaume François.*

Routledge, George (1812–1888) *See bookshops.*

Roux, Wilhelm (1850–1924) *See chromosomes.*

Rowland, Henry Augustus (1848–1901) *See concave diffraction grating, thermodynamics.*

Roxburgh, William (1751–1815) A Scottish botanist and surgeon from Ayrshire who served in the East India Company at Madras, South India. He became superintendent of the

Calcutta Botanical Gardens and 1793, and wrote several works on the plants of India.

Royal Institution of London Founded by an American-born physicist from Woburn, Massachusetts, **Benjamin Thompson, Count Rumford** (1753–1814) and an English botanist, **Sir Joseph Banks** (1743–1820), on 9th March 1799 at a house in Albermarle Street, Piccadilly. It was given a Royal Charter and made The Royal Institution of Great Britain in 1800. Its purpose was 'for diffusing knowledge and facilitating the general introduction of useful mechanical inventions and improvements, and for the teaching by courses of philosophical lectures and experiments, the application of science to common purposes of life'. The first lecture was given in 1801 by Garnett, who was the first professor of natural philosophy and chemistry in England. The second lecture was given in 1802 by **Thomas Young** (1773–1829). **Sir Humphry Davy** (1778–1829) became its director in the same year, and **Michael Faraday** (1791–1867) succeeded him in 1825.

Royal Society of London Started informally around 1645 by several learned scientists including **John Wilkins** (1614–1672) and **John Wallis** (1616–1703) who regularly met in London. The idea of weekly meetings seems to have been proposed by a German, Theodore Hawk. The founding members agreed to exclude theology and politics from their discussions. The group split in 1649 by the removal of Wilkins and Wallis to Oxford. The Oxford group was joined by **Seth Ward** (1617–1689) and **William Petty** (1623–1687). They first met at Wilkins' apartment at Wadham College, and later at the house of **Robert Boyle** (1627–1691). The Philosophical Society of Oxford was formed out of their meetings but only lasted until 1650. The London group continued to function with its members **Sir Christopher Wren** (1632–1723), **Laurence Rooke** (1622–1662), **Lord William Brouncker** (1620–1684) and several other important men. After the restoration of Charles II, it received its Royal Charter in 1662. In the same year **Robert Hooke** (1635–1703) was appointed curator to the society with a commitment for preparing two or three experiments of his own to be presented at the meetings. The Society's publication, *Philosophical Transactions of the Royal Society*, was started in 1665 by Henry Oldenburg at his own expense. **Sir Isaac Newton** (1642–1727) presented the manuscripts of his *Principia* in 1668 and it was published at the expense of **Edmund Halley** (1656–1742), who was clerk to the Society. Some of its distinguished presidents include: Sir Christopher Wren (1680), Samuel Pepys (1684), Sir Hans Sloane (1727), Sir John Pringle (1772), Sir Humphry Davy (1820) and Sir Benjamin Brodie (1858).

Royce, Sir Frederick Henry (1863–1933) An English pioneer of the motor car industry and airplane engines. He designed the engines for Spitfires and Hurricanes in World War II. *See car, Rolls, Stewart Charles.*

Rozier, François Pilâtre de (1757–1785) *See air balloon.*

Rubber A term first used by the English chemist **Joseph Priestley** (1733–1804), who used the substance to erase pencil marks. *See artificial rubber, Macintosh cloth, tire, vulcanization.*

Rubbia, Carlo (b 1934) *See antiproton, boson.*

Rubens, Heinrich (1865–1922) *See infrared radiation.*

Rubidium [Latin: *rubidus*, dark red] The second element to be discovered with the use of spectrum analysis, by **Gustav Robert Kirchhoff** (1824–1887) and **Robert Bunsen** (1811–1899), in 1861. Bunsen isolated it through electrolysis in 1863.

Rubik Cube A puzzle cube with millions of possible combinations, invented in 1974 by a Hungarian architect and inventor, **Ernö Rubik** (b 1944) of Budapest.

Rubik, Ernö (b 1944) *See Rubik cube.*

Rubin, Gerald Meyer (b 1950) *See cloning.*

Rücker, Sir Arthur William (1848–1915) *See surface chemistry.*

Rudaux, Lucien (1874–1947) *See astronomical paintings.*

Rudolf, Christoff (b 1500) *See accountancy, mathematical symbols.*

Rudolphine Tables The Danish astronomer **Tycho Brahe** (1546–1601) on his deathbed, requested **Johannes Kepler** (1571–1630) to use his planetary observations to compile a set of tables of planetary motion. The tables, known as the Rudolphine Tables, and named after the Austrian emperor, Rudolf II (1552–1612), were completed in 1627, while Kepler was at Ulm.

Rue, Warren de la (1815–1889) *See battery, celestial photography, eclipse, envelope.*

Ruffini, Paolo (1765–1822) *See Abel–Ruffini theorem.*

Ruhmkorff Coil A transformer for producing high-voltage direct current output from a low voltage. Invented in 1851 by a German mechanic from Hanover, **Heinrich Daniel Ruhmkorff** (1803–1877).

Ruhmkorff, Heinrich Daniel (1803–1877) A German mechanic from Hanover who lived in Paris. He invented a thermoelectric battery in 1844, and an induction coil in 1851. His induction coil formed the basis for the development of Geissler's tube which was used for the discovery of cathode rays. *See X-rays.*

Rumford, Count (1753–1814) *See Thompson, Benjamin.*

Rumsey, James (1743–1792) *See jet engine, steamships.*

Runge, Carl David Tolme (1856–1927) A German physicist from Bremen who was professor of physics at Hanover, and later at Göttingen. He was one of the first to investigate magnetic resolution in spectroscopy.

Runge, Friedlib Ferdinand (1795–1867) *See aniline, chromatography, coffee plant, dyes, pyrrole.*

Rush, Benjamin (1745–1813) An American physician and chemist who was one of the first to teach and publish on chemistry in America. He was appointed to the chair of chemistry at the College of Philadelphia in 1869.

Ruska, Ernst August Friedrich (1906–1988) *See electron microscope.*

Russell, Henry (1877–1957) *See Hertzsprung–Russell diagram.*

Russell, Bertrand Arthur William (1872–1970) A British philosopher and mathematician from Monmouthshire who is regarded as one of the founders of modern logic. He was educated at Trinity College, Cambridge and wrote *Introduction to the Philosophy of Mathematics* (1918) while he was serving a prison sentence for his pacifist views regarding the war. His most significant work, *Principia Mathematica* in three volumes, was published from 1910 to 1913.

Russell, Frederick Stratten (1897–1984) *See plankton.*

Russell, John Francis Stanley (1865–1931) *See motoring.*

Russell, John Scott (1808–1882) *See coaches, steamships.*

Russell, Sir John Edward (1872–1965) *See agriculture.*

Ruthenium A rare element discovered in 1845 by a Russian professor of chemistry at the University of Dorpat, **Karl Karlovich Klaus** (1796–1864), and named after Ruthenia in Russia.

Rutherford, Daniel (1749–1819) *See air, nitrogen.*

Rutherford, Lord Ernest (1871–1937) A Nobel Prize winner for chemistry in 1908, born in Nelson, New Zealand. He obtained his doctorate in mathematical physics from the University of New Zealand in 1893, and invented a detector for radio waves in 1895. He was awarded a scholarship to Cambridge, and worked under **John Joseph Thomson** (1856–1940), before he started his experiments on radioactivity in 1898. He was appointed professor of physics at McGill University, Montreal, in 1898, and worked with **Frederick Soddy** (1877–1965) in formulating the atomic theory of radioactivity, in 1902. *See alpha rays, artificial transmutation, atomic bomb, atomic disintegration, atomic theory, gamma rays, neutron, nuclear fusion, proton, tritium.*

Ruysch, Frederik (1638–1731) *See staining.*

Ruzicka, Leopold (1887–1976) A Swiss organic chemist from Croatia, who shared the Nobel Prize for chemistry in 1939 with **Adolf Friedrich Johann Butenandt** (1903–1995), for his work on the synthesis of sex hormones.

Rydberg Constant Used in a mathematical expression for frequencies of spectral lines of elements. Proposed in 1890 by a Swedish physicist, **Johannes Robert Rydberg** (1854–1919) of Halmstad, who was professor of physics at the University of Lund. An American physicist, **Arthur Leonard Schawlow** (1921–1999) of Mount Vernon, New York, devised a method to calculate the Rydberg constant with unprecedented accuracy. He shared the Nobel Prize for physics in 1981, with a Dutch-born American physicist, **Nicolaas Bloembergen** (b 1920) and a Swedish physicist, **Kai Manne Börje Siegbahn** (b 1918).

Rydberg, Johannes Robert (1854–1919) *See Rydberg constant.*

Ryle, Martin (1918–1984) *See pulsar, radio telescope.*

S

Sabatier, Paul (1854–1941) *See hydrogenation, hydrogen sulfide, soap.*

Sabine, Sir Edward (1788–1883) *See sunspots.*

Sabine, Wallace Clement Ware (1868–1919) *See acoustics.*

Saccharin (2-sulfobenzimide) The first artificial sweetener, obtained in 1879 from coal tar, by two Americans, **Constantin Fahlberg** (1850–1910) and **Ira Remsen** (1846–1927). It remained as a prescription product until the Food and Drug Administration allowed it to be used as an industrial food additive in 1938.

Sachs, Julius von (1832–1897) *See chlorophyll, chloroplasts, photosynthesis, plant physiology.*

Safety Matches *See matches.*

Safety Pin Invented in 1849 by an American, Walter Hunt.

Safety Razor The razor for shaving was one of man's earliest inventions, to prevent his hair from covering his face. During early civilization iron and bronze razors were used. The first safety razor was invented in 1762 by Jean Jacques Perret of France. He used a guard at one edge to stop the razor from cutting into the skin. A similar device was used in Sheffield, England around 1825. The modern safety razor with a disposable blade was invented in 1901 by **King Camp Gillette** (1855–1932) from Fond Du Lac, Wisconsin. Around 1915, G.P. Appleyard, in England, invented a hand-operated razor for dry shaving. The electric shaver was patented in 1923 by Jacob Schick. *See Gillette blade.*

Saha, Meghnad (1894–1956) An Indian physicist and pioneer in astrophysics from Dacca. He was professor of physics in Calcutta and published several papers on stellar atmospheres. In 1920 he showed that elements in stars are ionized in proportion to their temperature. *See Saha's equation.*

Saha's Equation Relates the ionization of elements in stars to their temperature. Proposed in 1920 by an Indian astrophysicist, **Meghnad Saha** (1894–1956) of Dacca.

Sailing Ships Sailing ships were used in Mesopotamia (now Iraq) around 5000 BC, and in Egypt in 3500 BC. Minoan craftsmen around 2200 BC were skilled at ship building. The Phoenicians later ousted the Minoans as the dominant sea power. Their ships were lightly built and had straight keels and high end posts. Known as *biremes,* they were the first to have two banks of oars on either side. The later Roman versions had three decks of oarsmen and were known as *triremes.* The early Egyptian sailing ships were made of reed. The Vikings developed a sophisticated system by which their ships were able to sail close to the wind. Around AD 1000 the Arabs used triangular or lateen sails, fixed to a pole placed at an angle to the mast, and made voyages to India, Ceylon and the rest of the east. A system of square and lateen sails was used in Europe in the 1500s. The *Cutty Sark* had sails of many different sizes and shapes. The fighting ships of Sir Francis Drake (1540–1596), and the Spanish galleons used triangular fore-and-aft and square sails in various combinations. The first modern three-decked sailing ship, *The Sovereign of the Seas,* was built in England in 1637. A Scottish-born naval architect, **Harry Eckford** (1775–1832), built several modern speedy sailing ships in America. In 1843 the Americans began building full-rigged ships that became known as clippers. *See boats, ships.*

Saint Joseph, John Kenneth Sinclair (b 1912) *See aerial photograph.*

Saint Vincent, Gregorius de (1584–1667) *See conics.*

Saint-Gillies, L. P. de (1832–1863) *See velocity of chemical reactions.*

Saint-Hilaire, Geoffry Etienne (1772–1844) *See homology.*

Saint-Hilaire, Isidore Geoffrey (1805–1861) *See animal husbandry.*

Sakharov, Andrey Dmitriyevich (1921–1989) *See H bomb.*

Salam, Abdus (b 1926) A Pakistani nuclear physicist, educated in Punjab and Cambridge, England. In 1957 he became professor of theoretical physics at the Imperial College of Science and Technology, London, and was instrumental in establishing the International Center of Theoretical Physics, in Trieste, in 1964. *See quantum chromodynamics.*

Salisbury, Edward James (1886–1978) *See British Ecological Society.*

Salisbury, Richard Anthony (1781–1829) An English botanist from Leeds who published *Paradisus Londinesis* (1805–1808), *Prodromus Stirpium* (1796) and several other works.

Sallo, Denys de (1626–1669) *See scientific journals.*

Salt, Sir Titus (1803–1876) *See textile industry.*

Samarium A rare earth element with the atomic number of 62, discovered in 1879 by **Paul Emile Lecoq de Boisbaudran** (1838–1912) of Cognac, France.

Sanctorius (1561–1636) *See nutrition, thermometer.*

Sand Dunes The first important study on the physics of sand dunes was done by a British scientist, **Ralph Alger Bagnold** (1896–1990), who published *Libyan Sands* (1935) and *Physics of Blown Sands and Desert Dunes* (1941). His work played an important role in the development of desert warfare. The factors leading to a persistent desert state were studied by an American meteorologist from San Francisco, **Jule Gregory Charney** (1917–1981).

Sandage, Allan Rex (b 1926) *See oscillating theory, quasars.*

Sandby, Thomas (1729–1809) *See architecture, British.*

Sanders, Howard Lawrence (b 1921) *See marine biology.*

Sangallo, Antonio Giambert da (1485–1546) *See military engineering.*

Sanger, Frederick (b 1918) *See deoxyribonucleic acid, insulin.*

Sanmichele, Michele (1484–1559) *See military engineering.*

Sap Pressure *See plant physiology.*

Saponification *See Chevreul, Michel Eugene.*

Sarich, Ralph (b 1938) *See internal combustion engine.*

Sarnoff, David (1891–1971) *See color television.*

Sarpi, Pietro (1552–1623) A clergyman of Venice who discovered the dilatation of the uvea in the eye, valves in human veins and the circulation of blood, which was later demonstrated by **William Harvey** (1578–1757). He experimented on electricity, and wrote on mathematics, astronomy, physics and architecture.

Sars, Michel (1805–1869) *See marine biology.*

Sarton, George Alfred Leon (1884–1956) *See ISIS.*

Satellite [Latin: *satelles*, guard or an attendant] A term initially used for a body orbiting a planet. Of the nine major planets that revolve around the sun, only Venus and Mercury have no natural satellites. Nearly 60 natural satellites in the solar system have been discovered to date. A science fiction writer from Minehead in Somerset, **Arthur Charles Clarke** (b 1917), who was a radar instructor in the Second World War, suggested the idea of satellite communication, in 1946. The US Vanguard project for launching artificial satellites was announced in 1955. The first artificial satellite, *Sputnik 1,* was launched by the Russians in October 1957. The first crewed space flight in history, planned by Korolev and led by **Yuri Alekseyevich Gagarin** (1934–1968), in *Vostok I,* took place on 12 April 1961. The first American satellite, *Explorer I* for space exploration, was launched in 1958. In 1960, an American electrical engineer, **John Robinson Pierce** (b 1910) of Des Moines, Iowa, was mainly instrumental in the launch of *Echo,* which reflected microwave signals to earth. He also contributed to the development of the communication satellite Telstar, which enabled the transmission of live television pictures across the Atlantic in 1962. The weather satellite *Tiros 7,* launched in America in 1963, served as the first spy satellite. *See astronauts, Jupiter, Mars, Neptune, Saturn, Uranus, Venus.*

Saturn The second largest of the planets and sixth in order of distance from the sun. Its motion was explained by the French astronomer, **Pierre Simon Marquis de Laplace** (1749–1827) in his *Traité de Mécanique Céleste* (1799–1825). Saturn's rings were observed by **Galilei Galileo** (1564–1642). An American astronomer, **James Edward Keeler** (1857–1900) of Illinois, used the Doppler displacement of spectral lines and proved that these rings are composed of small fragments. Its different satellites were discovered by several astronomers including **Giovanni Domenico Cassini** (1625–1712) of Nice (Rhea, 1672, Dione and Thetys, 1684), **Christian Huygens** (1629–1695) of the Hague (Iapetus, 1671), **William Cranch Bond** (1789–1859) of Portland, Maine (Hyperion, 1848), **William Henry Pickering** (1858–1938) of Boston, Massachusetts (Phoebe, 1898) and **Audoin Charles Dollfus** (b 1924) of Paris (Janus, 1966). An American astronomer from Connecticut, **Asaph Hall** (1829–1907), discovered a white spot on Saturn and used it as a marker to calculate its rotation period.

Saturn's Rings *See Saturn.*

Sauerbon, Karl Draise von (d 1851) *See bicycle.*

Saunders, Howard (1835–1907) *See ornithology.*

Saunderson, Nicholas (1682–1739) An English professor of mathematics at Cambridge who became blind during his early childhood. In his *Elements of Algebra* published posthumously in 1740, he described palpable arithmetic, which he called a computer for those without sight.

Saussure, Horace Benedict de (1740–1799) *See electrometer, geology, hygrometer.*

Saussure, Nicholas Theodore de (1767–1845) *See photosynthesis, plant nutrition.*

Sauveur, Joseph (1643–1716) *See acoustics.*

Savart, Felix (1791–1841) *See acoustics, polarization, Savart-Biot law.*

Savart-Biot Law Relates to the force or intensity in a magnetic field around a long straight current. Proposed by two French physicists, **Felix Savart** (1791–1841) and **Jean Baptiste Biot** (1774–1862).

Savart's Quartz Plate *See polarization.*

Savart's Wheel *See acoustics.*

Savery, Thomas (1650–1715) *See steam engine.*

Saville, Sir Henry (1549–1622) Warden of Merton College, Oxford and tutor of Greek and mathematics to Queen Elizabeth I, who established the Savillian chairs of astronomy and mathematics at Oxford University in 1619. **Henry Briggs** (1561–1631), a mathematician from Warley Wood, Halifax, was appointed as the first Savillian professor of mathematics in 1619.

Savillian Professorship *See Saville, Sir Henry.*

Saw According to **Pliny, the Elder** (AD 29–79), Talos designed the saw to resemble the jaw of a serpent. An Egyptian tomb built around 1450 BC illustrates the use of a saw by a man on a vertical wooden block.

Saxton, Christopher (1542–1611) *See cartography.*

Sayers, James (b 1912) *See radar.*

Scaliger, Joseph Justus (1540–1609) *See Julian day count.*

Scamozzi, Vincenzo (1552–1616) *See architecture, Italian, theater.*

Scandium An element with an atomic number of 21 discovered in 1879 and named after Scandinavia.

Scanning Electron Microscope (SEM) An electron microscope capable of producing three-dimensional images of 10 to 200 000 times magnification. The first scanning electron picture was produced in 1935 by Max Knoll of the German company Telefunken. The first commercial SEM produced by the Cambridge Instrument Company in the UK went on sale in 1965.

Scanning Tunneling Microscope The most powerful microscope, with a magnification of 100 million, and capable of resolving up to 15 nanometers, invented in 1981 at the IBM Zurich research laboratory. *See electron microscope.*

Schaafhausen, Hermann (1816–1893) *See Neanderthal man.*

Schaefer, Vincent Joseph (1906–1993) *See artificial rain.*

Schawlow, Arthur Leonard (1921–1999) *See Electron Spectroscopy For Chemical Analysis (ESCA), laser, Rydberg constant.*

Scheele, Carl Wilhelm (1742–1786) A Swedish chemist who learnt chemistry as an apprentice under an apothecary at Gothenburg at the age of 14 years. He moved to Uppsala in 1770, and in 1775 purchased an apothecary shop in Köping. He demonstrated the phosphorus content of bone, with **Johan Gottlieb Gahn** (1745–1818), in 1710. Scheele discovered chlorine gas, nitrous acid and barium (1774), molybdenum (1778) and glycerol (1779) which he named 'sweet principle of fats'. He studied the action of light on silver chloride in 1777, and his investigation of Prussian blue in 1782 led to the discovery of hydrocyanic acid. He was the first to prepare lactic acid from sour milk. His work on combustion predated that of **Joseph Priestly** (1733–1804) and **Antoine Lavoisier** (1743–1794). *See acids, air, atmosphere, barium, oxygen, photochemistry, photography, silicon.*

Scheubel, Johann (1494–1570) A professor of mathematics at Tübingen who edited some of the books of Euclid's *Elements.*

Scheutz, Pehr Georg (1785–1873) *See calculating machine.*

Schiaparelli, Giovanni Virginio (1835–1910) *See comet, Mars.*

Schickardt, Wilhelm (1592–1635) *See calculating machine.*

Schimper, Andreas Franz Wilhelm (1856–1901) *See chlorophyll, chloroplasts, ecology, photosynthesis, starch.*

Schimper, Wilhelm Phillip (1808–1880) A German botanist and father of **Andreas Franz Wilhelm Schimper** (1856–1901). He became the director of the Natural History Museum at Strasbourg in 1835 and published several works on botany. He was an authority on mosses.

Schlegel, Friedrich von (1772–1829) *See philology.*

Schleiden, Matthias Jacob (1804–1881) *See cell, cell division.*

Schliemann, Heinrich (1822–1890) *See Mycenae, Troy.*

Schmidt, Bernhard Voldemar (1879–1935) *See reflecting telescope, telescope.*

Schmidt, Ernst Johannes (1877–1933) *See marine biology, oceanography.*

Schmidt, Johann Friedrich Julius (1825–1884) *See Moon.*

Schmidt, Maarten (b 1929) *See quasars, radioastronomy.*

Schmidt Telescope *See telescope.*

Schneider, Friedrich Anton (1831–1890) *See mitosis.*

Schoeffer, Peter (1425–1502) *See color printing, printing.*

Schoengauer, Martin (1450–1491) *See engraving.*

Schoenheimer, Rudolf (1898–1941) *See isotopes, radioisotope studies.*

Schönbein, Christian Friedrich (1799–1868) *See chromatography, explosives, gun-cotton, ozone.*

Schoner, Johanes (1477–1547) *See globe.*

Schott, Kasper (1608–1666) *See air pump.*

Schrieffer, John Robert (b 1931) *See Bardeen–Cooper–Schrieffer theory, superconductivity.*

Schrödinger Equation A wave equation to describe the behavior of electrons in atoms, which formed the basis for wave mechanics. Proposed in 1926 by an Austrian physicist, **Erwin Schrödinger** (1887–1961) of Vienna. A Soviet theoretical physicist, **Vladimir Alexandrovich Fock** (1898–1974) and Oskar Klein independently generalized it to the relativistic case, resulting in the equation known as the Klein–Fock equation.

Schrödinger, Erwin (1887–1961) *See antimatter, atomic structure, matrix mechanics, positron, quantum mechanics, Schrödinger equation.*

Schrotter, Anton (1802–1875) *See matches.*

Schultz, Max Johann Sigismund (1825–1874) *See cell.*

Schumann, Stokes Victor (1841–1913) *See spectroscopy.*

Schuster, Sir Arthur (1851–1934) *See electricity, spectroscopy.*

Schwabe, Samuel Heinrich (1789–1875) *See sunspots.*

Schwann, Theodor (1821–1902) *See cell, cell theory, fermentology.*

Schwartz, Bertholet Michael or **Berthholdus** (c. 1320) *See firearms, gunpowder, military engineering.*

Schwartz, Melvin (b 1932) *See neutrino.*

Schwarz, Harvey Fisher (1905–1988) *See radio.*

Schwarzschild, Karl (1873–1916) *See Black Hole, photographic photometry.*

Schweigger, Johann Salomo (1779–1857) *See galvanometer.*

Schwinger, Julian (1918–1994) *See Feynman diagrams, quantum electrodynamics.*

Science Books *See early science books.*

Science Fiction The first writer on the subject was a mathematican and founder of the Royal Society, **John Wilkins** (1614–1672). His *Discovery of the World in a Moon* (1638) gave an account of a journey to the moon and a description of its inhabitants. One of the first science fiction books, *Voyage au Centre de la Terre* (Journey to the Center of the Earth) was published by a French novelist, **Jules Verne** (1828–1905) of Nantes, in 1864. His *De la Terre à la Lune* (From the Earth to the Moon), the first modern fiction on space travel, appeared in 1865, followed by *Vingt mille lieues sous les mers* (Twenty Thousand Leagues Under the Sea) in 1870. **Herbert George Wells** (1866–1946), an English pioneer of science fiction from Bromley, Kent, published *The Time Machine* (1895), *The War of the Worlds* (1898) and several other science fiction novels. **Frederik Pohl** (b 1919) of Brooklyn, New York, was a science fiction writer for various magazines and he published *Space Merchants* in 1953. **Clifford Donald Simak** (1904–1988) of Milville, Wisconsin started publishing science fiction in 1931, and produced a story sequence *The City* (1952), where robots took over the abandoned world.

Scientific Instruments *See early scientific instruments.*

Scientific Journals One of the first publications in science was by a German astronomer, **Johannes Muller** (1436–1476) from Konigsberg. He established his own printing press at his house in Nuremburg in 1471 and published *Ephemerides* which gave the position of stars, from 1474. The first scientific journal *Journal des Scavans* was published in 1665 in Paris at the initiation of **Denys de Sallo** (1626–1669). Three months after its publication, the secretary of the Royal Society in London, **Henry Oldenburg** (1615–1667) from Bremen, began publishing the monthly *Philosophical Transactions* at his own expense. In 1787, **William Curtis** (1746–1799) founded the *Botanical Magazine,* under the editorship of **Sir William Jackson Hooker** (1785–1865) in England. The Linnean Society started publishing its *Transactions* in 1791. The earliest important biological journal in France, *Annales du Musée d'Histoire Naturelle,* began in 1802. In Germany, the *Archiv für die Physiologie* edited later by the physiologist, **Johannes Peter Muller** (1801–1858), appeared in 1795. The *Proceedings* of the Royal Academy of Sciences of Amsterdam appeared in

1812, followed by *Müller's Archiv* in 1834. The *Magazine of Zoology and Botany* was founded in 1837 by a Scottish naturalist and physician, **Sir William Jardine** (1800–1874). A German professor of chemistry at Berlin, **Johann Christian Poggendorf** (1796–1877), founded and edited the journal *Annalen der physik und Chemie* from 1824 to 1874. The French mathematics journal *Journal des Mathématiques Pures et Appliqués* was founded in 1836 by a French mathematician, **Joseph Liouville** (1809–1882). One of the first English journals on electricity, the *Annals of Electricity*, was started by **William Sturgeon** (1783–1850) in 1836, and it ended in 1843. An early English mathematical journal *Quarterly Journal of Pure and Applied Mathematics* was started in 1855 with a London mathematician, **James Joseph Sylvester** (1814–1897) as its first editor. The scientific journal *Nature* was founded by an English astronomer, **Sir Norman Joseph Lockyer** (1836–1920) in 1869. A British natural philosopher from Bristol, **John Herapath** (1790–1868), published *The Railway Magazine and Annals of Science* from 1836 to 1839. A London molecular physicist and chemist, **Sir William Crookes** (1832–1919), founded the *Chemical News* in 1859. One of the early English periodicals on meterology, *Symon's Monthly Meteorological Magazine,* was founded as a circular in 1860 by an English meteorologist, **George James Symons** (1838–1900). The popular scientific magazine *Knowledge* was founded in 1881 by a London astronomer **Richard Anthony Proctor** (1837–1888). The English botanist **Arthur George Tansley** (1871–1955) founded *The New Phytologist* in 1902, and served as its editor for 30 years. The mathematical journal *Fundamenta Mathematicae* was founded in 1919 by a Polish mathematician, **Wactaw Sierpinski** (1882–1969) from Warsaw, who published over 700 papers on topology, number theory and mathematical logic. *See American Scientific Journals.*

Scientist [Latin: *scio*, to know] A term coined by a British scholar, **William Whewell** (1794–1866) of Lancaster, at a meeting of the British Association for the Advancement of Science at Glasgow in 1833. He popularized the new term through his work *The philosophy of inductive sciences*, in 1840.

Scintillation Count *See Geiger counter.*

Scopas of Ephesus (*c.* 430 BC) *See architecture, ancient.*

Scoresby, William (1789–1857) *See Arctic regions, North Pole.*

Scott, Dunkinfield Henry (1854–1934) *See paleophytology.*

Scott, Sir George Gilbert (1811–1878) *See architecture, British.*

Scott, Sir Giles Gilbert (1880–1960) *See architecture, British.*

Scott, Michael (*c.* 1175–1230) A Scottish astrologer and writer who studied at Oxford. He translated Arabic versions of Aristotle's works.

Scott, Sir Walter (1771–1832) *See bookshops.*

Screw *See Archimedian screw, lathe, Whitworth screw.*

Screw Propeller *See steamships.*

Scripps, James Edmund (1835–1906) *See newspapers.*

Scrolls Long sheets of parchment or papyrus usually attached at each end to a wooden rod. Ancient libraries contained thousands of these scrolls. *See cave exploration, libraries, writing materials.*

Scrope, G. Poulett (1787–1876) *See volcanoes.*

Scuba (**S**elf-**c**ontained **u**nderwater **b**reathing **a**pparatus). *See aqualung.*

Scudder, Samuel Hubbard (1837–1911) *See entomology.*

Sea *See oceanography.*

Seaborg, Glenn Theodore (1912–1999) *See americium, berkelium, californium, curium, einsteinium, mendelevium, plutonium.*

Seaplane An American inventor, **Glen Hammond Curtiss** (1878–1930) from Hammondsport, New York, designed and flew the first practical seaplane in 1911.

Secchi, Pietro Angelo (1818–1878) *See astrophysics, Milky Way, spectroscopy, stars.*

Sedgwick, Adam (1785–1873) *See Cambrian period, Devonian period, Paleozoic period, Sedgwick Museum.*

Sedgwick Museum Museum of Geology at Cambridge, named after **Adam Sedgwick** (1785–1873), a geologist from Yorkshire. He identified the Devonian and Cambrian systems in England and published *British Paleozoic Fossils,* in 1854.

Seebeck, Thomas Johan (1770–1831) *See thermocouple.*

Seebohm, Henry (1832–1895) *See ornithology.*

Seeds The founder of botany, **Theophrastus** (380–287 BC), in his *Historia Plantarum* (History of plants) described the process of germination of plants from their seeds. His description includes morphology of different species of seedlings and their duration of germination. A classification based on single-leafed seeds (monocotyledons) and two-leafed seeds (dicotyledons) was proposed by

Lobelius or **Matthias de l'Obel** (1538–1616) of the Netherlands, in his *New Note-book of Plants*. *See vernalization.*

Seeliger, Hugo (1849–1924)   A German professor of astronomy at Munich and director of the observatory there. He proposed the nebula theory for the birth of a nova.

Sefström, Nils Gabriel (1787–1854)   *See vanadium.*

Segre, Emilio (1905–1989)   *See antiproton, masurium.*

Seguin, Marc (1786–1875)   *See suspension bridges, thermodynamics.*

Seismograph [Greek: *seismos*, earthquake + *graphein*, to write]   *See earthquakes, seismology.*

Seismology [Greek: *seismos*, earthquake + *logos*, discourse] An early version of a seismograph, which indicated the direction of an earthquake by dropping a ball from the mouth of a bronze dragon into the mouth of a bronze frog, was invented in AD 132 by **Zhang Heng** (AD 78–139) of China. An English geologist, **John Michell** (1724–1793), following the major earthquake in Lisbon in 1755 in which 70 000 people died, suggested that earthquakes set up wave motions in the earth. A modern instrument for measuring these movements was invented in 1854 by an Italian meteorologist and a professor at Naples, **Luigi Palmieri** (1807–1896), who served as the director of the Vesuvius observatory. Another was described by Robert Mallet in 1858, and an American model was installed at the Lick Observatory, in California, in 1888. In 1892, an English mining engineer, **John Milne** (1859–1913) from Liverpool, developed a seismometer for precision measurement of the horizontal movements of the earth, and published *Earthquakes and other Earth Movements* (1886) and *Seismology* (1898). He established a private seismological observatory on the Isle of Wight, from where he issued regular seismological data. The inverted pendulum type of seismometer was invented by Emil Weichart in 1900. An Irish geologist and seismologist, **Richard Dixon Oldham** (1858–1936) of Dublin, distinguished between primary and secondary seismic waves in 1897, and established the existence of the earth's core, using seismographic records, in 1906. The Richter scale was invented in 1930 by **Charles Francis Richter** (1900–1985) of Hamilton, Ohio, and it was developed and named after him in 1954. A system of unprecedented seismographic accuracy of 0.1 second was devised by an American geophysicist, **Victor Hugo Benioff** (1899–1968) of Los Angeles. In 1974 a Japanese-born US seismologist, **Keiiti Aki** (b 1930), developed seismic tomography with a three-dimensional aspect, which gave the first quantitative estimate of the earth's tremors during volcanic eruptions. An American geophysicist, **Leon Knopoff** (b 1925) of Los Angeles, devised the first representation theorem for a full seismic wave equation, in 1956. *See earthquake, Wadati–Benioff zones.*

Selby, Prideaux John (1788–1857)   *See ornithology.*

Selenium [Greek: *selene*, moon]   Discovered by a Swedish chemist **Johan Gottlieb Gahn** (1745–1818). Another Swedish chemist, **Jons Jacob Berzelius** (1779–1848), observed it to be a new element in 1818. Its importance in photochemistry was discovered by W. Smith in 1873.

Semaphore [Greek: *sema*, sign + *phoros*, bearer]   An optical device for transmission of messages or images. The first, consisting of a series of discs and shutters, was devised in England in 1767 by an Anglo-Irish inventor, **Richard Lowell Edgeworth** (1744–1817) from Bath, and it was used to transmit the results of horse races. An improved model was invented in 1793 by a French engineer, **Claude Chappe** (1763–1805) of Brulon, Sarthe, and it continued to be used extensively in France up to 1851. Semaphore capable of transmitting words from a semaphore alphabet was invented around 1890.

Semenov, Nikolay Nicolaevich (1896–1986)   The first Soviet Nobel Prize winner and a physical chemist who studied the velocity of accelerated branched-chain reactions. He shared the Nobel Prize for chemistry in 1956, for his work, with **Cyril Norman Hinshelwood** (1897–1967).

Semiconductors   Crystalline material with a degree of electrical conductivity between that of metals and poor conductors such as insulators. They are made of materials such as selenium, germanium and silicon, the conductivity of which can usually be improved by minute additions of different substances or by other factors. The first attempt to replace thermionic valves with semiconductor devices was made by **John Bardeen** (1908–1991) of Madison, Wisconsin, and **Walter Houser Brattain** (1902–1987). *See Esaki diode, transistor.*

Semipermeable Membrane   The first artificial membrane for determination of osmotic pressure was made by a German wine merchant and physiologist, **Moritz Traube** (1826–1894). *See osmosis.*

Semper, Gottfried (1803–1873)   *See architecture, British.*

Senderens, Jean Baptiste (1856–1936)   *See hydrogenation, soap.*

Senebier, Jean (1742–1809)   *See photosynthesis.*

Seneca, Lucius Annaeus (d AD 65) *See convex lens, earthquake, gravity, optics, spectacles.*

Sennefelder, Alois (1771–1834) *See lithography.*

Serlio, Sebastiano (1475–1554) *See architecture, Italian.*

Sertürner, Friedrich Wilhelm (1783–1841) *See morphine.*

Seward, Sir Albert Charles (1863–1941) *See paleophytology.*

Sewing Machine The first sewing machine, made of wood and brass, was patented in 1790 by Thomas Saint in England, but it proved to be of no practical use. A French tailor, **Bathelèmy Thimonnier** (1793–1857), built a practical machine in 1830, but it was destroyed by workmen who considered it to be a threat to their livelihood. An American invention by Walter Hunt in 1832 met with the same fate. Prior to the 1840s sewing was a laborious process, as it had to be entirely done by hand. **Elias Howe** (1819–1867), the son of a poor farmer from Spencer, in Massachusetts, started working on a device to overcome this difficulty in 1841, and after five years of work he invented the sewing machine and patented it in 1846. As it was not a success in America, he sold the rights to an Englishman, Thomas, for a sum of 250 GBP, and came to England to adopt it for making corsets. On his return to America he found that his patent had been pirated by **Isaac Merrit Singer** (1811–1875) of Pittstown, New York, and several others. He then fought a legal battle and in 1854 won the sole rights to the machine for the next 13 years. He patented his continuous-stitch sewing machine in 1851. An American inventor, **John Wesley Hyatt** (1837–1920) from Starkey, New York, invented a multiple-needle sewing machine. The first electric sewing machine was introduced in 1889.

Sextant [Latin: *sextus,* sixth] A navigational instrument that utilizes an arc of one-sixth of a circle for determining latitude. It was developed from the reflecting quadrant, which used 90 degrees, by the Danish astronomer **Tycho Brahe** (1546–1601), who used it to calculate the motions of planets. The modern octant, using one-eighth of a circle, was developed by **Sir Isaac Newton** (1642–1727) around 1700, and it was improved by **John Hadley** (1682–1774) in 1731. An English navy captain, John Campbell, extended its arc to 120 degrees in 1757.

Seyfert Galaxies A special group of galaxies with bright bluish star-like nuclei, first studied by an American astronomer, **Carl Keenan Seyfert** (1911–1960) of Cleveland, Ohio. They were later identified as a type of low-luminosity quasars.

Seyfert, Carl Keenan (1911–1960) *See Seyfert galaxies.*

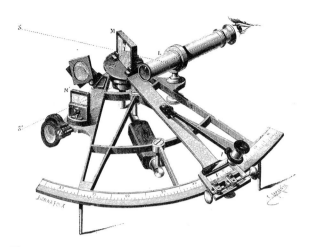

Figure 72 A mid-19th century sextant. Guillemin, Amédée. *The Application of Physical Forces.* London: Macmillan and Co, 1877

Shackleton, Sir Ernest Henry (1874–1922) *See magnetic poles.*

Shannon, Claude Elwood (b 1916) *See computers.*

Shapley, Harlow (1885–1972) *See cepheid variables, Milky Way,*

Sharman, Helen (b 1963) *See astronauts.*

Sharp, Phillip Allen (b 1944) *See ribonucleic acid.*

Sharp, William (1749–1824) *See engraving.*

Sharpe, Richard Bowdler (1847–1909) A Scottish ornithologist and one of the founders of the British Ornithology Club. He compiled most of the British Museum's *Catalogue of Birds* (1874–1898) while he was a member of staff there.

Sharpey-Schafer, Sir Edward Albert (1850–1935) *See insulin.*

Shaw, Sir William Napier (1854–1945) *See meteorology, tephigram.*

Shen Kua (1031–1095) *See canals, compass (1), shipping.*

Shepard, Alan Bartlett (1923–1998) *See astronauts.*

Shepard, Francis Parker (1897–1985) *See oceanography.*

Sheraton, Thomas (1751–1806) An English furniture designer from Stockton-on-Tees, who settled in London. He made furniture designing an art as well as a craft with his *The Cabinet-Maker and Upholsterer's Drawing Book* (1791–1794) and the *Cabinet Dictionary* (1803).

Sherman, Henry Clapp (1875–1955) *See nutrition.*

Shillibeer, George (1797–1866)   *See coaches, omnibus.*

Shipping   The use of a magnetic compass for navigation was first suggested by a Chinese scientist, **Shen Kua** (1031–1095) in 1086. The Arabians used the magnetic needle for navigation around 1300. An English scholar, **Alexander Neckham** (1157–1217) of St Albans, in his *De Naturis rerum* and *De utensilibus*, was the first in Europe to describe the use of a magnetic needle by sailors. The phenomenon of the magnetic deflection of a needle in relation to navigation was first studied in Europe by a London navigator and naval instrument maker, **Robert Norman** (1550–1600), in 1576. He published *Safeguard of Saylors*, translated from the Dutch, in 1590. This contained maps of the coast as seen from the sea. The first mention of the practice of insuring ships is found in Guicciardini's account of the Netherlands in 1567. In this, he referred to merchants from Antwerp who were accustomed to insuring their ships. The ship's log for keeping a record of the speed of the ship is supposed to have been invented by Humphry Cole in 1573. **Christian Huyghens** (1629–1693), a Dutch physicist from the Hague, designed a marine clock for reading the standard time at sea and for the purpose of determining longitude. The first practical marine chronometer was invented by a London instrument maker, **John Harrison** (1692–1776) from Foulby, Yorkshire, and his device won the British Board of Longitude Prize, for finding a practical way for determining longitude at sea. A Swiss clockmaker, **Ferdinand Berthoud** (1727–1807), improved it and published *Traité des l'Horloges Marines* (1773). A mathematician based in London, **William Jones** (1680–1749) from Anglesey, published *Art of Navigation* in 1702. A practical guide for mariners, *The British Mariner's Guide* (1763), was published by a London astronomer, **Nevil Maskelyne** (1732–1811), who initiated the *Nautical Almanac* in 1766. The lifeboat was invented by Lionel Lukin, a coach builder from Dunmow, Essex. It consisted of a series of airtight chambers to give buoyancy and was patented in 1785. **Henry Greathead** (1787–1816), a boatbuilder from Richmond, Yorkshire, after hearing of the tragic wreck of the *Adventure* at the mouth of the River Tyne in 1789, built an admirable lifeboat in 1789, which was bought by the Duke of Northumberland and presented to the people of North Shields. In 1869, **Samuel Plimsoll** (1824–1898), a member of parliament for Derby, England, known as the sailor's friend, introduced a compulsory mark on every ship indicating maximum load, and published *Our Seamen* (1873). This line, later known as the Plimsoll line, was made obligatory through the Merchant Shipping Act of 1876, which was enacted for the purpose of improving the safety of passengers and the crew. A patent slip for docking vessels,

as a substitute for the dry dock, was invented in 1819 by a Scottish ship-builder **Thomas Morton** (1781–1832). An American engineer, **Robert Bowie Owen** (1870–1940) of Maryland, invented electromagnetic direction control for navigation. The gyrocompass to overcome the inaccuracy of the magnetic needle in iron or metal ships, was introduced around 1900. *See atomic ships, boats, sailing ships, ships.*

Ships   *See atomic ships, marine engineering, sailing ships, shipping, steamships, warships.*

Shklovsky, Josef Samuilovich (1916–1985)   *See synchroton radiation.*

Shockley, William Bradford (1910–1989)   *See radio, transistor.*

Shorthand   The ancient Egyptians, the Persians and the Greeks used symbols or pictures to represent words and phrases. The first intentional shorthand was invented by **Marcus Tullius Tiro** (*c.* AD 100), who was a friend and biographer of the Roman orator and philosopher, Cicero. His method, known as the Tironian system, was taught in Roman schools, and continued to be used widely for several centuries up to AD 900. An English physician, **Timothy Bright** (1551–1615), proposed a method of shorthand in his *An Arte of Shorte, Swifte* and *Secrete writing by Character*. A system was invented by **Sir Isaac Pitman** (1813–1897), a teacher from Trowbridge, Wiltshire, who published *Stenographic Sound Hand* (1837). In 1839 he established the Phonetic Institute at Bath for teaching shorthand. His brother **Benjamin Pitman** (1822–1910) introduced the system into America in 1852, and formed the Phonetic Institute in Cincinnati in 1853. The German system was invented by a civil servant, **Franz Xavior Gabelsberger** (1789–1848) of Munich, around 1830. A new system was developed by an Irishman, **John Robert Gregg** (1867–1948) from Shantonagh, Monaghan, who wrote the *Gregg Shorthand Manual* (1888). He emigrated to America in 1893 and established a publishing house there. His other works include *Gregg Speed Studies* (1917) and *American Shorthand Teacher* (1920).

Shrapnel Shell   An artillery shell fused and filled with small spheres with a small charge of gunpowder for exploding at a predetermined time. Invented in 1784 by a British artillery officer, **Henry Shrapnel** (1761–1842) of Bradford-on-Avon, Wiltshire.

Shrapnel, Henry (1761–1842)   *See Shrapnel shell.*

SI Units (Système International d'Unités)   Standard system of scientific units proposed in 1960. By international agreement, seven base quantities, regarded as being dimensionally independent, were agreed: the meter, kilogram, second, ampere, kelvin, mole and candela.

Siderostat An astronomical telescope with its optical axis invariably fixed in a horizontal position, in order to keep the celestial object fixed to the eye-piece, to avoid the effect of motion caused by diurnal rotation. It was first suggested by **Robert Hooke** (1635–1703), and constructed by **Jean Bernard Léon Foucault** (1819–1868).

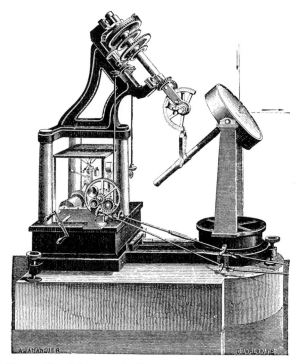

Figure 73 Siderostat. Guillemin, Amédée. *The Application of Physical Forces*. London: Macmillan and Co, 1877

Sidgwick, Nevil Vincent (1873–1952) *See valency.*

Siebold, Carl Theodor Ernst von (1804–1885) *See protozoa.*

Siebold, Philipp Franz von (1796–1866) *See horticulture.*

Siegbahn, Kai Manne Börje (b 1918) *See electron spectroscopy for chemical analysis, laser, Rydberg constant.*

Siegbahn, Karl Manne Georg (1886–1978) *See X-ray spectroscopy.*

Siegen, Ludwig von (1609–1675) *See engraving, mezzotint process.*

Siemans, Friedrich (1826–1904) *See steel.*

Siemen Unit An SI unit of electrical conductance named after **Ernst Werner von Siemens** (1816–1892) of Berlin, who determined the electrical resistance of different substances.

Siemens, Sir Charles William, originally **Karl Wilhelm Siemens** (1823–1883) *See locomotive, steel, tram car, Xerox copier.*

Siemens, Ernst Werner von (1816–1892) *See dynamo, siemen unit, tram car.*

Siemens, Wilhelm (1855–1919) A son of **Ernst Werner von Siemens** (1816–1892), and pioneer of the incandescent lamp.

Sierpinski, Wactaw (1882–1969) *See scientific journals.*

Signals *See flag signalling, heliograph, Morse code, railway signals, semaphore, traffic signal.*

Sikorsky, Igor Ivan (1889–1972) *See helicopter.*

Silicon [Latin: *silex*, flint] A German chemist, **Johann Joachim Becher** (1635–1682) studied its presence in earth, and its use in glass-making. Silicon tetrafluoride was obtained by a Swedish apothecary and chemist, **Carl Wilhelm Scheele** (1742–1786) in 1771. Two French chemists, **Joseph Louis Gay-Lussac** (1778–1850) and **Louis Jacques Thenard** (1777–1857) used the compound to obtain a combustible form in 1809. **Jons Jacob Berzelius** (1779–1848) discovered the basic element in 1823. **Henri Étienne Saint-Claire Deville** (1818–1881), a French chemist of West Indian origin, obtained crystalline silicon, in 1854. Silicon carbide was discovered in 1879 by a French chemist **Ferdinand Frederic Henri Moissan** (1852–1907), who was a demonstrator at the École de Pharmacie, Paris.

Silicon Chip *See computers, semiconductor.*

Silicones [Latin: *silex*, flint] *See polymer.*

Silk *See artificial silk, silkworms.*

Silkworms First cultured in China. The wife of the Emperor Huang-ti is supposed to have been the first to unroll a cocoon, and she made silk cloth around 2700 BC. Silkworms were first brought from India to Europe in the 6th century. The first microscopic dissection of an invertebrate (silkworm) was performed by **Marcello Malpighi** (1628–1694), in 1669. **Agostino Bassi** (1773–1856), an Italian lawyer and farmer, was the first to demonstrate fungi as the cause of muscardine disease of the silkworm in 1835.

Silliman, Benjamin (1779–1864) *See American Journal of Science.*

Silliman, Benjamin (1816–1885) *See American Journal of Science, petroleum.*

Silurian Period A geological era of mostly marine forms and limestone, starting around 439–409 million years ago, and lasting for 40 milllion years. It was identified and named after a Celtic tribe, the *Silures,* in 1835, by a Scottish geologist, **Roderick Impey Murchison** (1792–1871) of Tarradale, who published *The Silurian System* (1839). A study of fossils in Devon, between the Silurian and Carboniferous periods, was carried out in 1837 by a geologist from Bath, **William Londsdale** (1794–1871).

Silver [Anglo-Saxon: *soelfor*] The most malleable and ductile metal next to gold. It was more expensive than gold during predynastic times in Egypt up to 1500 BC, and it was used for coin making in the 8th century during the reign of the King of Argos. The Goggerdan mines in Aberystwyth, Wales, were an important source in Great Britain around the 16th century. The symbol *Ag* is taken from the latin term *argentum* for silver.

Silver Plating In 1742, an English cutler of Sheffield, Thomas Bolsover, noticed that copper and silver could be made to adhere firmly, by being beaten and rolled together. Following his observation he developed a process of silver plating or veneering on a copper base. This remained a major industry for nearly a century, until commercial electrodeposition of silver was introduced in 1840. In 1825, a German chemist, **Justus von Liebig** (1803–1873), noticed that when ammoniacal silver nitrate was warmed with acetaldehyde, it resulted in a deposit of brilliant metallic silver on the surface of the vessel, and his discovery formed the basis for silvering mirrors. *See electroplating.*

Simak, Clifford Donald (1904–1988) *See science fiction.*

Simon, Sir Francis Eugen (1893–1956) *See thermodynamics.*

Simpson, Sir George Clark (1878–1965) *See Beaufort scale, lightning, meteorology, wind.*

Simpson, George Gaylord (1902–1984) An American paleontologist from Chicago who proposed an important classification for mammals. He published *Tempo and Mode in Evolution* (1944), *The Meaning of Evolution* (1949) and several other books.

Simpson, James Y. (1811–1870) *See chloroform.*

Simpson, Robert (1687–1768) *See Euclid.*

Simpson, Thomas (1710–1761) *See Simpson's rule.*

Simpson's Rule Used for calculation of areas under graphic curves, devised by an English mathematician, **Thomas Simpson** (1710–1761) of Leicestershire.

Sinclair, Sir John (1754–1835) *See agriculture.*

Sines The Hindu mathematician **Aryabhata** (AD 475–550) of Patna gave a table of natural sines of the angles in trigonometry. **Georg von Peuerbach** (1423–1461) of Austria used sines in trigonometry and compiled a sine table, but he died before completing it. His pupil and a German astronomer, **Regiomontanus** (1436–1476) from Konigsberg, completed his table of sines.

Singer, Isaac Merritt (1811–1875) An inventor from Pittstown, New York, who founded the Singer Sewing Company. He developed a single-thread chain-stitch sewing machine in 1852. *See sewing machine.*

Siren Invented and named by a French Chemist and physicist, **Charles de la Tour Cagniard** (1777–1859), who used it to study the vibrations of various pitches.

Sirius The brightest star in the nothern sky with a luminosity 26 times that of the sun. The Ancient Egyptians knew it as *Sothis,* and used its appearance to calculate time and dates. Their calendar of 12 months was pegged to it. The British astronomer **Edmund Halley** (1656–1742) described its position, in 1718. Its companian star, Sirius B, was discovered in 1841 by a German astronomer, **Friedrich Wilhelm Bessel** (1784–1846), who was the first to measure the distance of a star.

Sitter, Willem de (1872–1934) A Dutch cosmologist and physicist who proposed an expanding universe of constantly decreasing curvature, as an alternative solution to Einstein's equations on general relativity. His theory was based on the concept of 'motion with no matter', as compared to Einstein's static concept 'matter with no motion'.

Skraup, Zdenko Hans (1850–1910) *See quinoline.*

Slater, Samuel (1768–1835) *See textile industry.*

Slide Rule The forerunner of the slide rule, Gunter's line, was invented by an English astronomer and mathematician, **Edmund Gunter** (1581–1626) of Hertfordshire. **William Oughtred** (1575–1660) of Eton, in England, invented the modern slide rule in 1621.

Slipher, Vesto Melvin (1875–1969) *See galaxy.*

Sloane, Sir Hans (1660–1753) *See museum.*

Smagorinsky, Joseph (b 1924) *See weather forecast.*

Smeaton Club For engineers in London. Named after an English engineer, **John Smeaton** (1724–1792) from Austhorpe, near Leeds. He designed Ramsgate Harbour in 1774 and improved **Thomas Newcomen's** (1663–1729) steam engine. He improved the air pump in 1752.

Smeaton, John (1724–1792) *See canals, cement, civil engineering, lighthouses, Smeaton Club, waterwheels.*

Smelting Extraction of a metal from its ore. **Anacharasis** of Scythia who lived around 569 BC is supposed to have invented the bellows for the purpose of smelting. **Theodorus** (*c.* 530 BC), from the Greek island of Samos, has also been credited with the invention of smelting, for the purpose of making objects such as locks and keys.

Smirke, Sir Robert (1781–1867) *See architecture, British.*

Smirke, Sydney (1799–1877) *See architecture, British.*

Smith, Francis Graham (b 1923) *See pulsar.*

Smith, Hamilton Othanel (b 1931) *See genetic engineering.*

Smith, Henry John Stephen (1826–1883) *See law of quadratic reciprocity, number theory.*

Smith, Horace (1808–1893) *See firearms.*

Smith, James (1789–1850) *See agricultural instruments.*

Smith, James Edward (1759–1828) *See Linnean Society.*

Smith, Michel (b 1932) *See polymerase chain reaction.*

Smith, Sir Francis Petit (1808–1874) *See steamships.*

Smith, Walter Sydney (1876–1956) *See Mount Wilson Observatory.*

Smith, William (1769–1839) *See fossils, geological map, geology, petrology, stratigraphy.*

Smith, William Henry (1792–1865) *See bookshops.*

Smithsonian Institution Founded by an English mineralogist and geologist, **James Lewis Macie Smithson** (1765–1829), who was an illegitimate son of Sir Hugh Smithson Percy (1715–1786), first Duke of Northumberland. His mother was a descendent of King Henry VII. He published a few treatises in the *Philosophical Transactions of the Royal Society* up to 1817. His intention to start a rival institution may have been triggered by the rejection of one of his treatises by the Royal Society of London in 1826. He bequeathed a sum of 105 000 GBP to his nephew, Henry James Hungerford, but stipulated that if he died without an heir the money was to be used to found 'at Washington, under the name of the Smithsonian Institution, an Establishment for the increase and diffusion of knowledge among men'. Accordingly the institution was established by an Act of Congress in 1846, with the American physicist and inventor of the first electromagnetic motor, **Joseph Henry** (1797–1878) of Albany, New York, as its first secretary.

Smithson, James Lewis Macie (1765–1829) *See Smithsonian Institution.*

Smoluchowski, M. (1872–1917) *See Brownian movement.*

Smythson, Robert (1534–1614) *See architecture, British.*

Snell, Willebrord (1591–1626) *See law of refraction, Snell's law, surveying.*

Snell's Law Law of refraction which states that the ratio of the sines of the angles of the incident and refracted rays to the normal is a constant. Discovered in 1624 by Snellius or **Willebrord Snell** (1591–1626), a professor of mathematics at Leyden. It was first made known by **Christian Huygens** (1629–1695) in his *Dioptrica*.

Snowflakes The hexagonal nature of the snowflake was known to the Chinese as early as 200 BC. This was first observed in Europe in 1591 by an English mathematician and astronomer, **Thomas Harriot** (1560–1621) of Oxford.

Snowmobile Motorized sled invented in 1959 by Canadian J Armand Bombardier.

Soane, Sir John (1753–1837) *See architecture, British.*

Soap According to **Pliny the Elder** (AD 28–79) it is a Gallic invention. It was probably made earlier in Germany, using goat tallow and beechwood ashes. Initially used as an ointment, it was used as a detergent in AD 100. A legend attributes its origin to a mixture of fat obtained from animals sacrificed on Sapo Hill, Rome. Marseilles became the center of soap manufacture in Europe around AD 1000, and soap making commenced in England in the 14th century. The process of hydrogenation of oil used in the large-scale production of soap was invented by two French chemists, **Paul Sabatier** (1854–1941) and **Jean Baptiste Senderens** (1856–1936). Sabatier was awarded the Nobel Prize for chemistry with **François Auguste Victor Grignard** (1871–1935), in 1912. Around 1886 an English industrialist, **William Hesketh Lever Leverhulme** (1851–1925), started producing soap from vegetable oils, instead of tallow. Fritz Gunter of Germany made the first soapless detergent in 1907. The physical chemistry of soap solutions, based on ions or ionic micelles, was explained in 1910 by a Canadian physical chemist, **James William McBain** (1882–1953).

Soap Bubble *See surface chemistry.*

Soap Film *See surface chemistry.*

Sobrero, Ascanio (1812–1888) *See explosives.*

Societas Ereunitica First German scientific academy founded at Rostock in 1622.

Socrates (470–399 BC) An Athenian philosopher who is regarded as the founder of inductive reasoning and abstract definitions. He left no writings and most of his works were made known through Plato (428–347 BC) and Xenophon. Plato met Socrates at the age of 20, and remained his pupil for eight years. Socrates was a censor of public wrongs and private follies and opposed state tyrants, which eventually earned him a death sentence.

Soda A Scottish chemist **James Keir** (1735–1820) of Edinburgh, who is regarded as the founder of the scientific chemical industry, began making caustic soda from sulfates of waste products in his Tipton Alkalie Works, in 1780. A British industrial chemist, **James Mushett** (1793–1886) from Dublin, started making soda on a large scale at Liverpool, using the Leblanc process. Following his success he opened several factories in other parts of Britain. *See Kellner process, Leblanc process, Solvay process.*

Soddy, Frederick (1877–1965) An English physicist from Eastbourne, who studied radioactivity with **Lord Ernest Rutherford** (1871–1937) at McGill University, Montreal. Working with **William Ramsay** (1852–1916) in 1903 he demonstrated that helium was produced by the decay of radium. He was awarded the Nobel Prize for chemistry in 1921. *See atomic disintegration, helium, isotopes, protactinium, radioactivity.*

Sodium The symbol Na for sodium or *natrium* was adopted according to the nomenclature proposed in 1811 by **Jons Jacob Berzelius** (1779–1848). **Pliny the Elder** (AD 28–79) was probably the first to use the term *natrium* for sodium carbonate. An Irish physicist and professor of mathematics at Cambridge, **Sir George Gabriel Stokes** (1819–1903), during his pioneering experiments, using a prism on the flame produced by the spirit lamp, identified the characteristic spectrum of sodium. A method for isolating sodium from brine, by electrolysis, was invented by a New York chemist, **Hamilton Young Castner** (1859–1899), who moved to Britain in 1886 and established a chemical factory at Oldbury.

Soil Erosion An English naturalist, **John Ray** (1628–1705) in 1692 suggested that erosion would reduce the land to sea level. The first systematic study of the cycle of erosion was done by an American professor of geology at Harvard, **William Morris Davis** (1850–1935). He introduced the concept of cycles of erosion.

Soil Science The study of soil in relation to plant growth. Multiple cropping in the same year was practiced in China around 1400 BC, and their farmers used manure as a fertilizer around 500 BC. The first conference on biological problems related to the soil (agrogeology) was held in 1909 at Budapest, and it led to the establishment of the International Society of Soil Science in Rome in 1924. The American journal *Soil Science* appeared in 1916. *See agriculture, agronomy, fertilizers, soil erosion.*

Solar Eclipse The first recorded date of a solar eclipse was probably 28th May 585 BC. The Medes and Lydians who fought a war on this day became frightened by the eclipse and called off hostilities. A solar eclipse was recorded by the Babylonians in 763 BC and the Chinese recorded a solar eclipse in 720 BC. The Greek philosopher **Anaxagoras** (*c.* 500–428 BC) correctly explained lunar and solar eclipses. An English astronomer, **Francis Baily** (1774–1844) from Newbury, Berkshire, observed the solar eclipse in 1842 and described the solar corona. The first photograph of a solar eclipse was taken in 1860 by **Warren de la Rue** (1815–1889) of Guernsey, with his invention of the photoheliographic telescope.

Solar Energy In 1748 a French astronomer and mathematician, **Pierre Bouguer** (1698–1758), invented a heliometer for measuring the light from the sun. A device that produced an electrical output when exposed to light was invented in 1896 by a German physicist, **Johann Phillip Julius Elster** (1854–1920) and his colleague **Hans Friedrich Geitel** (1855–1923), who was a professor at the Brunswick Technical Institute. Their invention formed the basis of the solar-powered photoelectric cell. An American physicist from Wilton, New Hampshire, **Charles Greely Abbot** (1872–1973), invented a device for converting solar energy to power and published *The Sun* in 1907. The largest solar power plant consisting of 1818 concentric mirrors, the *Solar I*, was tested in California, in 1982. The *Solar Challenger*, flown by the American aircraft designer **Paul MacCready** (b 1925) in 1980, was the first plane to fly entirely under solar power, and it made a cross-Channel flight in the following year.

Solar Magnetograph A device for making detailed observations of the sun's magnetic field. Invented in 1951 by an

American physicist, **Harold Delos Babcock** (1882–1968) of Wisconsin.

Solar Power *See solar energy.*

Solar System Refers to the sun and all the bodies orbiting around it. A Greek philosopher from the island of Samos, **Aristarchos** (*c.* 320–250 BC), initiated the heliocentric theory that the sun is the center of the solar system and the planets revolve around it. The modern study of the origin of the earth as part of the solar system was commenced in 1640 by **René Descartes** (1596–1650). According to his *Principles of Philosophy* (1644), the origin of the earth was a glowing mass, like the sun. A French mathematician, **Pierre Simon Marquis de Laplace** (1749–1827), proposed that the planetary bodies in the solar system were formed by the condensation of nebulous, diffuse primordial matter that was previously distributed in space. **Thomas Chrowder Chamberlin** (1843–1928), a professor of geology at Chicago, did fundamental work on the geology of the solar system and published *The Origin of the Earth* (1916), *Two Solar Families* (1928), *Sun's children* (1928) and several other books. In 1944 a German physicist, **Baron Carl Friedrich von Weizsäcker** (b 1912), suggested that multiple vortices, formed by a spinning gaseous mass, preceded the solar system. An American astronomer, **Fred Lawrence Wheeler** (b 1906), who was an expert on the solar system, published *Earth, Moon and Planets* in 1941. The US spaceprobe *Pioneer 10* was the first human-created object to achieve a velocity adequate to leave the solar system, in 1983.

Solar Wind Continuous stream of high-speed particles from the sun, which serve as a driving force behind the tails of comets. Predicted in 1951 by a German astronomer, **Ludwig Bierman** (1907–1986), and later confirmed by Russian space probes.

Soldering A method of joining two metals with the use of an alloy that melts easily, invented by Glaucus of Chios in 700 BC. In 1839 Isaac Babbit prepared a solder made of an alloy of tin, antimony and copper. Most of the present alloys used for soldering consist mainly of tin and lead.

Sollas, William Johnson (b 1849) *See petrology.*

Solute A term for the dissolved solid in a solution, introduced by an English mineralogist, **Mervyn Herbert Nevil Story-Maskelyne** (1823–1911) of Wiltshire, who published *Morphology of Crystals* (1895).

Solvay Process Also known as the ammonia–soda process. An economical way of producing soda (sodium carbonate) by passing carbon dioxide through a solution of common salt saturated with ammonia. Invented in 1863 by a Belgian industrial chemist, **Ernest Solvay** (1838–1922).

Solvay, Ernest (1838–1922) *See Leblanc process, Solvay process.*

Somerset, Edward (*c.* 1601–1667), the second Marquis of Worcester. *See steam engine.*

Somerville, Mary Greig (1780–1872) A Scottish astronomer and mathematician in London who wrote on physics, astronomy and other subjects. Somerville College at Oxford was named after her in 1879.

Sommerfeld, Arnold Johannes Wilhelm (1868–1951) *See conductivity, gyroscope.*

Sommerville, Duncan Maclaren Young (1879–1934) *See non-Euclidean geometry.*

Sonar *See ultrasound.*

Sopwith, Thomas Octave Murdoch (1888–1989) *See warplanes.*

Sorby, Henry Clifton (1826–1908) *See microscope, petrology.*

Sørenson, Søren Peter Lauritz (1868–1939) *See acidity or pH, buffer, osmosis,*

Sosigenes (*c.* 100 BC) *See Julian calendar.*

Soufflot, Jacques Germain (1713–1780) *See architecture, European.*

Sound A Greek mathematician, **Archytas of Tarentum** (428–347 BC), stated that there cannot be sound without one body striking another. He also realized that there are many sounds that the human ear cannot hear. **Aristotle** (384–322 BC) in his treatises, *On the Soul* and *De Audibulis*, dealt with the production, nature, conduction and perception of sound. The importance of consonance in sound to music was pointed out by a Roman philosopher, **Anicus Manlius Severinus Boethius** (AD 480–524) in his *De Institutione Musica*. *See acoustics, musical theory of sound, ultrasound, velocity of sound, Wood, Robert Williams.*

Sound Barrier The resistance met by an aircraft when it approaches the speed of sound. The speed of sound in aviation is known as Mach 1, and any faster speed is expressed as a ratio of this factor. *See supersonic flight.*

Sound Navigation and Ranging System (SONAR) *See ultrasound.*

South Pole One of the two diametrically opposite points (geographic poles) at which the earth's axis cuts the earth's surface. It is covered by the land mass of Antarctica. The

English navigator Captain **James Cook** (1728–1779) and his crew were the first to cross the Antarctic region in their ship, *Adventure,* in 1773. The first steamship to cross the Antarctic Circle was the *Challenger*, one of the first ships of the British Admiralty to be assigned in 1872 to conduct an oceanic exploration. A Russian explorer, **Fabian Gottlieb Benjamin von Bellinghausen** (1778–1852) of Oesel, was the first person to sight the Antarctic ice shelf in 1820. An Irish explorer **Ernest Shackleton** (1874–1922), with three others sledded to 88.38°S on 9 January 1909. The South Pole was first reached on 14 December 1911 by a team of five men from Norway, led by **Roald Engelbrecht Gravning Amundsen** (1872–1928). A Yorkshire-born English geologist in Australia, **Sir Douglas Mawson** (1882– 1958), who in 1907 joined the scientific staff of Shackleton's Antarctic expedition, mapped the position of the South Magnetic Pole. The British explorer Robert Falcon Scott, with four others, reached the South Pole in 1912, but all of them perished on the return journey. An American aviator, **Richard Evelyn Byrd** (1888–1957) of Winchester, Virginia, made the first flight over the South Pole, in 1929. In 1956 Conrad Shin of USA landed by air and established a station there. *See magnetic poles.*

South, James (1785–1867) A London astronomer who graduated in medicine and surgery and became a member of the Royal College of Surgeons. His main interest was in astronomy; while working with **John Herschel** (1792–1871), he charted over 380 double stars. He published a second catalog of double stars in 1826.

Sowerby, James (1757–1822) *See conchology.*

Sowerby, James de Carle (1787–1871) *See conchology.*

Space Art *See astronomical drawings.*

Space Station A permanent station in space that remains in orbit as a satellite. Such a station was first proposed by R.A. Smith and H.E. Ross to the Interplanetary Society in 1949. **Wernher von Braun** (1912–1977) proposed an elaborate, detailed plan for a space station in 1952, and published *Conquest of the Moon* (1953) and *Space Frontier* (1967). *See space travel.*

Space Travel The French writer Savinien Cyrano de Bergerac (1619–1655) in the 17th century suggested several ways of travelling from the earth to the Moon. Out of the seven methods he proposed in 1650, only the seventh method, which suggested the use of rockets, was practical. The physical laws governing the flight of artificial satellites were proposed by **Sir Isaac Newton** (1642–1727). A French novelist, **Jules Verne** (1828–1905) of Nantes, published *De*

la Terre à la Lune (From the Earth to the Moon), the first novel on space travel, in 1865. A Russian astrophysicist, **Konstantin Eduardovich Tsiolkovsky** (1857–1935), mentioned the possibility of space flight in 1895, and three years later he suggested the development of liquid-fuel rocket engines for such flights. His work *Exploration of Cosmic Space by means of Reaction Devices* (1903) was one of the first publications on the subject. A German rocket engineer, **Wernher von Braun** (1912–1977), founded a society for space travel and developed rockets at a site near Berlin in 1930. The first crewed spacecraft, planetary probes and soft lunar landings were designed by a Russian engineer, **Seregi Pavlovich Korolev** (1906–1966) of the Ukraine. The English science fiction writer **Arthur Charles Clarke** (b 1917) published a futuristic work *Interplanetary Flight* in 1950. The first crewed space flight in history, planned by Korolev, and led by **Yuri Alekseyevich Gagarin** (1934–1968) in *Vostok I,* took place on 12th April 1961. The first soft landing on the moon was achieved in 1966 by the Soviet spaceprobe *Luna IX,* and in the same year the Soviet spaceprobe *Venera III* reached Venus. The first casualty of space travel was a Soviet astronaut in *Soyuz I* who died in 1967 during his re-entry from orbit. The US spaceprobe *Surveyor VII* landed undamaged on the Moon in 1968 and sent 21 000 photographs of the lunar surface. In the same year the Soviet spacecraft *Zond 5* travelled around the Moon and safely returned to the earth. The first transfer of crew in space occurred between two Soviet spacecrafts, *Soyuz 4* and *Soyuz 5,* in 1969. The historical landing on the moon was achieved by the American astronauts **Neil Armstrong** (b 1930), **Edwin Eugene Aldrin** (b 1930) and **Michael Collins** (b 1930) in their *Apollo 11,* on 20th July 1969. The subsequent *Apollo 12, 14, 15* and *16* spacecrafts made successful landings on the moon and returned to the earth. The final successful *Apollo 17* flight took place in 1972. The first space station, *Salyut I,* was set up by the Soviets in 1971. In 1974, American astronauts stayed in space for 84 days in their spacecraft *Skylab* which was fitted with cameras, telescopes and special equipment. The US spaceprobe *Pioneer 10* was the first human-created object to leave the solar system, in 1983. *See astronauts.*

Space Walk A Russian cosmonaut, **Aleksey Arkhipovich Leonov** (b 1934) from the space probe *Voskhod 2,* was the first man to walk out of a space vehicle into space, in 1965. In 1984 **Bruce McCandless** (b 1937) from the space shuttle *Challenger* walked in space at a distance of 164 miles above the earth. A Russian cosmonaut, Svetlana Savitskaya, was the first woman to walk in space, in 1985. *See astronauts.*

Spallanzani, Lazzaro (1729–1799) *See canned food, fertilization, nutrition.*

Species [Latin: *species,* appearance]   *See binomial nomenclature, botany.*

Specific Heat   The concept was proposed in 1772 by a German-born Swedish physicist, **Johan Carl Wilcke** (1732–1796). The Dulong and Petit law, that the product of specific heat and atomic weight is constant for all elements, was proposed in 1818 by a French physician, **Alexis Thérèse Petit** (1791–1820) and a Parisian chemist, **Pierre Louis Dulong** (1785–1838). An Irish physician, **Adair Crawford** (1748–1795), was the first to measure the specific heats of gases. The ratio of the specific heats of gases was determined in 1819 by a French physicist, **Charles Bernard Desormes** (1777–1862) of Dijon and his son-in-law, **Nicolas Clement** (1779–1841). A special form of calorimeter for measuring specific heat at low temperatures was designed in 1911 by a German physicist, **Walther Hermann Nernst** (1864–1941) and a German-born British physicist, **Frederick Alexander Lindemann Cherwell** (1886–1957). Charles Bernard Desormes and Nicolas Clement Desormes proposed a method for directly measuring specific heat. A German-born French physical chemist, **Henri Victor Regnault** (1810–1878), devised an apparatus for measuring specific heat, using a method of mixtures. *See ice calorimeter.*

Spectacles [Latin: *specio,* to look]   The first authentic men-

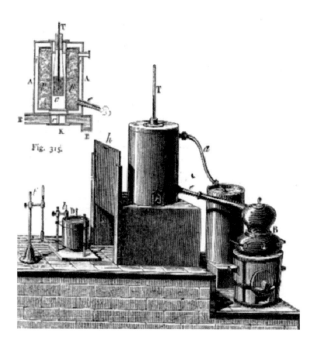

Figure 74   Renault's method of mixtures for determining specific heat. Atkinson, E. *Elementary Treatise on Physics.* London: Longmans, Green, and Co, 1872

tion of the use of lenses for reading was made by Meissner (AD 1260–1280), who stated that they would be advantageous to old people. The archives of the old Abbey of Saint-Bavlon-le-Grand contains a statement that a priest, Nicolas Bullet, used spectacles for signing an agreement in 1282. However, the use of magnifying glasses was probably known to Tyre and Sidon as far back as 1800 BC. **Nero** and **Lucius Annaeus Seneca** (d AD 65) were thought to have used ground and polished gems to help their defective sight. The Arabian mathematician, **Alhazen** or **Ibn Al-Haitham** (AD 965–1038) of Basra, wrote a book on optics entitled *Kitab Al-Manazir* which included refraction, reflection and the study of lenses. This work was the first step towards the invention of spectacles. In 1270 the English Franciscan monk **Roger Bacon** (1214–1298) of Ilchester suggested the use of lenses to aid the sight of old people. The term spectacle was first used in 1307 by a Scottish professor at Montpellier, Bernard de Gordon. The device is said to have been invented around 1250 by **Savinus Aramatus** or Salvino degli Aramati of Pisa. The earliest illustration of it, a Dominican friar using it for writing, painted in 1360 by Tomaso de Modena, is found in the church of San Nicola in Treviso. A record of a church sermon given in 1305 by Giordano da Rivolta, contains a statement 'it is only twenty years since the art of making spectacles was discovered'. Spectacles were prescribed for short-sighted people by Hollorius in 1550. Spectacles for the near-sighted were made in 1450 by **Nicholas Krebs** (b 1401) of Germany, who is also known as **Nicholas of Cusa**. The spectacles during this time were cumbersome and ugly, as they had to be mounted on wood, metal or leather. **Giovanni Battista della Porta** (1535–1615) of Naples mentioned the construction and use of spectacles in his book on natural magic in 1589. The modern form of spectacles, with hinged side pieces, came into use towards the latter half of the 18th century. A combination of two short- and long-focus convex lenses, to bring distant objects nearer, was invented by a Dutch lens maker, **Hans Lippershey** (1571–1619). The term optician first came into use in 1770. The use of prismatic and cylindrical lenses in the production of spectacles was introduced by a Dutch ophthalmologist and physiologist, **Franciscus Cornelis Donders** (1818–1889) of Utrecht.

Spectroscopy [Latin: *spectrum,* appearance + *skopein,* to view]   In 1752 **Thomas Melvill** (1726–1753), a Scottish scientist of Glasgow University, observed that colored flames of different metals and salts gave characteristic spectra when passed through a glass prism. In 1823 **Sir John Fredrick William Herschel** (1792–1871) suggested the use of this discovery for analysis of certain metals. An American physicist, **David Alter** (1807–1881) from West-mooreland, Pennsylvania, was one of the first to demonstrate in 1854 that each element had a specific spectrum. The prism spectroscope was invented in 1859 by **Robert Bunsen** (1811–1899) and **Gustav Robert Kirchhoff** (1824–1887). **Sir William Huggins** (1824–1910) attached a spectroscope to a telescope and studied the prominent lines seen around 40 stars in 1862. He also noted that when a star receded, its spectral lines were displaced towards the red end. An English astronomer, **Sir Norman Lockyer** (1836–1920) of Rugby, used the same method and predicted a new element, helium, which was discovered by **William Ramsay** (1852–1916) in 1895. Spectroscopy was first used to determine the chemical composition of the sun and stars, around 1845, by an Irish physicist, **Sir George Gabriel Stokes** (1819–1903) who was professor of mathematics at Cambridge. During his pioneering experiments with a prism, on the flame produced by the spirit lamp, he identified the characteristic spectrum that represented sodium. His discovery laid the foundation for the spectroscopic analysis of metals and other substances. The first spectroscopic survey of stars was done by the Roman astronomer **Pietro Angelo Secchi** (1818–1878), who used the method to catalog over 4000 stars in 1868. A Scottish physicist, **Balfour Stewart** (1828–1887) of Edinburgh, was another pioneer in spectrum analysis. An engineer from Leipzig, **Stokes Victor Schumann** (1841–1913), extended spectroscopy to the ultraviolet part of the spectrum, in 1892. The use of spectroscopy in astronomy was further developed by a French astronomer, **Pierre Jules César Janssen** (1824–1907), who in 1868 invented a spectrohelioscope for observing the bright light spectrum of the solar atmosphere. The Nobel Prize for physics in 1907, for studies on spectroscopic measurement of light, was awarded to **Albert Abraham Michelson** (1852–1931) of America. A Frankfurt-born British physicist, **Sir Arthur Schuster** (1851–1934), used spectroscopy to study the electrical conductivity of gases. The infrared rapid-scan spectrometers used in space probes were developed by an American physical chemist, **George Claude Pimental** (1922–1989) in the late 1960s. The Nobel Prize for chemistry in 1971, for early work on the spectroscopic study of the electronic structure and geometry of molecules, was awarded to a German-born Canadian physicist, **Gerhard Herzberg** (b 1904). *See absorption spectra, dispersion of light.*

Spectrum Analysis *See spectroscopy.*

Spedding, Frank Harold (1902–1984) *See chain reaction.*

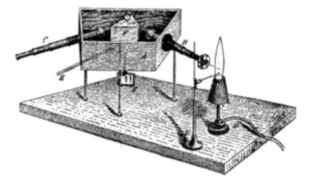

Figure 75 The first form of spectroscopy. Moore, F.J. *A History of Chemistry*, International Chemical Series. New York: McGraw-Hill Book Inc, 1918

Speed of Chemical Reactions *See velocity of chemical reactions.*

Speed of Electricity *See velocity of electricity.*

Speed of Light *See velocity of light.*

Speed of Sound *See velocity of sound.*

Speed, John (1542–1629) *See cartography.*

Speedometer *See odometer.*

Spence, Peter (1806–1883) A Scottish industrial chemist from Forfarshire who invented an improved method for making alum from coal shale in 1845. His plant at Pendelton, near Manchester, became the largest alum factory in the world.

Spencer, Herbert (1820–1903) A British philosopher from Derby who worked as a railway engineer, teacher and journalist. He wrote on ethics and sociology and was an advocate of 'social Darwinism', the idea that societies evolve in competition for resources and that survival of the fittest was morally justifiable. He suggested the evolutionary theory four years before Darwin published his *Origin of Species*. Spencer wrote: *System of Synthetic Philosophy*, *Principles of Biology*, *Principles of Psychology*, *Principles of Sociology* and *Principles of Ethics*. *See biology, evolution.*

Sperry, Elmer Ambrose (1860–1930) *See gyroscope, gyrostabilizer.*

Sperry, Roger Wolcott (1913–1994) *See vision.*

Speusippus (407–339 BC) *See Pythogorean Society.*

Spinning Mule A machine capable of spinning several threads at once, used in the cotton industry. It was invented in 1779 by **Samuel Crompton** (1753–1827) of Bolton,

Lancashire. It was called a mule because it was a cross between **James Hargreaves'** (1720–1778) jenny and **Sir Richard Arkwright's** (1732–1792) water-frame.

Spinning The conversion of fibers into yarn. A wooden hand-spindle was the earliest instrument used for spinning since Middle Ages. This resembled a knitting needle and was used for spinning a continuous thread from short fibers. The bobbing-wheel, consisting of a large wheel with a belt and a spindle, was introduced into England in the 14th century. Another implement, called a flyer, which twisted the yarn before winding it on the spool, was used in the 16th century. **Leonardo da Vinci** (1452–1519) gave a drawing of it around 1490. *See textile industry, spinning mule.*

Spinoza, Baruch (1632–1677) *See metaphysics.*

Spinthariscope An apparatus for demonstrating the emission of alpha particles, invented by **Sir William Crookes** (1832–1919).

Spitzer, Lyman (1914–1997) *See thermonuclear fusion.*

Spode, Josiah (1754–1827) *See porcelain.*

Spörer, Gustav Friedrich Wilhelm (1822–1895) *See Spörer's law.*

Spörer's Law The mean latitude of sunspots varies throughout the solar cycle. The phenomenon was observed independently by a London astronomer **Richard Christopher Carrington** (1826–1875) and a German astronomer **Gustav Friedrich Wilhelm Spörer** (1822–1895) of Berlin. **Vilhelm Friman Koren Bjerknes** (1862–1951) gave a theoretical explanation of the law in 1926.

Spottiswoode, William (1825–1883) A London physicist who carried out pioneer studies on electrical discharge in rarefied gases and polarization of light. In 1851, he published the first elementary mathematical treatise on determinants.

Sprague, Frank Julian (1857–1934) *See tram car.*

Sprengel, Christian Conrad (1750–1816) *See pollination.*

Sprengel, Hermann Johann Phillip (1834–1906) *See vacuum.*

Spruce, Richard (1817–1893) An English botanical explorer from Yorkshire, who published *Palmae Amazonicae* (1869), *Notes of a Botanist in the Amazon* (1908) and several other botanical treatises.

Spurr, Josiah Edward (1870–1950) *See Tertiary period.*

Sputnik [Russian: *sputnik*, fellow traveller] The first artificial satellite, *Sputnik I*, was launched by the Russians on 4th

October 1957. *Sputnik II*, which carried the first animal into space, a dog named *Laika*, followed on 3rd November 1957. The third *Sputnik* was launched in May 1958. *See space travel.*

Stahl, Franklin William (b 1929) *See genetic engineering.*

Stahl, Georg Ernst (1660–1734) *See acetic acid, oxygen.*

Staining A method introduced into microscopy by a Dutch microscopist, **Anthoni van Leeuwenhoek** (1632–1723), who described the use of the crocus or saffron to stain muscle fibers, to the Royal Society of London in 1714. **Frederik Ruysch** (1638–1731), professor of anatomy in Amsterdam, used cinnabar in tallow and wax to demonstrate the blood vessels of human specimens. Cochineal substances were used by an English botanist, **John Hill** (1716–1775), in 1770. Controlled standardized methods of staining in histology were introduced in 1858 by **Joseph von Gerlach** (1820–1896), professor of anatomy and physiology at Erlangen.

Stainless Steel First developed in 1904 by a French scientist, Leon Guillet, but he failed to recognize its property of corrosion resistance. In 1914, Harry Brearley of Sheffield was the first to note that the alloy stainless steel sheets when accidentally exposed to chromium did not corrode. In 1882, an English industrial chemist, **Robert Abbot Hadfield** (1858–1940) of Sheffield, Yorkshire, invented a method of producing stainless steel, and published *Metallurgy and its influence on Modern Progress* (1925).

Standard Deviation *See statistics.*

Stanhope, Charles (1753–1816) *See printing.*

Stanier, William Arthur (1876–1965) *See locomotive.*

Stanley, Wendell Meredith (1904–1971) *See Northrop, John Howard.*

Stanley, William (1858–1916) *See alternating current, electric transformer.*

Stannius, Hermann (1808–1883) *See protozoa.*

Stapler A device used for book binding, invented in 1868 by Charles Henry Gould of England.

Starch [Anglo-Saxon: *stearc*, flour] The Dutch microscopist, **Anthoni van Leeuwenhoek** (1632–1723), was the first to observe starch granules in concentric form in plants. In 1833, a French chemist **Anselme Payen** (1795–1871), extracted a substance from germinated barley seeds that was capable of breaking down starch to sugar, and named it amylase. **Antoine Jerome Balard** (1802–1876), a French chemist and apothecary, discovered that iodine turned blue in the presence of starch, and this formed the basis for the commonly used test for starch. In 1811 a German chemist, **Gottlieb Sigismond Kirchhof** (1764–1833) first produced glucose by treating starch with sulfuric acid. In 1880 **Andreas Franz Wilhelm Schimper** (1856–1901) showed that it was a source of stored energy for plants.

Stark Effect   *See quantum theory.*

Stark, Johannes (1874–1957)   *See quantum theory.*

Starley, James (1831–1881)   *See bicycle, differential gear, tricycle.*

Starling, Ernest Henry (1866–1927)   *See digestion, hormones.*

Starr, J.W. (1822–1847)   *See electric lighting.*

Stars   A philosopher and astronomer, **Anaximander** (611–547 BC) of Miletus (now Turkey), was the first Greek to draw a map of the earth giving details of its surface, and to speculate on the size and distances of the heavenly bodies. The method of describing and naming stars with Greek letters and by their constellation was introduced in 1572 by a German astronomer Johann Bayer, who published a complete celestial atlas *Uranometria*. In 1560 **Tycho Brahe** (1546–1601), a Danish astronomer, cataloged over 1000 stars. **Galilei Galileo** (1564–1642) made one of the first telescopes to be used in astronomy, with which he found the black spots on the sun and hills and valleys on the moon, and demonstrated that the Milky Way was composed of a multitude of stars. A German astronomer, **Johannes Hevelius** (1611–1687), cataloged over 1500 stars. In 1712 **John Flamsteed** (1646–1719), the first Astronomer Royal in England, prepared a new catalog of 3000 stars. His star map, published after his death in 1725, was the first map of the teloscopic age. A listing of the positions of 47 000 stars was given in 1801 by a professor of astronomy at the Collège de France, **Joseph Jerome Le François de Lalande** (1732–1807), who published *Traité d'astronomie* in 1764. The first spectroscopic survey of stars was done by the Roman astronomer **Pietro Angelo Secchi** (1818–1878), who used the method in 1868 to catalog over 4000 stars. Spectral analysis of stars was advanced by a German astronomer, **Hermann Carl Vogel** (1842–1907) of Leipzig, who discovered the spectroscopic binary stars. He was appointed as the first director of the Potsdam Observatory, in 1882.

Stas, Jean Servais (1813–1891)   A Belgian chemist and professor of chemistry at Brussels who developed some early methods for chemical analysis and estimation of atomic weights.

Statistics   A physician from Hampshire and a pioneer in the field of statistics, **William Petty** (1623–1687), first applied statistics to economy, and proposed the first statistical department for recording deaths, births, marriages, age, sex and all other aspects such as economy, trade and education. The earliest life tables were published by the British astronomer **Edmund Halley** (1656–1742). A clergyman and a London mathematician, **Thomas Bayes** (1702–1761), was one of the first to study the idea of statistical inference. His book *Essay towards solving a problem in the Doctrine of Chances* was published two years after his death, in 1763. **Sir Ronald Aylmer Fisher** (1890–1962), a professor of genetics and statistician from East Finchley, London, published *Statistical Methods for Research Workers* (1925), which became the first standard work on the application of statistics in research. The field of statistics was established as a specialty by a London mathematician, **Karl Pearson** (1857–1936), who invented the chi-square test of statistical significance, and the concept of standard deviation. An English industrial scientist, **William Sealy Gosset** (1876–1937) from Canterbury, applied the principles of statistics to industry. Mathematical principles and statistics were first applied to the study of genetics by **Gregor Johann Mendel** (1822–1884), and these tools were used by an English geneticist from Hampshire, **Lancelot Thomas Hogben** (1895–1975), who was director of Army Medical Statistics in England. A 20th century classic widely used in the medical field, *Principles of Statistics*, was published in 1937 by Austin Bradford Hill (1897–1991). *See normal distribution curve, probability theory.*

Staudinger, Hermann (1881–1965)   *See polymer.*

Staudinger's Law   *See polymer.*

Steady-State Theory   An alternative theory to the Big Bang theory and oscillating theory for the origin of the universe. It requires matter to be continuously created in order to maintain a constant density in the universe, and maintains that the universe is eternal and has always existed. Proposed in 1948 by an Austrian-born British scientist, **Sir Hermann Bondi** (b 1919), an Austrian-born American astronomer **Thomas Gold** (b 1920) and an English astrophysicist **Fred Hoyle** (b 1915) of Yorkshire.

Steam [Anglo-Saxon: *steam,* vapor]   *See steam engine, steam hammer.*

Steam Boat   *See ships.*

Steam Engine   The principle behind the steam engine dates back to about AD 100 when **Hero of Alexandria** demonstrated the first steam turbine. His instrument, *Aeliophile*, was essentially a hollow bronze ball with a narrow opening that emitted a blast of steam when the water inside the ball was heated. An instrument activated by air, compressed with heated water or steam, is recorded to have been constructed in AD 1125 by a man named Gerbert. The power of steam was mentioned by **Girolomo Cardan** (1501–1576) in the middle of the 16th century. The principle of the steam engine was expressed by an English Huguenot inventor, **Salomen de Caulx** (1576–1626), in his *Les Raisons des forces mouvantes avec diverse machines* (1615). In 1663 **Edward Somerset** (*c.* 1601–1667), the second Marquis of Worcester, outlined a machine capable of raising water to a height of 40 feet, and it is supposed to have been used at Vauxhall, London, from 1663 to 1670. The first steam gas-engine with a cylinder and piston was invented by **Christian Huygens** (1629–1695) in 1680. The indispensable safety valve for the steam engine, which prevented the steam from escaping and secured the due intensity of heat, was invented by **Denis Papin** (1674–1712), a French physician and physicist in 1682. He used steam to move a piston in 1690. Papin came to England and worked with **Robert Boyle** (1627–1691). Sir Samuel Moreland, master mechanic to Charles II (1630–1685), wrote on steam engines and invented a variety of models in 1680. A Cornish military engineer, **Thomas Savery** (1650–1715) of Devon, was the first to use steam power to operate the pumps in the Cornish tin mines in 1698. An entirely different form of the self-acting atmospheric or steam engine was developed by **Thomas Newcomen** (1663–1729) in 1707. **James Watt** (1736–1819), a mathematical instrument maker from Greenock, reviewed Newcomen's engine and improved it by adding a jacket for the cylinder. He patented it in 1775. His engine was six times more effective than that of Newcomen. Watt also patented a steam engine with a rotary motion instead of a back-and-forth motion in 1781, and his double-acting steam engine, invented in 1780, allowed steam to move alternately to both sides of the piston. A separate condenser, which kept the engine permanently hot, was invented by **Joseph Black** (1728–1799) and John Anderson in 1765. In 1770 a French army engineer, **Nicholas Joseph Cugnot** (1725–1804), developed a three-wheeled steam-powered road tractor capable of 6 kilometers per hour, which became the first automobile. The first steam engine carriage on iron rails, capable of hauling 10 tons of iron, was demonstrated at Coalbrookdale, Shropshire in 1803 by a Cornish engineer, **George Trevithick** (1771–1833). **George Stephenson** (1781–1848), a railway engineer from Wylam near Newcastle, developed the steam locomotive by adding a draught to the firebox, and operated it from Stockton to Darlington in 1821. It was the first practical passenger railway in the history of steam power. A pioneer of the steam engine in America, **Oliver Evans** (1755–1819) of Newport,

Delaware, constructed the first American steam-powered road vehicle in 1804. An early monograph, *The Steam Engine* (1827), was published by an English engineer, **Thomas Tredgold** (1788–1829), who advocated the use of steam for central heating. A compound steam engine, which effectively used the steam twice, was invented by a Scottish engineer, **William McNaught** (1813–1881) from Paisley. A New York engineer, **George Henry Corliss** (1817–1888), improved the steam engine by adding a system of rocking valves for steam and other devices. His engines, known as Corliss engines, were imported into Scotland for use in cotton mills in 1859 and became very popular. *See railway.*

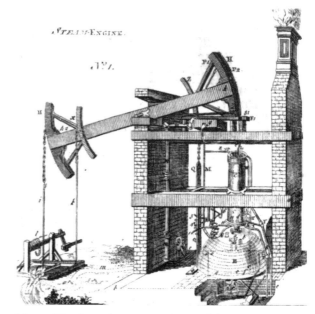

Figure 76   An early steam engine used for pumping water. Owen, W. *Dictionary of Arts and Sciences.* London: Homer's Head, 1754

Steam Hammer   A hammer propelled by steam, invented in 1838 by a Scottish engineer **James Nasmyth** (1808–1890) of Edinburgh. He also invented a cylinder-boring machine, a slotting and planing machine, a floating mortar used in warfare and several other tools.

Steam Heating   *See heating.*

Steam Navigation   *See ships.*

Steamships   The first steam boat propelled by the ejection of water from the stern was built by an American engineer, **James Rumsey** (1743–1792) from Maryland, and it was exhibited on the Potomac in 1787. In 1783 **Marquis Jouffroy d'Abbans** (1751–1832) used steam propulsion for his boat, *Pyroscaphe,* to ascend the River Saône near Lyon. An American inventor, **John Fitch** (1743–1798) from Windsor, Connecticut, built four steamships propelled by reciprocating paddles, from 1786 to 1790. The first practical steam boat, *Charlotte Dundas,* was built in 1802 by a Scottish inventor, **William Symington** (1763–1831) of Leadhills. In 1812 another Scottish pioneer, **Henry Bell** (1767–1830), built a 25-ton ship, the *Comet,* which was propelled by a three-horse-power engine, and it became the first steamship regularly to carry passengers. In 1803 **John Stevens** (1749–1838) of New York, built the *Little Juliana* propelled by archimedean screws, driven by a high-pressure steam engine. An American engineer of Irish origin, **Robert Fulton** (1765–1815) of Pennsylvania, designed another paddle ship, the *Clermont,* in 1807, and it operated a passenger service on the Hudson River between New York and Albany. The first steam warship, *Fulton the First,* was built by him in 1814. The first steamship to cross the Atlantic was the Dutch vessel *Curaçao,* a wooden paddler that left Rotterdam in April 1827, and took one month to cross. HMS *Rhabdamanthus* was the earliest steamship to make the entire transatlantic crossing under steam power, and it made a journey from Plymouth, Devon to Barbados in 1832. The *Great Western,* launched in 1832, made its first transatlantic voyage to New York in 1838. It was the largest ship in the world at that time, and was designed by **Isambard Kingdom Brunel** (1806–1859). The first successful screw-propelled steamer, *Archimedes,* was built by **Sir Francis Petit Smith** (1808–1874) of Hythe, in 1839. He also built screw-propelled warships for the Royal Navy in 1842. The first steamer with engine and boilers entirely below the water line, *Princeton,* was built by a Swedish-born American inventor, **John Ericsson** (1803–1889) in the same year. The 'wave-line system' of ship building was invented in 1855 by **John Scott Russell** (1808–1882), a Scottish engineer from Glasgow, and one of the founders of the Institution of Naval Architects in 1860. A London engineer, **Sir Charles Algernon Parsons** (1854–1931), developed a steam turbine in 1884, and patented a turbo-generator for a ship in 1894. The first such ship, the *Turbinia,* was launched in 1897. High-efficiency steam turbines using convergent and divergent nozzles were developed by a Swedish engineer, **Carl Gustav Patrick de Laval** (1845–1913), who also invented a high-speed turbine to drive the propellor for marine use. *See shipping.*

Stebbins, George Ledyard (b 1906)   *See hybridization.*

Stebbins, Joel (1878–1966)   *See photoelectric cell.*

Steel   The production of steel swords was known to the ancients and were used in Rome around 100 BC, and at Damascus in the 4th century. The first industrial treatise on iron, *L'art de convertir le fer forgé en acier* (The art of converting iron into steel) was published in 1722 by the French naturalist **René Antoine Ferchault de Reaumer** (1683–1757). He suggested the use of an open hearth process in his above treatise. An English inventor of Dutch descent, **Benjamin Huntsman** (1704–1776) from Lincolnshire, was one of the first to make high-quality steel suitable for making knives and razors, in 1745. The Bessemer process for large-scale manufacture of steel was introduced in 1856 by an English ironmaster, **Sir Henry Bessemer** (1813–1898). It was first used in America under a patent taken out by **William Kelly** (1811–1888) of Pittsburgh, Pennsylvania, who successfully claimed priority for the discovery. The open-hearth process was introduced in 1863 by **Sir Charles William Siemens,** originally **Karl Wilhelm Siemens** (1823–1883) of Germany, and his brother **Friedrich Siemens** (1826–1904). A magistrate's clerk, **Sidney Gilchrist Thomas** (1850–1885) of Lyme Regis in England, and his cousin **Percy Carlyle Gilchrist** (1851–1935), improved the process, and their method provided a cheap way of making steel. A French owner of iron and steel works, **Pierre Emile Martin** (1824–1915) from Bourges, developed the open-hearth furnace, under the licence of Bessemer, and exhibited it at the Great Paris Exhibition in 1867, for which he was awarded a gold medal. The addition of nickel to steel (nickel steel or Invar), to make the steel more elastic, was an invention of a Swiss physicist, **Charles Edouard Guillaume** (1861–1938), who served as director of the Bureau International des Poids et Mesures at Sèvres. He was awarded the Nobel Prize for physics in 1920.

Steenstrup, Johannes Lapetus (1813–1897)   *See alternation of generations, prehistory.*

Stefan Law   The amount of energy radiated from a black body is proportional to the fourth power of the absolute temperature. Proposed by an Austrian physicist, **Josef Stefan** (1835–1893), who was director of the Institute of Experimental Physics in Vienna. It was verified by two German professors of physics at Breslau, **Ernst Pringsheim** (1859–1917) and **Otto Richard Lummer** (1860–1925). In 1884, a former student of Stefan, **Ludwig Boltzmann** (1844–1906), gave a theoretical explanation for the Stefan law which became known as the Stefan–Boltzmann law.

Stefan, Josef (1835–1893)   *See black body radiation, quantum theory, Stefan law.*

Stein, William Howard (1911–1980)   *See chromatography, ribonucleic acid.*

Steinberger, Jack (b 1921) *See neutrino.*

Steiner, Jakob (1796–1863) *See projective geometry.*

Steinheim Man Name given to a primitive man of the middle Pleistocene Period (200 000–100 000 years ago) whose skull was found at Steinheim near Stuttgart in 1933.

Steinmetz, Charles Proteus (1865–1923) *See alternating current.*

Stellar Evolution *See helium.*

Steno, Nicolaus or Niels Stenson (1638–1687) A Danish geologist from Copenhagen who recognized the organic nature of fossils and proposed the principle behind their formation, in his work *Sample of the Elements of Myology* (1667). He was also an eminent anatomist but gave up his medical career for the church and became the bishop of Titiopolis in 1667. *See academy, crystallography.*

Stephenson, George (1781–1848) *See locomotive, railway, steam engine, Stephenson's lamp.*

Stephenson, Robert (1803–1859) *See bridges, railway.*

Stephenson's Lamp A safety lamp for miners which allowed air to enter along narrow tubes to prevent explosion. Devised by the English pioneer of locomotives, **George Stephenson** (1781–1848).

Stereochemistry [Greek: *stereos*, solid] A term coined by **Viktor Meyer** (1848–1897), a German professor of chemistry at Zurich, Göttingen and Heidelberg, to denote the chemical study of the spatial arrangement of atoms in molecules and the effect of these arrangements on molecular properties. A Scottish physicist, **William Nicol** (1768–1851), constructed a prism of Iceland spar in 1828, and used it in 1844 to make a polarimeter for studying optically active substances. The ability of various substances to rotate a plane of polarized light was studied by an English physicist, **Sir Gabriel Stokes** (1819–1903). **Louis Pasteur** (1822–1895) related optical activity and chemical structure in 1848; stereochemistry originated from his work on tartaric acid in the same year, following the identification of three tartaric acid isomers. An explanation was given independently in 1874 by a Dutch chemist, **Jacobus Henricus van't Hoff** (1852–1911), who suggested that the four bonds of carbon are directed towards the points of a tetrahedron, and a French chemist **Joseph Achille Le Bel** (1847–1930) from Alsace, who wrote on the three-dimensional structure of atoms in relation to optical activity in molecules. The migration of molecules in stereochemistry was studied by an English organic chemist, **Joseph Kenyon** (1885–1961) of

Lancashire. A French-born Swiss chemist and Nobel Prize winner in 1913, **Alfred Werner** (1866–1919), proposed the modern theory of coordination bonds between molecules and published *Lehrbuch der Stereochemie* (1904). Another London chemist, **Sir William Jackson Pope** (1870–1939), made an important study of stereochemistry in compounds in which asymmetry was due to elements other than carbon. He showed that compounds containing no asymmetric carbon atoms could still be optically active. A London chemist, **William Hobson Mills** (1873–1959), made significant advances in optical isomerism. Another English organic chemist, **Sir Derek Harold Richard Barton** (1918–1998) from Gravesend, during his work on the stereochemistry of natural compounds, showed that their biological activity depended on the shape of their molecules. He shared the Nobel Prize for chemistry in 1969, with a Norwegian chemist, **Odd Hassel** (1897–1981). The Nobel Prize for chemistry in 1975 for work on the stereochemistry of biochemical compounds was shared by a British organic chemist, **John Warcup Cornforth** (b 1917), and a Bosnian-born Swiss chemist, **Vladimir Prelog** (1906–1998).

Stereophonic Record [Greek: *stereos*, solid + *phone*, sound] Production of sound that can be reproduced through two speakers, giving different and complementary sounds, according to their spatial positions. The idea was initiated by an American, Samuel Waters, who in 1920 suggested that a record could be played back through two pickup cartridges in different grooves. His idea was developed by Bell Telephone Laboratories, who gave a demonstration of it at a symphony concert in Philadelphia in 1933. A British company, EMI, developed the technology in the same year. In 1951, Emery Cook of America made double-groove records with a stereophonic effect.

Stereophonic Sound *See musical recording, stereophonic record.*

Stereoscope [Greek: *stereos*, solid + *skopein*, to see] An instrument to unite two images of an object with the help of mirrors so as to produce one apparently solid image with depth. Invented in 1838 by **Sir Charles Wheatstone** (1802–1875), and improved by **Sir David Brewster** (1781–1868).

Stern, Otto (1888–1969) *See electron diffraction, molecular beams.*

Stevens, John (1749–1838) *See steamships.*

Stevens, Robert Livingston (1787–1856) Son of **John Stevens** (1749–1838). *See locomotive.*

Stevenson, Robert (1772–1850) *See lighthouses.*

Stevinus, Simon (1548–1620) *See car, decimal notation, gravity.*

Stewart, Balfour (1828–1887) *See spectroscopy.*

Stewart, Ralph Randles (b 1890) An American botanical explorer and plant collector from West Hebron, New York, who collected over 60 000 specimens in Pakistan and the Himalayan region, and published several books on botany.

Stieltjes, Thomas Jan (1856–1894) *See mathematics.*

Stifel, Michael (1487–1567) *See algebra, logarithms.*

Stirling Engine A hot-air engine in which heat is applied at one end of the cylinder continuously from an external source, to heat the working fluid or air. It was invented in 1816 by a Scottish clergyman, **Robert Stirling** (1790–1878) of Cloag, Perthshire. Theoretically it is supposed to be more efficient and less polluting than the internal combustion engine.

Stirling, James (1692–1770) A Scottish mathematician who studied at Glasgow and Oxford before he taught mathematics in London. He published *Methodus Differentialis* (1730), an important contribution towards the theory of infinite series.

Stirling, James (1835–1917) *See locomotive.*

Stirling, Patrick (1820–1895) *See locomotive.*

Stirling, Robert (1790–1878) *See Stirling engine.*

Stoic School A philosophical school established around 320 BC at a painted porch in Athens (*stoa poecile*) by the Greek philosopher **Zeno** (362–264 BC) **of Citium.**

Stokes' Law Relates the force of movement of a body through a fluid to the viscosity of the fluid and velocity and size of the body. Proposed by an Irish physicist, **Sir George Gabriel Stokes** (1819–1903).

Stokes, Sir George Gabriel (1819–1903) *See fluorescence, sodium, spectroscopy, Stokes' law.*

Stommel, Henry Melson (1920–1992) *See oceanography.*

Stone Age The earliest known period of human culture, characterized by the use of stone tools. Identified in 1758 by a French magistrate, Gouget. Evidence of Paleolithic [Greek: *palaeos,* old + *lithos,* stone] or Old Stone Age culture was found in Abbeville, France, by **Jacques Boucher de Perthes** (1788–1868), in 1805. His finding provided evidence for the existence of Stone Age culture over 30 000 years ago. In 1865, **Sir John Lubbock** (1834–1913) used the terms Paleolithic and Neolithic [Greek: *neos,* new + *lithos,* stone] to divide the Stone Age on the basis of the nature of stone artifacts found in Western Europe. Rough stone implements were assigned to the Paleolithic Age, and polished stone implements were thought to be of Neolithic origin. The Paleolithic Age was further divided into the period of Neanderthal man, and the time of appearance of *Homo sapiens* or modern man. According to evidence from sites at Parpallo (Spain) and the Sahara, the bow and arrow were invented around 25 000 BC, and evidence remains for their use in the Mississippi valley in North America around 800 BC. Stone arrowheads belonging to the Neolithic Period were observed and described by **Georgius Agricola** (1558) and **Conrad Gesner** (1565), but they offered no adequate explanation for their origin. A Danish archaeologist, **Christian Jörgensen Thomsen** (1788–1865) and Jacques de Perthes identified them as implements of the Stone Age. A Paleolithic hand-axe factory recently found at Box Grove, in East Sussex, England, is believed to be about 400 000 years old. *See prehistory.*

Stoney, George Johnston (1826–1911) *See electromagnetic theory, electron.*

Störmer A unit of momentum at which a particle circles around the equator, near the earth's surface. Described and named by a Norwegian astrophysicist, **Carl Fredrik Mulertz Störmer** (1874–1957), who became a professor at the Institute of Theoretical Astrophysics at the University of Oslo, in 1903.

Störmer, Carl Fredrik Mulertz (1874–1957) *See Störmer.*

Storms The American statesman and scientist **Benjamin Franklin** (1706–1790) described the course of storms over the North American continent. A German naturalist, **Friedrich Heinrich Alexander von Humboldt** (1769–1859), studied the nature of tropical storms. **William Redfield** (1789–1857) of New York, studied the origin of storms, and in 1831 published a chart of the hurricane of 1821. One of the early meterological studies of storms and winds was done by a German climatologist, **Heinrich Wilhelm Dove** (1803–1879) who published *The Law of Storms* (1857), in which he discussed the mechanism of production of storms. **Robert Fitzroy** (1805–1865), the commander of the *Beagle,* which carried **Charles Robert Darwin** (1809–1882), published *The Weather Book* (1863), which contained sophisticated pictures of storms, similar to present satellite pictures. **James Pollard Espy** (1785–1860) of Pennsylvania, who joined the Washington Observatory in 1843, published the *Philosophy of Storms* (1841) which earned him the nickname 'the Storm King'. *See climatology, clouds, cyclone, meteorology, wind.*

Story-Maskelyne, Mervyn Herbert Nevil (1823–1911) *See crystallography, solute.*

Stothard, Thomas (1755–1834) *See engraving.*

Strabo (*c.* 63 BC–AD 21) *See geography.*

Strasburger, Eduard Adolf (1844–1912) *See anaphase, cell division, cytology, cytoplasm, fertilization, metaphase, mitosis, prophase.*

Strassmann, Fritz (1902–1980) *See nuclear fission.*

Stratigraphy A branch of geology dealing with the formation, conditions and effects of various layers of rock. An English geologist **William Smith** (1769–1839) is regarded as the founder of the field. A German geologist born in Silesia, **Abraham Gottlob Werner** (1749–1817), in his work *On the External Characteristics of Fossils* (1774) dealt with the subject. *See petrology.*

Strato of Lampsacus (*c.* 330 BC) *See acceleration, dynamics, lever.*

Stratoscope [Latin: *stratum,* layer + Greek: *skopein,* to look] A space telescope that can be fixed onto a star via a control button on the ground control panel. Developed in the mid-20th century, it made it possible for astronomical observatories to be established in space.

Stratosphere [Latin: *stratum,* layer] A region of comparative calm and uniform temperature lying above an altitude of 10 kilometers, or the troposphere, discovered in 1898 by a French meteorologist, **Léon Philippe Teisserenc** (1855–1913). In 1931 a Swiss physicist, **Auguste Antoine HPiccard** (1884–1962), made pioneering studies of it, at a height of over 15 000 meters in a special balloon that he built. *See atmosphere, cyclone.*

Strickland, Hugh Edwin (1811–1853) *See ornitholgy, zoology.*

String Galvanometer *See galvanometer.*

String Theory *See superstring theory.*

Stringfellow, John (1799–1883) *See airplane.*

Stromeyer, Friedrich (1776–1835) *See cadmium.*

Strömgren, Bengt Georg Daniel (1908–1987) *See Strömgren spheres.*

Strömgren Spheres Zones of ionized hydrogen gas surrounding the hot stars, embedded in the gas clouds. Proposed in 1940 by a Swedish astronomer, **Bengt Georg Daniel Strömgren** (1908–1987) of Göttingen.

Strontium First noted in 1790 in a mineral from Strontian, Argylshire, by an Irish physician, **Adair Crawford** (1748–1795). A Scottish chemist **Thomas Charles Hope** (1766–1844) of Edinburgh, and a German chemist, **Martin Heinrich Klaproth** (1743–1817) of Berlin, independently identified it, in 1793. It was isolated by the English chemist **Sir Humphry Davy** (1778–1829).

Stroud, William (1860–1938) An English engineer from Bristol, who became Cavendish professor of physics at Leeds in 1885. *See Barr Stroud Ltd, military engineering.*

Structural Engineering The behavior of various materials under stress was first studied by **Leonardo da Vinci** (1452–1519). He looked at the load and strength of pillars and beams, and calculated the carrying power of pillars in relation to their height and diameter. Galileo's work on the strength of beams was experimentally tested in 1666 by a Swedish architect, P. Wurtz. In 1757 the Swiss mathematician **Leonhard Euler** (1707–1883) applied mathematics to the calculation of loads on pillars. The strength of different materials was studied by **Edmé Mariotte** (1620–1684) of France in the 17th century. The strength of wooden beams in construction was studied in England by an amateur mechanic, **Joseph Moxon** (1627–1700), who published *Mechanik Exercises* in 1677. The structural mechanics behind the construction of St Paul's and Westminster Abbey was first studied by **Sir Christopher Wren** (1632–1723) in the early 18th century. A French engineer, **Phillipe de la Hire** (1640–1718), wrote *Traité de Mécanique* (1695) in which he correctly analyzed the forces acting on various sections of the arch. A French civil engineer, **Hubert Gautier** (1660–1737) of Nîmes, summarized the ancient and contemporary practices in structural engineering in his *Traité des Ponts* (1716). An Italian civil engineer, **Alberto Castigliano** (1847–1884), introduced strain energy methods of structural analysis, in 1873.

Strum, Jacques Charles François (1803–1855) *See polynomial equation, Strum theorem, velocity of sound.*

Strum Theorem Deals with real roots of a polynomial equation. Proposed by a French mathematician, **Jacques Charles François Strum** (1803–1855).

Strutt, Jedediah (1726–1797) *See ribbing machine, waterframe.*

Struve, Friedrich Georg Wilhelm (1793–1864) A German astronomer and director of the Dorpat Observatory (1817) who made early observations on double stars and nebulae. He was the first to measure stellar parallax. His son

Otto Wilhelm Struve (1819–1905) was an eminent astronomer, who discovered over 500 new double stars.

Struve, Herman (1854–1920) Son of **Otto Wilhelm Struve** (1819–1905) and director of the Berlin Observatory (1904). He made micrometric studies of Mars, Uranus and Neptune.

Struve, Otto (1897–1963) An American astronomer and grandson of **Otto Wilhelm Struve** (1819–1905). He emigrated to America and became the first director of the National Radio Astronomy Observatory there in 1959. He was made director of the Yerkes Observatory in 1932 and founded the McDonald Observatory at the University of Texas in 1939.

Struve, Otto Wilhelm (1819–1905) Son of **Friedrich Georg Wilhelm Struve** (1793–1864). He discovered over 500 new double stars and a satellite of Uranus (1847).

Stubblefield, Nathan B. (d 1923) *See wireless telegraphy.*

Sturgeon, William (1783–1850) *See battery, electricity, scientific journals, tangent galvanometer.*

Sturrock, Archibald (1816–1919) *See locomotive.*

Sturtevant, Alfred Henry (1891–1970) *See chromosomes.*

Subatomic Particles Fundamental particles of an atom. *See antiproton, electron, meson, neutron, photon, pion, proton.*

Submarines The first one was demonstrated by **Cornelis Jacobson Drebbel** (1570–1633), a Dutch inventor from Alkmaar, who emigrated to England. In 1620 he tested his submarine. powered by rowers, and capable of carrying 24 passengers, for the first time in the River Thames, London. A four-person submarine was built in 1798 by an American engineer of Irish origin, **Robert Fulton** (1765–1815) of Pennsylvania. **David Bushnell** (1742–1824) of Westbrook, Maine, was a pioneer in the field of submarine engineering who suggested combining the submarine and torpedo into one unit. Bushnell's one-man submarine known as the *American Turtle* was developed in 1775. The first modern submarine capable of taking part in naval warfare was designed and launched by a Bavarian corporal, Wilhelm Bauer, in 1851. A Frenchman, Claude Desire Goubet, invented the electrically driven submarine around 1880. An Irish-born US inventor, **John Phillip Holland** (1840–1914), built and demonstrated a modern submarine, *Fenian Ram,* on the Hudson River in 1881. His more advanced *Holland IV* was launched in 1898. The first significantly longer submarine, the *Gustave Zédé* of 160 feet in length, was launched by the French in the same year. A Dutch geophysi-

cist, **Felix Andries Vening Meinesz** (1887–1966), was one of the first to conduct submarine expeditions to study gravity measurements under the sea, in 1929. The first U-boat submarine was introduced by the Germans in 1905, and the first atomic powered submarine, *Nautilus,* was launched in 1954 following the work of a Russian-born US naval officer, **Hyman George Rickover** (1900–1986). An Irish scientific instrument maker, **Sir Howard Grubb** (1844–1931) of Dublin, developed the periscope for submarines. The first British nuclear submarine, HMS *Dreadnought,* was launched at Barrow-in-Furness in 1960.

Suess, Eduard (1831–1914) *See tectonic theory.*

Suez Canal *See canals.*

Sugden, Samuel (1892–1950) *See surface tension.*

Sulfur [Latin: *sulfur,* brimstone] Known to the ancients and mentioned in the Old Testament. The use of pungent fumes of sulfur for cleansing was mentioned by **Homer** (*c.* 800 BC), **Pliny the Elder** (AD 28–79) and **Ovid** (43 BC–AD 17). The book *Cordex Germanicus* (*c.* AD 1350) states that pure sulfur will crackle if held in a warm hand, while impure sulfur will not. A method of obtaining sulfur from earth deposits or petroleum with the use of superheated steam was invented by a chemical engineer, **Herman Frasch** (1851–1914) from Württemberg, who emigrated to America and joined the laboratory of the Standard Oil Company at Cleveland.

Sulfuric Acid First produced by Basil Valentine in the 15th century. A Dutch inventor from Alkmaar, **Cornelis Jacobson Drebbel** (1570–1633), invented a method of making it. A German alchemist, **John Rudolph Glauber** (1604–1668), obtained a pure form of sulfuric acid in 1640. In 1831 **Peregrine Phillips** (*c.* 1800–1831) of Bristol, in England, discovered a method of manufacturing sulfuric acid by passing sulfur dioxide and oxygen over platinum. A German industrial chemist, **Rudolph Messel** (1848–1920), invented a similar but more advanced process in 1875.

Sulfurous Acid First produced by an English clergyman and chemist from Leeds, **Joseph Priestley** (1733–1804).

Sullivan, Louis Henri (1856–1924) *See architecture, American.*

Sumner, James Batcheller (1887–1955) *See Northrop, John Howard.*

Sundial Device used for reading the time by interpreting the movement of a shadow. The first sundial, known as a *gnomon* – a stick, struck upright on horizontal ground – was known in Mesopotamia and Egypt. It was introduced into Greece by **Anaximander** (611–547 BC), a pupil of Thales. A hemispherical sundial was invented by the Greek philosopher **Aristarchus** (*c.* 300 BC), who wrote a treatise *On the Sizes and Distances of the Sun and Moon,* which is extant. Several versions of sundials have been found in the remains of Pompeii and Tusculum, and they have been in use since the time of the Athenian statesman Pericles (*c.* 490–429 BC). Berosus, a Chaldean philosopher and priest at the temple of Belus, is supposed to have invented a hollow sundial, cut in a block of stone, in 300 BC. A sundial made by a Munich-born instrument maker and astronomer at Oxford, **Nicolas Kratzer** (1486–1550), and presented to Cardinal Wolsey (1471–1530), is still preserved. The world's largest sundial with a height of 118 feet was built in 1724 in Jaipur, India.

Sunspots   Dark spots on the sun's photosphere caused by a comparatively cool depression, were first recorded by Chinese astronomers in 165 BC. The first Western reference to sunspots was made around AD 820 by a historian, **Eginhard** (*c.* AD 770–840) of East Franconia, in his *Life of Charlemagne.* They were observed independently by **Simon Marius** (1573–1624) of Germany, **Galilei Galileo** (1564–1642) and **Johannes Fabricius** (1587–1615). The association between sunspots and terrestrial magnetic disturbances was discovered by a British physicist from Dublin, **Sir Edward Sabine** (1788–1883). Daguerreotype photographs of sunspots were taken in 1845 by **Jean Bernard Léon Foucault** (1819–1868). The ten-year periodicity of the sunspot cycle was discovered in 1843 by a German astronomer, **Samuel Heinrich Schwabe** (1789–1875). The sunspot cycle of 11 years was studied in detail in 1853 at Redhill, in Surrey, by a London astronomer, **Richard Christopher Carrington** (1826–1875). A London astronomer, **Edward Walter Maunder** (1851–1928), established the pattern of latitude drift in sunspots during the course of the sunspot cycle. The duration of the sunspot cycle was estimated by an American professor of physics and astronomy at Arizona, **Andrew Ellicott Doughlass** (1867–1962) from Windsor, Vermont.

Super Proton Synchrotron Accelerator   (SPS) The most powerful particle accelerator, installed at the Fermi National Accelerator Laboratory in Batavia, Illinois, around 1985. *See antiproton, boson.*

Superconductivity   Phenomenon of low electrical resistance in certain metals, when cooled to very low temperatures. In 1911 a Dutch physicist, **Heike Kamerlingh Onnes** (1853–1926), observed that the resistance of

mercury disappeared when it was cooled below a certain temperature, and his finding led to the discovery of superconductivity. In 1882 he became professor of experimental physics at Leyden, and in 1894 established the famous Cryogenic Laboratory there for studying low-temperature physics. The Bardeen–Cooper–Schrieffer theory of superconductivity, based on the movement of electrons, was developed in 1957 by three American physicists, **John Bardeen** (1908–1991) of Madison, Wisconsin, **Leon Niels Cooper** (b 1930) of New York, and **John Robert Schrieffer** (b 1931) of Oak Park, Illinois. The study of superconductivity in relation to insulators exposed to a magnetic field (DC Josephson effect) and current (AC Josephson effect) was carried out by a British physicist, **Brian David Josephson** (b 1940) from Cardiff. A new family of superconducting compounds at a higher temperature was discovered by a German physicist, **Johannes Georg Bednorz** (b 1950) and a Swiss physicist, **Karl Alex Muller** (b 1927) of Basel. They shared the Nobel Prize for physics for their work in 1987. A Norwegian-born US physicist, **Ivar Giaever** (b 1929), studied the tunneling effect in superconductors and his work led to the technique of measuring superconductor energy gaps. For his work on microelectronics he shared the Nobel Prize for physics in 1973, with a Japanese physicist, **Leo Esaki** (b 1925) and Brian David Josephson. In 1935, two German-born brothers and physicists in Britain, **Fritz Wolfgang London** (1900–1954) and **Heinz London** (1907–1970) derived the London equations that described the electromagnetic behavior of superconductors. Fritz London continued his research on superconductivity at Duke University in the USA. Heinz London worked on the atomic project and joined the Atomic Energy Research unit at Harwell, Berkshire, in 1946. The London equations were further advanced in relation to superconductivity and electromagnetic properties by a London physicist, **Brian Pippard** (b 1920). A German-born US physicist, **Bernard Teo Matthias** (b 1918), discovered that alloys with metals of five or seven valency electrons were the most effective. As a result of his work several new metal alloys came to be used as supeconductors until they were replaced by ceramic materials in the 1990s.

Supernova   A brilliant explosion of a massive star with a large burst of energy, leaving behind a gas cloud. Chinese astronomers recorded one in 1054. **Tycho Brahe** (1546–1601) described the supernova of 1572 in his *Astronomia instauratae progymnasmata* published posthumously in 1602. **Johannes Kepler** (1571–1630) recorded another in 1604 and published *The New Star* (1606).

Supersonic Flight Pioneer work on supersonic projectiles and jets was carried out in 1887 by an Austrian physicist, **Ernst Mach** (1838–1916). **Lawrence Dale Bell** (1895–1956), an aircraft designer from Indiana, launched the first jet-propelled aircraft in 1942, followed by the first manned aircraft to exceed the speed of sound in 1947. A test pilot, **Charles Elwood Yeager** (b 1923) of Myra, West Virginia, achieved supersonic flight by breaking the sound barrier at 670 miles per hour at the Edwards Air Force Base, Muroc, California in the same year. He later reached 2.5 times the speed of sound in 1953. In 1948 **John Derry** (d 1952) reached supersonic speed in England. An American pilot, **Jacqueline Cochran** (1910–1980), became the first woman to exceed the sound barrier, in 1953, and in 1964 she flew faster than twice the speed of sound. The first Russian supersonic aircraft intended for commercial use, the *Tupolev 144*, was demonstrated by the Soviets in 1968. The first supersonic passenger plane to go into service, Aérospatiale *Concorde,* with a speed of 1450 miles per hour, and designed for 100 passengers, was flown in 1969. It was built as a result of a 1.5 billion GBP joint venture started in 1962 between France and Great Britain. Its first regular passenger flights were to Bahrain in 1976, before it commenced its transatlantic flights to New York in 1977. The *Tupolev 144*, popularly known as *Concordski,* boasted a faster speed of 1518 miles per hour (Mach 2.3). It went out of control at the Paris Airshow in 1973 and crashed, killing the entire crew. In 2000, the *Concorde* was withdrawn from service following a crash, also in Paris, in which all crew and passengers perished. *See airplane, sound barrier.*

Superstring Theory Based on the idea that the ultimate constituents of nature, when inspected at very small scales, do not exist as point-like particles, but as strings in more than three dimensions. The theory attempts to unify general relativity with quantum mechanics, and was developed by a London physicist, **Michael Boris Green** (b 1946), John H. Schwarz and **Edward Witten** (b 1952).

Surface Chemistry The English chemist **Robert Boyle** (1627–1691) mentioned the iridescence of metallic films and soap bubbles in his *Experiments and Considerations touching Colors* (1664). **Robert Hooke** (1635–1703) investigated soap bubbles, oil on water and transparent films. The second small drop following the main drop of a liquid falling from a surface was first described by a Belgian chemist and professor of physics at Ghent, **Joseph Antoine Ferdinand Plateau** (1801–1883) and it was named after him. His main interest was the study of surface properties of fluids. The bursting of soap-films was photographically studied by the English physicist, **Lord John William Strutt Rayleigh** (1842–1919). Two English physicists, **Arnold William Reinhold** (1843–1921) and **Sir Arthur William Rücker** (1848–1915), measured the thickness of soap film with an interferometer. Surface chemistry was initiated as a special science in 1917 by an American chemist, **Irving Langmuir** (1881–1957) of Brooklyn, New York, who was awarded the Nobel Prize for chemistry for his work, in 1932. His work was advanced by an English chemist, **Neil Kensington Adam** (b 1891), who worked on unimolecular surface films of water from 1920 to 1939. He published a series of *The Physics and Chemistry of Surfaces* (1930, 1938, 1941). Further important research on the subject was done by an English physicist, **Sir John Edward Lannard-Jones** (b 1894), who became professor of theoretical chemistry in 1932. An English chemist from Lancashire, **Sir Hugh Stott Taylor** (1890–1974), who moved to the USA in 1914, carried out important research on the kinetics of reactions on surfaces, around 1920. *See emulsification, surface tension.*

Surface Tension The tension exihibited by the surface of a liquid, giving the surface some elastic charateristics. Whenever a free surface of a liquid is produced it tends to form the smallest possible area, owing to the mutual attraction of molecules. This phenomenon was known since **Thomas Graham's** (1805–1869) research on solutions in 1835, and was used in the process of emulsification and the production of soap. Early work in England was carried out by **Samuel Sugden** (1892–1950), a chemist from Leeds, who became professor of chemistry at University College London, in 1937. A simple experiment to demonstrate surface tension was devised by van der Mensbrugghe in 1866 and the apparatus to measure it was devised by Röntgen and Schneider in 1886. The Eötvös law, describing the relationship between surface tension, molar volume and the temperature of liquids, was proposed around 1870 by a Hungarian physicist, **Baron Roland von Eötvös** (1848–1919) of Budapest.

Surveying The Egyptian rope-stretchers known as *harpedonaptae* used ropes to measure distances. Their ropes knotted in certain ratios were probably the earliest devices in surveying. The diopter, an ancient form of theodolite, was suggested for land surveying by the Greek inventor, **Hero of Alexandria** (*c.* AD 100). His instrument consisted of a straight bar fitted with a movable indicator. He also devised an odometer for measuring distances. The astrolabes used in Babylonia and Greece were astronomical as well as surveying instruments. Metal parts of an ancient surveying instrument, the *groma,* were found at Pompeii in 1912. The original *groma* consisted of a six-foot long wooden staff with a metal foot that could be thrust into the ground. Its wooden arm swung on a pivot, at the top of the staff. The Roman surveyors, known as *agrimensores* [Greek: *agros,* field + Latin: *mensus,* measure] used simple geometrical methods for their work. The simple carpenter's square was used from the Middle Ages up to the 17th century, for measuring the height of towers, the depth of wells and the breadth of rivers. The cross-staff or *baculum,* consisting of a wooden rod of about four feet, fitted with a perpendicular cross-piece of equal arms, was used in the 15th to 17th century. A method of surveying using the principle of triangulation, which accurately located the points inaccessible to the surveyor, was introduced by a Dutch geographer, **Reiner Gemma Frisius** (1508–1555) of Dokkum. The modern theodolite, a telescope adapted to surveying, was invented in 1551 by an Oxford mathematician, **Leonard Digges** (1520–1571). His invention was published in 1571 by his son **Thomas Digges** (d 1595). An odometer used for the purpose of land surveying was invented by Paul Pfinzing of Nuremberg in 1554. An Italian mathematician, **Niccolò Fontana Tartaglia** (1499–1557) of Venice, invented a surveying compass called a circumferentor, which was described by a London mathematician, **William Leybourn** (d 1696) in his *Compleat Surveyor* (1674). Leybourn also described the plaintable which combined the features of a theodolite and circumferentor. A Dutch mathematician, **Willebrord Snell** (1591–1626), developed the use of triangulation in surveying. An important early treatise on surveying, *Geodartes Practicus: or, the art of surveying* (1664) was published by an English astronomer **Vincent Wing** (1619–1668). His nephew John Wing published *Geodartes Practicus Redivivus* in 1770. *See astrolabe, diopter, odometer, theodolite.*

Suspension Bridges An American civil engineer, **James Finley** (1762–1828) of Pennsylvania, proposed the idea of building suspension bridges, with the use of wrought-iron chains and masonry towers. His first such bridge was completed in 1801, and built the second one at Newburyport, over the Merrimack River, in 1810. The first practical suspension bridge in Europe, made of cables of wire, was built in Geneva by a French engineer, **Marc Seguin** (1786–1875) from Annonay. A Scottish engineer from Dumfries, **Thomas Telford** (1757–1834), built a bridge suspended by metal chains, over the Menai Strait connecting the island of Anglesey and the mainland, and it opened to traffic in 1826. A German-born US engineer, **John Augustus Roebling** (1806–1869), started using wire ropes in 1846, and built the suspension bridge at Niagara Falls in 1855. He designed the Brooklyn Bridge at New York which was completed in 1883 by his son **Washington Augustus Roebling** (1837–1926). The first wire-cable suspension bridge in America was built by **Charles Ellet** (1810–1862) of Pennsylvania, over the Ohio River in West Virginia. The highest suspension bridge in the world, having a height of 1053 feet, over the Royal Gorge of the Arkansas River, Colorado, was built in 1929. A Swiss-born American engineer, **Othmar Hermann Amman** (1879–1965), designed some of America's greatest suspension bridges, including the George Washington Bridge (1931) in New York, and the Golden Gate Bridge (1937) of San Francisco. The long-span suspension bridges over the Forth, Severn and Humber rivers were built by a London engineer, **Sir Ralph Freeman** (1880–1950), who also designed the Sydney Harbour Bridge in 1932.

Sutherland, Earl Wilbur Jr (1915–1974) A US physiologist who discovered cyclic AMP, a chemical messenger made by an enzyme in all living cells. He was awarded the Nobel Prize for Physiology or Medicine in 1971.

Sutherland, Gordon (1907–1980) A Scottish physicist from Caithness who used infrared spectroscopy to study molecular structure. At Michigan, USA, he was one of the first to use spectroscopy to study biophysical problems.

Sutton, Walter Stanborough (1877–1916) *See chromosomes.*

Svedberg, Theodor (1884–1971) *See centrifuge.*

Sverdrup, Harald Ulrik (1888–1957) *See oceanography.*

Swammerdam, Jan (1637–1680) *See entomology.*

Swan, Sir Joseph Wilson (1828–1914) *See artificial silk, electric lighting, photography, textile chemistry.*

Swedenborg, Emanuel (1688–1772) *See airplane, metallurgy.*

Swinburne, Sir James (1858–1958) *See celluloid.*

Swineshead, Richard (*c.* 1350) *See motion.*

Swinton, Alan Archibald Campbell (1863–1930) *See television.*

Sylow Theorem A fundamental theorem related to special types of subgroups in mathematics. Proposed by a Norwegian mathematician, **Ludwig Mejdel Sylow** (1832–1918) of Oslo. *See bridges.*

Sylow, Ludwig Mejdel (1832–1918) *See Sylow theorem.*

Sylvester, James Joseph (1814–1897) An English mathematician who developed the theory of algebraic variants. *See American Journal of mathematics, scientific journals.*

Symbiosis [Greek: *sym*, together + *bios,* life] The association of two different types of living things which results in mutual benefit. First demonstrated in 1860 in forms such as lichens, associations between an alga and a fungus, by a German botanist, **Heinrich Anton de Bary** (1831–1888).

Symbolic Algebra The first work on uniformly symbolic algebra, *In artem analytica isogoge* (1591), which used letters for both unknown and known quantitites, was published by the French mathematician **François Viète** (1540–1603).

Symbolic Logic *See mathematical logic.*

Symbols *See chemical symbols, mathematical symbols.*

Syme, James (1799–1870) *See Macintosh cloth.*

Symington, William (1763–1831) *See steamships.*

Symons, George James (1838–1900) *See scientific journals, weather forecast.*

Synchrotron A particle accelerator for accelerating electrons along a circular path. *See antiproton, boson, particle accelerator, super proton synchrotron accelerator.*

Synchrotron Radiation A polarized form of radiation produced by high-speed electrons in a magnetic field. In 1953 a Soviet astronomer, **Josef Samuilovich Shklovsky** (1916–1985), indicated the Crab nebula and other nebulae as possible sources in astronomy.

Synge, Richard Laurence Millington (1914–1994) *See chromatography.*

Synthesis [Greek: *syn,* together + *thesis,* placing] A term first used in chemistry by a German chemist, **Adolf Wilhelm Hermann Kolbe** (1818–1884), professor of chemistry at Leipzig. He is regarded as the founder of organic chemistry and synthesized the first organic compound, acetic acid, from inorganic materials.

Szilard, Leo (1898–1964) *See atomic bomb.*

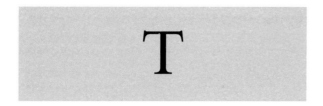

Tabor, David (b 1913) *See polymer.*

Taczanowski, Ladislaus (1819–1890) *See ornithology.*

Tait, Peter Guthrie (1831–1901) A Scottish mathematician and physicist from Dalkeith, who became professor of mathematics at Belfast in 1854, before his appointment in 1860 as professor of natural philosophy at Edinburgh. He wrote a treatise on quaternions, and his work on vortices and smoke rings contributed to the development of the topology of knots. He discovered the importance of underspin in the motion of the golfball, and published a number of books on physics. *See knot theory.*

Takayanagi, Kenjiro (b 1899) *See television.*

Talbot, William Henry Fox (1800–1877) *See photography, talotype process.*

Talotype Process or calotype process. A negative-to-positive process which revolutionized photography. It was invented by an English Victorian squire, **William Henry Fox Talbot** (1800–1877) from Wiltshire, who used the method to produce the first photographically illustrated book in the world, *The Pencil of Nature* (1844). Talbot's process was patented in Britain in 1841, and in the USA in 1847. *See photography.*

Tamm, Igor Yevgenyevich (1895–1971) *See Cherenkov effect.*

Tan The term was first used in trigonometry by a Dutch mathematician, **Albert Girard** (1595–1632) in his book on the subject published in 1626.

Tangent A line that touches a curve at one point only without cutting the curve. A German astronomer, **Regiomontanus** (1436–1476) from Konigsberg, wrote an astrological work *Tabulae Directionum* (1475), which contained a valuable table of tangents. The term tangent was first used by a Danish mathematician, **Thomas Finck** (1561–1646), in his book on geometry published in 1583. The theory of tangents was developed by **René Descartes** (1596–1650). **Isaac Barrow** (1630–1677), a teacher of **Sir Isaac Newton** (1642–1727) at Cambridge, suggested a method for drawing a tangent at a given point on a curve.

Tangent Galvanometer The first practical moving coil galvanometer was constructed by **William Sturgeon** (1783–1850) of Whittington, Lancashire, in 1836. Another early device used for measuring electric current was invented in 1837 by a French physicist, **Claude Servais Matthias Pouillet** (1790–1868), who was professor of physics in Paris. A German physicist and physiologist, **Hermann Ludwig Ferdinand von Helmholtz** (1821–1894), improved the instrument by adding two co-axial cables. This was followed in 1840 by an electrodynamometer invented by a German physicist, **Wilhelm Eduard Weber** (1804–1891). Weber's instrument was further developed by **William Thomson, Lord Kelvin** (1824–1907) and **James Prescott Joule** (1818–1889), in 1883. An improved form of the galvanometer was built in 1880 by **Jacques Arsène d'Arsonval** (1851–1940), and it was named after him.

Tansley, Arthur George (1871–1955) *See ecology, scientific journals.*

Tantalum [Greek: *tantalos,* symbol of eternal torment] An element with atomic number 73 discovered in 1802 by a Swedish chemist, **Anders Gustat Ekeberg** (1767–1813) of Stockholm. It was so named because of the tantalizing search for a substance to react with it.

Taoism An early scientific and philosophical movement in China which originated around the 5th century BC. The goal was to seek a hypothetical state or order of nature called Tao, and several methods were tried to achieve physical immortality. Around the 2nd century AD, it had developed into a religion.

Tape Recorder An American of French origin, Leon Scott de Martinville, was the first to make graphic recordings of speech with the use of a vibrating membrane and a stylus, in 1856. The first patent for an apparatus which transmitted recorded speech was obtained in 1877 by **Thomas Alva Edison** (1847–1931). The forerunner of the magnetic tape recorder, a telegraphone with a wire recording device, was invented by a Danish engineer, **Valdemar Poulsen** (1869–1942) of Copenhagen, in 1898. The first magnetic tape recorders were introduced into Germany by Fritz Pfleumer in 1928. Plastic tapes for recording were developed by BASF of Germany in 1934. *See magnetic recording, musical recording, video tapes.*

Tartaglia, Niccolò Fontana (1499–1557) Also known as Nicholas the stammerer, he was born in Brescia and died in Venice. He was appointed to the chair of mathematics in Venice in 1535, and discovered the solution of the cubic, and studied the fall of bodies under gravity and projectiles. His published works include *Della nova scienza* (1537), *Questi et invenzioni diverse* (1546) and *Trattato de numeri e misuri* (1556). *See accountancy, ballistics, Euclid, military architecture, military engineering, permutation, probability theory, surveying.*

Tatum, Edward Lawrie (1909–1975) An American biochemist from Boulder, Colorado who worked with **George Wells Beadle** (1903–1989) of Wahoo, Nebraska at Stanford University, to develop the concept that specific genes controlled specific enzymes. He shared the Nobel Prize for Medicine or Physiology in 1958, for his work on biochemical genetics, with Beadle and **Joshua Lederberg** (b 1925).

Taube, Henry (b 1915) A Canadian-born professor of chemistry at Stanford who was awarded the Nobel Prize in Chemistry, for his work on ionic inorganic reactions, in 1983.

Tautomerism [Greek: *tautos,* the same] A type of isomerism where a compound exists as a mixture of two interconvertible isomers in equilibrium. The concept was proposed by **Alexandr Mikhailovich Butlerov** (1828–1886), an organic chemist from Prussia. A German organic chemist, **Johann Friedrich Wilhelm Adolf von Bayer** (1835–1917) of Berlin, was one of the first to recognize the phenomenon.

Taxonomy [Greek: *taxis,* arrangement + *nomos,* law] A systematic classification of plants and animals on a morphological basis. The term taxonomy was coined independently by **Carolus Linnaeus** (1707–1778) in Sweden, and in 1813 by a Swiss botanist, **Augustin Pyrame de Candolle** (1778–1841). Linnaeus used a sexual system for classification of plants while Candolle considered morphology as the sole basis of taxonomy. The son of Pyrame de Candolle, **Alphonse Louis Pierre Candolle** (1806–1893) studied the processes governing the distribution of plants on the earth, and published *Géographie botanique raisonée* (1855) and *Origine des plantes cultivées* (1883). A German physician and naturalist, **Peter Simon Pallas** (1741–1811) of Berlin, who emigrated to England in 1761, did work on comparative anatomy, which formed the basis for modern taxonomy. He published *Miscellania Zoologica* in 1766. A French botanist and physician, **Antoine Laurent de Jussieu** (1748–1836) of Lyons, and his uncle **Bernard de Jussieu** (1699–1777) were pioneers in the field. Antoine published *Examen de la Famille des Renoncules* (1773), *Exposition d'un nouvel ordre de Plantes* (1774), *Genera Plantarum* (1789) and several other important works in botany.

Taylor, Brook (1685–1731) A mathematician from Edmonton in London, who received his education at St John's College, Cambridge, and graduated in law. He published a *Treatise on the Centre of Oscillation* (1703) and his *Methodus Incrementorum Directa et Inversa* (1715) formed the basis for the calculus of finite differences. In 1715 he gave the first analytical solution for the vibrating string, and a mathematical series is named after him.

Taylor, Edward Story (1903–1991) *See internal combustion engine, turbine.*

Taylor, Frederick Winslow (1856–1915) *See management.*

Taylor, John Edward (1791–1884) *See newspapers.*

Taylor, Joseph Hooton (b 1941) *See pulsar.*

Taylor, Richard Edward (b 1929) *See quarks.*

Taylor, Sir Geoffrey Ingram (1886–1975) *See meteorology.*

Taylor, Sir Hugh Stott (1890–1974) *See surface chemistry.*

Tea [Latin: *thea*] An infusion from the dried leaves of *Camellia sinensis,* introduced into Europe from the East by the Dutch in 1610. A Scottish botanist, physician and paleontologist, **Hugh Falconer** (1808–1865), carried out the first experiments on growing tea in India. A botanical investigations of tea plant in India and China were carried out in 1848 by another Scottish botanist and plant collector, **Robert Fortune** (1813–1880), at the request of the East India Company. He published *Two Visits to the Tea Mountains of China* in 1853.

Tebbutt's Comet First observed by an Australian astronomer John Tebbutt (1834–1916) from his home in Windsor, near Sydney. He published more than 300 scientific papers.

Technetium [Greek: *techne,* craft] *See masurium.*

Technicolor *See cinema.*

Tectonic Theory [Greek: *tecton,* joiner] Evidence suggests that the land surface of the earth was a single primeval continent or *Pangaea.* The tectonic theory is based on the concept that the earth's outer surface or crust is made up of a number of plates which move horizontally up to a few inches per year. The Greek philosopher **Xenophanes of Colophon** (*c.* 560–478 BC) believed that the surface of the earth changed with time. **Francis Bacon** (1561–1626), the Lord Chancellor of England and philosopher, thought that the continents may have drifted about the earth's surface. A London-born Austrian geologist, **Eduard Suess** (1831–1914), proposed that once there was a large supercontinent which became the present southern continents. He published *Das Antliz der Erde* (1885–1909), which was translated into English as *The Face of the Earth.* His work formed the basis of subsequent theories on continental drift. The theory of continental drift (Wegener hypothesis) was proposed by a German geophysicist, **Alfred Lothar Wegener** (1880–1930) of Berlin, in his *Die Enstehung der Kontinente und Ozeane* (Origins of Continents and Oceans) in 1912. A South African geologist, **Alexander Logie Du Toit** (1878–1948) contributed to continental drift theory and plate tectonics. In 1937, in his *Our Wandering Continents* he pointed out that the southern continents had, in earlier times, formed the supercontinent. An American paleontologist, **Edwin Harris Colbert** (b 1905) provided the paleontological evidence for Wegener's theory. Colbert's popular account for the evidence on continental drift, *Wandering Land and Animals,* was published in 1973. A general interest in continental drift was promoted by an English geologist, **Arthur Holmes** (1890–1965) of Newcastle upon Tyne. A study of plate tectonics in relation to geology was carried out by an American oceanographer and geologist, **William Maurice Ewing** (1906–1974) from Texas, who was professor of geology at the Columbia University. Tectonic theory in relation to oceanography was advanced by a New York geologist, **Harry Hammond Hess** (1906–1969). A French earth scientist, **Louis Antonin François Lliboutry** (b 1922), studied plate tectonics and derived a predictive theorem for plate velocities. In 1967, an English geologist, **Dan Peter McKenzie** (b 1942), developed a theory of plate tectonics that led to the understanding of Wegener's theory.

Teisserenc, Léon Philippe (1855–1913) *See stratosphere.*

Telegraphy *See electric telegraphy, Morse code, wireless telegraphy.*

Telephone [Greek: *tele,* far + *phone,* sound] The theory was suggested in 1849 by Antonio Meucci of Italy, and it was invented by **Alexander Graham Bell** (1847–1922) from Edinburgh. An English philologist and phoneticist, **Alexander John Ellis** (1814–1890), demostrated to Bell the important principle that the vibration of a tuning-fork could be influenced by electric current. In 1876 Bell succeeded in transmitting a vocal message to his assistant, Thomas Watson, in another room. His work on vocal physiology led to the invention of the telephone, which he patented on 4th February 1876. **Elisha Gray** (1835–1901), an inventor from Barnesville in Ohio, independently built a telephone around the same time, without being aware of Alexander Graham Bell's work. When Gray visited the patent office to register his invention, he found that Bell had already patented the device a few hours earlier. The first long-distance telephone call was made between between Alexander Graham Bell in New York and Thomas A. Watson in San Francisco in 1915. The first transatlantic call from

Arlington, Virginia to the Eiffel Tower in Paris took place later in the same year. The first dial telephones were installed in New Jersey, in 1914. *See facsimile machine, microphone, telephone exchange.*

Telephone Exchange The first telephone switchboard was installed in 1878 at New Haven, Connecticut. Early telephone exchanges involved manual connection of plugs and sockets. The automatic system was invented in 1892 by a Kansas undertaker, Alman B. Strowger, and it was installed at La Poste, Indiana. A Welsh electrical engineer, **Sir William Henry Preece** (1834–1913) introduced telephones into Britain. The electronic exchanges were introduced in the 1960s, and direct dialing across the Atlantic (London to Paris) commenced in 1967. The fiberoptic system for telephone lines was introduced in 1977. A single optical fiber capable of sending 300 000 simultaneous telephone conversations was developed at the AT&T Bell Laboratories in 1985. GEC Plessy Comunications demonstrated a telephone exchange capable of handling over 1 558 000 calls per hour, at Beeston, Nottingham, in 1989.

Telephotography *See facsimile machine.*

Telescope [Greek: *telos,* distance + *skopein,* to view] **Roger Bacon** (*c.* 1214–*c.* 1298) suggested the principle of the telescope around 1250. An Oxford mathematician, **Leonard Digges** (*c.* 1520–1571), constructed a telescope that was described later by his son **Thomas Digges** (d 1595). The first practical telescope was probably invented in 1608 by Dutch lensmaker, **Hans Lippershey** (1571–1619). A spectacle maker, Zacharias Jensen of Middelberg, is also credited with the invention, in 1604. According to **René Descartes** (1596–1650), it was invented by James Metius. The term telescope was coined in Italy around 1611. **Galilei Galileo** (1564–1642) heard of the invention in 1609, and constructed his own telescope, consisting of a concave eyepiece and a convex objective, with which he was able to make several important discoveries in astronomy. His findings were published in the *Sidereal Messenger* in 1610. An improved telescope with a wider field of view for astronomical use, was suggested by **Johannes Kepler** (1571–1630) in his *Dioptric* (1611). A telescope on the principles suggested by Kepler, was constructed by Christoph Scheiner of Vienna around 1614, and it superseded the Dutch model. A reflecting telescope for overcoming the spherical aberration, was proposed by **James Gregory** (1638–1675) in 1663, and it was built by **Sir Isaac Newton** (1642–1727), in 1668. **Chester Moor Hall** (1703–1771) invented the achromatic lens which produce images free of color fringes (chromatic aberration) in 1733. The Schmidt telescope, which eliminated the aberrations produced by spherical mirrors, was invented by an Estonian optical instrument-maker, **Bernhard Voldemar Schmidt** (1879–1935) in 1932. The world's largest Schmidt telescope is currently at Karl Schwarzschild Observatory in Tautenberg, Germany. The next largest was installed at the Palomar Observatory in California in 1948. *See reflecting telescope.*

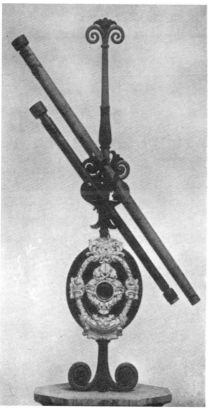

Figure 77   Galileo's telescopes. Singer, Charles. *Studies in the History and Method of Science.* Oxford: Clarendon Press, 1921

Television [Greek: *telos,* distance + *vision,* see]   A mechanical scanning device consisting of a revolving disk (Nipkow's disk), which formed the basis of television, was patented in 1884 by a German, **Paul Nipkow** (1860–1940) of Lauenberg. His device was based on the principle of photoconductivity of selenium discovered in 1873, and from the idea of television proposed in 1875 by an American, George Carey. The concept of television was promoted in 1880 by W.P. Sawyer of America, and a Frenchman, Maurice Leblanc. The first commercial cathode ray tube was devised in 1897 by a German physicist, **Karl Ferdinand Braun** (1850–1918) from Fulda in Prussia. Braun shared the Nobel Prize for physics with Marconi for his work in 1909. A Russian professor at St Petersburg, **Boris Rosing** (d 1918),

linked it to electric-vision in 1907. A Frenchman, Vichard, improved the process of focusing with a concentric electrode. **Alan Archibald Campbell Swinton** (1863–1930) published an early paper entitled *Distant Electric Vision* in the journal *Nature* in 1908. Televisions were produced only on an experimental basis, until the Bell Telephone Company managed a direct transmission from New York to Washington in 1927. The television was patented in 1928 by a Scottish electrical engineer, **John Logie Baird** (1888–1946), a graduate of Glasgow University. He gave up his position as an electrical engineer at the Clyde Valley Electric Power Company because of ill health, and started his research on television in 1922. The first public demonstration of his television image was given in 1924, and he launched his first television service through a BBC transmitter in 1929. The image of Baird and another person was transmitted in 1928 from Coulsdon, Surrey, to Hartsdale, New York. His commercial models, Baird Televisors, were marketed in 1930. The first all-electronic television camera tube with no moving parts, the iconoscope, was invented in 1928 by a Russian-born American electronic engineer, **Vladimir Kosma Zworykin** (1889–1982). In 1926 **Kenjiro Takayanagi** (b 1899) transmitted a 40–line electronic picture, with the help of Braun's tube and the Nipkow disk, in Japan. The first television transmitter in France was installed in 1935 on the Eiffel Tower, and the world's first commercial television transmitter was set up in 1936 on the Empire State Building, New York by the Radio Corporation of America. The world's first high-definition television pictures with 405 lines were transmitted from Alexandra Palace, London, in the same year. A television camera similar to the iconoscope, the *Emitron,* designed by J.D. McGee, was used for this transmission. By 1939 London BBC had transmitted television to 20 000 homes in England. The first live television pictures across the Atlantic via a satellite were transmitted through the telecommunication satellite *Telstar* in July 1962.

Television Camera   *See iconoscope.*

Telex   The first teleprinter was invented by a Canadian, **Frederick George Creed** (1871–1957). He perfected the system, which was named after him and first used in 1921 in Fleet Street, the headquarters of the British press. It was rapidly adapted in offices throughout the world and came to be known as Telex.

Telford, Thomas (1757–1834)   *See bridges, canals, Institute of Civil Engineers, roads.*

Teller, Edward (b 1908)   *See H bomb.*

Tellurium [Latin: *tellus*, earth] Discovered in 1782 as an impurity in a gold-bearing ore, by an Austrian minerologist, **Franz Joseph Muller** (1740–1825), also known as **Baron von Reichenstein**. A Hungarian chemist, **Paul Kitaibel** (1757–1817), discovered it independently in 1789. A German chemist, **Martin Heinrich Klaproth** (1743–1817) of Berlin, gave the metal its present name.

Telpherage A surface contact overhead electrical system for railways first installed at Glydde, Sussex in England. It was invented in 1881 by a London electrical engineer, **William Edward Ayrton** (1847–1908) and John Perry.

Temminck, Coenraad Jacob (1778–1858) *See ornithology.*

Temperate Zone *See climatic zones.*

Tennant, Smithson (1761–1816) *See diamond, iridium, osmium.*

Tennant, Charles (1768–1838) *See bleaching powder.*

Tephigram A thermodynamic diagram used in meteorology, devised in 1915 by an English meteorologist, **Sir William Napier Shaw** (1854–1945) of Birmingham.

Terbium An element discovered in 1843 by a Swedish chemist, **Carl Gustav Mosander** (1797–1858). It derives its name from Ytterby in Sweden.

Tereshkova, Valentina Vladimirovna (b 1937) *See astronauts.*

Terpenes The first important work on this group of organic compounds was carried out by professor of chemistry at Göttingen, **Otto Wallach** (1847–1931) of Konigsberg. He elucidated the structure of the key compound α-terpineol in 1895, and was awarded the Nobel Prize for chemistry in 1910.

Terrestrial Globe *See globe.*

Terrestrial Magnetism *See aurora borealis, dip, magnet, magnetic poles.*

Tertiary Period Geological age divided into five epochs: Paleocene, Eocene, Oligocene, Miocene and Pliocene. An American geologist, **Josiah Edward Spurr** (1870–1950) of Gloucester, Massachusetts, estimated it to be 45 to 60 million years ago. A French geologist, **Alexandre Brogniart** (1770–1847), studied the strata in tertiary rocks and classified the tertiary formations.

Terylene *See polymer, textile chemistry.*

Tesla Coil An air core transformer with primary and secondary coils, for producing high-voltage electricity at high frequency. Invented in 1891 by **Nikola Tesla** (1856–1943), an American electrical engineer of Croatian origin.

Tesla, Nikola (1856–1943) *See alternating current, direct current, inductiuon current, radar, Tesla coil, torpedo.*

Tessin, Nicodemus (1615–1681) *See architecture, European.*

Tessin, Nicodemus (1654–1728) *See architecture, European.*

Textile Chemistry As early as 1664, **Robert Hooke** (1635–1703) in his *Micrographia* suggested that it was possible to make an artificial glutinous compound resembling silk. The first such filaments were produced in 1883 by **Sir Joseph Wilson Swan** (1828–1914) of Sunderland, by extruding solutions of nitrocellulose. His method was adopted commercially by a French chemist, **Hilaire Bernigaud Comte de Chardonnet** (1839–1924), and he exhibited his material which had a remarkable resemblance to the fibers of the silkworm, in 1889. A modern way of producing artificial forms of silk, viscose or rayon, was invented by two English chemists, **Frederick Charles Cross** (1855–1935) of Brentford, Middlesex and **Edward John Bevan** (1856–1921) of Birkenhead. The first direct cotton dye that needed no mordant was discovered in 1884 by a German industrial chemist, **Peter Johann Griess** (1829–1888). An English physicist and director of Textile Physics Research Laboratory at Leeds University, **William Thomas Astbury** (1898–1961), used X-rays to examine wool and other fibers used in industry. Nylon was developed in the 1930s by **Wallace Hume Carothers** (1896–1937) and his team at the Du Pont company and launched in 1939. The Swiss chemist **Hermann Paul Muller** (1899–1965), the inventor of the insecticide DDT, worked on moth-proofing of fabrics at the Basel dye research laboratory of Johan Rudolf Geigy, in 1939. Another major development in synthetic fabrics was the synthesis of Terylene in 1941 by **John Rex Whinfield** (1901–1966) of Sutton, Surrey.

Textile Industry Spinning and weaving is of Neolithic origin. Fine linen woven from flax obtained from the banks of the River Nile was used by the Egyptians to cover their dead, around 3000 BC. Manual methods with primitive looms were used to produce this linen. Simple yarn-making has been practiced by the Australian Aborigines since prehistoric times. Modern inventions mainly came after the 15th century. Wool cards, wooden instruments with copper-wire teeth set in leather, for converting short fibers into a fluffy mass in the woollen industry, were used in England during the reign of Queen Elizabeth I (1558–1603). The flying shuttle for producing textiles was invented in 1733 by an English engineer, **John Kay** (1704–1780) from Walmersley in Lancashire. His invention doubled production and improved the textile quality. He also patented a machine for twisting and cording mohair and worsted. **Jacques de**

Vaucanson (1709–1782) of Grenoble, France, invented the first self-acting mechanical loom while he was inspector of silk factories in 1745. An English handloom weaver, **James Hargreaves** (1720–1778) of Lancashire, developed the spinning jenny in 1764. He also invented a preparatory carding process before spinning, which helped to double the output. **Richard Arkwright** (1732–1792) of Preston, Lancashire, invented the water-frame for the first cotton factory in 1771. It was the first water-powered machine that could produce cotton thread of such a good quality and strength that it could be used as a warp. A spinning machine (spinning mule) for use in the cotton industry was invented in 1779 by **Samuel Crompton** (1753–1827) of Firwood near Bolton, Lancashire. **Paul Lewis** (d 1759) invented a rolling spinning machine for use in his factories in Birmingham and Northampton. He invented a carding machine in 1738, and patented another spinning machine in 1758. In 1830 a Welsh engineer, **Richard Roberts** (1789–1864) of Montgomeryshire, improved it by adding a radial arm for winding the yarn. In 1793 an American inventor from Westboro, Massachusetts, **Eli Whitney** (1765–1825) invented the gin, a machine that gathered cotton while simultaneously separating it from the seed. Automatic textile production systems were developed independently by an American engineer, **Oliver Evans** (1755–1819) of New Port, Delaware, and a French engineer, **Joseph Marie Jacquard** (1752–1834) of Lyons. Textile technology in Europe was developed by a British engineer, **William Cockerill** (1759–1832). After working in Russia he set up his company with his sons in France, where he made carding machines, spinning frames and looms for the French woollen industry. In 1788 a French industrialist, **Étienne Calla** (1760–1835), established a factory in Paris to make machines for spinning mills, and invented a mechanical loom for which he was awarded a gold medal in 1827. A knitting machine that advanced the production of hosiery was invented in 1864 by a British inventor, **William Cotton** (1786–1866) of Leyton, Sussex. An English chemist, **John Mercer** (1791–1866), invented the process of treating cotton with caustic soda, and produced mercerized cotton. In 1824 a Swiss inventor, **Johann Georg Bodmer** (1786–1874) from Zurich, established a factory in England, which made cotton carding and spinning machines. The export of textile technology and emigration of textile workers was banned in Britain in the 18th century. **Samuel Slater** (1768–1835) from Derbyshire, who managed to emigrate under a false name in 1789, revolutionized the textile industry in America. He built spinning machines for the cotton industry and laid the foundation for the modern American cotton industry. The first power loom for weaving ingrain carpets was invented by an American engineer, **Erastus Bigham Bigelow** (1814–1879) of West Boylston, Massachusetts. He was also an economist and wrote two books on the subject. Complicated lace-making machinary was invented by an English inventor, **John Heathcoat** (1783–1861) from Duffield, near Derby in 1798. He also invented a ribbon- and net-making device. A New York engineer, **George Henry Corliss** (1817–1888), imported his steam engines known as Corliss engines into Scotland for use in cotton mills in 1859. Their smooth running and sensitive controls prevented the fine threads from being broken. **Sir Titus Salt** (1803–1876) of Leeds was a pioneer of mechanized textile manufacture in England, and he established a wool spinning factory at Bradford in 1834. Another English textile industrialist, **Samuel Cunliffe Lister** (1815–1906) of Bradford, invented a successful wool-combing machine (1839) and a waste-silk spinning machine (1855), and took out 12 other patents for various machines in the textile industry. *See knitting, spinning, textile chemistry.*

Textile Technology *See textile industry.*

Thalen, Tobias Robert (1927–1905) A Swedish physicist and pioneer in the spectroscopic study of the rare earths who published an important work on spectrum analysis.

Thales (640–546 BC) A merchant from the city of Miletus in Asia Minor who is regarded as the first Greek philosopher. He was one of the first to devote his time to the study of mathematics. He measured the height of a pyramid by its shadow. He founded the field of geometry by proposing many basic concepts. He stated that a circle is bisected by its diameter and defined the isosceles triangle. He also studied astronomy and is said to have predicted the exact date of an eclipse, and determined the number of days in a year as 365. Thales proposed water as an essence and the origin of all things, and observed the electrical properties of amber. Although he did not leave any writings, most of his teachings have been conveyed through Aristotle's works. *See air, astronomy, clock, eclipse, electricity, geometry, magnet, mathematics, philosophy, physics.*

Thallium [Greek: *thallos,* dim] A London physicist, **Sir William Crookes** (1832–1919) discovered the element in 1861. A French professor of physics at Lille and later at Paris, **Claude Auguste Lamy** (1820–1873), discovered it independently in 1862. It has an atomic number of 81.

Theater First used by the Greeks for perfomance of drama as early as 500 BC. The first stone theater erected in Rome in 55 BC had a capacity for 40 000 spectators. The

Colosseum of Rome with a capacity for 876 000 was completed in AD 80. The earliest in London, near Finsbury Field, was built by an actor, James Burbage in 1576. The oldest preserved indoor theater in the world, Teatro Olimpico, in Vienza, Italy, was designed by Andrea de Pietro (1508–1590) and completed by his pupil, Vicenzo Scamozzi (1552–1616) in 1583. The Rose theater built by an English stage manager, Philip Henslowe (d 1616) in 1584, was unearthed by archaeologists at Bankside, Southwark in London in 1989.

Thenard Blue Used for coloring porcelain. Discovered by a French chemist, **Louis Jacques Thenard** (1777–1857). In 1804 he succeeded **Louis Nicolas Vauquelin** (1763–1829) as professsor of chemistry at the École Polytechnique and became chancellor of the University of Paris in 1825. *See porcelain.*

Thenard, Louis Jacques (1777–1857) *See boron, catalysis, Thenard blue.*

Theodolite [Arabic: *athelida*] An ancient form, diopter, for surveying was suggested by the Greek inventor, **Hero of Alexandria** around AD 100. The modern theodolite, a telescope adapted to surveying, was invented in 1551 by an Oxford mathematician, **Leonard Digges** (d 1571). His invention was published in 1571 by his son **Thomas Digges** (d 1595). It consisted of a horizontal circle divided into 360 equal parts, and mounted on a vertical semicircle of 180 parts. It was greatly improved in 1763 by an English mathematical instrument maker from Halifax, **Jesse Ramsden** (1735–1800).

Theodoric of Freiberg (1250–1310) *See rainbow.*

Theodorus of Cyrene (*c.* 400 BC) *See irrational numbers.*

Theodorus of Samos (*c.* 530 BC) *See lock, metallurgy.*

Theon of Smyrna (*c.* AD 250) *See musical theory, perfect number.*

Theophrastus (380–287 BC) Regarded as the father of botany, he was born on the Greek island of Lesbos, and studied under Plato. He was later a pupil of Aristotle, whom he succeeded at the Lyceum in 323 BC. His two treatises, describing over 500 varieties of plants, are the first known surviving works on botany. He classified plants and studied flowers in detail. The words *carpos* and *pericarp* were coined by him. *See botanical classification, botany, biology, flower, germination, plant pathology, roots.*

Thermal Conductivity Expressed as a mathematical formula in 1822 by a French physicist, **Jean Baptiste Joseph**

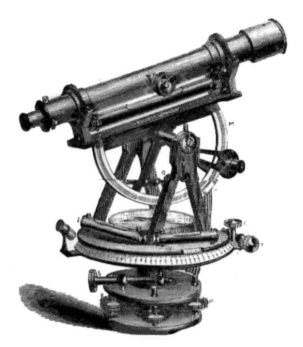

Figure 78 A mid-19th century theodolite. Guillemin, Amédée. *The Application of Physical Forces.* London: Macmillan and Co, 1877

Fourier (1768–1830) from Auxerre, France. His formula was used by a Swedish physicist, **Anders Jonas Ångström** (1814–1874), to determine the conductivity of a long bar. The thermal conductivity of a gas was predicted by **James Clerk Maxwell** (1831–1879).

Thermionic Valve [Greek: *therme*, heat + *eimi*, to go] The forerunner of the triode valve and transistor, which consisted of an evacuated glass or metal container, enclosing a system of two electrodes. It was invented in 1904 by an English electrical engineer, **Sir John Ambrose Fleming** (1849–1945) of Lancaster. An improved form of it, the triode, was invented in 1907 by an American physicist and pioneer in radio and wireless telegraphy from Iowa, **Lee de Forest** (1873–1961). He placed a metal grid between the filament and anode, to produce the triode, which acted as an amplifier as well as a rectifier. De Forest also invented the audion or the four-electrode valve.

Thermionics [Greek: *therme*, heat + *eimi*, to go] A term coined by an English physicist from Dewsbury, Yorkshire, **Sir Owen Willans Richardson** (1879–1959), to describe the phenomenon of emission of electricity (or electrons) from hot bodies (or a heated cathode). He published *The Emission of Electricity from Hot Bodies* (1916).

Thermocouple [Greek: *therme*, heat] A device in which an electric potential is created at the junction of two metals at different temperatures. The production of electricity by heating a junction of two dissimilar metals was discovered in 1822 by a German physicist of Estonian origin, **Thomas Johan Seebeck** (1770–1831). The method of measuring radiant heat based on this principle was invented by an Italian physicist, **Leopoldo Nobili** (1784–1835). A French physicist, **Jean Charles Athanase Peltier** (1785–1845), demonstrated the opposite effect or thermoelectric effect (Peltier effect), where a rise of temperature occurs when a current is passed through the junction of two different metals. Another Italian scientist, **Macedonio Melloni** (1798–1854) of Parma developed the thermocouple in 1850. A sensitive thermocouple for astronomical studies was invented in 1922 by an American physicist, Coblentz.

Thermodynamics [Greek: *therme*, heat + *dynos*, power] The term was coined in 1850 by **William Thompson, Lord Kelvin** (1824–1907), to denote the study of laws governing heat. A Swiss philosopher and scientist, **Pierre Prévost** (1751–1839), introduced the concept of dynamic equilibrium for heat in his *Sur l'équilbre du feu* (1792). Pioneer work was done by **Nicolas Leonard Sadi Carnot** (1796–1831), who proposed the first law (considered by some as the second law) of thermodynamics in 1824. His work was demonstrated experimentally by Clayperon (1799–1864) in 1834. The second law of thermodynamics, which states that energy in a closed system tends to become unusable as it gradually becomes uniform heat, was proposed in 1849 by **Rudolf Julius Emmanuel Clausius** (1822–1888), professor of physics at Bonn. In 1837 Karl Friedrich Mohr described heat as an oscillatory motion of small particles, and considered it to be a force similar to that described by Carnot. The first work on the relationship between heat and work was published in 1842 by **Julius Robert von Mayer** (1814–1878), a medical practitioner from Heilbronn, Bavaria. **James Prescot Joule** (1818–1889), a brewer from Salford, began a long series of experiments on heat in 1839, and demonstrated the relationship between work done and the generation of heat. He was the first accurately to determine the mechanical equivalent of heat, although **Marc Seguin** (1786–1875) made a rough estimate in 1839. One of the earliest textbooks on thermodynamics, *Théorie Mécanique de la Chaleur* (1862), was published by a French physicist, **Gustav Adolphe Hirn** (1815–1890). Joule's work was advanced by an American physicist, **Henry Augustus Rowland** (1848–1901) of Honesdale, Pennsylvania, in 1881. The third law of thermodynamics was verified experimentally by a German physicist, **Sir Francis Eugen Simon** (1893–1956) from Berlin, who left Germany because of its Nazi policies, and in 1935 became

reader in thermodynamics at the Clarendon Laboratory at the invitation of the English physicist, **Lord Frederick Alexander Lindemann** or **Viscount Cherwell** (1886–1957). An American physicist, **Josiah Willard Gibbs** (1839–1903), applied the principles of thermodynamics to chemistry. A Moscow-born Belgian chemist, **Ilya Vicomte Prigogine** (b 1917), made major contributions to the field of thermodynamics and applied it to 'dissipative' or non-equilibrium structures frequently found in biological and chemical reactions. Earlier theories had only considered systems at or about equilibrium. Prigogine's ideas have been applied to examine how life originated on Earth, to ecosystems and to the preservation of world resources. He received the Nobel Prize for chemistry in 1977 for his work.

Thermoelectricity The phenomenon was discovered by an Estonian-born German physicist, **Thomas Johann Seebeck** (1770–1831), who named it thermomagnetism in 1822. The changes in temperature at the junction of two dissimilar metals, when a current is passed through was observed in 1834 by a French physicist, **Jean Charles Athanase Peltier** (1785–1845). This principle is now used in thermocouples used for fine temperature measurement.

Thermometer [Greek: *therme*, heat + *metron*, to measure] The word thermometer was first used by J. Leurechon, a French Jesuit priest, in his work *Récréation Mathématique* (1624). The expansion of air due to heat was observed by ancient scientists including **Hero of Alexandria** (*c.* AD 100). **Philo of Byzantinium** appears to have constructed a thermoscope or air thermometer around 200 BC. An English physician, **Robert Fludd** (1574–1637), gave an account of a thermoscope, quoting a 500-year-old manuscript. An air thermometer for measuring temperature was invented by **Galilei Galileo** (1564–1642) in 1592. **Francis Bacon** (1561–1626) described a thermometer or thermoscope similar to that of Galileo in his *Novum Organon* (1620). The first suggestion of a liquid thermometer was made in 1632 by a French physician, John Rey, and the first such thermometer was constructed in 1650 by the Grand Duke of Tuscany, Ferdinand II (b 1610), the founder of the Academia del Cimento in Florence. He used a column of spirit in a sealed glass tube; his method was introduced into England by **Robert Boyle** (1627–1691). The first mercury thermometer was constructed by a French scientist, **Ismael Boulliau** (*c.* 1650), and it was developed by **Gabriel Daniel Fahrenheit** (1686–1736). Several workers including **Olaus Roemer** (1644–1710), Boyle and **Sir Isaac Newton** (1642–1727) proposed two fixed points in thermometry, and this was achieved in 1736 by **Anders Celsius** (1704–1744), who assigned two points to the melting point of ice and the boiling point of water. An improved air thermometer with the use of a copper sphere containing air attached to a U tube was designed in 1672 by **Otto von Guericke** (1602–1686), Mayor of Magdeburg in Prussia. **Sanctorius** (1561–1636), a professor at Padua, invented the first clinical thermometer for the study of metabolism. The familiar type of mercury thermometer was introduced by **Gabriel Daniel Fahrenheit** (1686–1736) in 1714. The scale of 80 degrees between the freezing and boiling points of water was introduced by **René Antoine Ferchault de Reaumer** (1683–1757), a mathematician and naturalist from La Rochelle in 1730. A differential thermometer containing two glass bulbs with air, separated by a liquid column, was described in 1803 by a Scottish physicist, **Sir John Leslie** (1766–1832) from Largo, Fifeshire, who published *An Experimental Inquiry into Heat* (1804). He became professor of natural philosophy at Edinburgh in 1819. A constant-pressure air thermometer (1891) that could measure up to 450 degrees Celsius and an accurate platinum thermometer (1886) were constructed by an English physicist, **Hugh Longbourne Callendar** (1863–1930) of Gloucestershire.

Thermonuclear Fusion The investigations in the 1930s into how the sun and the stars produced such vast energy led to the discovery of thermonuclear fusion. In 1938 a German physicist, **Baron Carl Friedrich von Weizsäcker** (b 1912), and a German-born US physicist, **Hans Albrecht Bethe** (b 1906), independently proposed that chain nuclear fusion reactions were the source of energy in the stars. The process involved a complicated cycle where four hydrogen atoms fused to create helium. A large amount of energy was released during the process, as the mass of the final helium atom was less than the total mass of four hydrogen atoms. This process is opposite to nuclear fusion, where a heavier nucleus such as uranium breaks up into lighter nuclei, releasing a large amount of energy. An American physicist, **Lyman Spitzer** (1914–1997) of Toledo, Ohio, following his research on the generation of energy in stars, attempted controlled thermonuclear fusion. In 1956, a Soviet physicist, **Igor Vasilevich Kurchatov** (1903–1963) obtained previously unattained high temperatures by passing an electric current through a tube containing deuterium; this formed the basis for further thermonuclear research. The first controlled major fusion experiment with ZETA (Zero Energy Thermonuclear Apparatus) was performed at Harwell, Berkshire in Britain around 1957. *See H bomb, pinch effect.*

Thermopile A number of thermocouples joined in series, and used in conjunction with a galvanometer, for measuring radiant heat. Invented by an Italian physicist, **Leopoldo**

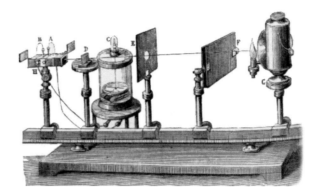

Figure 79 Thermopile of Leopoldo Nobili. Lardner, Dionysius. *Handbook of Natural Philosophy, Electricity, Magnetism, and Acoustics.* London: Walton and Maberly, 1856

Nobili (1784–1835) who was professor of physics at Florence. *See radiation of heat, thermocouple.*

Thiele, Friedrich Karl Johannes (1865–1918) *See valency.*

Thimonnier, Bathelèmy (1793–1857) *See sewing machine.*

Thiout, Antoine (1692–1767) *See horology, lathe.*

Throckmorton, Peter (1928–1990) *See marine archaeology.*

Thoma, Richard (1847–1923) *See microtome.*

Thomas, Clark (1801–1867) *See hard water.*

Thomas, Sidney Gilchrist (1850–1885) *See Bessemer process, steel.*

Thomason, George (d 1666) *See bookshops.*

Thompson, Benjamin, Count Rumford (1753–1814) An American-born physicist from Woburn, Massachusetts, who came to London in 1776. He was one of the first to suggest that heat is a form of energy, in 1796. He founded the Royal Institution in London in 1799, and established the Rumford Medals at the Royal Society, London, and the Rumford Chair at Harvard. *See clothing, cookers, gunpowder, heat.*

Thompson, John Taliaferro (1860–1940) *See firearms.*

Thompson, Sir D'Arcy Wentworth (1860–1948) *See ichthyology.*

Thompson, Sivanus Phillips (1851–1916) The first professor of physics at the University of Bristol in 1878, who published *Caluculus Made Easy* (1910) and several biographies of important scientists.

Thomsen, Christian Jörgensen (1788–1865) *See arrow, prehistory.*

Thomson, Sir Charles Wyville (1830–1882) *See Challenger, oceanography*.

Thomson, Elihu (1853–1937) An English-born US inventor who patented the arc light in 1881. He developed the three-phase alternating current generator, with **Edwin James Houston** (1847–1914), and founded the Thomson-Houston Electric Company in 1883.

Thomson, Sir George Paget (1892–1975) *See electron diffraction, electron microscope*.

Thomson, James (1822–1892) A Scottish engineer and brother of **William Thomson,** Lord Kelvin (1824–1907). He invented a turbine and discovered the effect of pressure on the freezing point of water.

Thomson, Robert William (1822–1873) *See Dunlop, John Boyd*.

Thomson, Sir John Joseph (1856–1940) An English physicist from Manchester who succeeded **Lord John William Strutt Rayleigh** (1842–1919) as Cavendish professor of experimental physics. He was awarded the Nobel Prize for physics in 1906 and was knighted in 1908. *See electric charge, cathode rays, electron, isotopes*.

Thomson, Thomas (1773–1852) A Scottish professor of chemistry at Glasgow in 1818 who published *System of chemistry* (1807) and established the first chemistry laboratory in Britain, in Glasgow, in 1817. *See pyridine*.

Thomson, William, Lord Kelvin (1824–1907) An eminent Scottish physicist, born in Belfast. In 1832 he came with his father to Glasgow, where he attended Glasgow University at the age of 10. He designed the first successful transatlantic cable system, which was installed in 1866. *See ampere, Diesel, Rudolph Christian Karl, electric telegraphy, electrical resistance, energy, heat pump, Joule–Thomson effect, knot theory, tangent galvanometer, thermodynamics*.

Thor The first American surface-to-surface intermediate-range ballistic missile, launched in 1958. Propelled by a liquid-fuel rocket engine, it was used for launching several space probes.

Thorarinsson, Sigurdur (1912–1983) *See glaciology*.

Thorium [*Thor,* god of thunder] An element of atomic number 90, discovered by a Swedish chemist, **Jons Jacob Berzelius** (1779–1848). The radioactivity of thorium, uranium and other possible minerals in pitchblende was demonstrated by **Marie Curie** (1867–1934) and **Pierre Curie** (1859–1906) in 1898. *See ionium*.

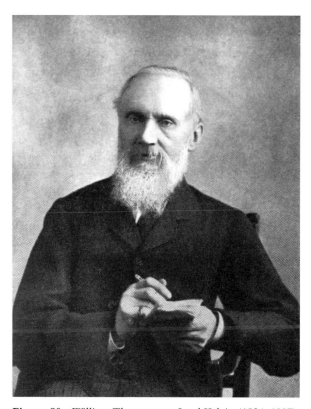

Figure 80 William Thomson, or Lord Kelvin (1824–1907). Snyder, Carl. *New Conceptions in Science*. London: Harper and Brothers, 1903

Thornycroft, John (1843–1928) *See hovercraft*.

Thorpe, Sir Thomas Edward (1845–1925) *See phosphorus, viscosity*.

Thorpe, William Homan (1902–1986) *See ethology*.

Thorson, Gunnar Axel (1906–1971) *See marine biology*.

Threshing Machine The Romans used a machine called a *tribulum*, a sledge loaded with stones and drawn by horses, for threshing corn. The first attempt to construct a modern machine was made by Michael Menzies of Edinburgh in 1732. The threshing machine was invented in 1776 by a Scottish millwright, **Andrew Meikle** (1719–1811), and it became one of the most useful instruments to farmers. *See agricultural instruments*.

Thulium A metallic element of atomic number 69, discovered in 1879 and named after Thule in Greenland.

Thurnberg, Carl (1743–1828) A Swedish botanical explorer who became professor of botany at Uppsala in 1778, and published several books on the flora of Japan and Capetown, South Africa.

Tides A Greek philosopher, **Pytheas of Marseilles** (360–290 BC), interpreted the tides in relation to the moon and its phases. **Posidonus of Apamea** forecast the tides from the motions of the moon in 79 BC. **Pliny the Elder** (AD 28–79) wrote on tides in relation to the rising of the moon. A Latin writer, **Ambrosius Aurel Macrobius** (*c.* AD 400), wrote on tides and oceans. A monk, the **Venerable Bede** (*c.* 673–735) from Jarrow, in the north of England, studied the effect of local conditions on the tides at the mouths of rivers. An Arabian astonomer, **Abu-Masher** or **Albumazer** (787–885), wrote an important work on the nature of tides. They were first explained on a scientific basis by a German astronomer, **Johannes Kepler** (1571–1630) in 1598. A modern study was carried out by **William Ferrel** (1720–1760), an oceanographer and meteorologist from Pennsylvania, who invented a tide-predicting machine. *See oceanography.*

Tieghem, Phillipe van (1839–1914) *See botanical classification.*

Tiemann, Johann Karl Ferdinand (1848–1899) *See dyes.*

Tilden, Sir William Augustus (1842–1926) *See artificial rubber.*

Time A Greek philosopher and mathematician, **Zeno of Elea** (463–425 BC), was the first to question the nature of time and apply logic to its concept. He believed that he could prove time and movement did not exist, and for this purpose he created the well known paradox of Achilles and the tortoise. **Galilei Galileo** (1564–1642) was the first to link time and motion by studying the pendulum and falling objects. **Albert Einstein** (1879–1955) created the idea that both space and time are relative. *See atomic clock, clepsydra, clocks, horology, quartz clock, sundial, watch, waterclock.*

Tin The metal was probably known to the Babylonians around 2800 BC. Around 1000 BC the Phoenicians obtained it from mines in Cornwall in Britain, which remained an important source for over eight centuries. Homer (*c.* 800 BC) used the term *cassiteros* for the metal. Tin cans for packing and preserving meat were introduced independently by an English scientist, **Bryan Donkin** (1768–1855) and Peter Durand around 1813. They were found to be invaluable on sea voyages and military campaigns, and were introduced into the USA in 1820. Tinned or canned beer appeared around 1935.

Tinbergen, Nikolaas (1907–1988) *See ethology, imprinting.*

Ting, Samuel Chao Chung (b 1936) *See particle accelerator.*

Tintype *See photography.*

Tire The pneumatic tire was invented and patented by a Scottish engineer, **Robert William Thomson** (1822–1873) in 1845. However, Thomson's invention was not a success, owing to the scarcity and expense of obtaining India rubber. Unaware of Thomson's invention, a Scottish inventor, **John Boyd Dunlop** (1840–1921) of Dreghorn in Ayrshire, reinvented it in 1888. The pneumatic tire was adapted to the bicycle in 1891, and wire edges for it were invented in 1892 by A.T. Brown and G.F. Stillman of New York City. André Michelin and Edouard Michelin of France fitted pneumatic tires to the car in 1895.

Tiro, Marcus Tullius (*c.* AD 100) *See shorthand.*

Tiselius, Arne Wilhelm Kaurin (1902–1971) *See electrophoresis.*

Tissandier, Gaston (1835–1899) *See air balloon.*

Tissue [French: *tissu*, woven] The term was first introduced into microscopic anatomy by a French physician, **Marie François Xavier Bichat** (1771–1802).

Tissue Culture The growth of tissue outside the organism. First demonstrated in 1907 in nerve fibers by **Ross Granville Harrison** (1870–1959), who introduced the hanging-drop culture method for studying living tissues.

Titan Fourth and largest moon of Uranus. Discovered by **Christian Huygens** (1629–1695) in 1656. He published *The System of Saturn* or *Systema Saturnium* (1659) and made several important contributions to astronomy.

Titanium [Greek: *Titans*, A Greek mythical race of symbolic brute force] A metallic element of atomic number 22. First observed in 1791 as black magnetic sand or *menakite* in the earth by **William Gregor** (1761–1817), a Parish priest at Menachen in Cornwall. **Martin Heinrich Klaproth** (1743–1817) of Germany studied the substance in detail and named it titanium in 1795, and **Jons Jakob Berzelius** (1779–1848) isolated it in 1825. Titanium was independently discovered by a Swedish chemist **Anders Gustat Ekeberg** (1767–1813). The element being remarkable for its light weight was initially used for making artificial teeth. It is currently a popular metal for making spectacle frames.

Titius, Johann (1729–1796) *See Bode law.*

Titius-Bode Rule *See Bode law.*

Tizard, Sir Henry Thomas (1885–1959) *See octane rating.*

Tobias, Phillip Valentine (b 1925) *See Homo habilis.*

Todt, Fritz (1891–1942) *See roads.*

Toilets A water closet with mechanical means of disposal was proposed by **Sir John Harington** (1561–1612), an English writer from Kelston near Bath, who described it in his *The Metamorphosis of Ajax* (1596). It was installed at the Richmond palace of Queen Elizabeth I, who was his godmother. An improved model with an incorporated stink-trap was patented in 1775 by a London watchmaker, Alexander Cumming. An English inventor, **Joseph Bramah** (1748–1814) from Yorkshire, added further improvements in 1778. An advanced sewerage system for the disposal of excreta was designed by a London public health engineer, **Sir Joseph William Bazalgette** (1819–1891) in the 1850s.

Tolansky, Samuel (1907–1973) *See diamond.*

Tomanaga, Sin-Itero (1906–1979) *See Feynman diagrams, quantum electrodynamics.*

Tombaugh, Clyde William (1906–1997) *See Pluto.*

Tommy Gun *See firearms.*

Tompian, Thomas (1639–1713) *See watches.*

Tonson, Jacob (1656–1736) *See bookshops.*

Tonstall, Cuthbert (1474–1559) *See accountancy, arithmetic, early printed science books.*

Tonti, Lorenzo (1620–1690) *See insurance.*

Topology [Greek: *topos,* place + *logos,* discourse] A branch of mathematics dealing with geometric figures whose overall properties do not change despite deformation. Developed by a French mathematician, **Marie Ennemond Camille Jordan** (1838–1922) of Lyons. A German-born US mathematician, **Max Dehn** (1878–1952), made significant contributions to the field. A Dutch mathematician, **Luitzen Egbertus Jan Brouwer** (1881–1966), enunciated the fixed point theorem in topology. A German mathematician, **Felix Hausdorf** (1868–1942), who is regarded as the founder of point set topology, in his *Grundzüge der Mengenlehre* (1914), proposed some basic concepts. A Moscow-born US mathematician, **Solomon Lefschetz** (1884–1972), proposed an important theorem related to the existence of fixed points of mapping, which bears his name. A Moscow mathematician, **Pavel Sergeevich Aleksandrov** (1896–1982) and a German mathematician, **Heinz Hopf** (1894–1971) wrote an influential book, *Topologie* (1935). A standard work on the subject, *Topological Groups,* was written by a Russian mathematician, **Lev Semyonovich Pontryagin** (1908–1988).

Torpedo A war instrument named after the electric fish, the torpedo, by **Robert Fulton** (1765–1815). It was invented by an American, **David Bushnell** (1742–1824) of Westbrook, Maine in 1777. The first self-propelling torpedo was invented in 1866 by an English engineer, **Robert Whitehead** (1823–1905) of Bolton-le-Moors. A Croatian-born US electrical engineer, **Nikola Tesla** (1856–1843), designed a remote-controlled torpedo. An Irish inventor, **Louis Brennan** (b 1852), developed a new torpedo, which was bought by the British government. The gyroscope was first introduced into the torpedo by Ludwig Obry.

Torrey, John (1796–1873) A New York botanist who contributed to the establishment of the New York Botanical Gardens with over 50 000 of his specimens. He published *Flora of the State of New York* (1843) and several other books, and the genus *Torreya* of the yew family is named after him.

Torricelli, Evangelista (1608–1647) *See academy, barometer, mercury (metal), motion, vacuum, weather forecast.*

Torsion Balance An English geologist, **John Michell** (1724–1793) of Nottinghamshire, has been credited with its invention. A French physicist, **Charles Augustus Coulomb** (1736–1806), invented it independently in 1785. **Sir Charles Vernon Boys** (1855–1944), an English physicist and inventor from Wing in Rutland, improved the torsion balance with the use of fused quartz fibers.

Tournachon, Gaspard Felix (1820–1910) *See aerial photograph.*

Tournefort, Joseph Pitton de (1656–1708) A French botanist who served as a professor at the Jardin des Plantes, founded in 1626 in Paris by Cardinal Richelieu (1585–1642). He developed the binomial nomenclature of plants before **Carolus Linnaeus** (1707–1778), and proposed the concept of the genus in botany. His work *Institutiones rei Herbariae* was published in 1700. *See flower.*

Town Planning An ancient science as seen from the remains of Harrapa and Mohanjadaro in the Indus valley and other cities such as Rome and Athens. The oldest planned walled city is Jericho, dating back to about 10 000 BC. After the Great Fire of London in 1666, **Sir Christopher Wren** (1632–1723) drew up plans for rebuilding the whole city. A French town-planner, **George Eugene Hausmann** (1809–1891), modernized Paris with wider roads, boulevards, parks and bridges. Modern town planning in Britain was pioneered by **Sir Patrick Geddes** (1854–1932) of Perth, Scotland, who published *City Development* (1904) and *Cities in Evolution* (1915), and coined the term megalopolis. An English architect, **Sir Leslie Patrick Abercrombie** (1879–1957) was mainly responsible for post-Second World War town replanning of London, and was instrumental in creating several post-war new towns. Some important parts of London including Regent Street and Trafalgar Square were designed by a London architect and town planner, **John Nash** (1752–1835). An American architect, **Walter Burley Griffin** (1876–1937) from Maywood, Illnois, designed the new city of Canberra in New South Wales, Australia. *See architecture, building, roads, towns.*

Townes, Charles Hard (b 1915) *See laser, maser.*

Towns The oldest continuously inhabited city in the world, Damascus in Syria, was built around 2500 BC. Sun-dried bricks held by mortar were used to build houses in Jericho in the West Bank of Jordan in 10 000 BC. In Catal Hüyük, another ancient city (now Anatolia, Turkey), tightly packed houses were built in 6250 BC so that there were no streets. People had to walk along the roof tops to enter their homes. The city of *Uruk,* near the Euphrates River, in Mesopotamia, was one of the earliest walled cities. The towns around the Tigris and Eupharates in Mesopotamia around 3000 BC had metalled roads that were surfaced to prevent damage. The cities of Mohenjadaro and Harappa in the Indus Valley built around 2000 BC had a sophisticated system of roads and public health. Abdera, an ancient town of Hispania, on the shores of the Mediterranean, near the mouth of the Nessus, was supposed to have been built by Abderus, the son of Mercury. *See building, town planning.*

Townsend, Sir John Sealy Edward (1868–1957) *See electric charge, electron.*

Townshend, Charles (1674–1738) *See agronomy.*

Trace Elements Elements that are required only in minute quantities for metabolism in plants and animals. The importance of organic salts for the growth and function of yeast was demonstrated by **Louis Pasteur** (1822–1895) in 1860. Their importance in the diet of higher animals was established in 1919 by **Thomas Burr Osborne** (1859–1929) and Lafayette Benedict Mendel.

Tracer Elements Another term for isotopes used in radio-isotopic studies. *See isotopes.*

Tradescant, John (1567–1637) *See horticulture, museum.*

Tradescant, John (1608–1662) *See horticulture, museum.*

Traffic Signals Semaphore-type traffic signals were set up in Parliament Square, London, in 1868. Red and green gas lamps were used at night. The three-way automatic traffic signal was patented in America, Britain and Canada by an American inventor, **Garrett A. Morgan** (1875–1963) in 1923. These were introduced into England on a trial basis at

Wolverhampton in 1928, and a month later came into permanent operation at Leeds. The Road Traffic Act of 1930 made it an offence to violate traffic lights. *See motoring.*

Trains *See electric railway, locomotive, railway, steam engine, tram car.*

Tram Car A new type of electric motor railway developed by an American inventor, **Frank Julian Sprague** (1857–1934) of Milford, Connecticut, and first used in Richmond, Virginia in 1887. In 1883 a German-born British engineer, **Karl Wilhelm Siemens**, later **Sir Charles William Siemens** (1823–1883) independently established a tramway at Portrush, in Ireland. Electric traction for the tram car was demonstrated earlier in Berlin by his brother **Ernst Werner von Siemens** (1816–1892). A Scottish industrialist and electrical engineer, **George Balfour** (1872–1841), built and operated several tramway systems in the English Midlands and Scotland.

Transatlantic Communication The first sucessful transatlantic telegraphic cable, designed by **Lord Kelvin** or **William Thomson** (1824–1907), was installed from Ireland to Newfoundland in 1866. **Sir Samuel Canning** (1823–1908) served as the chief engineer for this project and the cables were laid from Brunel's ship the *Great Eastern.* The first message through this cable, over a distance of 1896 miles, was sent in 1858. The first transatlantic wireless telegraphic message, from Cornwall to Nova Scotia, was sent on 12th December 1901 by the Italian physicist, **Guglielmo Marchese Marconi** (1874–1937) of Bologna. The first transatlantic transmission of human speech by telephone, from Arlington, Virginia, to the Eiffel Tower in Paris, was achieved in 1915 by US radio-telephone engineers. The first television images across the Atlantic were transmitted in 1928 from Coulsdon, Surrey, in England, to Hartsdale, New York. They consisted of the images of the Scottish pioneer of television, **John Logie Baird** (1888–1946) and another person. The first live television satellite pictures across the Atlantic were transmitted in July 1962 by the telecommunication satellite, Telstar.

Transatlantic Flight In 1919 **Albert Cusion Read** (1887–1967) and his crew made the first crossing of the north Atlantic by air from Newfoundland, Canada, to Lisbon, in a US Navy/Curtiss flying boat. The first non-stop transatlantic flight from Newfoundland to Galway, Ireland, was achieved 18 days later by **John William Alcock** (1892–1919) of Manchester, and **Arthur Whitten Brown** (1886–1948) of Glasgow. **Charles Augustus Lindbergh** (1902–1974) of Detroit was the first to make a non-stop solo transatlantic flight, from New York to Paris, in his monoplane *Spirit of Saint Louis* in 1927. The English pioneer of aviation **Geoffrey De Haviland** (1882–1965) from High Wycombe, designed the first jetliner to fly the Atlantic, the *Comet 4*, in 1949. The Boeing 747, known as the jumbo jet, started its transatlantic flights in 1970. The fastest transatlantic flight, of 1 hour 55 minutes, at 1807 miles per hour, from New York to London, was achieved in 1974 by Noel F. Widifield in a Lockheed aircraft.

Transatlantic Voyage The US-built *Savannah* was the first steamship to cross the Atlantic but it used steam power for three days only, sailing for the remaining 20 days of its voyage. HMS *Rhabdamanthus* was the earliest steamship to make an entire transatlantic crossing under steam power, in 1832, from Plymouth, Devon, to Barbados. The largest steamship in the world at this time, *Great Western,* designed by **Isambard Kingdom Brunel** (1806–1859), was launched in 1832. It made its first transatlantic voyage to New York in 1838. It was the first screw-propelled, iron-hulled and double-bottomed transatlantic passenger ship. A Scottish merchant, **Macgregor Laird** (1808–1861) of Greenock, built the *Sirius,* which made the entire crossing under steam in 1854. Weekly crossings from New York to Liverpool were commenced in 1860 by the Inman Line founded by **William Inman** (1825–1881) of Leicester.

Transformer *See electric tranformer.*

Transistor A semiconductor capable of amplifying electric currents. As a tiny device it replaced the much larger and power-consuming triode or thermionic valve. It was invented in 1947 by **John Bardeen** (1908–1991), **Walter Houser Brattain** (1902–1987) and **William Bradford Shockley** (1910–1989) of the Bell Telephone Laboratories. The junction transistor, which miniaturized the circuits in the radio, was invented by Shockley, later in the same year. Bardeen, Shockley and Brattain shared the Nobel Prize for physics, for their invention, in 1956. The molecular transistor made of carbon-based materials was developed by L. E. Lyons and Hugh McDiarmid in the late 1970s.

Translocation [Latin: *trans,* across + *locus,* place] Change of position of part of a chromosome to another part, or to a different chromosome. Discovered by **Colin Blackman Bridges** (1889–1938) in 1923.

Transmission Electron Microscope (TEM) A powerful electron microscope having ten times greater magnification than a scanning electron microscope and a thousand times more than an optical microscope. The first prototype was built in 1931 by German scientists Max Knoll and Ernest Ruska of the Technische Hochschule, Berlin, Germany.

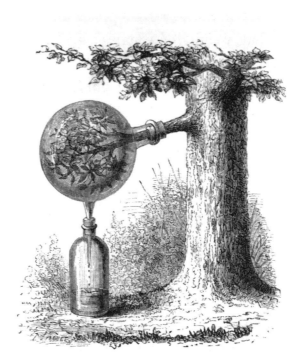

226. Transpiration in Plants. Guettard's experiment.

Figure 81 Experiments on transpiration in plants by Guettard. Pouchet, F.A. *The Universe.* London: Blacke and Son, 1871

Transmutation *See artificial transmutation, evolution.*

Transpiration [Latin: *trans,* through + *spirare,* breathe] A phenomenon of water loss in plants, discovered by the professor of physics at Gresham College and a pioneer in the field of experimental plant physiology, **John Woodward** (1665–1728). It was described independently by Muschenbroeck, a professor at Leyden. Further advances were made by a French physician and botanist, **Jean Etienne Guettard** (1715–1786). A British botanist, **H.H. Dixon** (1869–1953), related the sap pressure and pulling power of the leaf, to the tensile strength of the water column.

Transport *See airlines, airplane, car, coaches, electric railway, hovercraft, locomotive, omnibuses, railway, tram car, underground railway.*

Traube, Moritz (1826–1894) *See osmosis.*

Travers, Morris William (1872–1961) *See krypton, xenon.*

Tredgold, Thomas (1788–1829) *See heating, steam engine.*

Tresaguet, Pierre Marie Jerome (1716–1796) *See roads.*

Treviranus, Gottfried Reinhold (1776–1837) *See biology.*

Treviranus, Ludolf Christian (1779–1864) A German naturalist and brother of **Gottfried Reinhold Treviranus** (1776–1837), who discovered intercellular spaces.

Treviso Arithmetic Refers to one of the earliest printed works on arithmetic in 1478 by an anonymous writer, issued from a press in a town called Treviso, situated on the trade route to Venice from the north.

Trevithick, George (1771–1833) A pioneer of the steam engine, born in Illogan, Redruth. His steam engines developed higher steam pressures and gave greater power from smaller cylinders. He built a practical passenger-carrying road vehicle powered by steam in 1801. His first steam locomotive, which ran on an iron plateway, was demonstrated in 1803 at Coalbrookdale, Shropshire. His ventures were a commercial failure and he died in debt. *See steam engine.*

Triassic Period Geological time of the first period of the Mesozoic era, 245–208 million years ago, when the continents were fused and contained early dinosaurs. Identified in 1834 by Friedrich August von Alberti.

Triceratops [Latin: *tres,* three + Greek: *keros,* horn] A large plant-eating dinosaur about 20 feet in length. Its skeleton was reconstructed from its remains found in the Upper Cretaceous strata of the western USA. *See dinosaur.*

Tricycle A Scottish inventor, **Kirkpatrick Macmillan** (1813–1878) of Thornhill in Dumfriesshire, was the first to apply pedals to the tricycle in 1838. The first practical tricycle was invented by **James Starley** (1831–1881) from Albourne in Sussex. A tricycle propelled by a two-stroke single-cylinder motor was built in 1883 by a German automobile engineer, **Carl Friedrich Benz** (1844–1929). The first electric tricycle was built by a London engineer, **William Edward Ayrton** (1847–1908) in 1882. *See differential gear.*

Trigonometry [Greek: *tria,* three + *gonia,* angle + *metron,* to measure] The science of the triangle with reference to the problem of finding the value of unknown parts, when three independent parts are known. The Egyptians exhibited certain elementary knowledge of trigonometry in their construction of the pyramids. Some of the earliest works are found in the Egyptian mathematical papyrus written by **Ahmes** around 1650 BC. The science of trigonometry was established by **Hipparchus** of Bithynia (190–120 BC), who proposed the forerunner of trigonometric tables. Further contribution to the field was made two centuries later by **Ptolemy** (*c.* AD 127–151) of Alexandria. **Menelaus** (*c.* AD 100) wrote a treatise on spherical trigonometry

entitled *Sphaerica.* The Hindu mathematician **Aryabhata** (AD 475–550) of Patna, gave a table of natural sines of the angles in trigonometry. A Persian mathematician, **Albuzjani** or **Abdul Wafa** (AD 940–998), introduced some trigonometrical functions. An English mathematician and alchemist, **Robert of Chester** (*c.* AD 1200), was the first to use the word *sine* in the context of trigonometry. A German astronomer, **Regiomontanus** (1436–1476) from Konigsberg, was the first to give a trigonometrical formula for the area of a triangle. His teacher, **Georg von Peuerbach** (1423–1461) of Austria, used sines in trigonometry and compiled a sine table. In 1596 a German astronomer, **Georg Joachim Rheticus** (1514–1576), also known as **Georg Joachim von Lauchen**, worked out the trigonometrical tables to ten decimal places. The field of modern analytic trigonometry was established by a French lawyer and mathematician, **François Viète** (1540–1603), who was one of the first to represent numbers by letters, and apply algebra to geometry. The first use of the word trigonometry in print appeared in **Bartholomeus Pitiscus's** (1561–1613) work published in 1595. **John Bernoulli** (1667–1748), a professor of mathematics at Gröningen, treated trigonometry as a branch of analysis, and made several important contributions. The Swiss mathematician **Leonhard Euler** (1707–1783) contributed to the field and developed spherical geometry. A French mathematician, **Abraham de Moivre** (1667–1754) of Vitry, Champagne, was one of the first to use complex numbers in trigonometry. *See geometry, mathematics.*

Trinitrotoluene (TNT) An explosive invented in 1863 by a Swedish chemist, J. Wilbrand.

Triode An improvement to the diode or thermionic valve, the first step towards the invention of the triode, was made in 1904 by an English electrical engineer, **John Ambrose Fleming** (1849–1945) of Lancashire. It was invented in 1907 by a physicist and pioneer in radio and wireless telegraphy from Iowa, **Lee de Forest** (1873–1961). He placed a metal grid between the filament and an anode, and produced the triode, which acted as an amplifier as well as a rectifier.

Trippe, Juan Terry (1899–1981) *See airlines.*

Tritium An isotope of hydrogen with an atomic number of 1. It was discovered by **Lord Ernest Rutherford** (1871–1937), **I.M. Hunter** (1915–1975) and **Sir Mark Laurence Elwin Oliphant** (1901–2000) when they bombarded deuterium with deuterons in 1934.

Troostwijk, Van (1752–1837) *See electrolysis.*

Tropical Zone *See climatic zones.*

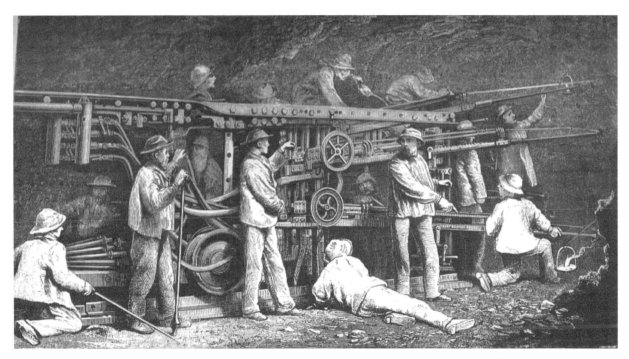

Figure 82　A mid-19th century French tunneling machine. Guillemin, Amédée. *The Application of Physical Forces*. London: Macmillan and Co, 1877

Tropism [Greek: *tropos,* turning]　The direction of movement of plants during germination, first demonstrated by an English physiologist, **Thomas Andrew Knight** (1759–1838), who was a friend of another English botanist, **Sir Joseph Banks** (1743–1820). The phenomenon was also studied by **Jacques Loeb** (1859–1924).

Troposphere　The lower layer of the atmosphere directly above the earth's surface extending for about 3 to 8 miles. *See atmosphere, cyclone.*

Troy　The City in Homer's *Iliad* (*c.* 800 BC), excavated in 1870 in Turkey by a German archaeologist, **Heinrich Schliemann** (1822–1890) of Berlin.

Trumpet　*See loudspeaker.*

Tschirnhaus, Ehrenfried Walter von (1651–1708)　A German member of the French Académie des Sciences, who constructed several powerful burning lenses, some of which are still extant. One of his lenses was used in 1695 in Florence for investigating the flammability of diamond.

Tsiolkovsky, Konstantin Eduardovich (1857–1935)　*See aerodynamics, space travel.*

Tswett, Mikhail Semenovich (1872–1919)　*See chromatography.*

Tu Shih (*c.* AD 31)　*See bellows.*

Tulasne, Charles (1816–1884)　*See mycology.*

Tulasne, Louis René (1815–1885)　*See mycology.*

Tull, Jethro (1674–1741)　*See agricultural instruments, animal husbandry.*

Tungsten　A metallic element of atomic number 74, discovered in 1783. In 1908 an American physicist, **William David Coolridge** (1873–1975) of Hudson, Massachusetts, used the element instead of a carbon filament for the electric light bulb. *See electric light bulb.*

Tunguska Event　An explosion that occurred at Tunguska, central Siberia, Russia, in June 1908, which is thought to have been caused by either a cometary nucleus or possibly an asteroid. The magnitude of the explosion was equivalent to a 10–20 megaton nuclear bomb.

Tunnel Diode　*See Esaki diode.*

Tunnel　The first tunnel below a river was built in 2200 BC by Queen Semiramis, below the River Euphrates, for linking the temple of Jupiter with her royal palace. The oldest navigable tunnel in Europe, on Canal du Midi, in south west France, was completed in 1681. The modern method of tunneling beneath water was devised by a French-born British inventor, **Sir Marc Isambard Brunel** (1769–1849). In 1825 he started building a tunnel under the River Thames between Rotherhithe and Wapping in London. It was the first public subaqueous tunnel and opened in 1843. The first trains used the tunnel in 1865 and it became part of the London Underground railway. The longest railway tunnel in Britain, the Severn Tunnel, connecting Avon and Gwent over a distance of 4 miles, was constructed between 1873 and 1886. The longest road tunnel in Britain, of 2.13 miles, the Mersey Queensway Tunnel, was started in 1925 and opened for traffic in 1934. A London civil engineer, **Sir Benjamin Baker** (1840–1907), was instrumental in building the Hudson Tunnel (1881–1891) in New York. *See Channel Tunnel.*

Tunneling Microscope *See electron microscope, scanning tunneling microscope.*

Tupolev, Andrei Nikolaevich (1888–1972) *See aerodynamics, warplanes.*

Turbine A system of a wheel with vanes powered by water, steam or wind. The first steam-powered turbine was invented by **Hero of Alexandria** around AD 100. The term *turbine* was invented in 1820 by a French mining engineer, Burdin, at the École de Saint-Étienne. The first commercially practical steam turbine was built in 1831 by an American, William Avery. **Charles Gorden Curtis** (1860–1953), a Boston engineer, invented the impulse steam turbine in 1896. A London engineer, **Sir Charles Algernon Parsons** (1854–1931), developed a steam turbine in 1884, and patented a turbogenerator for a ship in 1894. The first such ship, *Turbinia,* was launched in 1897. High-efficiency steam turbines, using convergent and divergent nozzles, were developed by a Swedish engineer, **Carl Gustav Patrick de Laval** (1845–1913), who also invented a high-speed turbine to drive the propellor for marine use. The principle of the turbine is employed in hydroelectric schemes and other types of engines. The concept behind modern gas turbines and jet engines was developed by an American aeronautical engineer, **Edward Story Taylor** (1903–1991), who founded the Gas Turbine Laboratory at the Massachusetts Institute of Technology in 1946. *See hydroelectric scheme, jet engine, steam engine, water turbine.*

Turbo Jet *See jet engine.*

Turing Machine *See computers.*

Turing, Alan Mathison (1912–1954) *See computers.*

Turner, Charles Henry (1867–1923) *See ethology.*

Turner, Edward (1798–1837) The first professor of chemistry at University College, London, in 1828. He determined atomic weights of several elements and published

Elements of chemistry including recent Discoveries and Doctrines of the Science and several other books.

Turner, William (1510–1568) An English physician from Northumberland who is regarded as the father of British botany. He published the first English botanical treatise *Liebellus de re Herbaria Novus* or *Names of Herbes* (1538) and *A New Herbal* (1551–1562). *See ornithology.*

Turriano, Juanelo (1500–1585) *See water pump.*

Twort, Frederick William (1877–1950) *See bacteriophage.*

Two-Stroke Engine In 1879 a German automobile engineer, **Carl Friedrich Benz** (1844–1929), developed a two-stroke internal combustion engine. In 1972 an Australian engineer, **Ralph Sarich** (b 1938) of Perth, built an orbital two-stroke reciprocating piston engine. *See internal combustion engine.*

Tyndall Effect The scattering of light by very small particles, suspended in a medium, resulting in a visible beam. A phenomenon described in 1869 by **John Tyndall** (1820–1893), an Irish physicist and professor at the Royal Institution in England. He used it to demonstrate the presence of bacterial spores in air. He succeeded **Michael Faraday** (1791–1867) as superintendent of the Royal Instituion in 1867.

Tyndall, John (1820–1893) *See calorescence, radiation of heat, Tyndall effect.*

Typesetting *See Gutenberg Bible, movable type printing, printing, typography.*

Typewriter In 1714 an American engineer at the New River Company, Henry Mill, took out a patent for a machine for impressing or transcribing letters as in writing. The first workable writing machine known as the typographer was invented by an American, William Austin Burt of Detroit, in 1829. His machine had type mounted on curved bars on a wooden frame. It also had a wheel to move the type and a lever. In 1833 a Marseille printer, Xavier Progin, obtained a French patent for his *Typhographique* which had a type bar. A machine with a cylindrical plate was designed in America by Charles Thurber, in 1842. The prototype of the modern typewriter with a wooden casing and two-bank keyboard was invented in 1858 by an Italian lawyer, Guiseppe Ravizza. One of the first typewriters to be mass produced was designed by an American printer and editor, Christopher Lathom Sholes of Milwaukee, Wisconsin in 1867. This was improved and mass produced by an American engineer, **Philo Remington** (1816–1889) of Litchfield, New York in 1874. In 1878 he produced the first typewriter with a shift key for upper and lower case letters. An Italian, **Camillo Olivetti** (1968–1943), founded the typewriter firm that was later developed by his son, **Adriano Olivetti** (1901–1960), and began mass producing typewriters. *See electric typewriter, electronic typewriter*.

Typography The forming of every letter or character separately so that they could be rearranged for producing different pages and text. It obliterated the need for the strenuous process of cutting a separate new block for printing every page. **Johannes Gutenberg** (1400–1468) invented the method around 1440. The Roman type letters in printing were introduced into Rome in 1465 by two professors, Conrad Sweinheim and Arnold Pannartz from Mayence. The Greek characters were cast by the Italians in 1476. The first book in Hebrew characters was printed at 1482. The italic type was invented in 1496 by a Roman, **Aldus Manutius** (d 1516), who set up a printing business in Venice. He first used it for entire volumes, which was not approved of by other typographers, who employed it only for specific words, prefaces and introductions. Alphabetical tables of the first words of each chapter were introduced as a guide to the binder in 1469. The 'old face' types used extensively in Europe were produced in London by **William Caslon** (1692–1766) of Worcestershire. In 1508 a French printer to King Henry VIII, **Richard Pynson** (d 1530), introduced the Roman type into England. **Ged Williams** (1690–1749) of Edinburgh, patented a process of stereotyping, which he used for printing prayer books and bibles for Cambridge University. The first book on typesetting and engraving, the *Manuel Typographique* (1764), was published by **Pierre Simon Fournier** (1712–1768) of France. An English printer, **John Baskerville** (1706–1775) from Worcestershire, set up his printing business at Birmingham in 1750, and started making special types in 1757, which were named after him. He also devised a method of pressing the paper between two hot copper plates, and in 1758 became printer to Cambridge University. In 1829 Claude Gennoux of Paris discovered a method of making molds for cast metal type. The first typesetting machine was patented in England by **William Church** (1778–1863) in 1822. The curved plates that could be used on a cylinder press were invented in 1849 by another Paris printer, Jacobs Warms, and his method was adopted by the New York papers in 1861. Two Americans, Charles Kastenbein and Robert Hattersley, independently invented a typesetting machine in 1866. A revolutionary type-forming and composing machine was invented in 1887 by an American, **Tolbert Lanston** (1844–1913) of Ohio, and it was first used in commercial printing in 1897. *See linotype printing, printing*.

Tyrannosaurus Enormous flesh-eating dinosaurs that lived in North America and Asia about 70 million years ago. The most complete skeleton of it was discovered in 1989 in Hell Creek, Montana, and is preserved in the Museum at Montana, USA.

Tyrrell, George Walter (1883–1961) *See petrology*.

Tyrrell, Joseph Burr (1858–1957) *See dinosaurs*.

U

Udine, Giovanni da (1487–1564) *See architecture, Italian.*

Uemura, Naomi (1941–1984) *See North Pole.*

UFO (**U**nidentified **F**lying **O**bjects) See *extraterrestrial life.*

Uhlenbeck, George Eugene (1900–1988) *See electron.*

Ulam, Stanislaw (1909–1985) *H bomb.*

Ulm, Charles Thomas Phillipe (1898–1934) *See airlines.*

Ultramicroscope [Latin: *ultra*, beyond + Greek: *mikros*, small + *skopein*, to view] Devised by H.F.W. Siedentopf and **Richard Adolf Zsigmondy** (1866–1930) of Vienna around 1848. Their instrument projected light from a source onto suspended particles in a solution which were then viewed on a dark background through the microscope. Zsigmondy was awarded the Nobel Prize for chemistry in 1925, for his work on colloids and the ultramicroscope.

Ultrasound [Latin: *ultra*, beyond + *sono*, sound] Sound waves beyond the frequency (more than 20 kilohertz) of human hearing. It was first applied in marine work for developing the Sound Navigation and Ranging System (SONAR) during World War I. The first sonar system was used in 1916 for locating submarines.

Ultraviolet Microscope [Latin: *ultra*, beyond; Greek: *mikros,* small + *skopein*, to look] A microscope of improved magnification using rays of shorter wavelength than those of visible light. Developed by a London scientist, **Joseph Edwin Barnard** (1870–1949), who published *Practical Photo-micrography* (1911).

Ultraviolet Rays Radiation beyond the spectrum of visible violet light. First observed in 1801 by a German physicist, **Johann Wilhelm Ritter** (1776–1810) from Silesia. The same phenomenon was independently observed by **William Hyde Wollaston** (1766–1822) in 1802.

Ulugh-Beg (1394–1449) The ruler of Turkestan whose real name was Muhammed Taragay. He became known by his title *Ulugh-Beg*, meaning the 'great prince'. He established Samarkand as a center of higher learning, especially for astronomy, in 1420. *See observatories.*

Umbrella [Latin: *umbra*, shade] Known to the ancients; carvings of it are seen in the remains of Persepolis. The modern form of umbrella was invented by the Chinese in AD 400; some of the prints on the old chinaware of this period show people shaded by the umbrella. It was first introduced into Europe in Italy. An English poet, Benjamin Jonson (1572–1637), used the term in one of his comedies in 1616. An Oxford mathematican and scholar, **John Kersey** (1616–1702), described it in his dictionary as a broad fan or screen used by women to shelter from the rain. The umbrella was defined in 18th-century dictionaries as 'a portable pent-house to carry in a person's hand to screen him from violent rain or heat'.

Underground Railways The earliest service opened in 1863 between Farringdon and Edgeware Road in London. The first tunnel beneath water in London, under the River Thames, between Rotherhithe and Wapping, was built in 1825 by a French-born English inventor, **Sir Marc Isambard Brunel** (1769–1849), and it was used for trains in 1865. It later became part of the London Underground railway. An English mining and railway engineer from Leeds, **John Hawkshaw** (1811–1891), designed the Inner Circle Underground railway in London, and further subways under the Thames in London were built by a South African-born British inventor, **James Henry Greathead** (1844–1896) in 1869. He invented an excavating device made of wrought iron tubing, and developed it, with the use of compressed air and hydraulic jacks, to build more subways around London in 1886. His tube or excavating device became known as a Greathead shield. A London civil engineer, **Sir Benjamin Baker** (1840–1907), was instrumental in laying many miles of London underground railways, and his contemporary **Sir John Fowler** (1817–1898) was responsible for building part of the London Underground. The New York City Transport Authority subway, with the most stations in the world, opened in 1904. One of the busiest in the world, the metro system in Greater Moscow, came into operation in 1935.

Undersea Exploration The earliest scientific novel on the subject *Vingt mille lieues sous les mers* (Twenty Thousand Leagues Under the Sea) was published by the science fiction writer **Jules Verne** (1828–1905) of Nantes in 1870. A French naval officer and undersea explorer **Jacques-Yves Cousteau** (1910–1997) invented the **s**elf **c**ontained **u**nderwater **b**reathing **a**pparatus (scuba) which allowed the diver to swim underwater without being attached to the boat for a supply of oxygen. In 1943, with Emile Gagnon of France, he used compressed air with valves to control oxygen delivery. Cousteau made the first underwater film in 1950, while he was commander of the oceanographic research ship, *Calypso,* and he also developed underwater television. He published *The Undersea Worlds of Jacques Cousteau* (1968–1976) and *The Living Sea* (1963). The bathysphere [Greek: *bathos,* depth + *sphaira,* a ball], a 4-foot 9-inch ocean-diving device to study deep sea marine forms, was invented by an American explorer, **Charles William Beebe** (1877–1962) of Brooklyn, New York. He reached a new record of 923 meters for diving with his invention in 1934. A Swiss physicist, **Auguste Antoine Piccard** (1884–1962), constructed another one in 1948, and investigated the possibilities of undersea living. *See oceanography, marine biology.*

Units and Measures The units of length, weight and capacity were legally fixed in Mesopotamia as early as 4000 BC. Weights of cylinders with rounded ends dating back to 3800 BC, known as *beqa,* were found at Naquada, Egypt. Many of the terms used for units of measurement came from body parts or easily obtainable materials. The oldest preserved standard of length, the foot, derives its origin from the foot of the statue of the ruler of Gudea in the Mesopotamian city of Lagash, in 4000 BC. It measured 10.41 inches and was divided into 16 parts. The royal foot was introduced as a unit of measure by the Emperor Charlemagne (AD 747–814) in 789. The inch probably comes from the Latin word *uncia* for thumb. The Sumerians developed standard weights for trade around 2500 BC. Their unit, the *shekel,* consisted of 129 grains, and the *mina* was 60 times as heavy. The oldest preserved weight is from the Mesopotamian city of Lagash, dating back to 2400 BC. The ounce was fixed as 640 dry grains of weight by King Henry III of England (1207–1272). The yard originally denoted the distance from the tip of the nose to the end of the fingers, when the right arm was outstretched. The French astronomer, **Jean Piccard** (1620–1682), was a pioneer in the standardization of units of length, and he proposed the length of a pendulum beating at one second at sea-level at a latitude of 45 degrees, as the standard unit of length. The Imperial Standards for measures in Britain was set by a commission in 1758. The carat [Greek: *keration,* horn-like pods] for measurement of diamonds and gold was originally obtained from the average weight of the seeds of the carob, a native tree of Africa and the southern Mediterranean. When diamonds were first discovered in India the seeds were transported there to be used as a measure. The English carat was fixed at 3.1683 grains by the Board of Trade in 1888, and was replaced by the metric carat in 1914. The kilogram was established as an official unit by the Bureau of Weights and Measures at the Pavilion de Bretail near Paris in 1875. *See metric system, SI units.*

Universal Joint Invented by **Robert Hooke** (1635–1703) in 1676.

Universe Named *mundus* in Latin because of the perpetual motion or *motu* of the sun, moon and other heavenly bodies. The age of the universe is currently estimated at 11 to 17 aeons (gigayears), each aeon being equivalent to 1000 million years. *See Big Bang theory, oscillating theory, Steady State theory.*

University The oldest teaching institutions were the schools of the Sumerians around 3500 BC. The first, the Alexandrian University, was established by **Alexander the Great** (356–323 BC) in 331 BC and it attracted scholars from all over the world, including **Euclid** the mathematician, **Archimedes** the physicist, **Herophilos** the anatomist and **Erasistratos** the physiologist. It had four departments: literature, mathematics, astronomy and medicine, and its library was the largest in the world with over 400 000 volumes. Cambridge University is said to have been founded by King Sigebert of East Anglia in AD 630. Oxford University was mentioned by Pope Martin in AD 802. One of the oldest existing universities, the University of Karueein in Morocco, was established in AD 859. The three oldest Scottish universities are St Andrew's University founded in 1411, the University of Glasgow founded in 1451 and Aberdeen University founded in 1494. The University of Bologna, Italy, was founded around AD 422, and is considered to be the oldest university in continental Europe. The dates of establishment of other important universities in Europe are as follows: Naples, Italy (1224); Toulouse, France (1229); Cologne, Germany (1385); Louvain, Belgium (1426); Toledo, Spain (1499); Venice, Italy (1592); Montpellier, France (1289); Vienna, Austria (1365); Cracow, Poland (1364), Geneva, Switzerland (1368); Heidelberg, Germany (1386); Leipzig, Germany (1409); Florence, Italy (1439); Basel, Switzerland (1460); Uppsala, Sweden (1496); Strasburg, Germany (1538); Königsberg, Germany (1544); Leiden, Holland (1575); Edinburgh, Scotland (1582); Dublin, Ireland (1591); Dorpat, Germany (1632); Utrecht, Holland (1636); Halle, Germany (1694); Erlangen, Germany (1743); Berlin, Germany (1810); Bonn, Germany (1818); Zurich, Switzerland (1832); Munich, Germany (1826); and Bern, Switzerland (1834). The largest university building in the world, part of the Lomonov State University, at Lenin Hills, south of Moscow, was built in 1949. *See Alexandrian Museum and Library.*

University Gown Worn by university students and graduates. An English traveller **Robert de Ketene** (*c.* AD 1143), who was the first to translate the Koran into English, wore

Arab robes that are supposed to have evolved into the present university gown.

Unverdorben, Otto (1806–1873) *See aniline, aromatic compounds.*

Ur A Sumerian town founded in Mesopotamia (now Iraq) in 4000 BC. Its inhabitants used sun-baked clay tablets for building houses and temples, and spoke the Babylonian language. The metal implements found at Ur by **Sir Flinders Petrie** (1853–1942) were metallurgically analyzed by a London metallurgist, **Cyril Henry Desch** (1874–1958). A London archaeologist, **Sir Leonard Charles Woolley** (1880–1960), carried out excavations (1922–1934) and discovered the royal cemetery. He published *Ur Excavations* (1934).

Uranium A metallic element named after the planet Uranus, by the German chemist, **Martin Heinrich Klaproth** (1743–1817). A Parisian chemist, **Eugene Melchior Peligot** (1811–1890), isolated uranium by heating tetrachloride with potassium in 1841. Natural uranium consists of two isotopes, uranium-235 and uranium-238. *See atomic bomb, atomic energy, fission, radioactivity.*

Uranium-235 Present in small quantities (0.7 per cent) in natural uranium. Its fission by the release of neutrons was observed in 1940 by a group of American physicists including **John Ray Dunning** (1907–1975) from Shelby, Nebraska, and German-born **Aristid V. Grosse** (b 1905).

Uranium-238 *See uranium.*

Uranus [Greek: *Ouranos,* god of heaven] The seventh major planet from the sun. **Pierre Charles Lemonnier** (1715–1799) of Paris made early observations of it before it was identified as a planet. It was discovered in 1757 by the

German-born British astronomer, **Sir William Herschel** (1738–1822), and was named by a German astronomer, **Johann Elert Bode** (1749–1826), who was director of the Berlin Observatory. The planet was observed earlier by **John Flamsteed** (1646–1719), but he failed to realize its significance. A French astronomer, **Alexis Bouvard** (1767–1843), believed that observational errors by Flamsteed and others led to the failure of Uranus to be recognized as a planet earlier. In 1851, an English astronomer from Bolton, **William Lassell** (1799–1880) discovered *Ariel* and *Umbriel*, the satellites of Uranus. A Scottish-born German astronomer, **Johan von Lamont** (1805–1879), calculated the mass of Uranus from the observations on the motions of its satellites. He cataloged over 34 000 stars while he was professor of astronomy at Munich.

Urbain, Georges (1872–1938) *See hafnium, lutecia.*

Ure, Andrew (1778–1857) A Scottish analytical chemist from Glasgow who published *Dictionary of chemistry* (1821), *Philosophy of Manufactures* (1835), *Cotton Manufactures of Great Britain* (1836) and *Dictionary of Art, Manufactures and Mines* (1839).

Urea The first organic compound to be obtained from the inorganic materials, potassium cyanate and ammonium sulfate, by a German chemist, **Friedreich Wöhler** (1800–1882) in 1829. John Davy (1790–1868), a brother of the English chemist **Sir Humphry Davy** (1778–1829), appears to have obtained it earlier, in 1811, by the action of ammonia gas on carbonyl chloride; however, he failed to realize the significance and did not document it.

Urey, Harold Clayton (1893–1981) *See deuterium, hydrogen.*

Utzon, Jörn (b 1918) *See architecture, Australian.*

V

Vacuum [Latin: *vaccus,* empty] The Greek philosopher **Aristotle** (384–322 BC) believed that a vacuum could not be created. **Albert of Saxony** (*c.* 1316–1390) denied the existence of a natural vacuum. The first vacuum was created by the Italian physicist, **Evangelista Torricelli** (1608–1647), during his experiments on the barometer in 1641. The invention of the air pump by **Otto von Guericke** (1602–1686), Mayor of Magdeburg in Prussia, helped to create a more practical vacuum, and he published *New Experiments concerning Empty Space* (1672). A German-born London chemist, **Hermann Johann Phillip Sprengel** (1834–1906), described a new type of vacuum pump without valves or pistons in his work *On the Vacuum* (1865). His device helped in the research on discharge tubes. In 1872 **Sir William Crookes** (1832–1919) developed a vacuum tube that advanced the study of cathode rays.

Vacuum Cleaner The first one, invented in America in 1859, consisted of bellows powered by hand. It needed two persons, one to work the bellows and the other to do the cleaning. The first model used in industry, based on the principle of an inverted propeller and powered by a steam engine, was developed in 1871 by an American, Ives W. McGaffey. In 1899 George S. Thurman of St Louis, Missouri, invented a powered model. In 1901 **Hubert Cecil Booth** (1871–1955) of Gloucester, England, devised a vacuum cleaner with an electric motor; due to its weight, it had to be pulled by an animal. His company offered a vacuum cleaning service on a commercial basis. In America a night security man, James Murray Spangler, invented a lighter model suitable for domestic use, and in 1907 he sold the rights to **William Henry Hoover** (1849–1932) of Ohio, who established the Electric Suction Sweeper Company in 1908 which was renamed the Hoover Company in 1910. The upright models were introduced in 1908, and the cylinder machines appeared in the 1920s. The Electrolux Company, which made vacuum cleaners on a commercial basis, was established in 1921 by a Swedish industrialist, **Axel Leonard Wenner-Green** (1881–1961).

Vail, Alfred Lewis (1807–1859) An American telegraphic engineer from Morristown, New Jersey, who worked with Samuel Morse and developed an improved design for the telegraph mechanism in 1838. He published *The American Electro Magnetic Telegraph* (1845).

Valency [Latin: *valens,* strength] The concept that every element has a defined capacity to combine with other elements was first proposed in 1852 by an eminent organic chemist, **Sir Edward Frankland** (1825–1899) of Churchtown, Lancashire. A similar theory was put forward independently in 1858 by a German chemist, **Friedrich August Kekulé von Stradonitz** (1829–1896) and a Scottish organic chemist, **Archibald Scott Couper** (1831–1892) from Kirkintilloch near Glasgow. The valency of an element was shown to depend on the number of electrons in the outer shell by a German chemist, **Richard Wilhelm Heinrich Abegg** (1869–1910) in 1897. Further research on the electronic theory of valency was carried out by an American physical chemist, **Gilbert Newton Lewis** (1875–1946) of Weymouth, Massachusetts, who received his education at Harvard University and worked with **Friedrich Wilhelm Ostwald** (1853–1932) at Leipzig, and **Walther Hermann Nernst** (1864–1941) at Göttingen. He published *Valence and the Structure of Atoms and Molecules* in 1923. The theory of partial valency, where two double-bonded atoms may preserve residual affinity, was proposed in 1899 by an organic chemist **Friedrich Karl Johannes Thiele** (1865–1918) of Silesia. Important contributions to the theory of valency were made by an English chemist from Oxford, **Nevil Vincent Sidgwick** (1873–1952), who published *The Electronic Theory of Valency* (1927) and *Some Physical Properties of the Covalent Link in Chemistry* (1933). A French physicist, **Paul Langevin** (1872–1946) of Paris, suggested that magnetic properties of an element depended on the valency electrons and his idea helped to explain magnetism in terms of electron theory. The terms univalent, bivalent and trivalent were coined by a German chemist, **Julius Lothar von Meyer** (1830–1895), who was appointed to the first chair of chemistry at Tübingen University in 1876. He published *Die modernen Theorien der Chemie* (Modern Chemical Theory) in 1864. **Walther Kossel** (1888–1956), professor of physics at Kiel (1921) and Danzig (1932), advocated the physical theory of valency. In England, **Charles Alfred Coulson** (1910–1974), the first professor of theoretical chemistry at Oxford, studied the application of molecular orbital theory to chemical bonds and published *Valence* (1952). A London-born Canadian chemist, **Ronald James Gillepsie** (b 1924) and an Australian chemist, **Sir Ronald Sydney Nyholm** (1917–1971), modified the valency shell electron theory of Sidgwick, stating that lone pairs of electrons have a greater repulsive effect than bonding pairs. This modified theory explained the distortion of bond angles of molecules such as water and ammonia. *See bonds.*

Valentine, Gabriel Gustav (1810–1883) *See cell, microtome.*

Valentinus, Basilus (*c.* AD 1500) *See alchemy.*

Vallisneri, Antonio (1661–1730) An Italian naturalist and professor of medicine at Padua. The waterweed *Vallisneria spiralis* is named after him. *See rivers.*

Van Allen Belts Two zones of high levels of radiation in the space around the earth. Discovered by an American physicist, **James Alfred van Allen** (b 1914) of Iowa, with the use of the first American satellite *Explorer I*, launched in 1958.

Van de Graaff Generator An electrostatic high-voltage generator built by an American physicist, **Robert Jemison van de Graaff** (1901–1967) of Alabama in 1929. It was used in medical research and was modified to give radiotherapy at the Boston Hospital in 1937. His generator was also adapted for use as a particle accelerator and became immensely useful in nuclear research.

Van Der Waals Equation Related to intermolecular forces and molecular volume of gases, derived by a Dutch physicist, **Johannes Diderik Van der Waals** (1837–1923) of Leiden, who became professor of physics at Amsterdam University in 1877. He published *On the Continuity of Liquid and Gaseous States* (1873) and was awarded the Nobel Prize for physics in 1910.

Van Der Waals Forces Weak attraction between molecules. Named after a Dutch physicist, **Johannes Diderik Van der Waals** (1837–1923) who served as professor of physics at Amsterdam University from 1877 to 1907.

Van't Hoff, Jacobus Henricus (1852–1911) An eminent chemist born in Rotterdam, who graduated from Utrecht in 1874. He was professor of chemistry at Amsterdam in 1878 and moved to Berlin in 1896. He proposed the tetrahedral structure of carbon in 1874 and came to be regarded as the founder of stereochemistry and physical chemistry. He stated that solutions and gases behaved similarly, proposed the dissociation theory related to electrolytes in solution in 1877, and published *Studies in Chemical Dynamics* (1884). *See Boyle–van't Hoff law, dissociation, electrolysis, gas laws, physical chemistry, stereochemistry.*

Vanadium [*Vanadis*, goddess of love] A hard white metal of atomic number 23 discovered in 1801 by a Spanish mineralogist, **Andrés Manuel del Río** (1764–1849) of Madrid. A Swedish chemist and physician, **Nils Gabriel Sefström**

(1787–1854), independently discovered it in 1831. It was first isolated in a pure metallic state in 1869 by a London chemist, **Sir Henry Enfield Roscoe** (1833–1915).

Vapor Density The density of gas or vapor in relation to that of hydrogen. In 1823 **Jean Baptiste André Dumas** (1800–1884), a French apothecary in Geneva, devised a method for its determination. A simpler and more practical method was described by a German chemist, **Viktor Meyer** (1848–1897) of Berlin.

Varenius or **Bernhard Varen** (1622–1650) *See geography.*

Variable Star A star whose luminosity changes over periods of time. The first, *Mira,* was discovered in 1592 by **David Fabricius** (1564–1617) of Essen, Germany. The relationship between intrinsic luminosity and the period of variability of the variable stars (Leavitt's period-luminosity law) was discovered in 1904 by an American astronomer, **Henrietta Swan Leavitt** (1868–1921). Her discovery helped to determine the distances of other galaxies and stars. A Buckinghamshire-born British astronomer, **Celia Helena**

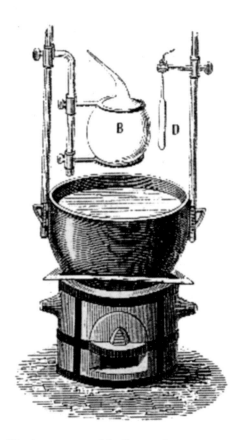

Figure 83 Apparatus used by Dumas for measuring vapor density. Akinson, E. *Elementary Treatise on Physics.* London: Longmans, Green, and Co, 1872

Payne-Gaposchkin (1900–1979), who emigrated to America to work at the Harvard College Observatory in 1922, did monumental work, measuring variable stars on photographic plates, with her husband Sergei Gaposchkin, and produced a catalog of variable stars in 1938. *See cepheid variables.*

Vauban, Sebastian le Prestre de (1633–1707) *See military engineering, water supply.*

Vaucanson, Jacques de (1709–1782) *See lathe, textile industry.*

Vauquelin, Louis Nicolas (1763–1829) *See asparagine, beryllium, chromium, Thenard blue.*

Vavilov, Nikolai Ivanovitch (1887–1943) *See agronomy.*

Velcro A fastening device for clothing and other purposes, invented in 1948 by a Swiss engineer, Georges de Mertral. He conceived the idea after trying to get rid of burs from plants from his socks and his dog's fur, after a walk in the woods. When he examined the seeds under the microscope he noticed that several hooks enabled them to hold onto clothes. After eight years of work, in 1957 he developed the final product made of two nylon surfaces where one had thousands of hooks, and the other a similar number of loops.

Vellum [French: *velin*, veal or calf] *See writing materials.*

Velocity [Latin: *velox*, swift] Rate of motion or speed in a given direction. *See velocity of chemical reactions, velocity of electricity, velocity of gas molecules, velocity of light, velocity of sound.*

Velocity of Chemical Reactions A mathematical formula for the velocity of the forward reaction between an alcohol and acid, giving an ester and water, was proposed in 1862 by **L.P. de Saint-Gillies** (1832–1863). Two Norwegian professors of chemistry at the University of Christiana (Oslo), **Cato Maximillian Guldberg** (1836–1902) and **Peter Waage** (1833–1900) did extensive work on the rate of forward and reverse reactions, and studied the effect of mass, concentration and temperature on the reaction rates.

Velocity of Electricity In 1747 a London physician and physicist, **Sir William Watson** (1715–1787), attempted to measure the velocity of electricity, but due to the lack of sensitivity of his experiments he came to the conclusion that electricity was instantaneous. In 1834 an English physicist **Sir Charles Wheatstone** (1801–1875) of Gloucester, made the first measurement by using a rotating mirror to measure the delay between sparks, as the current travelled through a wire. **James Clerk Maxwell** (1831–1879) dis-

covered electric waves and proposed that the velocity of electricity is identical to the velocity of light.

Velocity of Gas Molecules The English physicist **James Prescott Joule** (1818–1889), made the first determination of the velocity of gas molecules, which he described in his paper on the theory of kinetic gases in 1848.

Velocity of Light A Greek philosopher and physician, **Empedocles** (*c.* 490–430 BC) of Agrigentum, pointed out that there must be an interval of time involved, when light travels from one place to another. **Robert Hooke** (1635–1703) regarded the velocity of light as being too great for any experimental determination. The evidence that light has a definite velocity came from astronomical observations. The Danish astronomer **Olaus Roemer** (1644–1710) in 1675 observed the different intervals between the eclipses of the moons of Jupitor in relation to the movement of the earth. This phenomenon was later explained by the fact that light had a definite velocity. Although **René Descartes** (1596–1650) and **Sir Isaac Newton** (1642–1727) conceived light as a stream of particles, no satisfactory method of measuring the velocity of light was available until 1849, when a French physicist, **Armand Hippolyte Louis Fizeau** (1819–1896), devised an ingenious method without the use of astronomical distances. The idea of using a rotating mirror occurred to **Sir Charles Wheatstone** (1801–1875) during his attempts to measure the velocity of electricity in 1834, and this was demonstrated by a French physicist and physician, **Jean Bernard Léon Foucault** (1819–1868) of Paris, around 1855. Fizeau's method of measuring the velocity of light was improved by a Scottish physicist, **George Forbes** (1849–1936) of Edinburgh, who obtained an accurate result. In 1888 **Albert Abraham Michelson** (1852–1931) and **Edward Williams Morley** (1838–1923) jointly made an attempt to determine the velocity of the earth, by measuring the velocity of light in relation to the ether. Their work showed that the velocity of light was the same in all directions and was independent of the motion of the earth. Scientists in the late 1990s have suggested that the velocity of light has been slowing down since the origin of the universe.

Velocity of Sound Experimentally investigated by members of Accademia del Cimento in Florence in 1657. A French natural philosopher, **Marin Mersenne** (1588–1648), was the first to measure the velocity of sound through the timing of echoes. The propagation of sound through the air was demonstrated by **Otto von Guericke** (1602–1686), mayor of Magdeburg in Prussia. The evidence of propagation of sound through water was provided independently by an English physicist, **Francis Hawksbee** (d 1713) in 1705 and Arderon in 1748. In 1708 an English naturalist, **William Derham** (1657–1735), attempted to verify Newton's theoretical calculation of the speed of sound. In 1826 a French mathematician, **Jacques Charles François Strum** (1803–1855), measured the velocity of sound under water by using a bell submerged in Lake Geneva. The velocity of sound waves in air was measured by **Sir Isaac Newton** (1642–1727). The correct interpretation of Newton's mathematical formula used in the calculation was given by **Pierre Simon Marquis de Laplace** (1749–1827).

Vening Meinesz, Felix Andries (1887–1966) *See oceanography.*

Venn Diagram Used in logical teaching of elementary mathematics. Devised by a British logician and clergyman, **John Venn** (1834–1923) of Drypool, Hull, who published *The Logic of Chance* (1866), *Symbolic Logic* (1881) and *The Principles of Empirical Logic* (1889).

Venn, John (1834–1923) *See Venn diagram.*

Ventilation The German mining engineer and physician **Georgius Agricola** (1494–1555) described wind-scoops, centrifugal fans and bellows used for maintaining an underground supply of fresh air.

Venturi Effect *See hydraulics.*

Venturi, Giovanni Battista (1746–1822) *See hydraulics.*

Venus The hottest of the nine major planets of the solar system, and the nearest to the earth. It is also the brightest of the five planets visible to the naked eye. Its transit was first observed by an English astronomer, **Jeremiah Horrocks** (1618–1641) of Toxteth Park, near Liverpool, on 24th November 1639. Another method for observing its transit was devised by a French astronomer, **Joseph Nicolas Delisle** (1688–1768) of Paris. The atmosphere of Venus was discovered in 1761 by a Russian scientist, **Mikhail Vasilievich Lomonosov** (1711–1765). A well-documented account of the transit of Venus was given in 1769 by a French astronomer, **Joseph Jerome Le François de Lalande** (1732–1807) of Bourg-en-Bresse. The Soviet spaceprobe *Venera III* became the first object made by humans to reach another planet, Venus, in 1966. The first pictures of the surface of Venus were received in 1970 from the Soviet spaceprobe *Venera 7*.

Verbiest, Ferdinand (1623–1687) *See automobile.*

Vermuyden, Sir Cornelius (*c.* 1595–1683) A Dutch engineer from Thoren, Zeeland, who moved to England in 1621, where he became a waterworks and drainage engineer.

Vernadsky, Vladimir Ivanovich (1863–1945) A Russian mineralogist and one of the first to recognize the possibility of using atomic power as a source of energy. He served as professor of mineralogy at Moscow University before he moved to the Ukraine and founded the Ukrainian Academy of Sciences.

Vernalization [Latin: *vernalis,* of spring] Retardation of germination in the winter seed by freezing, in order to sow it in the spring. A method developed by a Soviet biologist, **Trofim Denisovich Lysenko** (1898–1976) from the Ukraine, who won the Stalin Prize in 1949 for his book *Agrobiology* (1948).

Verne, Jules (1828–1905) *See astronomical paintings, science fiction, undersea exploration.*

Vernier Scale A device for taking readings on a graduated scale to a fraction of a division. It has a movable auxiliary scale with subdivisions of the basic units of the main scale. A principle suggested by a Portuguese mathematician, **Pedro Nuñez** (1492–1577). The scale was devised in 1631 by a French instrument maker, **Pierre Vernier** (1584–1638) of Ornans. The slide calipers are based on its principle.

Vernier, Pierre (1584–1638) *See Vernier scale.*

Vertebrates Aristotle in his *Historia Animalium* used morphology or appearance for classification of animals into groups and subgroups. In his treatise *On the Generation of Animals* he stated that all sanguinous animals (animals with blood) have a backbone. An early comparative study of the structure of vertebrate animals was done by a Belgian biologist, **Gerard Blaes** (1646–1682), who published *Anatome Animalium* (1681). An eminent British comparative anatomist and paleontologist, **Richard Owen** (1804–1892), published an important work *Anatomy and Physiology of the Vertebrates* (1866–1868), based on his personal observations. A London zoologist, **St George Jackson Mivart** (1827–1900), published *The Cat: An Introduction to the Study of Backbone Animals* in 1886. An American zoologist from Connecticut, **Henry Fairfield Osborne** (1857–1935), did important work on fossil vertebrates and published *The Age of Mammals* (1910). Another American, **Libbie Henrietta Hyman** (1888–1969), published *A Laboratory Manual for Comparative Vertebrate Anatomy* (1929) and six volumes of *The Invertebrates* (1940–1968). An American vertebrate paleontologist, **Alfred Sherwood Romer** (1894–1973) of White Planes, New York, whose special interest was the evolution of vertebrates, published some importants books including

Vertebrate Paleontology (1933), *The Vertebrate Body* (1949) and *The Vertebrate Story* (1952).

Very, Frank Washington (1852–1927) *See Mars.*

Vespucci, Amerigo (1451–1512) *See America.*

Vicat, Louis Joseph (1786–1861) *See concrete.*

Video Game The first video game *Pong,* which worked on the principle of the liquid crystal screen (LCD), was invented in 1972 by an American, Norman Bushnell.

Video Tapes The first recording on video tapes (*Ampex* tapes) was demonstrated in 1956 by a US engineer, Alexander M. Pontiaff. The first home video recorder was developed by Norman Rutherford and Michael Turner of the Nottingham Electronic Valve Company, and it was demonstrated at the BBC studio in Alexandra Palace, London, in June 1963.

Video Telephone A video-telephone with a television screen was developed in the early 1970s by the Bell Telephone Company of the United States.

Viète, François (1540–1603) *See algebra, decimal notation, goniometry, trigonometry.*

Vignola, Giacomo Barozzi da (1507–1573) *See architecture, Italian.*

Vignoles, Charles Blacker (1793–1875) *See railway.*

Villard, Paul Ulrich (1860–1934) *See gamma rays.*

Viollet-le-Duc, Eugene Emmanuel (1814–1879) *See architecture, European.*

Virchow, Rudolph (1821–1902) *See cell.*

Virtanen, Artturi Ilmari (1895–1973) *See nitrogen-fixing bacteria.*

Virtual Reality One of the first models was developed by Edwin Link in 1929 to train pilots. His flight trainer had mock aircraft cockpits and flight instruments. The principle was further developed for space programs, and **Neil Armstrong** (b 1930) practiced landings on a virtual moon before his real landing in 1969. The new technology, called computer-generated imagery, combined with other techniques such as holography, has helped to produce more realisitic images. The term cyberspace for the world produced by virtual images, was coined by a science fiction writer William Gibson. Several advanced programs since then have been developed for training in defense and warfare. The world's first virtual air-traffic-control center is due to be opened at Nasa's Ames research center in California in summer 1999.

Virus [Latin: *virus,* poison] The first evidence for the existence of particles smaller than bacteria, capable of producing disease, was presented in 1892 by a Russian botanist, **Dmitri Iosifovich Ivanovski** (1864–1920). During his investigation of the mosaic disease of the tobacco plant, he discovered that the sap of the diseased plant was still capable of transmitting the disease despite its treatment through a bacterial filter. A Dutch botanist, **Wilhelm Martinus Beijerinck** (1851–1931), revived the interest in 1898 and coined the term virus.

Viscose *See textile chemistry.*

Viscosity [Latin: *viscidus,* sticky] The property of a fluid that causes it to resist motion. The physical properties of fluids in relation to their flow through a tube were studied in 1840 by **Jean Leonard Marie Poiseuille** (1799–1869). An early work was published by A. du Pre Denning and John H. Watson in the *Proceedings of the Royal Society* in 1906. An English chemist and science historian from Manchester, **Sir Thomas Edward Thorpe** (1845–1925), studied the viscosity of fluids and discovered a formula for its coefficient. Original work on plastic flow and viscosity was done by an American chemist, **Eugene Cook Bingham** (b 1878) from Vermont, who published *Fluidity and Plasticity* (1921). An American physicist, **Percy Williams Bridgman** (1882–1961) of Cambridge, Massachusetts, who was a pioneer in high-pressure physics, showed that viscosity increases with high pressure. He published *The Logic of Modern Physics* (1927) and *The Nature of Physical Theory* (1936), and was awarded the Nobel Prize for physics in 1946.

Vision A Polish cleric, **Witelo** (*c.* 1250–1275), in his *Perspectiva* (1270) rejected the previous belief that rays are emitted from the eyes. He also discussed the psychological aspects of vision. Other philosophers of the Middle Ages in England who discussed the mechanism of vision based on optics include **Adelard of Bath** (1090–1150) and **Alexander Neckham** (1157–1217), an Augustinian monk from St Albans, Hertfordshire. **Roger Bacon** (*c.* 1214–*c.* 1298) in his *Opus Majus* illustrated the internal structure of the eye on the basis of optics. The role of the retina in vision was elucidated by the German astronomer **Johannes Kepler** (1571–1630), in his *Dipotrice* (1611). **René Descartes** (1596–1650) studied the mechanism of vision and the eye in detail in 1637 and compared it to the camera obscura. A French priest, **Edmé Mariotte** (1620–1684), did away with the old belief that the eye was the cause of light, in 1671. The mechanism of accommodation and errors of refraction were studied by Christoph Scheiner of Vienna in 1619. Distortion of vision due to irregular refraction was described by the English physician, **Thomas Young** (1773–1829), in his treatise *On the Mechanism of Eye* (1801). Young's three-color theory was developed by the Scottish physicist, **James Clerk Maxwell** (1831–1879), who showed that color blindness was due to a defect in receptors. The biochemical processes involved in the retina were studied by a New York biochemist, **George Wald** (1906–1997), who in 1933 discovered the colorless protein opsin involved in vision. He also explained color blindness on the basis of retinal pigments and shared the Nobel Prize for Physiology or Medicine in 1967 with **Ragnar Granit** (1900–1991) and **Halden Keffer Hartline** (1903–1983) of Bloomsberg, Pennsylvania. A Canadian-born US neurophycist, **David Hunter Hubel** (b 1926), studied the mechanism of processing of visual information by the higher centers of the brain, for which he was awarded the Nobel Prize for Physiology or Medicine in 1981, with **Roger Wolcott Sperry** (1913–1994) of Hartford, Connecticut, and **Torsten Nils Wiesel** (b 1924).

Visual Telegraphy *See flag signalling, railway signals, semaphore.*

Vital Statistics [Latin: *vita*, life]   A statistical study of births, morbidity and mortality. The first book on the subject, *Natural and Political Observations Upon the Bills of Mortality* (1662) was published by **John Graunt** (1620–1674) of London. A valuable life table for the purposes of life insurance was published in 1693 by the British astronomer, **Edmund Halley** (1656–1742). **Sir William Petty** (1623–1687) from Hampshire, England, studied the mortality rates in the 17th century, and his work was further advanced by **Gregory King** (1648–1712). A French mathematician, **Pierre Simon Marquis de Laplace** (1749–1827) of Normandy, published *Théorie analytique des probabilités* (1812), an important landmark in the field. The study of vital statistics was established on a scientific basis in 1839 by an English physician and statistician, **William Farr** (1807–1883) of Kenley, Shropshire.

Vitamins [Latin: *vita*, life]   The concept of essential or accessory food factors, later known as vitamins, was proposed in 1906 by an English biochemist, **Fredrick Gowland Hopkins** (1851–1947) of Cambridge University. The first of these accessory food factors, which prevented the disease beri-beri, was discovered in 1911 by a Polish chemist, **Casimir Funk** (1884–1967) and he named it vitamine. **Elmer Verner McCollum** (1879–1967), an American biochemist from Fort Scott, Kansas, gave the first description of an accessory food factor, and discovered vitamin A in 1913. He detected the rickets-preventing factor (vitamin D)

in cod liver oil in 1922. **Sir Edward Mellanby** (1884–1955), an English pioneer in the study of vitamins, produced rickets in dogs by maintaining them on a deficient diet and suggested for the first time that the missing nutrient factor in the disease was a fat-soluble substance.

Vitello of Silesia (*c.* 1250)   *See optics.*

Vitruvius Marcus Pollio   A Roman architect who designed Rome at the time of Augustus in the 1st century, and wrote a book on architecture entitled *De Architectura, Libri Decem* in ten volumes. *See acoustics, architecture, ancient, catapult, cement, crane, dyes, odometer, water pump, water supply.*

Vivianni, Vincenzo (1622–1703)   *See Accademia del Cimento, barometer.*

Vleck, John Hasbrouck, Van (1899–1980)   An American physicist from Connecticut whose main interest was the magnetic properties of atoms. He published *The Theory of Electric and Magnetic Susceptibilities* (1932). The Nobel Prize for physics in 1977 for work on magnetic systems was shared by Van Vleck, **Phillip Warren Anderson** (b 1923) of Indianopolis and an English physicist, **Sir Neville Francis Mott** (1905–1996).

Voelcker, Augustus (1822–1884)   *See fertilizers.*

Vogel, Hermann Carl (1842–1907)   *See binary stars.*

Vogel, Hermann Wilhelm (1834–1898) *See color photography.*

Volcanic Eruptions   The largest known flow of volcanic lava in prehistoric times, the Roza basalt, in North America, took place 15 million years ago. Santorini in the Aegean Sea, north of Crete, erupted in 1628 BC. The eruption of Vesuvius in AD 79, accompanied by an earthquake, destroyed the city of Pompeii. A major eruption of Taupo in New Zealand took place in AD 130. The world's northernmost volcano, Beeren Berg, on the island of Jan Meyen, was discovered in 1607 by an English explorer, **Henry Hudson** (*c.* 1550–1611). The southernmost volcano, on Ross Island in Antarctica, was discovered in 1841 by the Scottish explorer, **Sir James Clark Ross** (1800–1862). A loss of 90 000 lives occurred during the eruption of Tambora on the island of Sunbawa in Indonesia in 1825. Nearly 40 000 people were killed in 1883 during the eruption of Krakatoa, an island between Java and Sumatra in Indonesia. The largest currently active volcano, Mauna Loa, in Hawaii, has been erupting since 1832. *See seismology, volcanoes.*

Volcanoes [Latin: *Vulcanus,* Roman god of fire]   A Jesuit priest, **Athanasius Kircher** (1601–1680) of Geysen, in his *Subterranean World* (1665), postulated that numerous volcanoes and thermal springs fed by the sea, existed under the earth's surface. **Sir James Hall** (1761–1832), a British geologist from Dunglass, Haddingtonshire, was one of the first to study volcanoes in detail. The modern theory of volcanoes was proposed by **G. Poulett Scrope** (1787–1876), who studied volcanic action for 20 years and published *Considerations on Volcanoes* (1825). **James Dwight Dana** (1813–1895), an American geologist from Utica, New York, published *Hawaiian Volcanoes* (1890). Photographic study of volcanic phenomena was pioneered by an English surgeon, **Tempest Anderson** (1846–1913), who published *Volcanic Studies in Many Lands* (1903). In 1974 a Japanese-born US seismologist, **Keiiti Aki** (b 1930), developed seismic tomography with a three-dimensional aspect that gave the first quantitative estimate of the earth's tremors during volcanic eruptions. A French geologist, **François Antoine Alfred Lacroix** (1863–1948), carried out studies immediately after the volcanic eruption of Mont Pelée, Martinique, in 1902, and published *La Montagne Pelée apres ses éruptions* (1908). *See seismology, volcanic eruptions.*

Volhard, Jacob (1834–1910)   *See Volhard method.*

Volhard Method   Quantitative analysis of an element, by titrating its chloride against silver nitrate, devised by a German chemist, **Jacob Volhard** (1834–1910) of Darmstadt.

Volta, Alessandro (1745–1827)   *See battery, electricity, voltage, voltaic pile.*

Voltage   An electrical effect between two different metals in contact with moisture. First observed around 1790 by **Alessandro Volta** (1745–1827).

Voltaic Pile   A device made of alternate piles of copper, zinc and paste board, capable of generating electricity, devised in 1800 by **Alessandro Volta** (1745–1827), professor of natural philosophy at the University of Pavia. He announced his discovery in a letter entitled *On the electricity excited by the mere contact of conducting substances of different kinds* addressed to **Sir Joseph Banks** (1743–1820). A London physicist, **William**

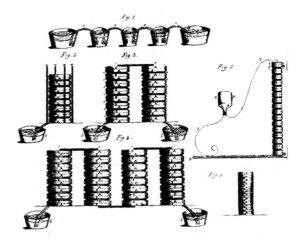

Figure 84   Voltaic pile. Moore, F.J. *A History of Chemistry*, International Chemistry Series. New York: McGraw-Hill Book Inc, 1918

Nicholson (1753–1815) from Portsmouth, used the principle to construct the first voltaic battery in England.

Vonnegut, Bernard (b 1914)   *See artificial rain.*

Vostok   *See astronauts.*

Vries, Hugo Marie de (1848–1935)   *See mutation, osmosis.*

Vulcanization [Latin: *Vulcanus*, Roman god of fire]   The first patent for making rubber more elastic and moldable was taken out in 1820 by an English inventor, **Thomas Hancock** (1786–1865) of Marlborough. In 1843 he took out another patent for a process very similar to vulcanization. The reaction of rubber with a sulfur solution was studied independently by **Nathaniel Hayward** (1808–1868) and **Alexander Parkes** (1813–1890) of Birmingham. In 1839 **Charles Goodyear** (1800–1860), a hardware merchant from New Haven, Connecticut, accidently rediscovered that a rubber mix containing sulfur when heated became tough and its tackiness disappeared. He developed this process and named it after the Greek god of fire.

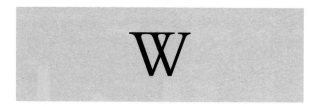

Waage, Peter (1833–1900) *See law of mass action, velocity of chemical reactions.*

Waals, Johannes Diderik van der (1837–1923) *See Van der Waals equation, Van der Waals forces.*

Wadati, Kiyoo (b 1902) *See Wadati–Benioff zones.*

Wadati–Benioff Zones Deep seismic zones that reveal the motion of descending oceanic crust. Described independently by a Japanese seismologist, **Kiyoo Wadati** (b 1902) and an American geophysicist, **Victor Hugo Benioff** (1899–1968) of Los Angeles.

Wager, Lawrence Rickard (1904–1965) *See carbon dating.*

Wagner, Otto (1835–1917) *See architecture, European.*

Wald, George (1906–1997) *See vision.*

Walden Inversion A phenomenon connected with the optical isomerism of carbon. Discovered in 1896 by a Russian chemist, **Paul Walden** (1863–1957) of Wenden, Latvia. He was professor of chemistry at St Petersburg (1910) and Riga (1918) and published *History of Organic Chemistry* (1941).

Walden, Paul (1863–1957) *See Walden inversion.*

Waldeyer-Hartz, Wilhelm (1836–1921) *See chromosomes, neuron.*

Waldseemuller, Martin (*c.* 1480–1521) *See America.*

Walker, John (1781–1859) *See matches.*

Walker, Sir James (1863–1935) *See physical chemistry.*

Wallace, Alfred Russell (1823–1913) A Welsh naturalist, born at Usk, in Monmouthshire. He commenced a study of species with his first trip of exploration to the Amazon in 1848, and independently thought of a mechanism for the origin of new species, one year before Darwin published his *Origin of Species* in 1859. He spent eight years in the Malay peninsula and made a remarkable comparative study of the flora and published *The Malay Archipelago* (1869). *See evolution.*

Wallace, Henry (1836–1916) *See American scientific journals.*

Wallace, William (1768–1843) Son of a leather merchant from Dysart, in Fifeshire. He became professor of mathe-

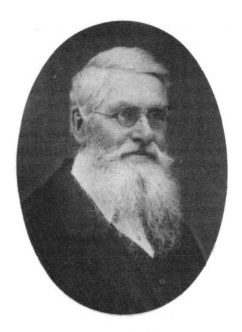

Figure 85 Alfred Russell Wallace (1823–1913). Wallace, Alfred Russell. *Darwinism*. London: Macmillan and Co, 1889

matics at the Royal Military College, Great Marlow in 1819, and played a vital role in establishing the Calton Hill Observatory. He contributed several important papers to the Transactions of the Royal Society of Edinburgh.

Wallach, Otto (1847–1931) *See terpenes.*

Wallis, John (1616–1703) *See algebra, arithmatic, calculus, law of conservation of momentum, mathematical symbols, momentum, Royal Society of London.*

Wallis, Sir Barnes Neville (1887–1979) *See airships, warplanes.*

Walschaerts, Égide (1820–1901) *See railway.*

Walter, John (1739–1812) *See newspapers.*

Walton, Ernest Thomas Sinton (1903–1995) *See cyclotron.*

Wang, An (1920–1990) *See computers.*

Wankel Engine *See rotary engine.*

Wankel, Felix (1902–1988) *See rotary engine.*

Warburg, Otto Heinrich (1883–1970) *See photosynthesis.*

Ward, Seth (1617–1689) An English astronomer and clergyman from Hertfordshire who became bishop of Salisbury in 1667. He proposed a theory of planetary motion in 1653. *See Royal Society of London.*

Warfare *See catapult, firearms, military engineering, torpedo, warplanes, warships.*

Warming, Johannes Eugenius Bülow (1841–1924) *See ecology.*

Warplanes The first air raid in history was carried out in 1849 against Venice by the Austrians who dropped bombs from a balloon. The German airship pioneer, **Count Ferdinand von Zeppelin's** (1838–1917) airships were used against the British during the First World War. The first British military airplane was built in 1906 by an English inventor and author **John William Dunne** (1875–1945). The first British aircraft manufacturing firm Handley-Page Ltd, founded in 1909 by an English aircraft designer, **Sir Fredrick Handley-Page** (1885–1962), built the first twin-engined bomber for the First World War. A British aircraft designer, **Robert Blackburn** (1885–1955), founded the Blackburn Aircraft Company in 1914, which built military biplanes. In 1912 **Thomas Octave Murdoch Sopwith** (1888–1989) founded the Sopwith Aviation Company at Kingston Upon Thames, Surrey, where he built several aircraft for World War I. **Glen Hammond Curtiss** (1878–1930) from Hammondsport, New York, produced several military aircraft for World War I. A Dutch-born German engineer **Anton Herman Gerard Fokker** (1890–1939), who built his first plane in 1911, later made warplanes for the German air force during the First World War at his factory in Schwerin. He also designed a method for firing machine guns through the revolving propeller blades. He emigrated to the USA in 1922 and became president of the Fokker Aircraft Corporation there. The British automobile and aircraft engineer, **Frederick William Lanchester** (1868–1948), published *Aircraft in Warfare* in 1914. **Sir Sydney Camm** (1893–1966) of Windsor, Berkshire, in England, designed several successful military aircraft including *Fury, Tornado, Sea Hawk* and *Harrier*. Another English engineer, **Roy Chadwick** (1893–1947), built the *Anson*, which was used in the Second World War, and the Lancaster heavy bombers. **Donald Willis Douglas** (1892–1971), an aeronautical engineer from Brooklyn, New York, produced the B-19 bomber during the Second World War. Naval aircraft were developed by an American engineer and navy pilot, **Leroy Randle Grumman** (1895–1982) of Huntingdon, New York, who designed important navy planes of World War II, such as the *Wildcat, Hellcat* and the *Tigercat*. The single-engined fighter plane the *Spitfire* was designed by an English aeronautical engineer, **Reginald Joseph Mitchell** (1895–1937). The fighter planes in Germany during the Second World War were mostly developed by **Wilhelm Emil Messerschmitt** (1898–1978) of Frankfurt-am-Main.

Another German, **Ernst Heinrich Heinkel** (1888–1958), built several bombers and fighter planes during the Second World War. The Russian fighter aircraft known as the *MiG* (Mi = Mikoyan + G = Gurevich) was designed by **Mikhail Iosifovich Gurevich** (1893–1976) and **Artem Ivanovich Mikoyan** (1905–1970). Another Russian aircraft designer, **Sergei Vladimirovich Ilyushin** (1894–1977), designed several bombers including *TSBK-30, IL-2 shturmovik* and *IL-2,* which were used in the Second World War. In 1943 **Leonard Clarence Johnson** (1910–1990) of the Lockheed Corporation designed the first US jet fighter to go into production, the *P-80*. An English aeronautical engineer, **Sir Barnes Neville Wallis** (1887–1979), developed the concept of a variable-geometry wing (swing-wing) to overcome the problems associated with trimming aircraft for flight in both super- and subsonic conditions. The first swing-wing aircraft, the US built Northrop *X-4*, led to the development of the *F-111* and *F-114* and, later, the *F-15* and Panavia *Tornado* also took advantage of the benefits of variable geometry. A Russian engineer, **Andrei Nikolaevich Tupolev** (1888–1972), designed several twin-engined miltary aircraft for the Second World War. His *ANT-20* had eight engines with a wing span of 260 feet.

Warships The world's first steam warship, *Fulton the First,* was designed in 1814 by an American engineer, **Robert Fulton** (1765–1815) of Pennsylvania. Initially named *Demologos* by Fulton, it was intended to defend the port of New York against the British fleet. The first British warship, the *Comet,* was designed by **Sir John Rennie** (1794–1874) and **Isambard Kingdom Brunel** (1806–1859), and launched in 1822. A Swedish-born American inventor, **John Ericsson** (1803–1889), designed screw-propelled warships for the Royal Navy in 1842. In 1858 **Sir Edwards James Harland** (1831–1896), a British shipbuilder, founded a firm in Belfast which built many warships. The earliest iron-clad warships including the *Black Prince* (1860) were designed by a Scottish ship-builder, **Robert Napier** (1791–1876) of Dumbarton. The thickest armor ever was installed on HMS *Inflexible* in 1881. The largest guns were first mounted on a light battle cruiser, HMS *Furious* in 1917. One of the fastest destroyers, *Le Terrible,* was built at Blainville, France in 1935. The US 'Liberty Ships' of World War II were designed by **William Francis Gibbs** (1886–1967) of Philadelphia.

Washing Machines The earliest invention related to clothes-washing, a mangle, was used in England in the 15th century. It consisted of a wooden structure with a large hand-turned wheel for pressing clothes. The handle brought a weighted tray over the rollers which pressed the clothes after washing. It was improved by adding heavy wooden rollers and an iron stand, and continued to be used until the middle of the 19th century. The first hand-operated washing machines appeared around 1840, and they consisted of simple wooden boxes on rockers. In 1850 an American, Joel Houghton, invented a hand-operated machine that agitated the water. Hand-operated models with gyrotype rotating blades appeared in 1869. The first electric washing machine was patented by Alva F. Fisher of America in 1907.

Watches   The first known pocket watch, a small spring-driven device, was invented by Peter Henlein of Nuremberg in 1502. The first watches with their dials protected by glass appeared around 1600. **Thomas Tompian** (1639–1713) from Northhill, Bedfordshire, is regarded as the father of English watchmaking; he devised the first English watch with a balance spring, under the supervision of **Robert Hooke** (1635–1703) in 1658. Tompian was appointed as the first clockmaker to the Royal Observatory in 1676. In 1704 two Swiss watchmakers in London, **Nicholas Faccio de Duiller** (1664–1753) and Peter Jacob Debaufe invented the first jewel-run watches, which had pivot-holes made of sapphires for a longer life. In 1755 **John Mudge** (d 1793), a physician and mechanic from Plymouth, invented a superior escapement mechanism that became known as the English lever. The first pocket chronometer was produced in 1766. The first standard wristwatches were made in Geneva in 1790 by Jacquet Droz and Paul Leschot. The first self-winding watch was invented by a Frenchman, **Peter Joseph Rivaz** (1711–1772), and another automatically winding watch was invented in 1770 by a Swiss watchmaker, **Abraham-Louis Perrelet** (1729–1826) of Le Locle. A gold colored alloy of copper and zinc used for producing imitation gold watches was invented by a London clockmaker *Christopher Pinchbeck* (1670–1732). His son **Christopher Pinchbeck** (1710–1783) was a maker of astronomical clocks and invented automatic pneumatic brakes. Some of the finest watches, still maintaining their tradition, were made by **Abraham-Louis Breguet** (1747–1823) of Neuchâtel. Wristwatches were introduced into England by J.W. Benson in 1886. The first self-winding wristwatch in England was patented in 1924 by John Harwood, who also designed the first electric watch. The first waterproof watch, *Oyster*, was made by Hans Wilsdorf at the Swiss watch firm Rolex, in 1926. The first commercial watch with electric batteries was introduced by the French company Lip, in 1956. The first electronic watch, *Accutron*, was developed by an American company, Bulova, around 1960; worked on a mercury cell that vibrated a tiny tuning-fork. The first quartz crystal wrist watch appeared in 1967.

Water   The composition of water was discovered in 1784 by the English chemist, **Henry Cavendish** (1731–1810), and it was accurately determined in 1895 by an American **Edward William Morley** (1838–1923), professor of chemistry at Western Reserve University, Ohio. The compressibility of water was demonstrated in 1762 by an English physicist, **John Canton** (1718–1772) of Stroud. The first electrolysis of water was performed in 1800 by an English waterworks engineer at Portsmouth, **William Nicholson** (1753–1815). A Scottish chemist, **Thomas Charles Hope** (1766–1844) of Edinburgh, designed an apparatus for determining the maximum density of water.

Water Immersion Objective   *See Amici, Giovanni Battista.*

Water Pump   The archimedian screw, which is still used in some parts of Egypt for raising water, is one of the earliest water pumps, invented by **Archimedes** (287–212 BC) during his visit to Egypt around 250 BC. Around AD 100, the Roman architect, **Marcus Pollio Vitruvius**, described a water pump. A Roman pump of a similar nature, based on the principle of the piston, was unearthed at Silchester in England. The German mining engineer and physician, **Georgius Agricola** (1494–1555), described several kinds of water pump. An English Huguenot engineer, **Salomen de Caulx** (1576–1626), described a steam engine for raising water in his *Les Raisons des forces mouvantes avec diverses machines* (1615). Bellows were used for pumping water during this period. A water machine based on a system of archimedian screws, in Augsburg, was mentioned in 1550 by **Girolomo Cardan** (1501–1576). In 1565, an Italian clock-maker, **Juanelo Turriano** (1500–1585), described a machine with a system involving a chain and metal buckets for raising water from the river in Alcazar. In 1698, a Cornish military engineer, **Thomas Savery** (1650–1715) of Devon, patented a steam engine for pumping water out of the mines.

Water Siphon   Its principle and construction was described by **Hero of Alexandria** (*c.*AD 100) in his treatise, *Pneumatics.*

Water Supply   The Cretan palace of Minos in 2000 BC had interior bathrooms fitted with a water supply. The first water-carrying tunnel, through a mountain in Greece, was built by a Greek architect, **Epalinus of Megara** in 503 BC. The first Roman aqueduct, bringing water from the springs, was built by **Appius Claudius Caecus** in 312 BC. The aqueduct at Pont du Gard at Nîmes, Provence, carrying water 155 feet above a valley, to the Roman city of Nemausus, was built by **Marcus Agrippa** (*c.* 63–12 BC) in 19 BC. **Sextus Julius Frontius** (*c.* AD 35–103), a water commissioner in the city of Rome in AD 97, left a manuscript, *De Aquis Urbis Romae*, which illustrated the water supply to the city during his time. The aqueduct at Carthage, Tunisia, was built by the Romans during the reign of Aelius Hadrianus (AD 117–138). A celebrated Roman architect, **Marcus Pollio Vitruvius**, who lived during the time of Julius Caesar and Augustus in the 1st century, was the first to point out the disadvantages in terms of health of using lead pipes for the water supply, and his work was first published in 1486. **Bernard Forest de Belidor** (1698–1761), a French pioneer in engineering, described various hydraulic mechanisms of use for dams in Europe in his *Architecture Hydraulique* (1737–1753). A French military engineer, **Sebastian le Prestre de Vauban** (1633–1707), designed two major aqueducts for the great Languedoc Canal, and the Maintenon aqueduct, which conveyed water from Eure to Versailles. An English engineer, **Sir William Edmund Garstin** (1849–1925), studied the hydrography of the River Nile in Egypt and designed the Aswan Dam. The longest water supply tunnel, the New York City West Delaware tunnel of 105 miles, was begun in 1937 and completed in 1944. *See canals, irrigation.*

Water Turbine The use of flow of water to turn a wheel was known to the ancients, and **Hero of Alexandria** constructed a steam turbine around AD 100. The first practical water turbine, which led to the development of hydroelectric schemes, was developed by a French engineer, **Benoit Fourneyron** (1802–1867). *See hydroelectric schemes.*

Waterclock An improvement on the primitive sundial as it did not rely on the sun. A preserved clepsydra or waterclock of the Egyptians during the reign of Amenhotep III (1397–1360 BC) exists. Its calendar depiction indicates that the instrument was known as early as 1540 BC. Around 245 BC **Ctesibius** of Alexandria constructed a device to measure the rate of flow of water through an aperture, and it was introduced into Rome around 157 BC. The simple waterclock of the Egyptians allowed water to escape from a hole in the bottom of a vessel at a fixed rate. The time was read from the sinking water level. An astronomical instrument maker, **Abu Ishaq al-Zalqali** (*c.* AD 1100) of Toledo, made astronomical and scientific instruments including a complex waterclock that showed the movements of the phases of the moon.

Waterframe A mechanical water-driven spinning mill, invented in 1771 by **Sir Richard Arkwright** (1732–1792) of Lancashire, in partnership with a hosier of Derby, **Jedediah Strutt** (1726–1797). It was the first water-powered machine that could produce cotton thread of good enough quality and strength to be used as a warp.

Waterglass Solidified glassy material consisting of sodium silicate, named in 1818, on the basis of its solubility in water, by a Bavarian chemist, **Johan Nepomuk von Fuchs** (1774–1856).

Waterhouse, Alfred (1830–1905) *See architecture, British.*

Waterson, John James (1811–1883) *See kinetic energy.*

Waterways *See canals.*

Waterwheels An important source of power before the invention of the steam engine. They were used in foundries, factories and sawmills. An English engineer, **John Smeaton** (1724–1792) from Austhorpe, conducted several experiments on the theory and functioning of waterwheels. The wood used in the construction of waterwheels started to be replaced by metal in 1830.

Watkin, Sir Edward (1819–1901) *See Channel tunnel.*

Watson, James Dewey (b 1928) *See deoxyribonucleic acid.*

Watson, Sir William (1715–1787) *See conductivity, velocity of electricity.*

Watson-Watt, Robert Alexander (1892–1973) *See radar.*

Watt SI unit (Système International d'Unités) of power, equal to one joule of energy expended in one second. Named after the Scottish mechanical engineer, **James Watt** (1736–1819) of Greenock.

Watt, James (1736–1819) Son of a joiner in Greenock, Scotland, who was apprenticed as an instrument maker and set up his business in Glasgow. During his duties as an instrument maker to Glasgow University he was called to repair Newcomen's steam engine, and in the process he improved the thermal efficiency of the machine by using a separate cylinder. Watt's original engine in 1765 is now exhibited in the Science Museum in London. Watt made further improvements to the steam engine by making it double acting in 1782. *See steam engine, watt.*

Watt, James (1769–1848) A marine engineer and son of **James Watt** (1736–1819). In 1817 he fitted a steam engine to the first English steamer, the *Caledonia*.

Wave Mechanics A special form of mechanics used in the theoretical study of wave-particles. *See matrix mechanics, quantum theory, Schrödinger equation.*

Wave Theory of Light *See light, quantum theory.*

Weapons *See catapult, firearms, military engineering, torpedo.*

Weather Forecast Attempts to forecast weather have been made since ancient times. The Greek naturalist and philosopher, **Theophrastus** (380–287 BC), wrote on the nature and directions of winds, and their use as weather signs. The invention of the barometer by **Evangelista Torricelli** (1608–1647) became a landmark in the field. **James Pollard Espy** (1785–1860) of Pennsylvania, who joined the Washington Observatory in 1843, laid the basis for the Weather Bureau in America. The meteorologist and commander of the ship, *Beagle*, **Robert Fitzroy** (1805–1865), was a pioneer in making weather charts and he started producing the first weather forecasts for the press. A telegraphic system for weather reporting was devised by an American physicist, **Joseph Henry** (1797–1878) at the Smithsonian Institution. A Dutch meteorologist, **Christoph Hendrik Diederik Buys Ballot** (1817–1890), founded the Royal Netherlands Meteorological Institute in 1854, and organized the first weather forecast and storm warnings in 1860. A London meteorologist, **George James Symons** (1838–1900), was instrumental in expanding the number of rainfall-reporting stations in England from 168 to 3500. **Sir William Napier Shaw** (1854–1945), the first professor of meteorology at the Imperial College, London, was instrumental in reorganizing the British Weather Service. A Norwegian-born American meteorologist, **Jacob Aall Bonnevie Bjerknes** (1897–1975), formulated a theory on the cyclone and published *On the Structure of Moving Cyclones* (1919). Modern weather forecasting is based on his work. His father **Wilhelm Firman Koren Bjerknes** (1862–1961) was also a pioneer in weather forecasting. **Lewis Fry Richardson** (1881–1953) of Newcastle upon Tyne, in Britain, made attempts to calculate weather with the help of some fundamental equations that he derived, but was unsuccessful. He published *Weather Prediction by Numerical Process* in 1922. Large-scale wave-like motions in the upper atmosphere (Rossby waves) of considerable reliability in weather forecasting were discovered by a Swedish-born US meteorologist, **Carl Gustav Arvid Rossby** (1898–1957). An American meteorologist, **Jerome Namias** (b 1910) of Bridgeport, Connecticut, discovered that these waves could be used for forecasting up to five days ahead. An English climatologist, **Hubert Horace Lamb** (b 1913) of Bedford, produced weather forecasts for transatlantic flights during World War II. He also produced daily weather classifications for Britain. Numerical weather prediction in America was developed by a New York meteorologist, **Joseph Smagorinsky** (b 1924). A German-born US climatologist, **Helmut Eric Landberg** (1906–1985), who was director of the Climatology Weather Bureau (1954–1965) and president of the World Meteorological Organization for Climatology (1969–1978), organized the first numerical weather prediction efforts. Meteorologists were able to observe and predict huge hurricanes for the first time through the American weather satellite *Tiros 7* launched in 1963. *See climatology, meteorology.*

Weather *See clouds, cyclone, meteorology, storms, weather forecast, wind.*

Weaving Mats and baskets were some of the first weaved products in Mesopotamia as early as 3000 BC. The Egyptians knew the art of weaving cloth and used the loom around 1200 BC. The Chinese invented a draw-loom around 300 BC. The loom was introduced in to Europe around AD 400. The ribbon-loom was invented in Holland in 1620, and came into use in England and the rest of Europe over the next century. In 1744 **Jacques de Vaucanson** (1709–1782) of Grenoble, France attempted to mechanize weaving. Thomas Barber in England made significant improvements to the loom in 1774. *See textile industry.*

Weber Unit An SI unit of magnetic flux density, named after the German physicist and professor of physics at Göttingen, **Wilhelm Eduard Weber** (1804–1891) from Wittenberg. He was the first to demonstrate that electricity consists of charged particles, and devised several instruments for measuring electricity and magnetism.

Weber, Ernst Heinrich (1795–1878) *See acoustics.*

Weber, Wilhelm Eduard (1804–1891) *See acoustics, bifilar magnetometer, electrical resistance, magnetic theory, tangent galvanometer, weber unit.*

Wedderburn Theorem The first Wedderburn theorem, relating to finite division algebra was proposed by a Scottish mathematician, **Joseph Henry Wedderburn** (1882–1948) from Forfar in his paper *On Hyper-Complex Numbers* (1907). His second theorem relates to semi-simple algebra and the finite number of elements.

Wedderburn, Joseph Henry (1882–1948) *See Wedderburn theorem.*

Wedgwood, Josiah (1730–1795) An English potter from a long established family of potters in Burslem, Stafforshire. He set up his own factory at Burslem in 1759. He developed the technique of green glazing and a new type of cream ware. He created jasper, a fine stone ware used for portraits and other intricate art work, and described a pyrometer for measuring high temperatures in furnaces.

Wegener, Alfred Lothar (1880–1930) *See tectonic theory.*

Wegener Theory *See tectonic theory.*

Weierstrass, Karl (1815–1897) A German professor of mathematics in Berlin who is known for his original work on the theory of functions. He published *Abhandlungen aus der Funktionlehre* (1886), and showed that every continuous function could be uniformly approximated by polynomials.

Weighing *See units and measures.*

Weighbridge The invention of the weighbridge did away with the need for large beam scales in steelyards and industry. John Wyatt in England used the principle of gearing forces to build a weighbridge in 1741. A Strasbourg mechanic, Alois Quintenz, developed the principle and took out a patent in 1822.

Weights and Measures The carat (Greek: *keration,* horn-like pods) for measurement of diamonds and gold was originally obtained from the average weight of the seeds of the carob, a native tree of Africa and the southern Mediterranean. The French Académie in the 18th century decided that the unit of weight should be represented by the weight of a cubic decimeter of distilled water in a vacuum at the temperature of melting ice. Attempts to measure this accurately were made by **René Just Haüy** (1743–1822) and **Antoine Lavoisier** (1743–1794). Giovanni Fabrino Valentino Fabroni repeated their experiments in 1799. The kilogram was established as an official unit by the Bureau of Weights and Measures at the Pavilion de Bretail near Paris in 1875. The English carat was fixed at 3.1683 grains by the Board of Trade in 1888 and was replaced by the metric carat in 1914. *See units and measures.*

Weil, André (1906–1998) *See Bourbaki group.*

Weinberg, Steven (b 1933) *See quantum chromodynamics.*

Weismann, August Friedrich Leopold (1834–1914) *See cell division, chromosomes, gamete, meiosis.*

Weizmann, Chaim (1874–1952) A Russian-born Jewish-German industrial chemist who, in 1912, discovered a bacteriological method of producing acetone. He became the first president of the new state of Israel in 1948.

Weizsäcker, Baron Carl Friedrich von (b 1912) *See cosmology, solar system, thermonuclear fusion.*

Weldon Process An improved process for soda manufacture, in which the expensive manganese is recycled. Invented in 1866 by an English industrial chemist, **Walter Weldon** (1832–1885) of Leicestershire.

Weldon, Walter (1832–1885) *See Weldon process.*

Wells, Herbert George (1866–1946) An English pioneer of science fiction from Bromley, Kent, popularly known as H.G. Wells, who studied biology under **Thomas Henry Huxley** (1825–1895). He published *The Time Machine* (1895), *The War of the Worlds* (1898) and several other science fiction novels.

Welsbach Mantle *See lamp .*

Welsbach, Carl Auer von (1858–1929) *See lamp, neodymium, praseodymium.*

Wenner-Green, Axel Leonard (1881–1961) *See monorail, vacuum cleaner.*

Wenzel, Carl Friedrich (1740–1793) *See law of mass action.*

Werner, Abraham Gottlob (1749–1817) *See petrology, stratigraphy.*

Werner, Alfred (1866–1919) *See affinity, bonds, isomerism, stereochemistry.*

Wesson, Daniel Baird (1825–1906) *See firearms.*

Westinghouse, George (1846–1914) *See air brake, alternating current, railway signals.*

Weston, Sir Richard (1591–1672) *See agronomy.*

Weyl, Hermann (1885–1955) *See quantum mechanics.*

Wheatstone Bridge A device for making accurate measurements of electrical resistance. It consists of a circuit that is divided into sections, enabling the relative resistances placed in the sections to be deduced. It was popularized in 1843 by an English physicist, **Sir Charles Wheatstone** (1801–1875) of Gloucester.

Wheatstone, Sir Charles (1801–1875) A physicist from Gloucester who was appointed as professor of philosophy at King's College in 1834. He invented a sound magnifier for which he coined the term microphone. *See chronoscope, dynamo, electric telegraphy, microphone, stereoscope, velocity of electricity, velocity of light, Wheatstone bridge.*

Wheel Neolithic man used rounded stones to move heavy stones for construction of megalithic structures. The next wheel to be invented was probably a potter's wheel. Four-wheeled carts were in use in Sumeria around 3500 BC. Wheels were used on a chariot in Mesopotamia around 3000 BC. A simple machine with a grooved wheel to lift heavy objects, the pulley, was developed by **Archytas of Tarentum** (Italy) around 410 BC.

Wheeler, Fred Lawrence (b 1906) *See micrometeorite, solar system.*

Wheeler, John Archibald (b 1911) *See atomic bomb, black hole.*

Whewell, William (1794–1866) *See Bridgewater treatises, British Association for the Advancement of Science, catastrophism, scientist.*

Whinfield, John Rex (1901–1966) *See polymer, textile chemistry.*

Whipple, Fred Lawrence (b 1906) *See comet.*

White, Canvass (1790–1834) *See canals, cement.*

White, Gilbert (1720–1793) *See ecology.*

Whitehead, Alfred North (1861–1947) *See mathematical logic.*

Whitehead, Robert (1823–1905) *See torpedo.*

Whitehurst, John (1713–1788) *See geology.*

Whitman, Charles Otis (1842–1910) *See ethology.*

Whitney, Eli (1765–1825) *See textile industry.*

Whitney, Josiah Dwight (1819–1896) *See gold.*

Whitney, William Dwight (1827–1894) *See philology.*

Whittaker, Sir Edmund Taylor (1873–1956) An English mathematician and science historian from Lancashire, who published *History of the Theories of Aether and Electricity* (1910), *A Treatise on the Analytical Particles and Rigid Bodies* (1904) and several other books.

Whittle, Frank (1907–1996) *See jet engine.*

Whitworth Screw The present standard screw thread was devised by an English engineer from Stockport, Cheshire, **Sir Joseph Whitworth** (1803–1887). He invented several devices including a screw-measuring machine, screw-cutting lathe, screw dies and tap, and a gun of compressed steel. Before his invention a screw-thread measurement of only 1/16 of an inch was possible, and he improved it to 1/10 000 of an inch in 1840. He founded the Whitworth Scholarship for the promotion of engineering.

Whitworth, Sir Joseph (1803–1887) *See Whitworth screw.*

Wiedemann, G. (1826–1899) *See conductivity.*

Wien, Wilhelm Carl Werner Otto Fritz Franz (1864–1928) *See black body radiation.*

Wiener, Christian (1826–1896) *See Brownian movement.*

Wiener, Nobert (1894–1964) *See automation, cybernetics.*

Wiesel, Torsten Nils (b 1924) *See vision.*

Wigglesworth, Vincent Brian (1899–1994) *See entpomology.*

Wigner Theorem Relates to the conservation of the angular momentum of electron spin. Proposed by a Hungarian-born US physicist, **Eugene Paul Wigner** (1902–1995) who was professor of mathematics at Princeton University from 1938 to 1971. His calculations were used by **Enrico Fermi** (1901–1954) for the construction of the first nuclear reactor in Chicago.

Wigner, Eugene Paul (1902–1995) *See atomic nucleus, Wigner theorem.*

Wilcke, Johan Carl (1732–1796) *See latent heat, specific heat.*

Wiles, Andrew (b 1953) *See Fermat's last theorem.*

Wilkes, Maurice Vincent (b 1913) *See computers, RAM.*

Wilkins, John (1614–1672) *See extraterrestrial life, Royal Society of London, science fiction.*

Wilkins, Maurice Hugh Fredrick (b 1916) *See deoxyribonucleic acid.*

Wilkinson, Geoffrey (1921–1996) An English organic chemist from Todmorden, Yorkshire, who researched on inorganic compounds and their use as catalysts. He shared the Nobel Prize for chemistry in 1973, with **Ernst Otto Fischer** (b 1918).

Wilkinson, John (1728–1808) *See blast furnace, lathe, machine tools.*

William of Moerbeke (c. 1215–1286) A translator of Greek works into Latin in the 13th century. The first printed works of Archimedes, in 1503, at Venice, were based on his translation.

William of Ockham (1300–1349) *See Ockham's razor.*

Williams, Ged (1690–1749) *See typography.*

Williams, Robley Cook (b 1908) A biophysicist from Santa Rosa, California, who improved the electron microscopy techniques for viewing viruses and other biological material.

Williams, Sir Frederic Calland (1911–1977) *See computers, RAM.*

Williamson, Alexander William (1824–1904) *See catalysis.*

Williamson, William Crawford (1816–1895) *See paleophytology.*

Willstätter, Richard (1872–1942) *See acidity, chlorophyll, photosynthesis.*

Wilson, Alexander (1766–1813) *See ornithology.*

Wilson, Allan Charles (1934–1991) *See molecular clock.*

Wilson, Charles Thompson Rees (1869–1959) *See alpha particles, cloud chamber, Compton effect, cosmic rays, electric charge, positron.*

Wilson, Sir Daniel (1816–1892) *See prehistory.*

Wilson, Edward Osborne (b 1929) *See entomology.*

Wilson, Horace Hayman (1786–1860) *See philology.*

Wilson, Kenneth Geddes (b 1936) A theoretical physicist from Waltham, Massachusetts, who was awarded the Nobel Prize for physics in 1982, for his theory of critical phenomena in relation to phase transitions. His work explained the behavior of substances under different pressure and temperature.

Wilson, Robert Woodrow (b 1936) *See background radiation, Big Bang theory, cosmic rays, helium, radioastronomy.*

Wind The Greek naturalist and philosopher, **Theophrastus** (373–287 BC), wrote on the nature and directions of winds, and their use as weather signs. The first map of the winds on earth's surface was published by **Edmund Halley** (1656–1742) in 1686. The English philosopher and scientist **George Hadley** (1685–1768) studied the northerly and southerly winds in relation to the earth's rotation and published on meteorology from 1731 to 1735. One of the earliest English treatises on hurricanes and wind entitled *A Discourse concerning the Origine and the Properties of Wind* was published by Ralph Bohun in 1671. **William Dampier** (1652–1751), an English navigator from Yeovil, wrote a classic work on meteorology entitled *Discourse on Winds*. The Beaufort scale, used for classification and description of wind force, was first proposed in 1805 by **Francis Beaufort** (1774–1857). It was revised and improved in 1921 by an English meteorologist from Derby, **Sir George Clark Simpson** (1878–1965). The anemometer, an instrument used for measuring the velocity of wind, was invented in 1846 by an Irish astronomer, **John Thomas Romney Robinson** (1792–1882) of Dublin. A Norwegian explorer and oceanographer, **Fridtjof Nansen** (1861–1930), explained the wind-driven sea currents and designed several oceanographic instruments. **Sir William Napier Shaw** (1854– 1945), the first professor of Meteorology at the Imperial College, London, wrote *Life-History of Surface Air Currents,* and was instrumental in reorganizing the British Weather Service.

Windmill The earliest known were built in Persia around AD 600. They consisted of a vertical shaft and horizontal sails and were used for grinding corn. The early windmills were called postmills as the sails and gears were fixed to a central post. The tower mill followed, around 1200. The earliest in England, at Weedley, Humberside, is dated at 1185. The oldest working windmill in England, at Outwood, near Redhill, Surrey, was built in 1665. The Netherlands' largest, Dijkpolder, at Maasland, was built in 1718. In 1750, a Scottish millwright, **Andrew Meikle** (1719–1811), invented shutters that could be operated without the sails having to be climbed. Metal started to be used for the building of windmills in the latter part of the 18th century. An English engineer, **John Smeaton** (1724–1792) from Austhorpe, and **Charles Augustus Coulomb** (1736–1806), built several experimental windmills that could use various shapes of sail. Steam power started to replace windmills around 1840.

Windscreen Wipers For use in automobiles, these were first introduced in America in 1916.

Wine According to Greek mythology, it is supposed to have been discovered by the god Dionysus. He learnt the method of making it during his extensive travels into Asia, Syria, Egypt and other countries, and introduced it into Greece. **Pliny the Elder** (AD 28–79) described 116 different types of wine around AD 50. The Greek historian and philosopher **Plutarch** (AD 46–120) mentioned wine as the most palatable table medicine. The largest quantity of wine brought into Greece came from the Aegean islands of Cos, Delos, Samos and Lesbos.

Wing, Vincent (1619–1668) *See surveying.*

Winkler, Clemens Alexander (1838–1904) *See germanium.*

Winthrop, John (1714–1779) *See Mercury (planet).*

Winzer, Frederick Albert (1763–1830) *See gas lighting.*

Wireless Telegraphy The earliest treatise on the subject, entitled *Telegraphy without Wires,* was presented in 1859 to the British Association by James Bowman Lindsay of Dundee, Scotland. His initial experiments in 1853 involved the use of water to conduct electricity. In 1866 an American, **Mahlon Loomis** (1826–1886), observed a potential difference between two kites, which were 14 miles apart, and obtained a patent for telegraphy without wires in 1872. **James Clerk Maxwell** (1831–1879) first noted electromagnetic waves in 1865, and suggested that they could be used for wireless telegraphy. A Welsh electrical engineer, **Sir William Henry Preece** (1834–1913), sent and received current between two points, a quarter of a mile apart, and published *Telegraphy* (1876) and *A Manual of Telephony* (1893). **Heinrich Rudolf Hertz** (1857–1894) of Bonn was the first person to observe radio waves, and in 1888 he demonstrated that these electromagnetic waves could be generated from one point and received at another point. In 1897 a Russian physicist, **Alexander Stepanovich Popov** (1859–1905), first used a suspended wire as an aerial during his experiments on wireless telegraphy and transmitted signals over a distance of 5 km with the help of his antenna. The first wireless telegraphic station in the world was set up at Alum Bay on the Isle of Wight in the same year, and it handled its first paid message in 1898. Wireless telegraphy was made possible with the invention of a coherer in 1890 by professor **Edouard Eugène Désiré Branly** (1844–1940) of the Catholic University in Paris. **Sir Oliver Joseph Lodge** (1851–1940), the first professor of physics at Liverpool, theoretically applied the coherer to the production of wireless telegraphy, and demonstrated that messages could be sent and received without wires, to the British Royal Society in 1894. The first paper on wireless telegraphy, *La telegrafia senza fila* (1903) was written by an Italian physicist, **Augusto Righi** (1850–1920) of Bologna and **B. Dessau**. A Hindu professor from Calcutta, Jagadis Chander Bose, was one of the first to demonstrate the process of wireless telegraphy. In 1892 **Nathan B. Stubblefield** (d 1923) gave a public demonstration of wireless transmission of speech at the town square in Murray, Kentucky. The Italian physicist, **Guglielmo Marchese Marconi** (1874–1937) of Bologna, improved Branly's coherer and used it for wireless telegraphy for the first time in 1896, over a practical distance of a few miles. He obtained a patent for his invention in the same year. The first transoceanic wireless telegraph was sent from Cornwall to Nova Scotia by Marconi on 12 December 1901. He shared the Nobel Prize for physics in 1909, for his work on wireless telegraphy, with **Karl Ferdinand Braun** (1850–1918). The first successful radio signal between England and Australia was sent from Marconi's transmitter from Caernarvon, North Wales, and received at Sydney by a radio engineer, **Ernest Thomas Fisk** (1886–1965) from Sunbury-on-Thames, in England. He made the first human voice contact between the two countries when he spoke to Marconi in 1924. *See coherer.*

Wislicenus, Johannes Adolf (1835–1902) *See isomerism.*

Witelo (*c.* 1250–1275) *See vision.*

Witten, Edward (b 1952) *See superstring theory.*

Wittig Synthesis A method of synthesizing olefins or alkenes. Devised by a German chemist, **Georg Wittig**

(1897–1987) of Berlin, who shared the Nobel Prize for chemistry in 1979, for his invention, with a London-born US chemist, **Herbert Charles Brown** (b 1912).

Wittig, Georg (1897–1987) *See Wittig synthesis.*

Wiveleslie, Sir William de (1844–1920) *See celestial photography, photography.*

Wöhler, Friedrich (1800–1882) *See acetylene, aluminum, beryllium, chemistry, organic chemistry, urea.*

Wolf Diagram A method for detecting interstellar dust by star counting. Invented by **Maximilian Franz Joseph Cornelius Wolf** (1863–1932) who became professor of astronomy at Heidelberg in 1893.

Wolf, Christian von (1679–1754) A German philosopher and mathematician from Breslau, Silesia. He was a pupil of **Gottfried Wilhelm Leibniz** (1646–1716) whose philosophy he popularized in his *Philosophia prima sive ontologia* (1729). He became professor of mathematics at Halle in 1707.

Wolf, Emil (b 1922) *See quantum optics.*

Wolf, Maximilian Franz Joseph Cornelius (1863–1932) *See celestial photography, Wolf diagram.*

Wolgemut, Michael (1435–1519) *See engraving.*

Wollaston, William Hyde (1766–1822) A British physician who devoted his time to chemistry. The dark bands in the spectrum of sunlight, later identified as ultraviolet rays, were first observed by him in 1802. He discovered the metallic element, palladium in 1803, and in 1804 identified a rare metal rhodium, in platinum ore. In 1807 he first used a camera lucida to project distant landscapes onto paper, in order to trace their outline. *See absorption spectra, astrophysics, Bunsen, Robert, camera lucida, hypsometer, palladium, rhodium, ultraviolet rays.*

Wollman, Elie Léo (b 1917) *See genetic engineering.*

Wood Engraving The first attempt at printing in Europe, by taking impressions from woodcuts, was for the purpose of making playing cards for the amusement of Charles VI of France in the 14th century. One of the earliest specimens of wood-engraving, a representation of St Christopher by an unknown artist and dated 1423, was discovered in a German convent, Chartreuse of Buxheim, near Augsburg. This method was superseded by metal engraving in the 18th century.

Wood, Robert Williams (1868–1955) An American physicist from Concord, Massachusetts, who served as professor

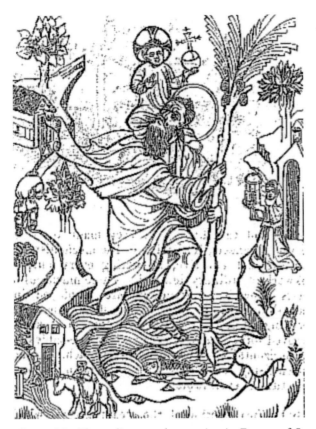

Figure 86 The earliest wood engraving in Europe of St Christopher in 1423. Partington, F. Charles. *The British Encyclopaedia of Arts and Sciences*. London: Orr & Smith, 1835

of experimental physics (1901–1938) at Johns Hopkins University. He obtained photographs of sound waves reflected from various surfaces and published *Physical Optics* (1905). *See optical pumping.*

Woodward, Arthur Smith (1864–1944) An English geologist from Macclesfield who served as the keeper of geology at the British Museum from 1901 to 1924. He published *Outlines of Vertebrate Palaeontology* (1898). *See Piltdown Man.*

Woodward, John (1665–1728) *See geogeny, geology, transpiration.*

Woodward, Robert Burns (1917–1979) *See chlorophyll.*

Woolley, Sir Leonard Charles (1880–1960) *See Ur.*

Woolley, Sir Richard van der Riet (1906–1986) *See eclipse.*

Wotton, Edward (1492–1555) *See zoology.*

Woulfe, Peter (1727–1803) *See explosives, picric acid.*

Wren, Sir Christopher (1632–1723) An English architect, astronomer and scientist, born in East Knoyle, Wiltshire. He was one of the original members of the Invisible College at Oxford, which later became the Royal Society, and Savillian professor of astronomy at Oxford. He designed the Greenwich Observatory, the new St Paul's Cathedral (1675–1710) and many other important buildings. Wren also constructed the first rain gauge for measuring rainfall in 1662, and served as the president of the Royal Society from 1680 to 1683. *See impact, Royal Society of London.*

Wright, Benjamin (1770–1842) *See canals.*

Wright, Frank Lloyd (1867–1959) *See architecture, American.*

Wright, Orville (1871–1948) *See aerodynamics, airplane.*

Wright, Sewall (1889–1988) *See animal husbandry.*

Wright, Thomas (1711–1786) *See cosmology.*

Wright, Wilbur (1861–1912) *See aerodynamics, airplane.*

Wrist Watch *See watches.*

Writing The use of symbols in a logical sequence for the purpose of expression. The earliest written language dating back to 5000 BC was found on Chinese pottery in the Shensi province of China in 1962. An early form of pictograph writing on clay tablets, consisting of 2000 pictures resembling arrowheads and symbols, known as cuneiform writing, was in use in Erech, Sumeria around 3500 BC. This was developed in Egypt into hieroglyphics with each picture representing an object. The Egyptians wrote on stone before they started using papyrus around 2600 BC. Thousands of clay tablets related to Assyrian culture were found in the remains of the royal library of the king of Assyria, Ashurbanipul (668–626 BC) at Nineveh in the late 19th century, and deciphered by Campbell Thompson in 1906. The use of symbols to represent sounds rather than objects, by the cuneiform writers, led to the more advanced system of phonetic writing. The Phoenicians used a 22-letter alphabet around 1700 BC, from which the Greeks developed their 24-letter alphabet. The oldest surviving printed writing from wooden blocks, dating to around AD 700, was found in 1966 at the Pulguk Sa Pagoda, in South Korea. The earliest known extant writing in the British Isles is a fragment of Irish ecclesiastical history, dating back to AD 630. *See hieroglyphics.*

Writing Devices The reed was the earliest writing device, used by the Egyptians and the Persians. The ancient Egyptians used a holder for their brushes, to write on sheets of papyrus, and a palette for their ink. **Philo** of Byzantinium (*c.* 200 BC) described an ingenious ink stand, which, regardless of its position, presented an opening on its upper face to receive the pen. The ancient Chinese used cochineal insects for ink, and by AD 300 they had developed ink from lamp-black and soluble gums. Quills were introduced around the 5th century and continued to be used for over 1000 years. Metal pens came into use in the late 18th century. The pencil was invented in 1792 by J.N. Conté of France. The early 19th century saw a rapid development of the pen industry, with nibs made of osmium, gold, iridium and steel. The annual production of pens was estimated to be over 220 million in the mid 19th century. A device with a continuous flow of ink for writing was patented in 1884 by Lewis E. Waterman. The Biro or ballpoint pen was invented by a Hungarian journalist, Laszlo Biro, during his search for a quick-drying ink, while he was in Argentina after escaping from the Nazis in 1938. It was patented in Argentina and sold in Buenos Aires in 1945. *See pen.*

Writing Machine　*See typewriter.*

Writing Materials　Clay provided the earliest source for permanent writing. The Sumerians, around 3500 BC, wrote on moist clay with a reed or piece of wood, and allowed it to dry in the sun. This provided a most effective way of preserving their work, some of which is still extant. Their method was subsequently copied by the Babylonians and Assyrians. Thousands of clay tablets related to Assyrian culture were found in the remains of the royal library of the king of Assyria, Ashurbanipul (668–626 BC) at Nineveh in the late 19th century. Writing on stone was more difficult and laborious and that method was mainly used in temples, monuments and tombstones. The Egyptians made sheets of papyrus for writing by cutting lengthwise sections of the

reed-like papyrus plant and joining them in two layers. The library at Pergamum in Asia Minor, established around 200 BC, had to resort to a different writing material, parchment, since Ptolemy V around 190 BC blocked the supply of papyrus from Egypt to this rival library established by King Eumenes II of Pergamum. Parchment, or *charta pergamena*, was made from the skin of animals such as goats, sheep and pigs, and the finest parchment was known as vellum. *See paper.*

Wroblewski, Zygmunt Florenty von (1845–1888)　*See nitrogen.*

Wu, Chien Shiung (1912–1997)　*See parity.*

Wurtz Reaction　The synthesis of hydrocarbons by reacting alkyl halides with sodium, invented by a French chemist, **Charles Adolphe Wurtz** (1817–1884). He became professor of chemistry at the Sorbonne in 1857, and published *Atomic theory* (1880) and *Modern Chemistry*.

Wurtz, Charles Adolphe (1817–1884)　*See bonds, glycol, Wurtz reaction.*

Wyatt, Benjamin Dean (1775–1850)　*See architecture, British.*

Wyatt, James (1746–1813)　*See architecture, British.*

Wyckoff, Ralph Walter Graystone (1897–1994)　A US biochemist who developed the ultracentrifugation technique for the purification and study of viruses. He became professor of microbiology at the University of Arizona in 1959 and worked with **Robley Cook Williams** (b 1908) to improve imaging methods in electron microscopy.

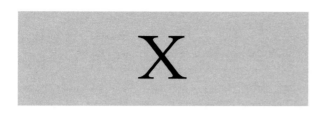

Xanthus Ancient capital of Lycia, discovered in 1838 by an English archaeologist, **Sir Charles Fellows** (1799–1860).

Xenocrates (395–314 BC) A Greek philosopher of Chalcedon who succeeded his teacher **Plato** (428–348 BC) at the academy.

Xenon [Greek: *xenos,* stranger] An inert gas was discovered by two London chemists, **Sir William Ramsay** (1852–1916) and **Morris William Travers** (1872–1961) in 1898. Its first chemical compound, xenon fluoroplatinate, was obtained in 1962 by a British chemist **Neil Bartlett** (b 1932) from Newcastle upon Tyne, who became professor of chemistry at Princeton University, New Jersey, in 1966.

Xenophanes of Colophon (*c.* 560–478 BC) A Greek philosopher who was exiled from Ionia. He brought philosophy to Elea and founded the Eleatic school. He considered earth to be the fundamental material, and made the first observations on fossils. *See fossils, tectonic theory.*

Xenophon (450–360 BC) An Athenian philosopher and disciple of Socrates. Some of his writings on history are extant.

Xerography [Greek: *xerox*; dry + *graphein*, to write] A copying process that electrically shuffles fine powder to form the printing image, and fuses it in place by heat. It was invented in 1938 by **Chester Floyd Carlson** (1906–1968) of Seattle, Washington, who patented it in 1940. He established the Xerox Corporation, through which he marketed his product on an international basis.

Xerox Copier [Greek: *xeros,* dry] The first mechanical copier was developed in 1844 by a German-born British engineer, **Karl Wilhelm Siemens**, later **Sir Charles William Siemens** (1823–1883). The modern copying process, using electroconductivity, was invented in 1938 by **Chester Floyd Carlson** (1906–1968) of Seattle, Washington. After being refused a patent by 20 companies he formed an agreement with a small company Haloid in 1947, and developed it into the Xerox Corporation. The first commercial Xerox copier (Xerox 914) came into use in 1959.

Xerox Printing [Greek: *xeros,* dry] See *xerography.*

X-Ray Astronomy A New York physicist, **Herbert Friedman** (b 1916), pioneered the use of detectors in rockets to study the X-rays in space. The first extrasolar source of X-rays was discovered by an Italian-born US astrophysicist, **Ricardo Giaconni** (b 1931) and his team in 1962. He also discovered the extragalactic background radiation and built the first orbiting X-ray detector. *See radioastronomy.*

X-Ray Crystallography The X-rays discovered in 1895 by the German physicist **Wilhelm Konrad von Röntgen** (1845–1923) of Würzberg, were proved to be a form of radiation in 1911, by a German physicist at Zurich, **Max Theodor Felix von Laue** (1879–1960). His work showed that crystals could be split up by the X-rays into a regular pattern of spots. His findings were explained and followed up by **Sir William Bragg** (1862–1942) and his Australian-born son **Sir Lawrence Bragg** (1890–1971), who used the X-rays to discover the positions of the layers of atoms in various crystals. They constructed the first X-ray spectrometer and established X-ray crystallography, which proved to be of immense value in research to many branches of science. Powdered crystals in X-ray crystallography were first used in 1916 by **Peter Joseph Wilhelm Debye** (1884–1966) of Maastricht, the Netherlands. He was awarded the Nobel Prize for chemistry in 1936, for his work on dipole moments and molecular structure. In 1929 **Dame Kathleen Lonsdale** (1903–1971), an Irish crystallographer at University College, London, used the method to elucidate the structure of hexamethylbenzene and hexachlorobenzene. Two New York physical chemists, **Herbert Aaron Hauptman** (b 1917) and **Jerome Karle** (b 1918) invented a direct method for interpreting measurements and data in X-ray crystallography, for which they shared the Nobel Prize for chemistry in 1985. X-ray diffraction photography of DNA molecules was first carried out around 1952 by **Elsie Rosalind Franklin** (1920–1958) of King's College, London.

X-Ray Diffraction A method of determining the structure of molecules or organic crystals, by the way in which they diffract a beam of X-rays. It is achieved by projecting X-rays at a small angle of incidence, to bring about diffraction at very short wavelengths. *See X-ray crystallography.*

X-Ray Spectroscopy A method that allows separation of X-rays and measurement of their different wavelengths. Developed by a Swedish physicist, **Karl Manne Georg Siegbahn** (1886–1978), director of the Nobel Institute for physics in Stockholm. He showed that X-rays could be diffracted with a prism as could light. He was awarded the Nobel Prize for physics in 1924, for his work on X-ray spectroscopy and for the discovery of the M series of the spectrum. An English physicist, **Henry Gwynn Jeffreys Moseley** (1887–1915) from Weymouth, introduced the method for determining the X-ray spectra of elements.

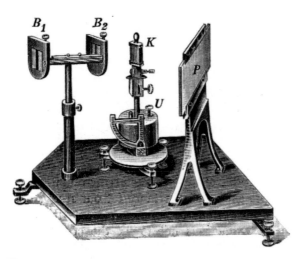

Figure 87 Siegbahn's apparatus for X-ray spectroscopy. Graetz, Leo. *Recent Developments in Atomic Theory.* London: Methuen & Co, 1923

X-Rays An induction coil for producing electricity was built in 1855 by a German physicist, **Heinrich Daniel Ruhmkorff** (1803–1877) of Hanover. In 1858, a German physicist, **Julius Pflucker** (1801–1868), used the induction coil to demonstrate that when electricity was passed through two metal electrodes, which were sealed at the end of a glass tube under reduced pressure, it produced sparks and underwent a series of changes. This phenomenon was exploited by **Heinrich Geissler** (1814–1879), a glass blower from Thuringia, for making tubes of various designs which lit up when electrically excited. On reducing the pressure, a number of dark spaces appeared around the electrodes. In 1869 a German physicist, **Johann Wilhelm Hittorf** (1824–1914), demonstrated that these dark spaces near the cathode were really a form of ray. These rays, known as cathode rays, were investigated in 1872 by **Sir William Crookes** (1832–1919), using a high-vacuum tube. He demonstrated that the fluorescence produced in the glass tube was due to the electrons striking its walls. The nature of these particles were further studied and explained in 1897 by **Joseph John Thompson** (1856–1940). Professor **Wilhelm Conrad Röntgen** (1845–1923) of Würzberg used the Crookes tube and found that the cathode rays, when brought into focus and allowed to impinge on a plate of dense metal, produced rays that could pass through the glass tube and affect a photographic plate, also rendering certain substances fluorescent. Röntgen announced his discovery under the name X-rays in 1895. **Charles Glover Barkla** (1877–1944), professor of physics at King's College London, established that the X-rays were of the same nature as light, but were shorter in wavelength. A German physicist, **Max Theodor Felix von Laue** (1879–1960), proved that the X-rays were a form of electromagnetic radiation, for which he was awarded the Nobel Prize for physics in 1914. The first diagnostic X-ray photograph in America was taken in 1896 by a Hungarian-born US physicist, **Michael Idvorsky Pupin** (1858–1935) of Columbia University, New York. The prototype of the modern X-ray vacuum tube (Coolridge tube) was invented in 1916 by an American physicist, **William David Coolridge** (1873–1975).

Xyloengraving *See wood engraving.*

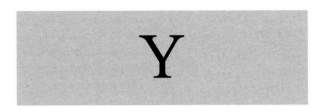

Yale, Linus (1821–1868) *See lock.*

Yang, Chen Ning (b 1922) *See parity.*

Yard A term used during ancient times to denote the distance from the tip of the nose to the end of the fingers when the right arm was outstretched. It was adopted as a measure of length in England by King Henry I. The modern yard is defined on the basis of the length of a pendulum with a period of one second, placed at the Greenwich Observatory, by a Royal decree in England in 1824. It was redefined as 0.9144 meters by the Weights and Measures Act of 1963.

Yarrell, William (1784–1856) *See ichthyology.*

Yeager, Charles Elwood (b 1923) *See supersonic flight.*

Year *See month.*

Yeast *See fermentology.*

Yerkes, Charles Tyson (1837–1905) *See Yerkes Observatory.*

Yerkes Observatory Presented in 1892 by an American railway magnate, **Charles Tyson Yerkes** (1837–1905) of Philadelphia, to the University of Chicago.

Young, Arthur (1741–1820) *See agriculture.*

Young, Charles Augustus (1834–1908) An American astronomer from Hanover, New Hampshire and one of the first to make spectroscopic investigations of the Sun. He was also the first person to observe the spectrum of the solar corona. He published *General Astronomy* (1888), *Lessons in Astronomy* (1891) and *Manual of Astronomy* (1902).

Young, James (1822–1883) The founder of the shale-oil industry in Scotland. In 1848 he established an oil refinery for using the oil from a coal mine in Derbyshire. He discovered a method of producing paraffin oil from shale, and established a factory for this purpose in West Lothian in 1856, which became a great commercial success. He founded the chair of technical chemistry at Anderson College in 1869.

Young, Matthew (1750–1800) An Irish mathematician and clergyman educated at Trinity College, Dublin, where he became professor of philosophy in 1786. He published *Analysis of the Principles of Natural Philosophy* and *The Method of Prime and Ultimate Ratios.*

Young, Thomas (1773–1829) *See contact lenses, energy, ether, heat, interference, light, quantum theory, relativity.*

Yttrium Silver-grey, metallic element with an atomic number of 39. It was first noted in a black mineral found in the quarry at a small town called Ytterby, by a Swedish mineralogist, Arrhenius, who named it yttrite in 1788. In 1804, a Finnish mineralogist, **Johan Gadolin** (1760–1852) of Helsinki, isolated the oxide of yttrium (gadolinite). In 1843 it was isolated in a pure state (ytterbium) by a Swedish chemist, **Carl Gustav Mosander** (1797–1858). Another Swiss chemist **Jean Charles Gallisard de Marignac** (1817–1894) isolated in 1878.

Yukawa, Hideki (1907–1981) *See meson.*

Yunus, Abul Hasan ibn (c. AD 950–1020) *See zij.*

Z

Zabaglia, Nicholas (1674–1750) An Italian architect in Rome who invented a method for transferring fresco paintings from plaster. He became architect to the Vatican.

Zahn, Johann (1641–1707) *See microscope.*

Zakaraya, al-Qazvini (*c.* 1350) *See rainbow.*

Zambeccari, Count Francesco (1756–1812) *See air balloon.*

Zassenhaus Groups One of the basis for the contemporary development of finite group proposed by a German-born US mathematician Hans Julius Zassenhaus (b 1912) whose main study was on group theory and number theory.

Zeeman Effect The splitting of spectral lines of a substance placed in an intense magnetic field. **Michael Faraday** (1791–1867) was aware of a relationship between light and electromagnetism around 1862, but was unable to demonstrate it. In 1896 a Dutch physicist, **Pieter Zeeman** (1865–1943), demonstrated the phenomenon, by spectroscopically observing a sodium flame in a strong magnetic field. The theory behind it was worked out by his teacher, **Hendrik Antoon Lorentz** (1853–1928), who shared the Nobel Prize for physics with him in 1902.

Zeeman, Erik Christopher (b 1925) A British mathematician who developed catastrophe theory and applied it to biological, physical and behavioral sciences. He was founder and director of the Mathematic Research Center at Warwick.

Zeeman, Pieter (1865–1943) *See Zeeman effect.*

Zeiss, Carl (1816–1888) A pioneer in the development of modern microscopes and lenses on a large scale. He was born in Weimar, East Germany, and established a firm for making optical instruments at Jena, in 1846. **Ernest Abbe** (1840–1905) joined his company in 1866 and became his partner in 1876. Their company helped to modernize the microscope and made it possible for microscopes to be produced on a commercial scale. They made the first ground spherical contact lenses for Sulzer in 1892, and in 1936 they started making contact lenses from individual casts of eyes. On the death of Carl Zeiss in 1888, Abbe became the owner of the optical works. *See microscope.*

Zendrini, Bernard (1679–1747) An Italian mathematician, physician and hydraulic engineer, who was superintendent of all the rivers and ports in Venice. He executed several water schemes for the Austrian government.

Zeno (362–264 BC) The founder of the Stoic sect was born at Citium, on the island of Cyprus. He was a pupil of **Xenocrates** (395–314 BC) and several other philosophers. He established a school of philosophy at a *stoa* or porch in Athens, where his followers became known as Stoics. He strangled himself to death.

Zeno of Elea (463–425 BC) A Greek philosopher and mathematician from Elea, a Greek colony in Italy. He was the first to question the nature of time and apply logic to its concept. He believed that he could prove time and movement did not exist, and for this purpose he created the well known paradox of Achilles and the tortoise. He proposed other paradoxes or questions to challenge some of his contemporaries who believed that quantities could be divided into an infinite number of particles. These are still considered to be fundamental to mathematics and philosophy.

Zeolite A water-softening silicate discovered around 1751 by a Swedish metallurgist, **Baron Axel Fredrik Cronstedt** (1722–1765) of Turinge, who anonymously published *Essay on New Mineralogy* (1758).

Zeppelin, Count Ferdinand von (1838–1917) *See airplane, airships, warplanes.*

Zermelo, Ernst Friedrich Ferdinand (1871–1953) A German mathematician, born in Berlin, who became a professor at Göttingen (1905–1910) and Zurich (1910–1916). He gave the first axiomatic description of set theory in 1908.

Zermelo-Fraenkel Theory An axiomatic description of set theory, related to modern mathematical logic, proposed in 1908 by a German mathematician, **Ernst Friedrich Ferdinand Zermelo** (1871–1953). An Israeli mathematician, **Abraham Fraenkel** (1891–1965) developed the theory and added an eighth axiom, to follow Zermelo's seventh.

Zernike, Fritz (1888–1966) *See phase contrast microscopy.*

Zero [Arabic: sifr, zero] According to a mathematical historian, Moritz Cantor, the Babylonians discovered the use of zero around 1700 BC. The symbol for zero was in use in India in 876 BC. The Mayan Indians of Yucatàn knew the sign in the first century. The goose egg sign for zero appeared in Cambodia and Sumatra in AD 680. It was introduced into Europe by an Italian mathematician, **Leonardo Fibonacci** (*c.* 1172–1250) of Pisa, in his *Liber Abaci* (Book of Abacus) in 1202.

Zeta (**Z**ero **E**nergy **T**hermonuclear **A**pparatus) See *thermonuclear fusion.*

Zeugmatography A method of coupling two fields to an object, in order to produce a magnetic resonance image. First described and named in 1973 by Paul Lauterbur, a professor at the University of Illinois in Chicago.

Zeuss, Johann Kasper (1806–1856) *See philology.*

Zhang Heng (AD 78–139) *See seismology.*

Ziegler, Karl (1898–1973) *See polymer.*

Ziggurat A pyramidal tower surmounted by a temple. The largest one known, the Ziggurat of Choga Zanbil, was built by the Elamite king Untash around 1250 BC in Iran. The largest surviving Ziggurat, at Ur, Iraq, was built during the reign of Ur-nammu (2133–2096 BC).

Zij Arabic term for astronomical tables. The *Zij al-sindhind*, containing a set of planetary and stellar positions, was prepared by an Arabian mathematician, **Alkarismi** or **Abu Jafar Mohammed ibn Musa Al-Khowarimi** in the 9th century, and is the earliest Islamic astronomical work to survive in its entirety. Another Arabian astronomer, **Abu Abduallah al-Battani** (*c.* AD 1100), wrote *Kitab al-Zij* (The Book of Astronomical Tables), which was an improvement on Alkarismi's work. **Abul Hasan ibn Yunus** (*c.* AD 950–1020) of Egypt wrote the *Zij,* a large astronomical table of over 81 chapters, and dedicated it to his Caliph, al-Hakim. An astronomical instrument maker, **Abu Ishaq al-Zalqali** (*c.* AD 1100) of Toledo, wrote a *Zij,* known in the west, as the Toledan Tables.

Zimmerman, Eberhard Augustus William von (1743–1815) *See zoogeography.*

Zinc (German: *zink*) Discovered and extracted by the Indians in the 14th century. The knowledge of the metal spread to China in the 16th century, and a primitive method of extracting the metal is mentioned in the Chinese book *Tien Kong Kai Wu* written in 1637. **Wilhelm Homberg** (1652–1715) identified it as a pure metal in 1695. Johann Kunckel or Kungelius, a metallurgist to King Charles of Sweden, obtained pure metallic zinc from calamine in 1721. The name *zinkum* was first used by a Swiss alchemist and physician, **Paracelsus** or **Theophrastus Bombastus von Hohenheim** (1493–1541), who introduced it into Europe in the early 16th century.

Zinc–Carbon Cell A forerunner of the dry cell and flashlight battery, in which the anode is in the form of a carbon rod in a single fluid mixture of manganese dioxide and carbon particles, in a porous pot. Invented in 1868 by a French chemist, **Georges Leclanché** (1839–1882) of Paris.

Zinder, Norton David (b 1928) *See genetic engineering.*

Zinjanthropus A hominid fossil skull, nearly 1.75 million years old, was found in 1959 in Tanzania by an English archaeologist, **Mary Douglas Leakey** (1913–1997).

Initially named *Zinjanthropus*, it was later reclassified as *Australopithecus robustus.* Mary's husband, **Louis Seymour Bazett Leakey** (1903–1972), was also an archaeologist who discovered several important hominid fossils in East Africa.

Zinn, Walter Henry (b 1906) *See atomic pile.*

Zip Fastener A device made of two rows of hooks, held together by a slidable zip. First demonstrated by an American, Whitcome L. Judson, at the Chicago Exhibition in 1893. It was improved in 1912 by a Swedish inventor in America, Gideon Sundback, and came into large-scale use in 1920.

Zircon The oldest fragments in the earth's crust, of zircon, in the form of crystals were discovered in 1984 in the Jack Hills, north of Perth, Australia. They are estimated to be 4276 million years old.

Zirconium [Persian: *zargun*] The attention to this metallic element was brought about through its compound zirconium silicate which shone like an orange gem. Various varieties of it were available in Ceylon and it was first studied by a German professor of chemistry, **Martin Heinrich Klaporoth** (1743–1817) in 1789. Zirconium was obtained in an impure form by **Jons Jacob Berzelius** (1779–1848) in 1829, and its structure and atomic weight were determined by Mixter and Dane in 1873.

Zittel, Karl Alfred von (1839–1904) *See paleontology.*

Zodiac The band of constellations, first known to the Chaldeans, through which the Sun, Moon and planets seem to move. The concept was brought to Egypt by the Greeks during their conquest in 300 BC. A circular Zodiac of 30 BC was found at the temple of Hathor at Dendera in Upper Egypt.

Zoetrope [Greek: *zoe*, life + *trope*, turning] See *cinema.*

Zoo [Greek: *zoon*, animal] An abbreviated term for a collection of animals or a zoological garden. The earliest known collection of animals was that of Shulgi, 3rd dynastic ruler of Ur, in south-east Iraq, around 2098 BC. The first zoo was established in China around 2000 BC. Collecting live exotic animals became a favorite pastime for many princes during the Renaissance period. A famous animal park in Europe was owned by Duke Ferrante (1433–1494) of Naples. Lorenzo (1449–1492) of Florence had a large collection of animals. A zoo at Schönbrunn, in Vienna, was built in 1752 by the Emperor Franz I, for his wife Maria Theresa. The Zoological Society of London was established in 1826, and it housed its collection of animals at Regent's Park, London. A Scottish zoologist, **Sir Peter Chalmers Mitchell** (1864–1945) from Dunfermline, who became secretary of the

Zoological Society in 1903, developed the London Zoo, and was instrumental in establishing the Whipsnade Zoo. The British colonial administrator **Sir Thomas Stamford Raffles** (1781–1826), founded the London Zoo and served as its first president. The first zoo without cages was established in 1907 by **Carl Hagenbeck** (1844–1913) at Stellingen, in West Germany. He used large pits and pens instead of cages. The largest zoological reserve in the world, the Etosha National Park, was established at Namibia in 1907.

Zoogeography [Greek: *zoon*, animal + *ge*, earth + *graphein*, to write] The study of the distribution of animals across the world. A German physician and naturalist, **Peter Simon Pallas** (1741–1811) of Berlin, is regarded as the first zoogeographer, owing to his studies on the relationship between animals and their environment. The first zoogeographic map was published in 1777 by a German naturalist, **Eberhard Augustus William von Zimmerman** (1743–1815).

Zoology [Greek: *zoon*, animal + *logos*, discourse] A set of seals from the Indus Valley city of Mohanjadaro around 2500 BC show detailed naturalistic representations of many animals. **Aristotle** (384–322 BC) is regarded as the first zoologist, owing to his study of various species of animals. His treatises include *On the Generation of Animals* (five books), *On the Parts of Animals* (four books), *On the Motion of Animals* (one book) and *On the Progression of Animals* (one book). **Galen** (AD 129–200) dissected higher animals such as apes and pigs and based his knowledge of anatomy and physiology on these dissections. An English physician and naturalist, **Edward Wotten** (1492–1555) of Oxford, in his Latin treatise *On the Difference of Animals* (1552), gave a survey of the animal kingdom and described several animal parts. **Ulysses Aldrovandi** (1522–1605) published one of the first important works on zoology, *Natural History*, in 1599. **John Ray** (1628–1705), an English biologist from Essex, was one of the first to attempt the classification of plant and animal kingdoms, and his system of zoology formed the basis for **Georges Cuvier's** (1769–1832) work. **Morton Thrane Brünnich** (1737–1827) of Copenhagen, who is regarded as the father of Danish zoology, published *Ornithologia Borealis, Zoologiae fundamenta* (1777) and several other works. **Martin Hinrich Carl Lichtenstein** (1780–1857), a physician and first professor of zoology at the new Berlin University in 1810, became the director of the Berlin Zoological Museum in 1815, and developed it into one of the leading institutions in the field. An American clergyman and naturalist, **John Bachman** (1790–1874) of Rhinebeck, New York, publish-

ed one of the early works in America entitled *The Viviparaous Quadrupeds of North America* (1845–1849). A Swiss-born American glaciologist and zoologist, **Jean Louis Rodolphe Agassiz** (1807–1873), founded the Museum of Comparative Zoology in 1859 to which he gave all his specimens. **Hugh Edwin Strickland** (1811–1853), a grandson of the inventor of the power loom, **Edmund Cartwright** (1743–1823), published *Rules of Zoological Nomenclature* (1841). The first chair of zoology and comparative anatomy at Cambridge was established in 1866 to which **Alfred Newton** (1829–1907) was appointed. Zoology became an established science during the 18th century, and several other chairs of zoology were created in Europe during the 19th century. *See entomology, ornithology, invertebrates, vertebrates.*

Zoopraxiscope A forerunner of cinematography, consisting of a series of photographs mounted on a rotating disc. Invented in 1880 by a photographer, **Eadweard Muybridge** (1830–1904) from Kingston-upon-Thames, Surrey, who emigrated to California in 1852. He used the device to study movements in animals and published *Animal Locomotion* (1887). His Zoopraxographical Hall in Chicago in 1893 became the world's first motion picture theater.

Zosimus (*c.* 400) A byzantine alchemist who proposed a formula for transmutation of base metals into gold. *See alchemy, hydrogen sulfide.*

Zsigmondy, Richard Adolf (1866–1930) Inventor of the ultramicroscope and a chemist at Göttingen. He was a pioneer in the study of colloidal solutions, for which he received the Nobel Prize for chemistry in 1925.

Zuse, Konrad (1910–1995) *See calculating machine.*

Zweig, George (b 1937) *See quarks.*

Zwicky, Fritz (1898–1974) A Bulgarian-born Swiss astronomer and one of the first to suggest a relationship between supernovae and neutron stars. He predicted the existence of neutron stars in 1934 and discovered 18 supernovae.

Zworykin, Vladimir Kosma (1889–1982) *See electron microscope, iconoscope, television.*

Zymase [Greek: *zyme*, leaven] An enzyme extracted from yeast and named in 1897 by professor of chemistry at Berlin, **Eduard Buchner** (1860–1917), for which he was awarded the Nobel Prize for chemistry in 1907. An English biochemist, **Arthur Harden** (1865–1940) of Manchester, demonstrated the complex nature of the enzyme.

Bibliography

Accum, Fredrick. *System of Theoretical and Practical Chemistry*. London: G. Kearsley, 1807

Allport, Noel L. *Chemistry and Pharmacy of Vegetable Drugs*. London: George Newnes Limited, 1943

Arthur, Thompson. *Heredity*. Revised Edition. London: John Murray, 1926

Atkinson E. *Elementary Treatise on Physics*. London: Longmans, Green and Co, 1872

Balfour, John Hutton. *Manual of Botany*. Edinburgh: Adam and Charles Black, 1875

Ball, Rouse W.W. *A Short Account of the History of Mathematics*. London: Macmillan & Co Ltd, 1927

Ball, Sir Robert Stanwell. *The Story of The Heavens*. London: Cassell and Company Ltd, 1888

Bateson, W. *Mendel's Principles of Heredity*. Cambridge: Cambridge University Press 1930

Beckman, John. *A History of Discoveries, Inventions and Origins*. London: Henry G. Bohn, 1846

Benjamin, Park. *The Intellectual Rise of Electricity*. London: Longmans, Green & Co, 1895

Berkenhout, John Clavis. *Anglica Lingue Botanicae or A Botanical Lexicon*, 1788

Bliss, Michael. *The Discovery of Insulin*. London: Faber and Faber, 1988

Bonavia, R. Michael. *The Channel Tunnel Story*. London: David & Charles Newton Abbot, 1987

Borradaile L.H. *Manual of Elements of Zoology*. Oxford: Oxford University Press, 1926

Boule, Pierre Marcellin. *Fossil Men, Elements of Human Palaeontology*. Edinburgh: Oliver and Boyd, 1923

Boyle, Robert. *Certain Physiological Essays, written at Different Times*. London: Henry Herringman, 1661

Bragg, W.H. and Bragg, W.L. *X-ray Crystals and Crystal Structure*. London: G. Bell and Sons Ltd, 1924

Brajendranath. *Positive Science of Ancient Hindus*. Delhi: Motilal Banarsidass, 1985

Brewster, David. *Analysis of Solar Light*. Edinburgh: Transactions of the Royal Society of Edinburgh, 1832

Brown, Wilbur Roland. *Composition of Scientific Words*. Published by the author, 1954

Bryan, S. *George Edison*. London: Alfred A. Knope, *c* 1935

Buckley, H. *Physics*. Sheffield: The Bennett College Reference Library, *c*. 1940

Bull, Henry B. *Physical Chemistry*. New York: John Wiley & Sons, 1945

Bury, J.B. *A History of Greece*. London: Macmillan & Co Ltd, 1956

Butterfield, H. *The Origin of Modern Science 1300–1800*. London: G. Bell and Sons Ltd, 1949

Carey, John. *The Faber Book of Science*. London: Faber and Faber, 1995

Chambers R. *Book of Dates*. London: R. Chambers, 1866

Chambers, William and Chambers, Robert. *Chambers's Information for the People*. London: W.S. Orr, 1948

Clarke, Hans Thacher. *Handbook of Organic Analysis*. London: Edward Arnold & Co, 1931

Cochrane, C. Rexmond. *The National Academy of Sciences, The First Hundred Years*. Washington: National Academy of Sciences, 1978

Cohen, Morris R. and Drabkin I.E. *A Source Book in Greek Science*. New York: McGraw-Hill Book Company, Inc, 1948

Cutler, D. *Evolution, Heredity and Variation*. London: Christophers, 1925

Dampier, Sir William Cecil. *A History of Science and its Relations with Philosophy and Religion*. Cambridge: Cambridge University Press, 1942

Darlington, C. D. and Mather K. *Elements of Genetics*. London: George Allen and Unwin Co, 1950

Darwin, Charles. *Autobiography of Charles Darwin*. London: Watts & Co, 1929

Darwin, Charles. *Naturalist's Voyage Round the World*. London: John Murray, 1879.

Dawes, Ben. *A Hundred Years of Biology*. London: Gerald Duckworth & Co, 1952

Dingle, Herbert, ed. *A Century of Science*. London: Hutchinson's Scientific and Technical Publications, 1951

Duckworth W.L.H. *Prehistoric Man*. Cambridge: Cambridge University Press, 1912

Durant W. *The Story of Philosophy*. London: Ernest Benn Ltd, 1946

Einstein, Albert. *Relativity, The Special and General Theory*. London: Methuen & Co Ltd, 1920

Einstein, Albert. *Sidelights on Relativity*. London: Methuen & Co Ltd, 1922

Encyclopaedia Britannica. *Year Book of Science*. Chicago: Encyclopaedia Britannica, 1992

Encyclopaedia Britannica. *Year Book of Science*. Chicago: Encyclopaedia Britannica, 1993

Evans, Charlotte, ed. *Illustrated History of the World*. London: Kingfisher Books, 1992

Faraday, Michael. *Chemical Manipulations*. London: John Murray, 1842

Findlay, Alexander. *The Spirit of Chemistry*. London: Longmans, Green and Co, 1930

Flood W.E. *Scientific Words, Their Structure and Meaning*. London: Oldbourne, 1960

Forbes, George. *History of Astronomy*. London: Watts & Co, 1909

Francis, G.E., Mulligan, W. and Wormall, A. *Isotopic Tracers*. London: Athlone Press, 1954

Friend, J. Newton. *Man and Chemical Elements*. London: Charles Griffin & Co Ltd, 1961

Fyfe, J. Hamilton. *Triumphs of Inventions and Discovery in Art and Science*. London: T. Nelson and Sons, 1878

Gibson, Harvey R.J. *Two Thousand Years of Science*, second edition. London: A. & C. Black Ltd, 1931

Gibson, R. Charles. *The Romance of Modern Electricity*. London: Seeley & Co Ltd, 1910

Glass, Justin. *The Earth Heals Everything. The Story of Biochemistry*. London: Peter Owen, 1964

Glenn, Lt.Col John, Carpenter, Lt Cmdr Scott and Shepard, Cmdr Alan. *Into Orbit*. London: Cassel, 1962

Goran, Morris. *The Modern Myth, Ancient Astronauts and UFOs*. New York: A.S. Barnes and Company, 1978

Gordon, Cook J. *Science for Everyman Encyclopaedia*. Watford, UK: Merrow Publishing Co Ltd, 1962

Graetz, Leo. *Recent Developments in Atomic Theory*. London: Methuen & Co, 1923

Graf, H. zu Solms-Laubach. *Fossil Botany*. Oxford: Clarendon Press, 1891

Graham, Thomas. *On the Law of Diffusion of Gases*. Edinburgh: Transactions of the Royal Society of Edinburgh, 1832

Grant, Edward. *A Source Book in Medievial Sciences*. Cambridge: Harvard University Press, 1974

Guillemin, Amédée. *The Applications of Physical Forces*. London: Macmillan and Co, 1877

Guynot, Arnold. *The Earth and Man or Comparative Physical Geography in relation to the History of Mankind,* New Edition, 1883

Haddon C. Alfred. *History of Anthropology*. London: Watts & Co, 1910

Haldane J.B.S. *Everything has a History*. London: George Allen and Unwin Ltd, 1951

Haldane J.B.S. *New Paths in Genetics*. London: George Allen & Unwin Ltd, 1941

Halliburton, William Dobinson. *The Essentials of Chemical Physiology*, 1922

Harré, Rom. *Great Scientific Experiments*. Oxford: Phaidon, 1981

Haslett, A.W., Ed. *Science News Series* 27. Melbourne: Penguin, 1953

Hebert, S. *The First Principles of Heredity*. London: Adam and Charles Black, 1910

Hellemans, Alexander. *The Timetables of Science*. Simon and Schuster, 1988

Henderson, I.F. and Henderson, W.D. *A Dictionary of Scientific Terms*. Edinburgh: Oliver and Boyd, 1949

Herschel F.W. *Popular Lectures on Scientific Subjects*. London: David Bogue, 1880

Hinshelwood, Cyril Norman. *The Chemical Kinetics of the Bacterial Cell*. Oxford: Clarendon Press, 1946

Hoernes, Dr Moriz. *Primitive Man*. London: Bedford Sheet, 1900

Hogg, Jabez. *The Microscope, Its History, Construction and Application*. London: George Routledge and Sons, 1887

Howard A.V. *Chamber's Dictionary of Scientists*. London: W & R Chambers, 1952

Hull L.W.H. *History and Philosophy of Science*. London: Longmans, Green and Co Ltd, 1960

Iltis, Hugo. *Life of Mendel*. London: George Allen & Unwin Ltd, 1932

Irving, Joseph. *The Book of Scotsman*. Paisley, UK: Alexander Gardner, 1882

Jinks, John. *Fifty Years of Genetics*. Edinburgh: Oliver and Boyd, 1969

Johnston, James S.W. *Chemistry of Common Life*, New edition. Edinburgh: William Blackwood and Sons, 1859

Jones, Bence. *Life and Letters of Faraday*. London: Longmans, Green and Co, 1870

Keesom, W.H. *Helium*. Amsterdam: Elsevier, 1942

Keith, Sir Arthur. *The Antiquity of Man*. London: Williams and Norgate, 1915

King, Robert C. *Genetics*. Oxford: Oxford University Press, 1965

Knight and Lacey. *The Worthies of the United Kingdom*. London: Knight and Lacey, 1828.

Laing, S. *Human Origins*. London: Chapman and Hall Ltd, 1892

Lardner, Dionysius. *Common Things Expained*. London: Walton and Maberly, 1856

Lardner, Dionysius. *The Microscope*. London: Walton and Maberly, 1856

Lardner, Dionysius. *Handbook of Natural Philosophy, Electricity, Magnetism, and Acoustics*. London: Walton and Maberly, 1856

Larson, Egon. *Inventors Cavalcade*. London: Lindsay Drummond Ltd, 1944

Lehmann, C.G. *Physiological Chemistry*. London: Cavendish Society, 1851

Lempriere, J. *Universal Biography; Containing Copious Account, Critical and Historical Account of the Life and Character, Labors and Actions of Eminent Persons in all Ages and Countries, Conditions and Professions*. London: T. Cadell and W. Davies, 1808

Lewis, William C. McC. *A System of Physical Chemistry*. London: Longmans, Green and Co, 1916

Libby, Walter. *An Introduction to the History of Science*. London: George G. Harrap & Co Ltd, 1918

Lubbock, Sir John. *Pre Historic Times as illustrated by Ancient Remains and the Manners and Customs of Modern Savages*. London: Frederic Norgate, 1878

Mackenzie, A. Donald. *Ancient Man in Britain*. London: Blackie and Sons Ltd, 1923

Magnusson, Magnus, ed. *Chambers Biographical Dictionary*. Edinburgh: Chambers Harrap Publishers Ltd, 1990

Malthus, A.M. *An Essay on the Principle of Population*. London: J. Johnson, 1806

The Mind Alive Encyclopedia, Technology. London: Marshall Cavendish, 1977

Maunder, Samuel. *The Biographical Treasury*. London: Longman, Brown, Green & Longmans, 1847

Maunder, Samuel. *The Scientific and Literary Treasury*. London: Longman, Brown, Green & Longmans, 1848

Mee, Arthur, ed. *Harmsworth Popular Science*. London: The Educational Book Co Ltd, *c*. 1930

Messadié, Gerald. *Great Modern Inventions*. Edinburgh: W. & R. Chambers Ltd, 1991

Miall, L.C. *History of Biology*. London: Watts & Co, 1911

Mitchell, Arthur. *The Past and the Present: What is Civilisation*. Edinburgh: David Douglas, 1880

Möller, C. and Rasmussen, Ebbe. *The World and Atom (Atomer og andre Smaating, 1938)*. London: George Allen & Unwin Ltd, 1940

Moore, F.J. *History of Chemistry*, International Chemical Series. New York: McGraw-Hill Book Company, 1918

Muir, Hazel, ed. *Larousse Dictionary of Scientists*. Edinburgh: Larousse, 1994

Muir, M.M. Pattison. *Heroes of Science. Chemists*. London: Society for Promoting Christian Knowledge, 1883

Murray, H. Robert. *Science and Scientists in the Nineteenth Century*. London: The Sheldon Press, 1925

Nechaev, I. *Chemical Elements*. London: Linsay Drummond Ltd, 1944

Universal Knowledge. London: Odhams Press Ltd., *c.* 1938

Overman, Michael. *Understanding Sound and Video Recording*. London: Lutterworth Press, 1977

Partington, F. Charles. *The British Encyclopaedia of the Arts and Sciences*. London: Orr & Smith, 1835

Pledge, H.T. *Science Since 1500*. London: His Majesty's Stationary Office, 1940

Popham, A.E. *The Drawings of Leonardo de Vinci*. London: Jonathan Cape, 1947

Porter, Roy, ed. *The Hutchinson's Dictionary of Scientific Biography*. Oxford: Helicon Publishing Ltd, 1994

Pouchet, F.A. *The Universe*. London: Blacke and Son, 1871

Powell, Davies A. *The Meaning of the Dead Sea Scrolls*. London: Frederick Muller Ltd, 1957

Presence, Peter, ed. *Purnell's Encyclopedia of Inventions*. London: Intercontinental Book Productions, 1976

Quatrefages, A. De. *Metamorphoses of Man and Lower Animals*. London: Robert Hardwicke, 1894

Ramsay, Sir William. *Essays Biographical and Chemical*. London: Archibald Constable & Co Ltd, 1908

Ramsay, Sir William. *Text-book of Physical Chemistry*. London: Longmans, Green and Co, 1919

Ramsay, Sir William. *The Gases of the Atmosphere and the History of Their Discovery*. London: Macmillan and Co Ltd, 1905

Rodwell, G.F. *A Dictionary of Science*. The Haydn Series. London: E. Moxon, Son, and Co, 1871

Rolt-Wheeler, Francis. *The Science-History of the Universe, Mathematics*. London: The Waverley Book Co Ltd, 1911

Ronan, Colin A. *The Cambridge Illustrated History of World's Science*. London: Book Club Associates, 1983

Routledge, Robert. *Discoveries and Invention of the 19th Century*. London: Braken Books, 1989

Russell, Bertrand. *The Scientific Outlook*. London: George Allen & Unwin Ltd, 1931

Rutherford, Ernest. *Radio-Activity*. Cambridge: Cambridge University Press, 1905

Rutherford, Ernest. *Radioactive Substances and their Radiation*. Cambridge: Cambridge University Press, 1913.

Sanford, Vera. *A Short History of Mathematics*. London: George G. Harrap & Co Ltd, 1930

Seifriz, William. *Protoplasm*. London: McGraw-Hill, 1936

Sidgwick, Neville Vincent. *The Electronic Theory of Valency*. Oxford: Clarendon Press, 1927

Singer, Charles. *A Short History of Biology*. Oxford: Clarendon Press, 1939

Singer, Charles. *A Short History of Scientific Ideas to 1900*. Oxford: Clarendon Press, 1959

Singer, Charles. *From Magic to Science*. London: Ernest Benn Ltd, 1928

Singer, Charles. *Studies in the History and Method of Science*. Oxford: Clarendon Press, 1921

Smith, Edward and Dallas, W.S. *Organic Nature*. Orr's Circle of Sciences Series. London: Houlston and Stoneman, 1859

Snyder, Carl. *New Conceptions in Science*. London: Harper and Brothers, 1903

Spencer, Herbert. *The Principles of Biology*. London: Williams and Norgate, 1899

Stewart, Alfred W. *Recent Advances in Organic Chemistry*. London: Longmans, Green and Co, 1931

Stormonth, Rev. James. *A Manual of Scientific Terms*. Edinburgh: Machlachlan and Stewart, 1885.

Taylor, F. Sherwood. *Science Past and Present*. London: William Heinemann Ltd, 1945

Taylor, F. Sherwood. *Century of Science*. London: Readers Union Ltd, 1942

Taylor, F. Sherwood. *Short History of Science*. London: William Heinemann Ltd, *c* 1940

Taylor, F. Sherwood. *Illustrated History of Science*. London: William Heinemann Ltd, 1960

Temple, Ralph. *Invention and Discovery*. London: Hodder and Stoughton, 1893

Thomson, Robert Young. *A Faculty for Science*. Glasgow: University of Glasgow, 1993

Thorpe, Sir Edward. *History of Chemistry*. Walls & Co, 1909

Tilden, William A. *Chemical Discovery and Inventions in the Twentieth Century*, revised by Glasstone, S. London: George Routledge and Sons Ltd, 1936

Timbs. *Curiosities of Science. Past and Present*. London: Kent & Co, 1859

Turner, Edward. *Elements of Chemistry Including Recent Discoveries and Doctrines of the Science*. Edinburgh, 1829

Turner, Edward. *Elements of Chemistry*. London: Taylor and Walton, 1847

Twyman, F. *Prism and Lens Making*. London: Adams Hilger Ltd, 1942

Tyndall, John. *Sound*. London: Longmans, Green and Co Ltd, 1875

Unsworth, A.V. *Chemistry*. Sheffield, UK: The Bennett College Reference Library, *c* 1940

Velikovsky, Immanuel. *Earth in Upheaval*. London: Victor Gollancz Ltd, 1956

Vincent, Benjamin. *Haydn's Dictionary of Dates*. London: Edward Moxon and Co, 1868

Vulliamy, C.E. *Our Prehistoric Forerunners*. London: The Bodley Head Ltd, 1925

Wallace, Alfred Russell. *Darwinism*. London: Macmillan and Co, 1889

Watkins, Arthur Ernest. *Heredity and Evolution*. London: John Murray, 1935

Watkins, John. *A Biographical Historical and Chronological Dictionary*. London: Richard Phillips, 1806

Weiner, J.S. *The Piltdown Forgery*. Oxford: Oxford University Press, 1955

Williams, Trevor I. *An Introduction to Chromatography*. London: Blackie & Son Ltd, 1946

Williams, Trevor I. *A Biographical Dictionary of Scientists*. London: Adams & Charles Black, 1969

Wilson, William. *A Hundred Years of Physics*. London: Gerald Duckworth & Co Ltd, 1950

Wolf, A. *History of Science Technology and Philosophy in the XVI and XVII centuries*. London: George Allen & Unwin Ltd, 1935

Woodward, B. Horace. *History of Geology*. London: Watts & Co, 1911

Wright, W.B. *Quaternary Ice Age*. London: Macmillan and Co Ltd, 1937

Young, John F. *Cybernetics*. London: Ilife Books Ltd, 1969